The Theory and Practice of Oncology

Historical evolution and present principles

Ronald W. Raven

O.B.E. (Mil.), O.St.J., T.D., F.R.C.S., Hon. F.R.S.M.

Consulting Surgeon, Royal Marsden Hospital and Institute of Cancer Research.
Consulting Surgeon, Westminster Hospital.
Member, Court of Patrons (late Council); Erasmus Wilson Lecturer; Arris and Gale Lecturer; Bradshaw Lecturer; and Hunterian Professor, The Royal College of Surgeons of England.
Founder President, Head and Neck Oncologists of Great Britain.
Founder President, British Association of Surgical Oncology.
Chairman, Marie Curie Memorial Foundation.

The Parthenon Publishing Group

International Publishers in Science, Technology & Education

Casterton Hall, Carnforth, Lancs, LA6 2LA, UK

120 Mill Road, Park Ridge, New Jersey, USA

Published in the UK by
The Parthenon Publishing Group Limited
Casterton Hall, Carnforth,
Lancs. LA6 2LA, England

Published in the USA by
The Parthenon Publishing Group Inc.
120 Mill Road,
Park Ridge,
New Jersey 07656, USA

British Library Cataloguing in Publication Data
Raven, Ronald W. (Ronald William)
The theory and practice of oncology: historical evolution
and present principles.
I. Title
616.99'4

ISBN 1-85070-179-2

Library of Congress Cataloguing-in-Publication Data
Raven, Ronald William.
The theory and practice of oncology.

Includes bibliographical references.
1. Oncology 2. Oncology—history.
I. Title. [DNML: 1. Medical Oncology—history.
2. Neoplasms—history. QZ 11.1 R253t]
RC254.R38 1989 616.99'2 89-23192

ISBN 0-940813-14-9 (U.S.)

First published 1990

Printed and bound in Great Britain by Butler and Tanner Ltd.,
Frome and London

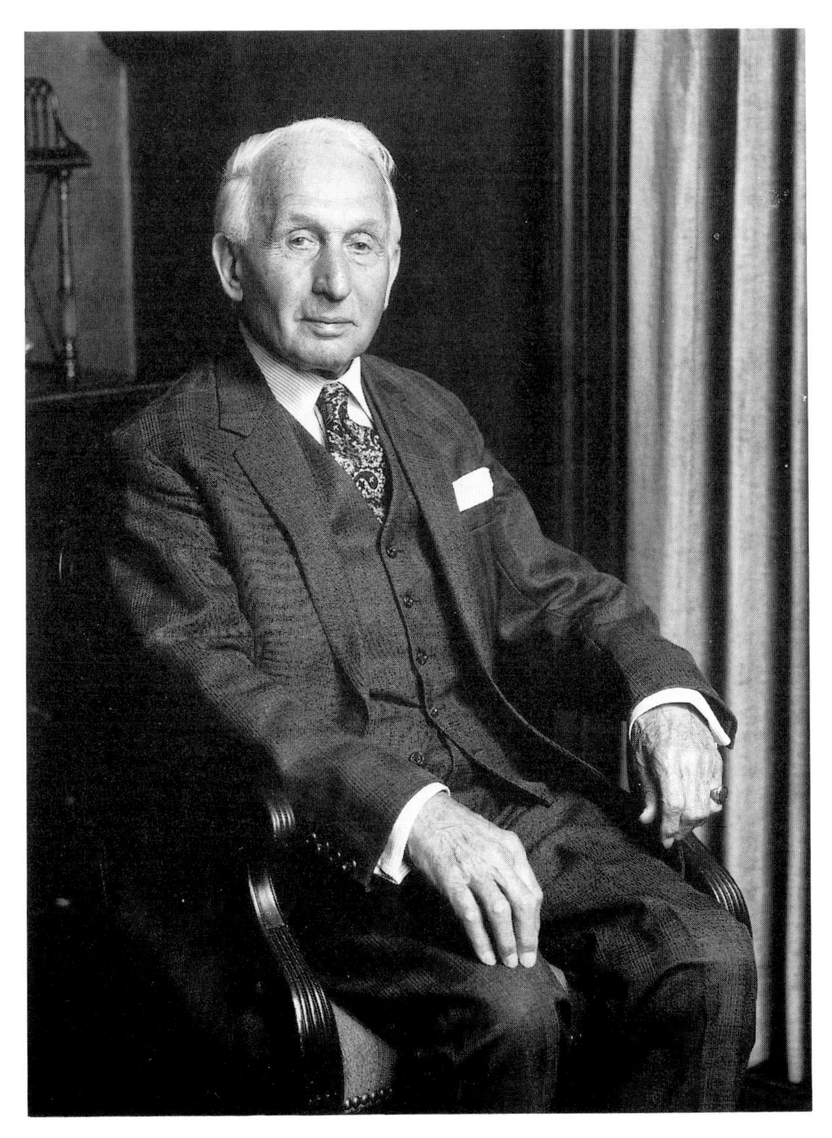

Ronald W. Raven, O.B.E. (Mil), O.St.J, T.D., F.R.C.S., Hon. F.R.S.M.

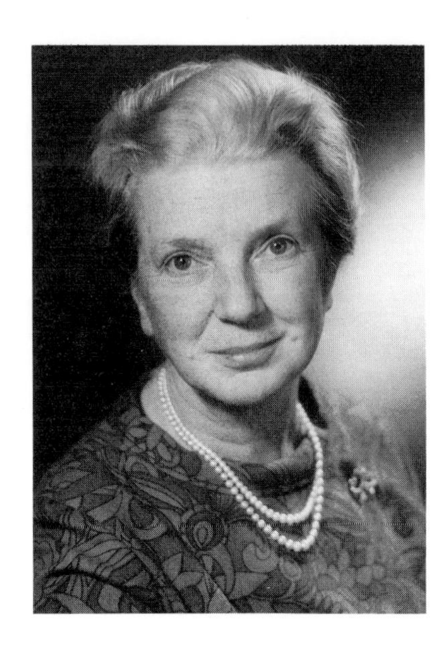

This book is dedicated to my sister,
Dame Kathleen A. Raven D.B.E., O.St.J., F.R.C.N., F.R.S.A.
— wife of Professor John T. Ingram M.D., F.R.C.P. —
who has dedicated her life to the profession of nursing

CONTENTS

PREFACE

Over a period of more than 50 years my professional life has been devoted to the problems of cancer, from its prevention and diagnosis to rehabilitation, including definitive treatment, and the continuing care of patients with malignant diseases. In this work I have witnessed many changes due to the important advances that have been made in our knowledge of the nature, aetiology, prevention, diagnosis and treatment of cancer. The growth of scientific knowledge and clinical practice has accelerated to a remarkable extent during recent decades and from its synthesis the multidisciplinary subject of oncology has emerged, which can now be clearly recognised.

The contemplation of the history of oncology and the evolution of the study and treatment of cancer which has occurred over many centuries is a rewarding exercise. In writing this book, not only has my personal experience with regard to cancer been crystallised, but the extensive research which I have had to do in the cancer literature has been very rewarding. Perusing many original contributions by outstanding scientists and clinicians has given me both considerable pleasure and enlightenment, which have been enhanced by reading about the work and recalling the comments of many of my own friends and colleagues.

I have been stimulated in my task by the words of Sir Ernest Kennaway, who wrote: "Many investigations are reported which appear to promise further results, and yet in say 10 years' time, if they are remembered at all, they are found to have no progeny. This may be because they are inherently infertile, or because the investigator has been diverted to other matters. Some person should be appointed to pick over the literature of say the last 20 years in the light of later knowledge, and to seek for anything worthy of resuscitation — now and then something useful may be disinterred." I am in full agreement that it is very rewarding to "pick over the literature" and I trust that by doing so I may have "resuscitated" some important information from the past. This, however, is an exercise of some magnitude, because the literature concerning cancer is international and very extensive; moreover, the scope and quantity increase daily.

The task of searching, reading and abstracting the cancer literature can be a full-time occupation for one person, and really requires a team of experts. I suggest, therefore, that ongoing research and review of the cancer literature should be organised and directed as a special section of literature studies in departments of oncology. There is an ever-increasing need to synthesise and correlate our knowledge of oncology, which is being constantly augmented by the enormous international research and clinical efforts being carried out today. There can be no doubt that much valuable information and data "worthy of resuscitation", to quote Kennaway, are lying entombed in the literature housed in our libraries.

My objective in writing this book is to show how "cancer" has become "oncology". This momentous transformation has taken place in the course of many decades through the furtherance of our knowledge by scientists and clinicians working in the laboratory, field and clinic. The basic sciences have made valuable contributions to the theory of oncology, whilst the art of oncology has been built up by clinicians and other members of the caring professions. The value of the work done by hospitals, hospices and special homes for patients with all varieties and stages of cancer must not be overlooked or forgotten; a great contribution has also been made by Voluntary Cancer Associations, whose members, in many cases, give freely of their talents and time.

Although the major part of this book is rightly concerned with the past, we must look to the future. The evolution of the study and treatment of cancer is a continuing process and doubtless important advances in knowledge will be made and changes in treatment will occur to give new hope, cure and relief to many people and patients. Light is now coming in to dispel some of the gloom caused by cancer; it seems that today we are witnessing a new dawn. However, we must not be complacent, for much work still remains to be done to wring all the oncological secrets from Nature. It is encouraging for us to realise that all the great killer diseases which caused such havoc in the past proved eventually to be preventable. There is strong evidence today that the oncological diseases will largely be prevented in the future; this is our greatest hope.

I wish to record my gratitude to Joan Gough-Thomas, M.A., for all her valuable help in my oncology work throughout many years.

I am very grateful to David Bloomer of the Parthenon Publishing Group for his collaboration in publishing this book.

I have been ably supported in all my professional work by splendid colleagues, both senior and junior, including the nurses who have cared for my patients by day and by night. The courage and gratitude of the patients it has been a privilege to serve have been my constant inspiration and support.

Ronald W. Raven
London

INTRODUCTION

The continued accretion of new knowledge during recent years has given us a much clearer understanding of the nature, causation and behaviour of the large group of serious diseases which for many centuries have been included under the general designation of "cancer". This new knowledge is being used in a practical way today for the prevention and diagnosis of those diseases and for the rehabilitation, including definitive treatment, and continuing care of patients with them.

Professional and public attitudes towards cancer are now changing, and increasing optimism is being generated by the institution of cancer prevention programmes on a national scale, the use of new methods of screening and diagnosis and the advances in treatment modalities. It is now possible to save the life of many more cancer patients than previously; some varieties of cancer which used to be fatal are being cured; and much of the suffering of patients is being ameliorated.

The emergence of oncology was an event of outstanding medical importance and significance. This is a multidisciplinary subject composed of the arts and sciences which are concerned with the nature, causation and management of cancer. Oncology is now recognised and accepted as the vehicle for our scientific and clinical knowledge about all the different serious diseases which for many centuries were indiscriminately grouped together under the term "cancer".

These diseases occur throughout the world; no nation can escape their ravages. Consequently, they are universally feared, as they cause morbidity with severe suffering and a high mortality. As a result, there is an intense international effort to "fight cancer" by marshalling and coordinating all our scientific and clinical forces against this enemy of mankind. The cancer campaign continues to attract considerable support in many different ways, from individuals, groups, institutions and governments, for scientific research and cancer care. The financial support which is required for work of this magnitude and importance is very considerable, but help from charitable sources is most encouraging. However, the whole concerted effort must be intensified, if malignant diseases are to be prevented and controlled in the foreseeable future.

We are constantly on the search for new ideas, concepts and scientific methodology to solve the abstruse problems of cancer, the secrets of which are closely guarded and controlled by Nature. Much new knowledge is being provided by the basic oncological sciences, which are expanding continuously. As work progresses it may be necessary to have recourse to knowledge provided by other scientific disciplines which at present may appear to have no relevance to the study of oncological diseases. The multi-disciplinary subject of oncology will widen our horizons and introduce more flexibility into our work. New ideas and concepts which now seem novel or unusual should not be discarded lightly as being perhaps too fanciful.

SCIENTIFIC REVOLUTIONS

It is very relevant to refer here to the review by Judson *(1982)* of the book by I. Bernard Cohen entitled *The Newtonian Revolution, with Illustrations of the Transformation of Scientific Ideas*, which was published by Cambridge University Press. In this stimulating review Judson explains how Cohen reaches "a genuinely new way to understand the process by which concepts emerge and develop in science", which is described as "the transformation of scientific ideas". Judson speaks of "scientific revolutions" and he describes how molecular biology emerged from the confluence of at least five disciplines, some of which are closely and obviously related: X-ray crystallography and physical chemistry are both concerned with the structure of molecules, but the other contributing subjects were not considered by most scientists to be in any way relevant. He cites the specific example of Watson, a trained geneticist working with micro-organisms, who was ridiculed by his colleagues when he announced that he was going to Cambridge to learn the discipline of X-ray crystallography, but nevertheless there emerged the important discovery of DNA, the genetic material.

Judson quotes the writing by Cohen about Watson's action as follows: "He did not create an artificial system to be superimposed upon nature and he certainly did not merely combine in a synthetic 'stew' the principles of Copernicus, Kepler and Galileo, Descartes, Hooke and Huygens. Rather he carefully selected certain ideas (concepts, principles, definitions, rules, laws and hypotheses) and transformed them, giving each of them a new form which only then was useful to him."

Perhaps a scientific revolution which could result in a breakthrough in our endeavours to solve the difficult problems of cancer is necessary today. There has certainly been an impressive accretion of knowledge about these dangerous diseases.

THE HISTORY OF ONCOLOGY

The history of oncology, which is the subject of this book, extends over many centuries during which increasing interest was displayed in lesions described as cancer. The growth in knowledge proceeded slowly on the whole, especially during those many decades when scientific methodology was either non-existent or meagre. There were periods of acceleration, however, which can clearly be recognised as being due to the work of individual scientists and the development of scientific instruments such as the microscope.

Scientific and clinical knowledge on all aspects of cancer is now being rapidly built up, correlated and sythesised in the new multidisciplinary subject of oncology. Opportunities are being created and arrangements made for research and clinical oncologists to be associated more closely to enable them to share their ideas and knowledge and to discuss their problems and work together. This new and constant feedback system which is being established between the laboratory and the clinic has great potential value, for it can aid discoveries to be made which will advance our knowledge regarding all aspects of cancer.

NEW NOMENCLATURE

Following the establishment of oncology, it is logical and appropriate to introduce new nomenclature. Thus the old term "cancer" is now outmoded and should not be used. It has no scientific meaning in the connotation of disease nomenclature, for it is given to a large number of different diseases with diverse aetiology, behaviour and manifestation, which require various forms of management and clinical care. Moreover, the prognosis of these diseases after treatment is very variable. In addition to these criticisms, the term "cancer" causes widespread fear in many people as it is associated in their minds with much suffering and ultimate death.

The proposal is now made that the diseases which hitherto have been designated "cancer" should henceforth be called "oncological diseases". This new terminology associates them in a logical way with oncology, which is the master subject. It also conforms with that of other large groups of diseases; good examples are the dermatological diseases associated with dermatology and gynaecological diseases associated with gynaecology.

Whilst the adoption of the new name would constitute an important modern advance and mitigate much of the fear and apprehension caused by "cancer" in the past, there still remain problems of nosology to solve, including the classification and arrangement of this heterogeneous group of diseases.

REFERENCE

Judson, H. F. (1982). On the shoulders of giants. *The Sciences*, January 1982. New York Academy of Sciences

CHAPTER ONE

Cancer in Antiquity and Later Centuries

Cancer appears to have been rare in the millennia which preceded the coming of Christ and ancient descriptions of conditions which were considered to be malignant tumours are confusing, for they included various swellings which were caused by injury and inflammation. The documentation of tumours that afflicted mankind in antiquity is very scanty and we are dependent largely on the Egyptian papyri for the information which is given about the tumours found in mummies. Special reference is therefore made here to two treatises which were written between the years 3000 and 1500 BC, based on sources even older.

The Edwin Smith Papyrus, which was written between 3000 and 2500 BC and dealt with various surgical conditions, was translated by J. H. Breasted in 1930. It contains the descriptions of eight cases of "tumours or ulcers of the breast" which were treated by the application of the cautery *(Bett, 1957)*. The Ebers Papyrus, dating from about 1552 BC and translated by Ebbell, deals with medical conditions and contains a warning against treating a large tumour occurring in a limb, because this might prove to be fatal *(Bett, 1957)*.

The rarity of descriptions of malignant tumours is notable until the times of Hippocrates (460–370 BC). This remarkable medical authority was born on the Greek island of Cos. His life and work have exerted an abiding influence on the profession of medicine. His clinical knowledge was based on the careful and skilled observations he made of disease processes, but his therapy was entirely empirical. It is obvious from his writings that he was familiar with cancer, as he described different varieties which affected the skin, breast, stomach, cervix uteri and rectum *(Haagensen, 1933)*. Hippocrates and his school contributed to man's early knowledge about cancer by their attempt to establish a classification of tumours based on the facts they derived from their clinical observations. This initial classification

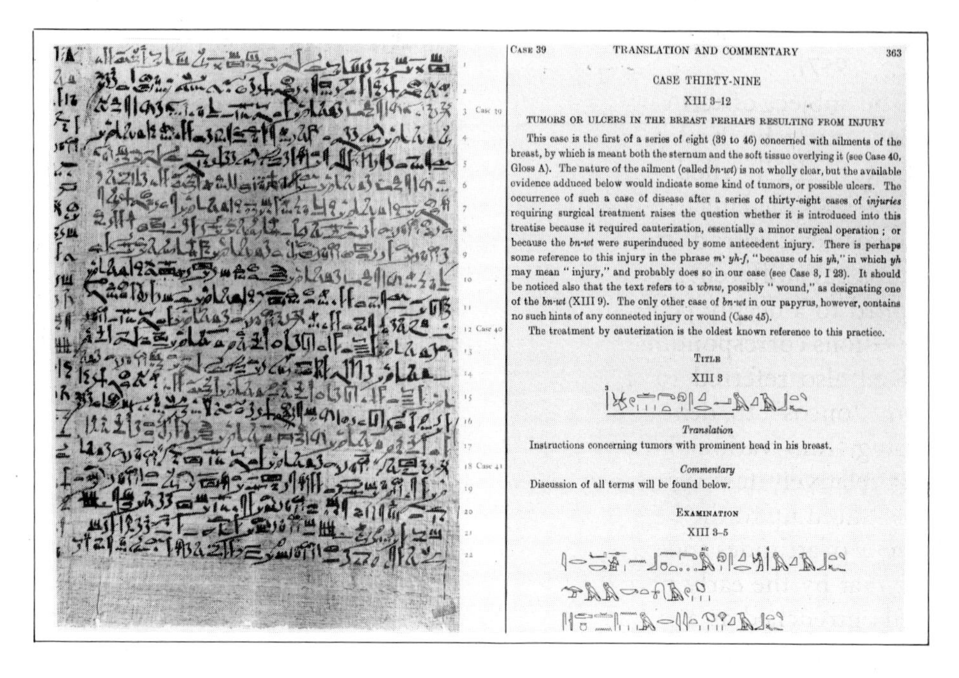

CASE 39 TRANSLATION AND COMMENTARY 363

CASE THIRTY-NINE

XIII 3–12

TUMORS OR ULCERS IN THE BREAST PERHAPS RESULTING FROM INJURY

This case is the first of a series of eight (39 to 46) concerned with ailments of the breast, by which is meant both the sternum and the soft tissue overlying it (see Case 40, Gloss A). The nature of the ailment (called *bn·wt*) is not wholly clear, but the available evidence adduced below would indicate some kind of tumors, or possible ulcers. The occurrence of such a case of disease after a series of thirty-eight cases of *injuries* requiring surgical treatment raises the question whether it is introduced into this treatise because it required cauterization, essentially a minor surgical operation; or because the *bn·wt* were superinduced by some antecedent injury. There is perhaps some reference to this injury in the phrase *m' yh-f*, "because of his *yh*," in which *yh* may mean "injury," and probably does so in our case (see Case 8, I 23). It should be noticed also that the text refers to a *wbnw*, possibly "wound," as designating one of the *bn·wt* (XIII 9). The only other case of *bn·wt* in our papyrus, however, contains no such hints of any connected injury or wound (Case 45).

The treatment by cauterization is the oldest known reference to this practice.

TITLE

XIII 3

Translation

Instructions concerning tumors with prominent head in his breast.

Commentary

Discussion of all terms will be found below.

EXAMINATION

XIII 3–5

Figure 1.1 An extract from the Edwin Smith Surgical Papyrus and the English translation of case 39.

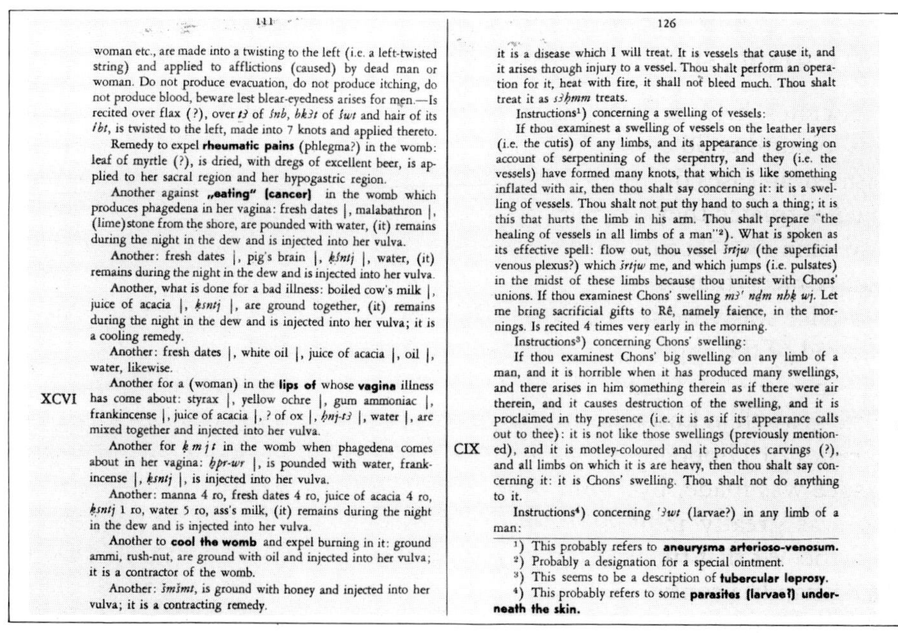

111

woman etc., are made into a twisting to the left (i.e. a left-twisted string) and applied to afflictions (caused) by dead man or woman. Do not produce evacuation, do not produce itching, do not produce blood, beware lest blear-eyedness arises for men.—Is recited over flax (?), over *t3* of *šnb*, *bk3t* of *šwt* and hair of its *ibt*, is twisted to the left, made into 7 knots and applied thereto.

Remedy to expel **rheumatic pains** (phlegma?) in the womb: leaf of myrtle (?), is dried, with dregs of excellent beer, is applied to her sacral region and her hypogastric region.

Another against **„eating" (cancer)** in the womb which produces phagedena in her vagina: fresh dates |, malabathron |, (lime)stone from the shore, are pounded with water, (it) remains during the night in the dew and is injected into her vulva.

Another: fresh dates |, pig's brain |, *ḳšntj* |, water, (it) remains during the night in the dew and is injected into her vulva.

Another, what is done for a bad illness: boiled cow's milk |, juice of acacia |, *ḳsntj* |, are ground together, (it) remains during the night in the dew and is injected into her vulva; it is a cooling remedy.

Another: fresh dates |, white oil |, juice of acacia |, oil |, water, likewise.

Another for a (woman) in the **lips of** whose **vagina** illness

XCVI has come about: styrax |, yellow ochre |, gum ammoniac |, frankincense |, juice of acacia |, ? of ox |, *ḥnj-t3* |, water |, are mixed together and injected into her vulva.

Another for *ḳmjt* in the womb when phagedena comes about in her vagina: *ḫpr-wr* |, is pounded with water, frankincense |, *ḳsntj* |, is injected into her vulva.

Another: manna 4 ro, fresh dates 4 ro, juice of acacia 4 ro, *ḳsntj* 1 ro, water 5 ro, ass's milk, (it) remains during the night in the dew and is injected into her vulva.

Another to **cool the womb** and expel burning in it: ground ammi, rush-nut, are ground with oil and injected into her vulva; it is a contractor of the womb.

Another: *šmšmt*, is ground with honey and injected into her vulva; it is a contracting remedy.

126

it is a disease which I will treat. It is vessels that cause it, and it arises through injury to a vessel. Thou shalt perform an operation for it, heat with fire, it shall not bleed much. Thou shalt treat it as *s3ḥmm* treats.

Instructions[1]) concerning a swelling of vessels:

If thou examinest a swelling of vessels on the leather layers (i.e. the cutis) of any limbs, and its appearance is growing on account of serpentining of the serpentry, and they (i.e. the vessels) have formed many knots, that which is like something inflated with air, then thou shalt say concerning it: it is a swelling of vessels. Thou shalt not put thy hand to such a thing; it is this that hurts the limb in his arm. Thou shalt prepare "the healing of vessels in all limbs of a man"[2]). What is spoken as its effective spell: flow out, thou vessel *šrtjw* (the superficial venous plexus?) which *šrtjw* me, and which jumps (i.e. pulsates) in the midst of these limbs because thou unitest with Chons' unions. If thou examinest Chons' swelling *m3' nḏm nhḳ wj*. Let me bring sacrificial gifts to Rê, namely faience, in the mornings. Is recited 4 times very early in the morning.

Instructions[3]) concerning Chons' swelling:

If thou examinest Chons' big swelling on any limb of a man, and it is horrible when it has produced many swellings, and there arises in him something therein as if there were air therein, and it causes destruction of the swelling, and it is proclaimed in thy presence (i.e. it is as if its appearance calls out to thee): it is not like those swellings (previously mention-

CIX ed), and it is motley-coloured and it produces carvings (?), and all limbs on which it is are heavy, then thou shalt say concerning it: it is Chons' swelling. Thou shalt not do anything to it.

Instructions[4]) concerning *'3wt* (larvae?) in any limb of a man:

[1]) This probably refers to **aneurysma arterioso-venosum.**

[2]) Probably a designation for a special ointment.

[3]) This seems to be a description of **tubercular leprosy.**

[4]) This probably refers to some **parasites (larvae?) underneath the skin.**

Figure 1.2 Extracts from Ebell's translation of the Ebers Papyrus, giving remedies for "eating" (cancer) in the womb and for "chons" (swelling on a limb).

was made two millennia ago, but it is not yet complete, for work on classification and staging of oncological diseases continues today.

TERMINOLOGY

The writers at the time of Hippocrates in the 5th and 4th centuries before Christ used the words "carcinos" and "carcinoma", meaning "crab", to describe indiscriminately chronic ulcerations and swellings that appear to have been malignant tumours. The word "cancer" occurs in old English medical terminology and it was reintroduced into middle English to denote the celestial constellation which is situated between Leo, the Lion, and Gemini, the Twins. About the year 1600 it began to be used in the medical sense, as it was considered to be more definite and technical than "canker" *(Bett, 1957)*.

The subject of terminology is considered in a very interesting and detailed article by Keil *(1950)*, which contains valuable references to the literature. Keil called attention to the work carried out on terminology by Celsus (see later), who translated the word "carcinos" into the Latin "cancer" and introduced the term "carcinoma" into the Latin language. Celsus gave different interpretations to these terms. "Cancer" was generally applied to a deeply penetrating type of ulcer, while he used "carcinoma" for lesions corresponding to our premalignant and malignant lesions.

Keil also referred to the concepts of Galen (see later), who used the term "oncos" to denote a swelling or tumour, pathological in nature, arising from various humors or combinations of humors. Keil observed that relatively few new terms relating to swellings or tumours had been introduced up to the beginning of the 18th century, but he gave a valuable review of attitudes and developments throughout many centuries, pointing out that by the early part of the 19th century the word "carcinoma" was well entrenched as a synonym for "cancer". In general he also discussed the ending "-oma" for a variety of lesions.

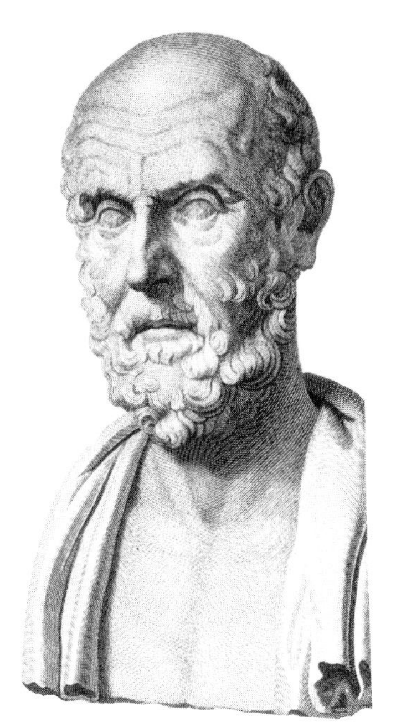

Figure 1.3 Hippocrates.

THE GROWTH IN KNOWLEDGE

Hippocrates held definite opinions concerning the treatment of cancer. Thus in number 38 of his *Aphorisms* he stated: "It is better not to apply any treatment in cases of occult cancer; for, if treated, the patients die quickly, but if not treated they hold out for a long time." Hippocrates did not define his meaning of "occult cancer", so some authorities have assumed that he meant cancer that is non-ulcerating or deep-seated *(Littré, 1839–1861)*. His advice was wise at that time, when the available methods of treatment consisted of the application of the cautery and various caustic pastes to the tumour.

The growth in knowledge about cancer continued to be very slow from the times of Hippocrates, so that three centuries elapsed before the next advance was made, by Aulus Cornelius Celsus (25 BC–50 AD), a Roman who was greatly influenced in his thinking by Greek and Alexandrian medicine. At that time Rome was the great centre of Western civilisation, but Alexandria continued to exert a considerable influence on scientific and medical thought and outlook. According to Castiglioni *(1940)*, Celsus was the founder of systematic teaching in medicine and the representative of the intellectual achievement of his time. He was a prolific writer, for his works include an encyclopaedia with a section devoted to medicine. His views about cancer are expressed in Book V, Chapter 28 of *De Medicina (Shimkin, 1977)*, where he states that this disease occurs mostly in the upper parts of the body in the region of the face, nose, ears, lips and in the female breast, but it may arise also in an ulceration, or in the spleen.

Celsus also described the development of cancer in stages. The first stage is called "cacoethes" by the Greeks; this is followed by a carcinoma without ulceration; and then a wart develops. He believed that only the cacoethes should be removed, because the other stages of the tumour would be irritated by treatment. He therefore advised against treating more advanced lesions with caustic medicaments, cautery application, or excision. It is

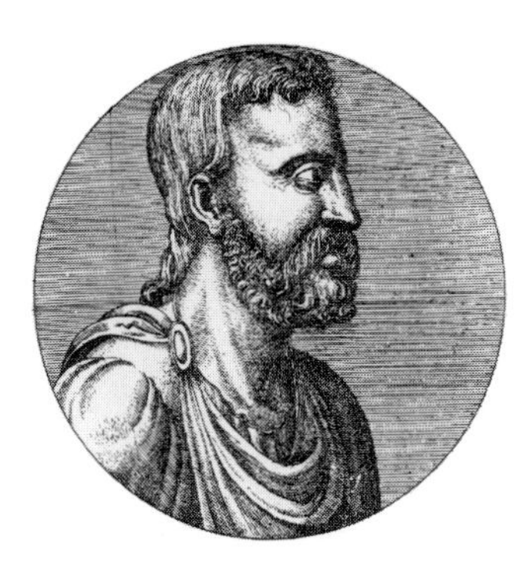

Figure 1.4 Aulus Cornelius Celsus.

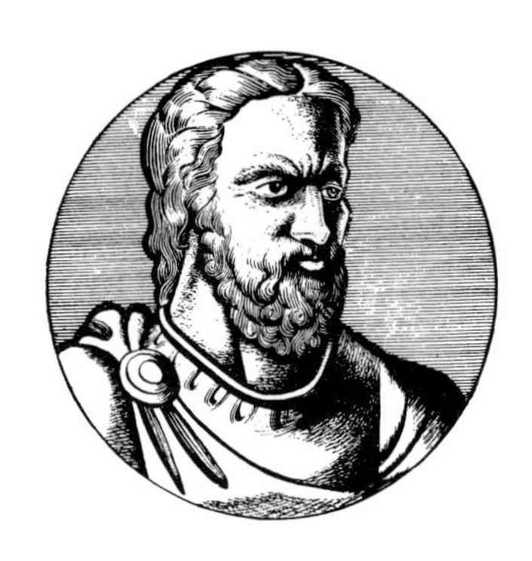

Figure 1.5 Aretaeus, the Cappadocian.

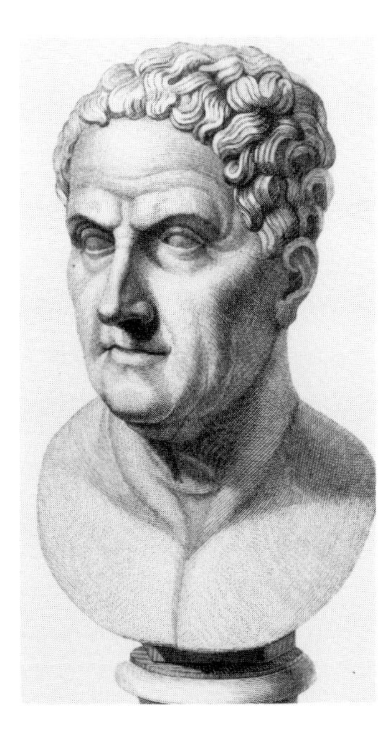

Figure 1.6 Clarissimus (Claudius) Galen.

thus interesting to learn that even in antiquity the treatment of cancer was correlated with the stage of the disease, which is the practice today, and that advice was given then not to employ treatment methods which could make the patient even worse than before therapy.

In the influential Alexandrian school in medical antiquity, Aretaeus, the Cappadocian, was outstanding for his important contributions to the literature. This authority lived in Alexandria during the 2nd or 3rd centuries AD *(Adams, 1856; Leopold, 1930)* and he described cancer of the uterus as superficial and deep ulcers, which infiltrate later into the uterus and either prove fatal after a lengthy period or become very chronic. He also described another variety of uterine cancer without any ulceration, which causes a hard, intractable swelling that distends the whole uterus. He distinguished between carcinoma of the cervix uteri and corpus uteri as being separate entities, and recognised that the ulcerative cancers caused the worst symptoms and prognosis.

Leonides of Alexandria (180 AD) described retraction of the nipple as an important sign of breast cancer. He performed the mastectomy operation, but advised against this treatment for advanced disease. The encircling incisions for mastectomy were made with the scalpel, care being taken that they were made in normal tissues around the tumour. After removal of the breast the open wound was cauterised to secure haemostasis and to destroy any residual cancerous tissue.

The abiding influence of Galen

From the time of Celsus many years elapsed without any further real advance being made in man's knowledge about tumours till Clarissimus (or Claudius) Galen (130–200 AD) appeared on the medical scene. Galen was born in Pergamon in Asia Minor, studied in Alexandria and later practised as a physician in Rome. He was a prolific writer on many subjects and he exerted a profound influence on medicine, which persisted for a millennium.

He enunciated his humoral theory of the causation of cancer, which no authority was competent to challenge at that time. He considered that tumours were caused by an excess of black bile which tended to solidify in certain parts of the body, including the lip, tongue and breast. He postulated that cancer was a disease which was caused by this condition of the bile and that the right treatment was to administer purgatives to dissolve the solidified bile, but that when this treatment failed the tumour should be excised.

Galen's humoral theory of cancer causation lasted for a thousand years, which doubtless explains the lack of any advance in man's knowledge of cancer throughout this long period of history.

There was a complete dearth of scientific methodology at that time, but a system of clinical cancer was gradually formed which was based upon accurate clinical observations and the compilation of records of the behaviour of different tumours.

The treatment of cancer remained very simple, being confined to the application of caustic pastes, the administration of various herbal preparations and the excision by the cautery of certain tumours, especially those located in superficial and accessible sites in the body.

The contributions of Arabian physicians

The valuable contributions to man's knowledge of clinical cancer which were made by various Arabian physicians around the end of the first millennium must not be overlooked. The most influential among these doctors was Avicenna (980–1037 AD), who lived in Baghdad, where he wrote his *Canon of Medicine (Gruner, 1930; Riesman, 1935)*. He described the way in which a cancer increases progressively in size, invades and destroys the contiguous tissues, and finally kills the tissues and eliminates sensation in the affected part.

Another important Islamic physician, called Albucasis (1013–1106), practised in Cordoba, where he wrote his book on surgery and surgical instruments *(Spink and Lewis, 1973)*. For the treatment of an early cancer which is situated in an accessible site, such as in the breast or thigh, he recommended complete excision of the tumour; he advised no treatment for advanced cancer. For the arrest of the development of an early cancer he advised treating the circumferential tissues of the tumour by the application of the circular cautery to stop it spreading and to ulcerate it out. Preoperative treatment consisted of purging the patient several times for the black bile, followed by blood letting when the patient's veins were distended. The patient was then placed in the most convenient position for performing the operation. If severe haemorrhage occurred by dividing an artery or vein, he advised that the blood vessel should be cauterised until the bleeding ceased and that the wound be dressed until it healed.

The other notable Cordoban physician was Averzoar (1070–1162), who described the clinical features of cancer of the oesophagus and stomach. For the treatment of stenosis of the oesophagus caused by cancer he used sounds for dilatation, and this procedure also confirmed the diagnosis.

THE CONTINUED INCREASE IN KNOWLEDGE

There was a continued increase in man's knowledge of cancer during the Middle Ages, and it is interesting to see the contributions made by surgeons.

The first outstanding surgeon in England was John of Arderne (1307–1390), who studied at Montpellier and gained much surgical experience during the Hundred Years War. He was a surgeon of the long robe, as distinct from the barber-surgeons of the short robe; the surgeons and the barber-surgeons were two separate guilds in London at that time, whose members were engaged in the practice of surgery. John of Arderne described the symptoms of carcinoma of the rectum as haemorrhage and obstruction, being familiar with this disease and realising its seriousness because he had never seen a patient with it who was cured *(Power, 1922; Millar, 1954)*.

Guy de Chauliac (1300–1370) of the school of Montpellier exerted considerable professional influence through his surgical text *Chirurgia Magna*, which was used throughout the 13th and 14th centuries. Although this surgeon undoubtedly was a highly competent clinician, he contributed little new knowledge about cancer and his treatment methods were those which had been recommended by his predecessors. Consequently, he performed a wide excision of operable tumours; more extensive disease was treated by the application of caustic paste as a palliative measure. The patient's general condition was built up with a dietary regimen and by purgation.

The famous military surgeon Ambroise Paré (1510–1590) made important contributions to surgery, but he wrote very little about cancer and he practised the traditional methods for its treatment. Thus he excised small, accessible tumours and a wide surrounding margin of healthy tissues and then cauterised the wound. For the treatment of other varieties of cancer he prescribed a dietary regimen and purgation for the patient.

The basic medical sciences

During the 16th century the basic medical sciences, which were then in their infancy, began to be recognised as important and developed. In the famous schools of Bologna, Padua and Pisa the teaching of anatomy was of outstanding quality and they attracted students from many countries. During this epoch Gabriele Fallopis (Fallopius) (1523–1562), who studied under the illustrious Vasallius, became Professor of Anatomy successively at Pisa and Padua. He was an observer of outstanding ability, who wrote many valuable descriptions of the different varieties of cancer. He suggested no new methods of treatment, however, and continued to use the traditional technique of excision and cauterisation of early cancers. More advanced cancers were treated by applying various caustic pastes, his favourites being those which contained arsenic. It is clear that he did not recognise the carcinogenic property of arsenic.

The discovery of the lymphatic system

The discovery and the development of our knowledge of the lymphatic system was a most important landmark in the evolution of oncology *(Leaf, 1898; Poirier and Charpy, 1909)*. This system plays a vital role in the dissemination of many forms of cancer, in addition to participating in other reactions of the body. Its discovery is attributed to Gaspare Aselli (1581–1625), who worked in Milan and illustrated the dilated lacteals in the mesentery of a well-fed dog. Later the thoracic duct was demonstrated by Jean Pecquet (1622–1674). Thereafter a considerable period elapsed before it was demonstrated that a main route for the dissemination of malignant disease is through the lymphatic system. This led to the realisation that the management of metastatic disease in the various regional lymph nodes is a major part of cancer therapy.

Case-records and illustrations

In the absence of the discipline of experimental research in cancer, due to the lack of scientific instruments and methodology, the main sources for acquiring new knowledge on this subject were the clinical observations of various human cancers and the recording of them. The importance of compiling clinical case-records was recognised by the outstanding German surgeon Wilhelm Fabry (Fabricius Hildanus, 1560–1634). His work resulted in the best collection of clinical records, which held that position of excellence for many years. These contained the descriptions of

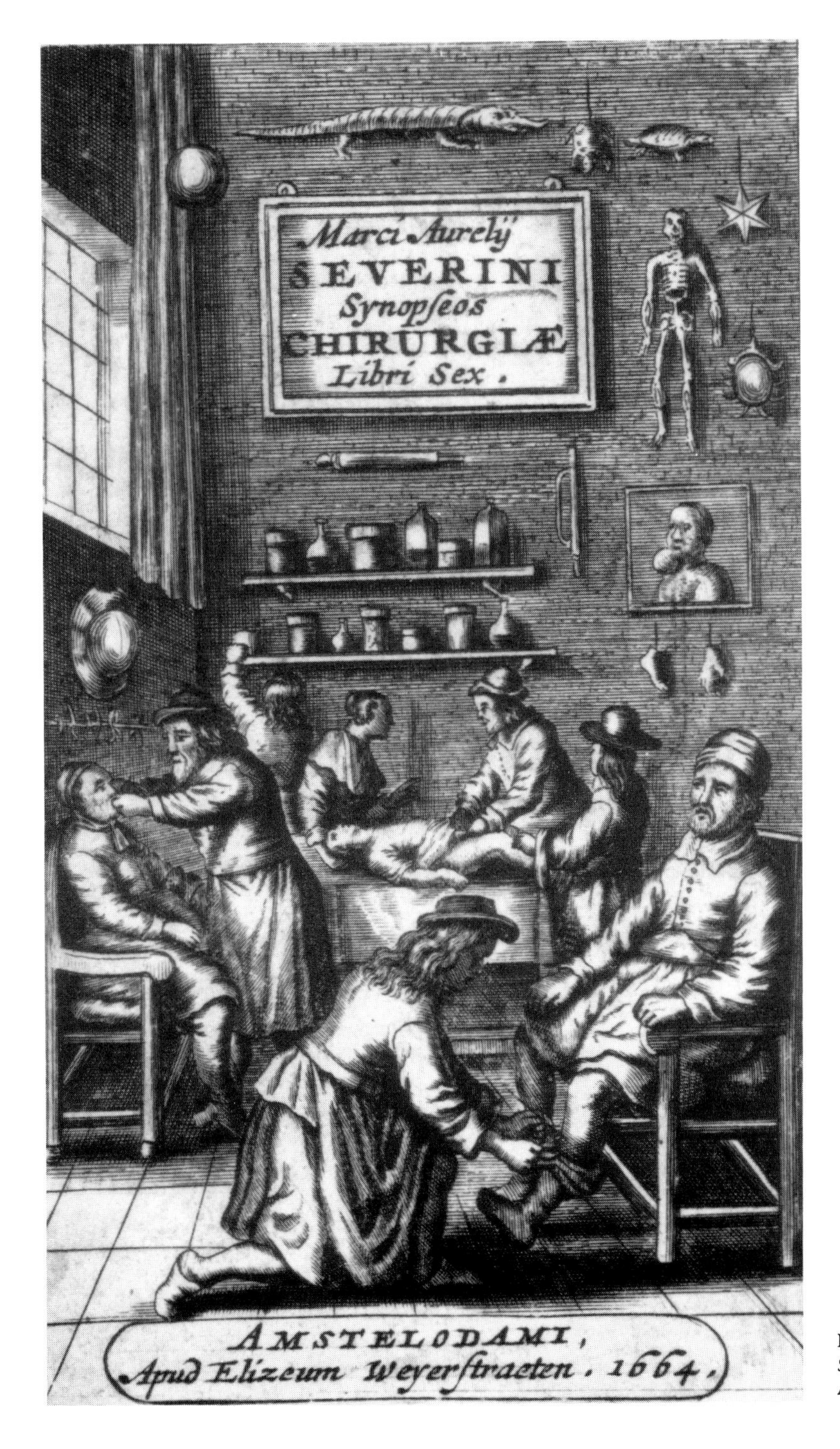

Figure 1.7 An illustration from the *Synopseos Chirurgicae* by Marcus Aurelius Severini.

patients with cancer who had been treated by extensive surgical operations. It is recorded that Fabry performed a dissection of the axillary lymph nodes in patients with breast cancer.

During these years breast cancer was attracting considerable interest, and it was the subject of one of the most important sections of the first text-book on surgical pathology, written by Marco Aurelio Severini (1580–1656). This was the first author to use illustrations of the various lesions described in the text. In his book he discussed the differential diagnosis of benign and malignant tumours of the breast and a clear description

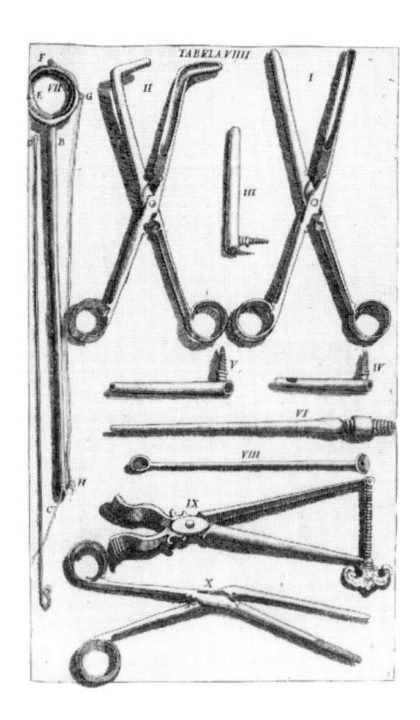

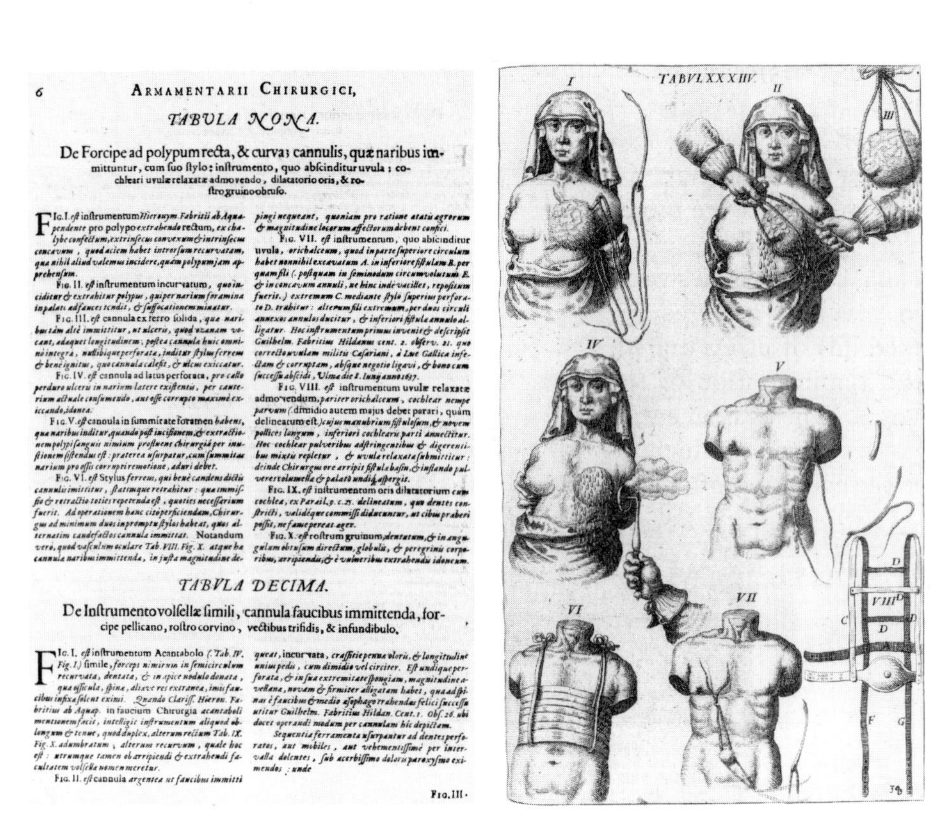

6 ARMAMENTARII CHIRURGICI,

TABVLA NONA.

De Forcipe ad polypum recta, & curva; cannulis, quæ naribus immittuntur, cum suo stylo; instrumento, quo abscinditur uvula; cochleari uvulæ relaxatæ admovendo, dilatatorio oris, & rostro gruino obtuso.

FIG. I. *est* instrumentum *Hieronym. Fabritii ab Aquapendente* pro polypo *extrahendo* rectum, *ex chalybe confectum, extrinsecus convexum & intrinsecus concavum, quod aciem habet introrsum recurvatam, qua nihil aliud valemus incidere, quàm polypum jam apprehensum.*

FIG. II. *est* instrumentum incurvatum, *quo inciditur & extrahitur polypus, qui per narium foramina in palati adfauces tendit, & suffocationem minatur.*

FIG. III. *est* cannula ex ferro solida, *quæ naribus tàm altè immittitur, ut ulceris, quod ozænam vocant, adæquet longitudinem; postea cannulæ huic omninò integræ, nullibique perforatæ, inditur stylus ferreus & benè ignitus, quo cannula calescit, & ulcus exiccatur.*

FIG. IV. *est* cannula ad latus perforata, *pro callo perduro ulceris in narium latere existentis, per cauterium actuale consumendo, aut osse corrupto maximè exiccando, idonea.*

FIG. V. *est* cannula in summitate foramen *habens, quæ naribus inditur, quando post incisionem, & extractionem polypi sanguis nimium profluens chirurgiâ per inustionem sistendus est: præterea usurpatur, cum summitas narium pro ossis corrupti remotione, aduri debet.*

FIG. VI. *est* Stylus *ferreus, qui benè candens dictis cannulis imittitur, statimque retrahitur: quæ immissio & retractio toties repetenda est, quoties necessarium fuerit. Ad operationem hanc citò perficiendam, Chirurgus ad minimum duos in promptu stylos habeat, quos alternatim candefactos cannulæ immittat.* Notandum *verò, quod vasculum oculare Tab. VIII. Fig. X. atque hæc cannula naribus immittenda, in justa magnitudine depingi nequeant, quoniam pro ratione ætatis ægrorum & magnitudine locorum affectorum debent confici.*

FIG. VII. *est* instrumentum, quo abscinditur uvula, *orichalceum, quod in parte superiore circulum habet nonnihil excavatum A. in inferiore fistulam B. per quam fili (postquam in seminodum circumvolutum E. & in concavum annuli, ne hinc inde vacillet, repositum fuerit.) extremum C. mediante stylo superius perforato D. trahitur: alterum fili extremum, per duos circuli annexos annulos ducitur, & inferiori fistulæ annulo alligatur. Hoc instrumentum primus invenit & descripsit Guilhelm. Fabritius Hildanus cent. 2. observ. 21. quo correctò uvulam militis Cæsariani, à Lue Gallica infectam & corruptam, absque negotio ligavi, & bono cum successu abscidi, Ulmæ die 8. Iunij anno 1637.*

FIG. VIII. *est* instrumentum uvulæ relaxatæ admovendum, *pariter orichalceum, cochlear nempe parvum* (dimidio autem majus debet parari, quàm delineatum est.) *cujus manubrium fistulosum, & novem pollices longum, inferiori cochlearis parti annectitur. Hoc cochlear pulveribus adstringentibus & digerentibus mixtis repletur, & uvulæ relaxatæ submittitur: deinde Chirurgus ore arripit fistulæ basin, & inflando pulveres columellæ & palatò undiq; aspergit.*

FIG. IX. *est* instrumentum oris dilatatorium *cum cochlea, ex Paræil. 9. c. 25. delineatum, quo dentes constricti, validéque commissi diducuntur, ut cibus præberi possit, ne fame pereat æger.*

FIG. X. *est* rostrum gruinum, *dentatum, & in angulum obtusum directum, globulis, & peregrinis corporibus, arripiendis, & è vulneribus extrahendis idoneum.*

TABVLA DECIMA.

De Instrumento volsellæ simili, cannula faucibus immittenda, forcipe pellicano, rostro corvino, vectibus trifidis, & infundibulo.

FIG. I. *est* instrumentum Acantabolo (*Tab. IV. Fig. I.*) simile, *forceps nimirum in semicirculum recurvata, dentata, & in apice nodulo donata, quæ ossicula, spinæ, aliæve res extraneæ, imis faucibus infixæ solent eximi. Quando Clariss. Hieron. Fabritius ab Aquap.* in faucium Chirurgia *acantaboli mentionem facit, intelligit instrumentum aliquod oblongum & tenue, quod duplex, alterum rectum Tab. IX. Fig. X. adumbratum; alterum recurvum, quale hoc est: utrumque tamen ob arripiendi & extrahendi facultatem volsellæ nomen meretur.*

FIG. II. *est* cannula *argentea ut faucibus immitti queat,* incurvata, *crassitie pennæ oloris, & longitudine unius pedis, cum dimidio vel circiter. Est undique perforata, & in sua extremitate spongiam, magnitudine avellanæ, novam & firmiter alligatam habet, qua ad spinas è faucibus & medio æsophago trahendas felici successu utitur Guilhelm. Fabritius Hildan. Cent. 1. Obs. 26. ubi docet operandi modum per cannulam hic depictam.*

Sequentia ferramenta usurpantur ad dentes perforatos, aut mobiles, aut vehementissimè per intervalla dolentes, sub acerbissimo doloris paroxysmo eximendos: unde

FIG. III.

Figure 1.8 Drawing *(left)* and description of surgical instruments *(centre)*, and *(right)* the different steps in the operation of mastectomy for carcinoma of the breast, reproduced from Johann Schultes' *Armamentarium Chirurgicum XLIII.*

of fibroadenoma was included. He advised excision of benign breast tumours because of the risk of malignant degeneration occurring in them. All varieties of swellings were described under the general term "abscess" and descriptions were included of tumours of the genital organs and bone sarcomas.

The value of using illustrations to demonstrate clearly the different steps of a surgical operation was recognised many centuries ago. Johann Schultes (Scultetus, 1595–1645) is famous for his pioneer work as an illustrator of operative surgery and for his descriptions of surgical instruments. He illustrated the steps of the operation performed at that time for breast cancer. A study of these early illustrations of the art of surgery demonstrates the enormous progress which has occurred in surgical techniques in recent decades.

PROGRESS IN THE 18TH CENTURY

During the 18th century important additions were made to our knowledge about cancer. One of the chief reasons for these advances was that the influence of Galen and the relevance of his humoral theory were waning. That theory had really hindered progress for many years, but now, having been accepted for several centuries, it was overthrown. The change that was taking place was stimulated by Henri François Le Dran (1685–1770), who wrote the most enlightened dissertation to date on the nature and treatment of cancer. He believed that cancer commenced as a local disease and that it later spread through the lymphatic vessels to the lymph nodes and then into the general circulation.

This new concept was of profound importance and significance because it explained the spread of breast cancer to other sites in the body, including the lungs. Since the treatment of cancer must be correlated with the pathology, Le Dran postulated that surgical treatment for early local cancer gave the only prospect of cure and that the operation of mastectomy should include the dissection of the associated lymph nodes in the axilla. He also recognised that the presence of axillary lymph node metastases warranted a grave prognosis.

Le Dran was a strong advocate of the surgical treatment of cancer, in which he believed, and he deprecated the use of the older treatment methods of using caustic pastes as local applications to the tumours and the administration of the various internal remedies which were then in vogue. This was an entirely new attitude towards the pathology and treatment of cancer, which made the work of Le Dran an important landmark in the evolution of oncology.

Advances in pathology

The firm foundations of pathology were established by the work of Giovanni Battista Morgagni (1682–1771), which is recorded in one of the most important books in the history of medicine. He completed his great work in his 79th year, which truly was a remarkable achievement. His famous book, called *De Sedibus et Causis Morborum* (1761), contains a series of 70 letters which report about 700 cases, together with the autopsy findings, which are correlated to the best of his knowledge. Morgagni had performed most of the autopsies, which were done on victims of cancers of the breast, stomach, rectum and pancreas. However, although he gave clear and detailed descriptions of the cancers affecting different organs, it is apparent that he failed to recognise and understand the pathology of metastasia.

The increasing study and investigation of autopsy material represented an important development which contributed greatly to man's knowledge of morbid anatomy. This subject received a vital stimulus from Matthew Baillie (1761–1823), the talented physician who was a nephew of William and John Hunter. He compiled a systematic and illustrated atlas on gross pathology, finding much of his material in the preparations in the Hunterian Museum. His book, entitled *The Morbid Anatomy of Some of the Most*

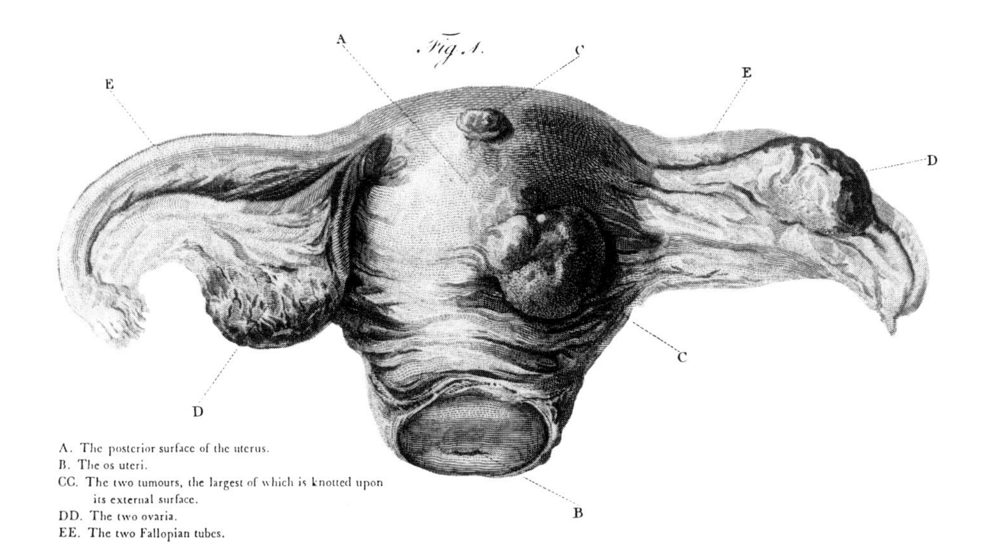

Figure 1.9 A pathology specimen of the uterus in the Hunterian Museum, with two tumours growing on the surface. (From Matthew Baillie's *A Series of Engravings with Explanations which Are Intended to Illustrate the Morbid Anatomy of Some of the Most Important Parts of the Human Body)*

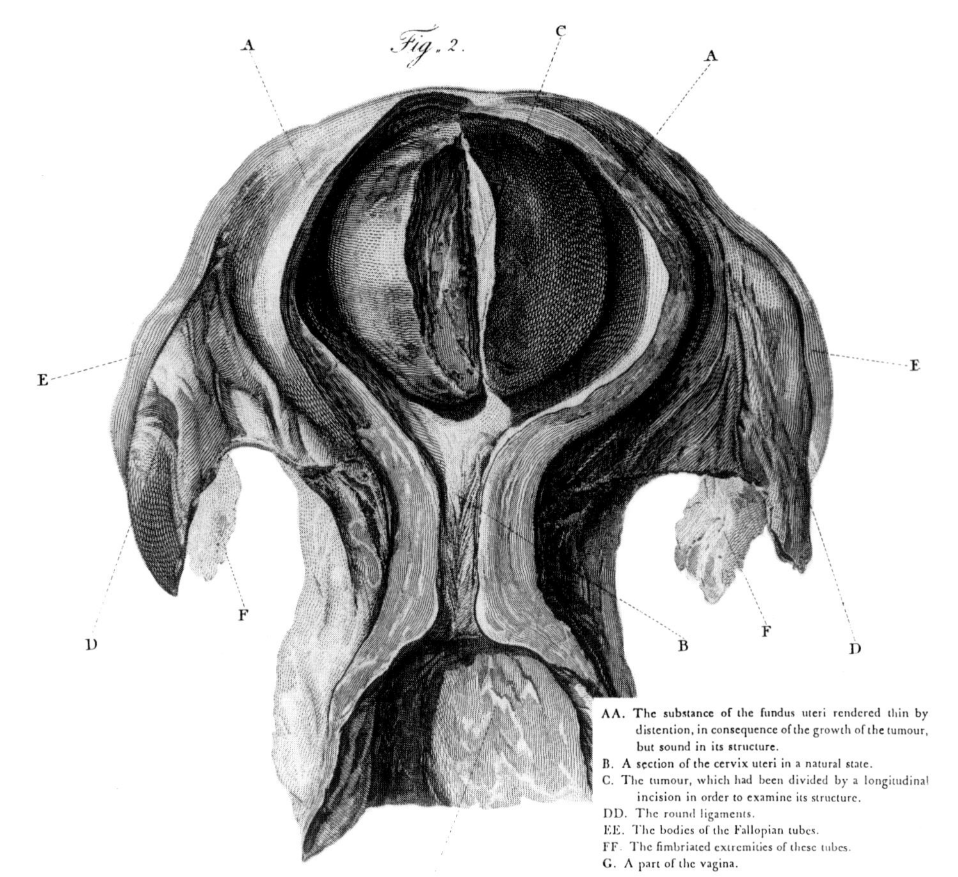

Figure 1.10 A tumour in the cavity of a specimen of a uterus in the Hunterian Museum. (From Matthew Baillie's *A Series of Engravings with Explanations which Are Intended to Illustrate the Morbid Anatomy of Some of the Most Important Parts of the Human Body)*

Important Parts of the Human Body, was published in 1793. It was followed at a later date, 1799–1802, by a series of engravings to illustrate it. Baillie's descriptions and engravings were of cancers affecting the oesophagus, stomach, bladder and testes and they reached a high standard of perfection. (In *A Series of Engravings with Explanations which Are Intended to Illustrate the Morbid Anatomy of Some of the Most Important Parts of the Human Body*, published by W. Bulmer & Co., London)

The dawn of experimental research in cancer

The 18th century witnessed the vital development of experimental research in cancer which has continued to increase in amount and scope in a remarkable way to the present time. The dawn was ushered in by Bernard Peyrilhe (1735–1804), when he performed his first experiment with cancer of the breast. He extracted fluid from a breast cancer and then injected it into a dog, but the animal howled so much that Peyrilhe's house-keeper objected to the experiment being done and the animal was therefore drowned *(Haagensen, 1933)*. Although this particular experiment was a failure, Peyrilhe wrote an important thesis about cancer, in which he pointed out that cancer is initially a local disease but later becomes a generalised disease due to tumour cells permeating the lymphatic system. He advocated that surgical treatment for breast cancer should include removal of the breast and the pectoralis major muscle and dissection of the lymph nodes in the axilla.

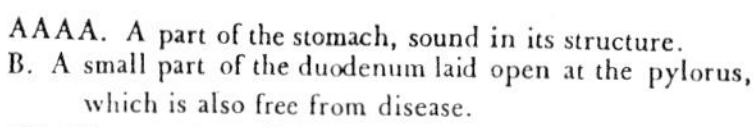
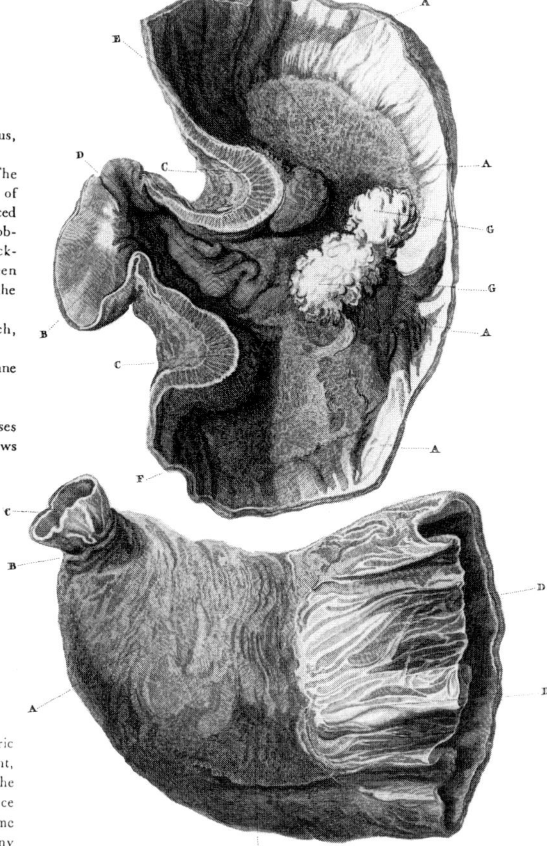

Figure 1.11 *Top:* A section of a stomach near the pylorus, affected with cancer, laid open to show the inner surface. *Bottom:* A section of the stomach inverted, with one part of its coats "a great deal affected by the action of the gastric juice". (From Matthew Baillie's *A Series of Engravings with Explanations which Are Intended to Illustrate the Morbid Anatomy of Some of the Most Important Parts of the Human Body)*

The development of scientific surgery

Another important development was taking place in the 18th century as the immortally renowned John Hunter (1728–1793) laid the basis of scientific surgery. Hunter's mind ranged throughout the whole realm of biology. His prodigious output of ideas and work and his indefatigable energy in the pursuit of knowledge were quite outstanding. He exerted a very profound influence on surgery, which has persisted to the present day. The historicity of John Hunter is enshrined in perpetuity in the Hunterian Museum, which is permanently housed in the Royal College of Surgeons of England in Lincoln's Inn Fields, London. There is a unique display in this famous museum, known all over the world, of the numerous actual dissections and specimens which were prepared so beautifully by John Hunter and which a constant stream of visitors from many countries comes to see and study.

Hunter had definite opinions about cancer, which he propounded in his *Lectures on the Principles of Surgery (1839)*. These writings have been examined by Jessie Dobson *(1959)*, the well-known authority on Hunter and a past Curator of the Hunterian Museum; she died in 1984.

Hunter stated that there are three predisposing causes of cancer, namely, age, heredity and perhaps climate. Although the disease may, of course, occur sooner or later, the "cancerous age" is from 40 to 60 years. When cancer develops in the breast of a woman aged less than 40, its course is

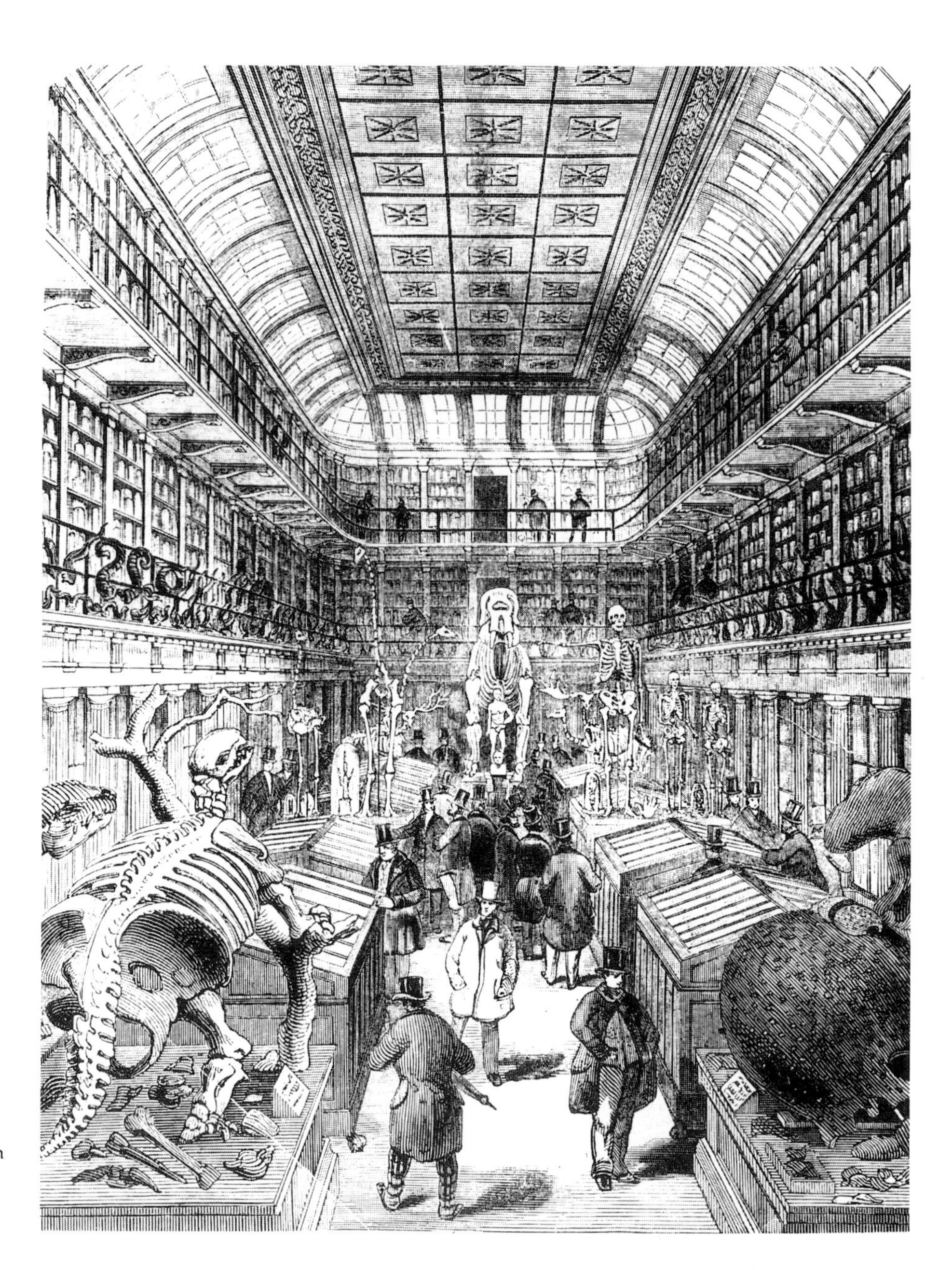

Figure 1.12 The original Hunterian Museum, which was destroyed in the aerial bombardment of London in 1941.

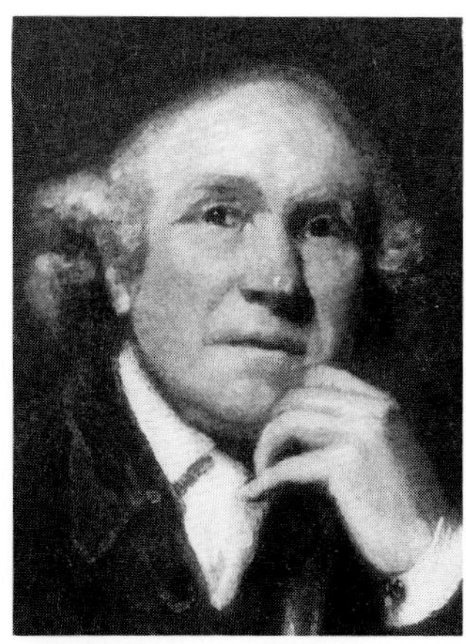

Figure 1.13 John Hunter (1728–1793).

more rapid than in older patients. Hunter found that the sites of the body chiefly affected by cancer were the breast, uterus, lips, external part of the nose, pancreas and the gastric pylorus, but he also pointed out that in addition to these the testicle was often affected. It is therefore most interesting to compare the site incidence of cancer in Hunter's time with the incidence today. For example, Hunter did not mention cancer of the lung, colon or rectum and it seems that the lymphomas and leukaemias were not known to him.

Describing the physical signs of cancer, Hunter stressed the importance of the fixity of the tumour, because mobile tumours can be excised. He stated that lymph nodes which appear to be mobile are often found on excision to run in a chain beyond the field of operation, which makes the operation unsuccessful. He advised that surgical treatment should not be carried out when the lymph nodes are considerably enlarged.

THE SUCCESSORS OF JOHN HUNTER

The abiding strong influence exerted by John Hunter on surgery lived on through the work of his distinguished successors. The Hunterian tradition is a perpetual and living force today.

Astley Paston Cooper (1768–1841) was a brilliant pupil of John Hunter and a great admirer of his work. He had much influence on the development of British surgery during the first part of the 19th century, and made many important contributions to several branches of surgery. He was very interested in diseases of the breast and described hyperplastic cystic disease of the breast *(1829)*.

Sir James Paget (1814–1899) was another distinguished surgeon in the line of succession to John Hunter. He held the important appointment of Sergeant-Surgeon to Queen Victoria and was Surgeon to the Royal Hospital of St Bartholomew in London. He made important contributions to the understanding of several diseases, including Paget's disease of bone (osteitis deformans). He was an outstanding surgical pathologist as well as an able practical surgeon. In 1874 he described the disease entity "Paget's disease of the nipple", a form of eczema of the nipple which is associated with deep-seated carcinoma of the breast (see Chapter 12).

The prevention and control of infection in the treatment of cancer and particularly in surgical operations are highly important. Special mention is made here of the great contribution made to the control of infections by Joseph Lister (First Baron Lister, 1827–1912). He applied Louis Pasteur's (1822–1895) great discoveries about bacteria to surgical practice and introduced antisepsis, which has had a profound influence on surgery. In his time infections caused considerable mortality from surgical operations, so he endeavoured to prevent the access of bacteria to wounds and to kill them on the surface or in the wound. He selected carbolic acid as the antiseptic for

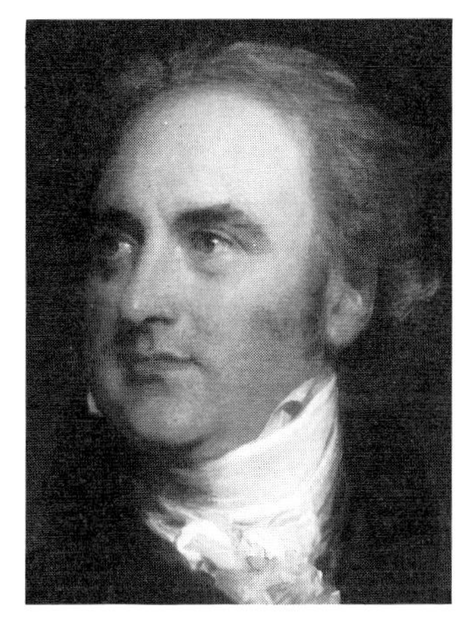

Figure 1.14 Sir Astley Paston Cooper (1768–1841), Surgeon to Guy's Hospital, London.

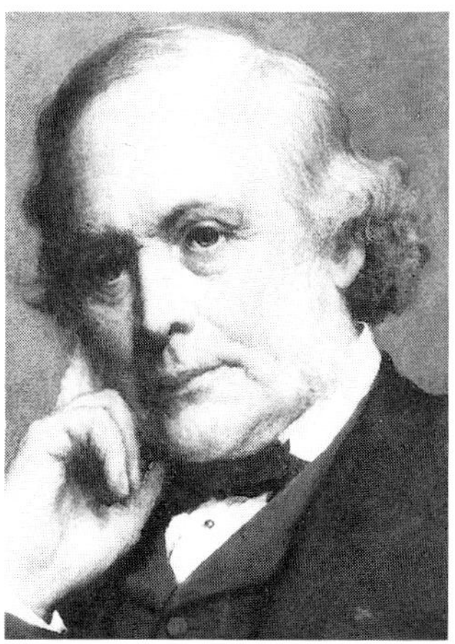

Figure 1.15 Joseph Lister (1827–1912), Professor of Surgery successively at Glasgow, Edinburgh and King's College, London.

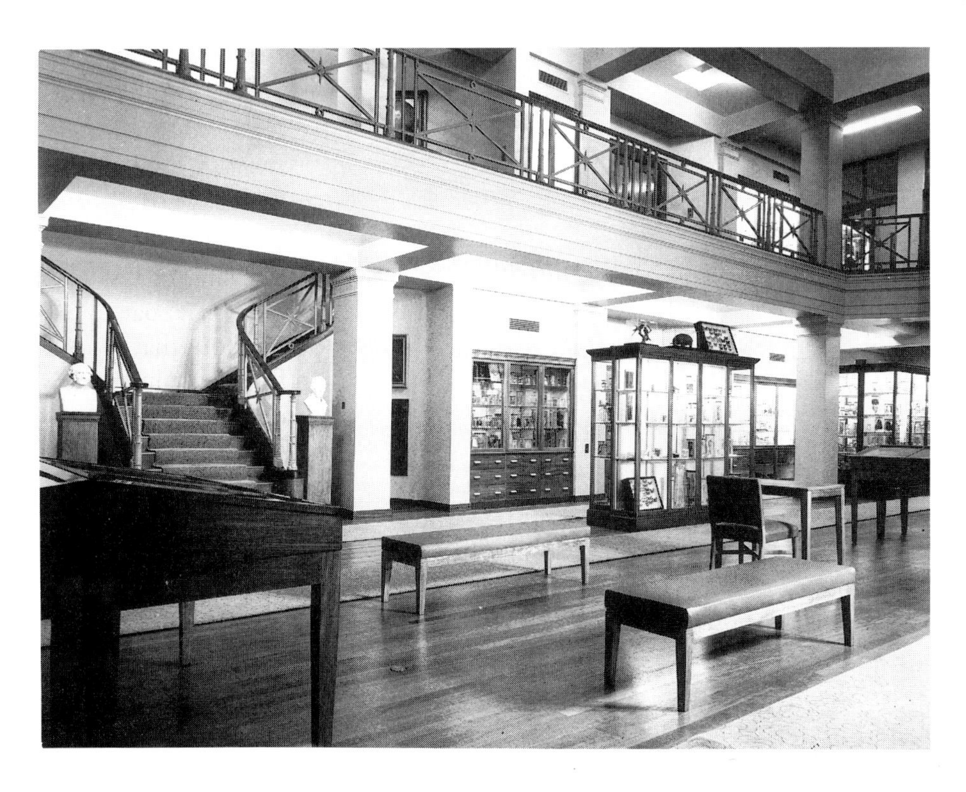

Figure 1.16 The new Hunterian Musem, built on the site of the original building, was opened in 1963.

treating everything that might touch the wound and used a carbolic spray to disinfect the surrounding air. The antiseptic principles were accepted and used by surgeons throughout the world.

Other chemical antiseptics soon became available and aseptic principles were introduced later into surgical work, especially in operation theatres, where sterilised gowns, caps and masks came to be worn by all taking part in surgical operations. Surgeons and nurses began to wear sterilised gloves after washing and disinfecting their hands. We now live in a new era in which powerful antibiotics are available for the control of bacterial infections and sterile areas are demarcated in the operating departments of our modern hospitals.

Since the time of Lord Lister impressive advances have been made in surgery, both in theory and in practice. The development of modern anaesthesia, postoperative and intensive care units, blood transfusion and fluid and electrolyte replacement therapy have all made valuable contributions. Surgery is team-work, with the surgeon, assistants, anaesthetist, nurses and other specialists in vital roles.

ACKNOWLEDGEMENT

The author acknowledges that the historical information in this chapter has been taken from Garrison and Morton (eds) *A Medical Bibliography, An Annotated Check-list of Texts Illustrating the History of Medicine by Leslie T. Morton*, (3rd edn), published by André Deutsch.

REFERENCES

Adams, F. (ed. and trans.) (1856). *The Extant Works of Aretaeus the Cappadocian*. Sydenham Society, London

Bett, W. R. (1957). Historical aspects of cancer. In Raven, R. W. (ed.) *Cancer*, Vol. 1, pp 1–5. Butterworth & Co., London

Castiglioni, A. (1940). Aulus Cornelius Celsus as a historian of medicine. *Bull. Hist. Med.*, **8**, 857–73

Cooper, A. (1829). *Illustrations of Diseases of the Breast*. Longman & Rees, London

Cooper, A. (1840). *On the Anatomy of the Breast*. Longman, Orme, Green & Longman, London

Cooper, A. (1841). *Observations on the Structure and Diseases of the Testis*. J. Churchill, London

Dobson, J. (1959). John Hunter's views on cancer. *Ann. Roy. Coll. Surg. Engl.*, **25**, 176–81

Galen (AD 130–200). De tumoribus praeter naturam. In his *Opera* edited by Kuhn, C. G. (1824), Vol. 7, pp 705–32

Gruner, C. C. (1930). *A Treatise on the Canon of Medicine of Avicenna*. Luzac & Co., London

Haagensen, C. D. (1933). An exhibit of important books, papers and memorabilia illustrating the evolution of knowledge of cancer. *Am. J. Cancer*, **18**, 42–126

Hunter, J. (1839). *Lectures on the Principles of Surgery*. Haswell, Barrington & Haswell, Philadelphia

Keil, H. (1950). The historical relationship between the concept of tumor and the ending -oma. *Bull. Hist. Med.*, **24**, 352–75

Leaf, C. H. (1898). *Anatomy of the Lymphatic Glands.* Archibald Constable & Co., London

Leopold, E. J. (1930). Aretaeus the Cappadocian. *Ann. Med. Hist.*, **2**, 424–35

Littré, E. (1839–1861). *Oeuvres Complètes d'Hippocrate* (10 vols), 572. Baillière, Paris

Millar, T. McW. (1954). John of Arderne, the father of British proctology. *Proc. Roy. Soc. Med.*, **47**, 75–84

Paget, Sir James (1874). On disease of the mammary areola preceding cancer of the mammary gland. *Saint Bartholomew's Hospital Reports*, Vol. 10, pp 87–9

Poirier, P. and Charpy, A. (1909). *Traité d'Anatomie Humaine.* Vol. 2: Les lymphatiques (Poirier, P. and Cunés, B.). Masson et Cie, Paris

Power, Sir D'Arcy (trans.) (1922). *De Arte Phisicali et de Cirurgia of Master John Arderne, Surgeon of Newark, dated 1414.* John Bale Sons & Danielson Ltd, London

Riesman, D. (1935). *The Story of Medicine in the Middle Ages*, pp 52–4. Paul B. Hoeber, New York

Shimkin, M. B. (1977). *Contrary to Nature — Cancer.* US Dept of Health, Education & Welfare, Public Health Service, National Institutes of Health

Spink, M. S. and Lewis, G. L. (1973). *Albucasis on Surgery and Instruments.* University of California Press, Berkeley

CHAPTER TWO

The First Society for the Study of Cancer

There are numerous well managed organisations throughout the world which are concerned with different aspects and problems of cancer. Their work includes research; prevention; treatment, with emphasis placed on rehabilitation and continuing care; and education, training and counselling. A major contribution is being made to this comprehensive programme by voluntary associations, which provide considerable professional and lay expertise and finance. Much financial support also comes from voluntary gifts.

This work has continued with ever-increasing momentum for nearly 200 years and has now reached a very considerable size internationally. It is therefore very interesting to study in outline the work of the First Society for the Study of Cancer and particularly the series of questions and answers which were formulated by the Medical Committee of this society. The series illuminates the state of knowledge about cancer in our country about 200 years ago.

In 1801 the Institution for Investigating the Nature and Cure of Cancer was established under the auspices of the Society for Bettering the Condition and Increasing the Comforts of the Poor. A Medical Committee was formed, whose distinguished members were Dr Matthew Baillie (nephew of John and William Hunter), Mr Sharpe, Mr Everard Home (brother-in-law of John Hunter), Mr Pearson, Mr John Abernethy (pupil of John Hunter), and Dr Denman as the Secretary.

In 1802 this committee published a small brochure which outlined the aims of the Society and listed a number of practical questions concerning cancer. They hoped that the medical profession would submit answers to the questions, so that a valuable series of observations would be obtained. It seems that this approach was well received, as 4 years later the brochure was republished in the *Edinburgh Medical and Surgical Journal* with "the hope both to preserve it and to forward the views of so laudable an Institution". The Society appears to have lapsed after this publication, for there is no record of any further activity. We may conclude that the members felt that their work was done once they had defined the current knowledge about cancer with their questions and answers. (See the *Edinburgh Medical Journal*, (1806), **2**, 382.)

The solution of a problem often depends on asking the right questions for which answers are sought. It is interesting to read the questions formulated by that early Society and to study the answers they received. Whilst additional questions about cancer are asked today and need to be answered, we have not yet answered all the questions which were posed in 1802. The position reached at that time merits our consideration. The present author has added his comments at the end of each answer.

Question 1: What are the diagnostic signs of cancer?

Answer: It is very much wished that we had an exact definition of cancer, those of the nosologists being very imperfect and insufficient. If a just and accurate definition of cancer cannot yet be found, we must be satisfied with such a description as a correct history of the disease will afford. This it appears has never yet been judiciously and accurately done, though it would probably enable us to discriminate the various forms of the disease and its distinction from other diseases. It is much to be wished that we may no longer be deceived by ambiguous words and phrases, or consider them as conveying to us any essential and practical knowledge.

Comment: The symptomatology depends on the variety of cancer and here today we regard cancer as the name given to a large group of diseases of different organs and tissues of the body which therefore cause different symptoms and signs. Accurate clinical descriptions of the different varieties of cancer are now available, which also differentiate them from other diseases. Important advances have occurred in methods of investigation for precise diagnosis and staging of these diseases for treatment programmes to be arranged. The recent introduction of non-invasive investigation techniques such as computer tomography, isotope imaging and ultrasonography has been of great value and these techniques are now used as a matter of routine. Computer tomography has stimulated the development of the latest imaging technique, called nuclear magnetic resonance, whose images depend on magnetic fields and radio frequency pulses. Immunodiagnosis is now developing, the alpha-fetoprotein test is being used to diagnose primary liver carcinoma and the carcinoembryonic antigen test is being used for colonic carcinoma. Cytology examinations, for example, for lesions of the cervix uteri, and aspiration biopsy of solid tumours, for example, of the breast, are of great practical value. Great progress has been made, too, in endoscopy examinations.

Question 2: Does any alteration take place in the structure of a part preceding the more obvious change which is called cancer? If there does, what is the nature of that alteration?

Answer: One great consequence of obtaining an answer to this query would be that though we are unable to cure cancer in an advanced stage, we might extinguish the disposition to it, or suppress it completely in an early stage. Some pains have been taken to discover, by the properties of the discharge from cancer, the nature of the disease.

Comment: In formulating this question, the members of the committee were querying whether precancerous changes might occur in organs and tissues, as well as hoping to identify other diseases which might predispose to malignant disease. Many precancerous conditions are now recognised in the body; for example, in the cervix uteri, where the epithelium is very active and squamous metaplasia occurs frequently, though it is not certain whether this is precancer. Dysplasia is more serious, for in about 7% of patients carcinoma *in situ*, or invasive carcinoma develops. Carcinoma *in situ* usually commences between the ages of 25 and 30 and invasive carcinoma develops in about 25% after 5–10 years.

In the buccal mucosa precancerous changes are well known and include leucoplakia, erythroplakia, which may become carcinoma *in situ*, chronic hyperplastic candidiasis and possibly submucous fibrosis.

Hormone-induced tumours are of great interest today. These neoplasms begin as tissue hyperplasia and advance gradually through stages, without any distinct separation, into malignant tumours. Other changes can occur which include discontinuous progression; regression, either spontaneous or hormone-induced; or a benign tumour may be formed. A small proportion of women with cystic hyperplasia of the breast develop carcinoma; a solitary papilloma in a large duct may show a highly differentiated structure with prominent myoepithelial cells, and multiple papillomas in small ducts deep in the breast are also found; a breast fibroadenoma can undergo malignant changes.

There are certain diseases and syndromes where the incidence of cancer is increased. Good examples are found in the gastrointestinal system, where

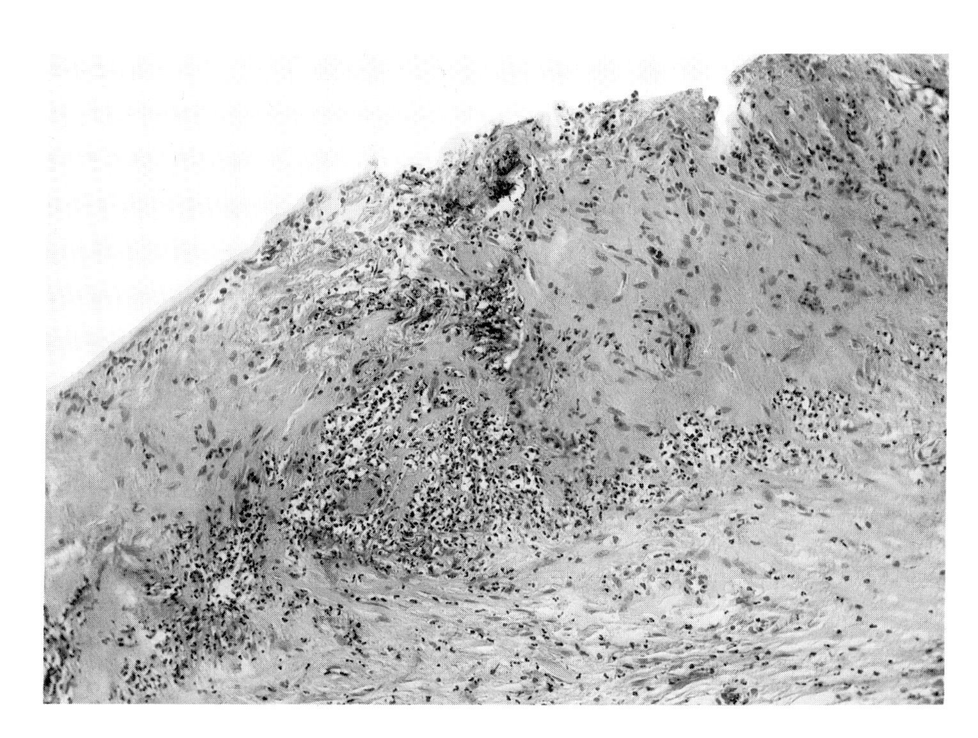

Figure 2.1 Histological specimen showing the base of a chronic gastric ulcer (X 160).

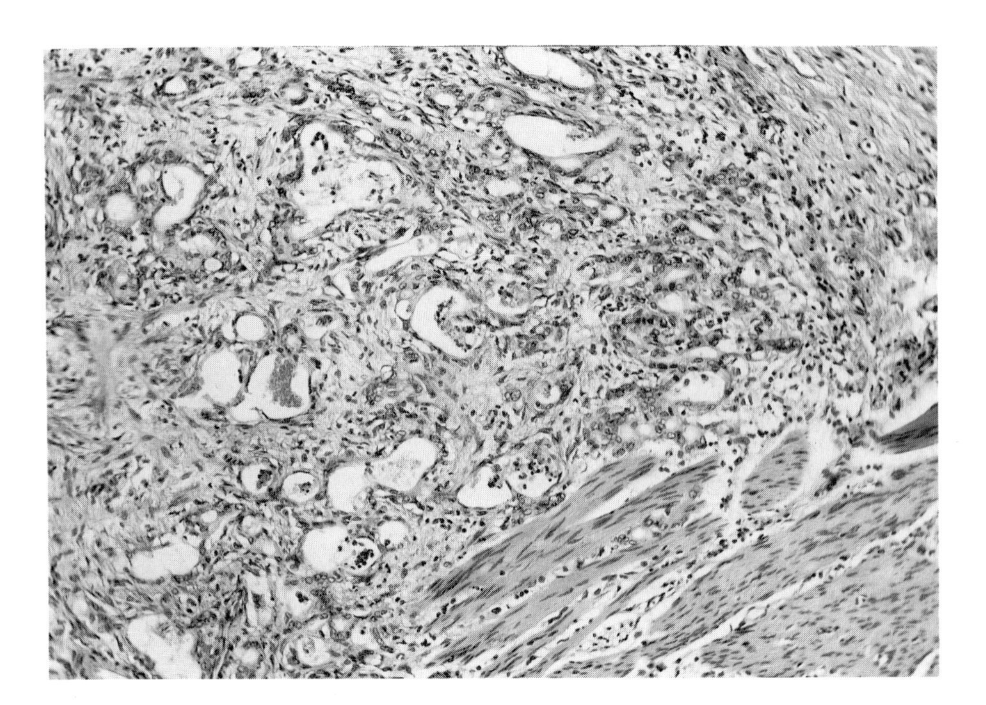

Figure 2.2 Histological specimen showing an infiltrating gastric carcinoma at the edge of a chronic peptic ulcer (X 160).

invasive cancer is frequent and dangerous. The increased risk of gastric carcinoma in patients with pernicious anaemia is well documented and the risk of carcinoma developing in the colon in patients with total chronic ulcerative colitis of 10 years' duration is 30 times greater than in the normal population. Carcinoma develops in a chronic gastric ulcer in about 1% of cases and adenomatous polyps in the stomach, colon and rectum can become carcinoma.

The high risk of carcinoma developing in the colon and rectum with familial adenosis of these regions is well known.

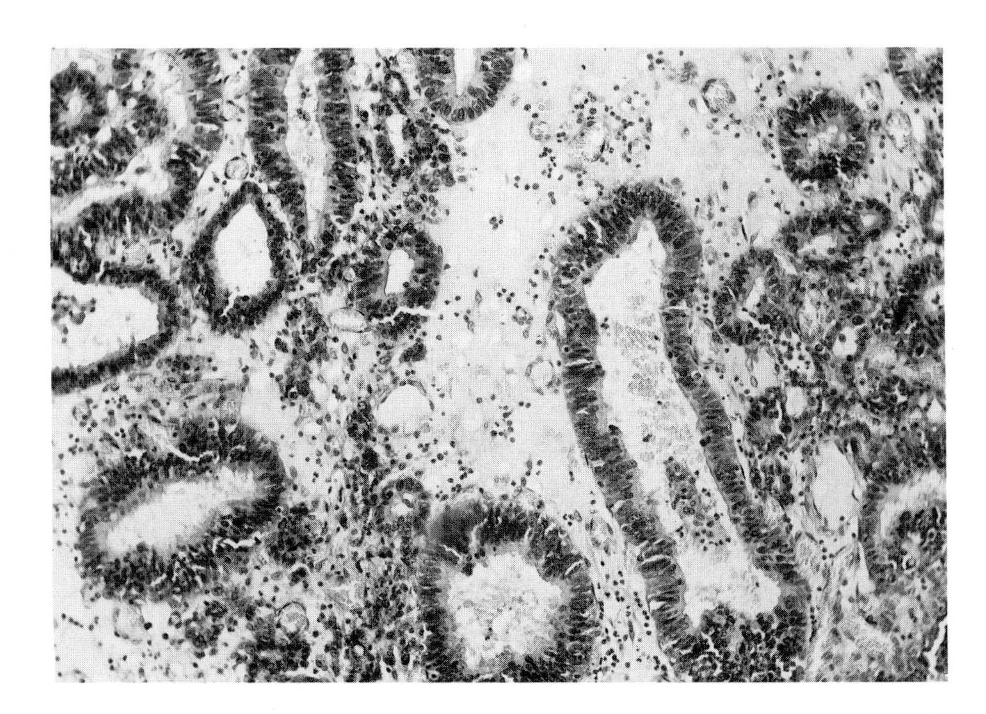

Figure 2.3 Histological specimen showing a benign gastric polyp (X 160).

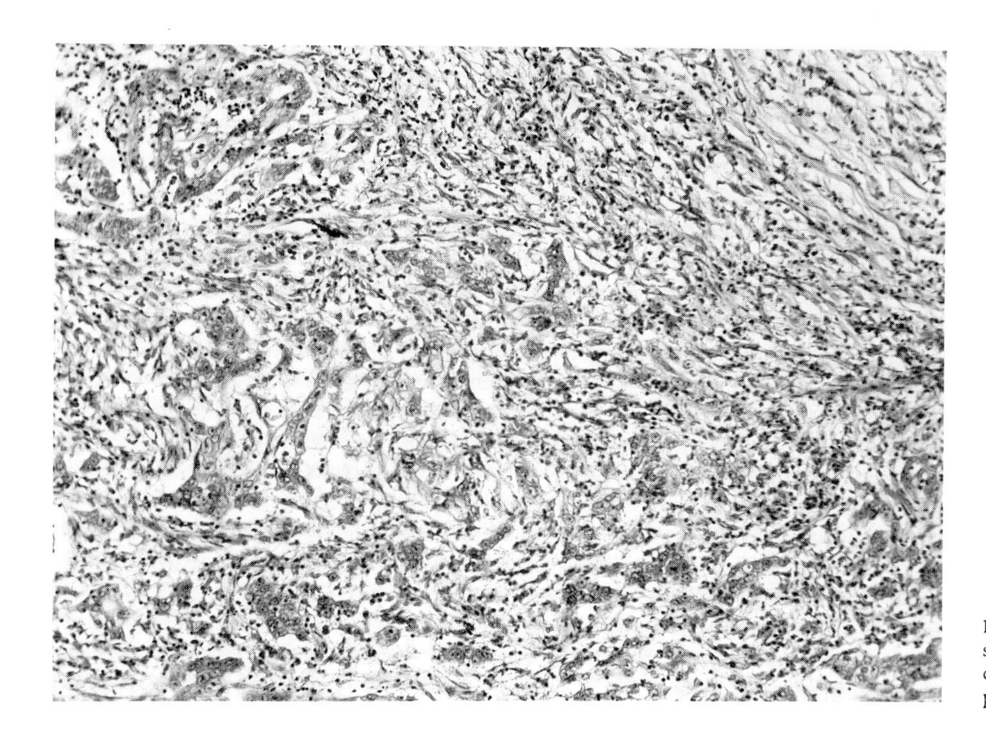

Figure 2.4 Histological specimen showing an infiltrating gastric carcinoma associated with a gastric polyp (X 160).

The development of carcinoma of the hypopharynx in females with the Paterson–Kelly syndrome has aroused much interest for many years. There is evidence associating the Peutz–Jeghers syndrome with gastro-intestinal carcinoma, especially of the small intestine, and the relationship of coeliac disease with subsequent abdominal reticuloses is strongly suggested.

Malignant bone tumours may arise in osteitis deformans; a chondrosarcoma may develop in diaphyseal aclasis, dyschondroplasia and Ollier's disease. Malignant changes occur in some patients with osteoclastoma.

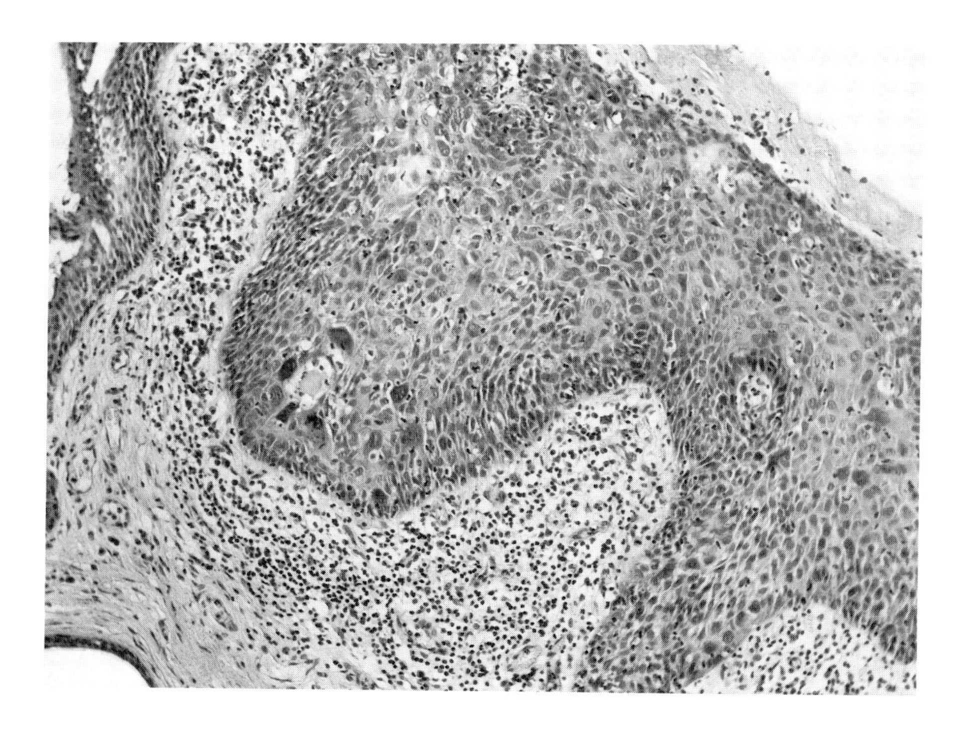

Figure 2.5 Histological specimen showing a carcinoma *in situ* of the larynx (X 160).

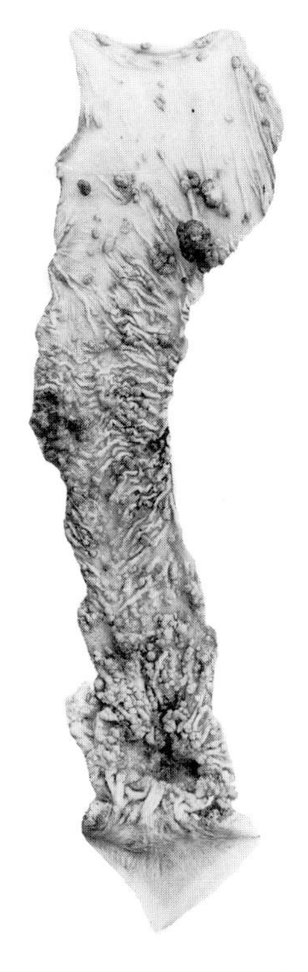

Figure 2.6 A rectum removed by an abdominoperineal excision (Miles' operation), showing polyposis with a carcinoma.

The increase in our knowledge of these premalignant conditions is impressive and important because of the practical possibility of cancer prevention. Early detection of cancer in its initial stages gives the patient the best chance of curative treatment.

The answer to the question also includes reference to the work being done at that time in investigations regarding the "properties of discharge from cancer", without giving details of any findings. The committee members were doubtless concerned with the discharges from external tumours which had been discussed in cytological investigations. They could hardly have had any knowledge of the hormonal secretions of many tumours that give rise to various syndromes which we recognise today.

Question 3: Is cancer always an original and primary disease, or may other diseases degenerate into cancer?

Answer: We must leave this query to be determined by future experience and observations; and if the latter should unexpectedly be decided in the affirmative we must then enquire what kind of disease and under what circumstances of the part, or of the constitution, there exists such aptitude to develop into cancer.

Comment: It is well recognised that cancer does develop as a primary disease, but there is a greater risk with certain conditions. This subject was considered in the comment under question 2. The circumstances under which cancer develops in other diseases remain largely unknown. Pernicious anaemia is an autoimmune disease which causes inflammation and atrophic

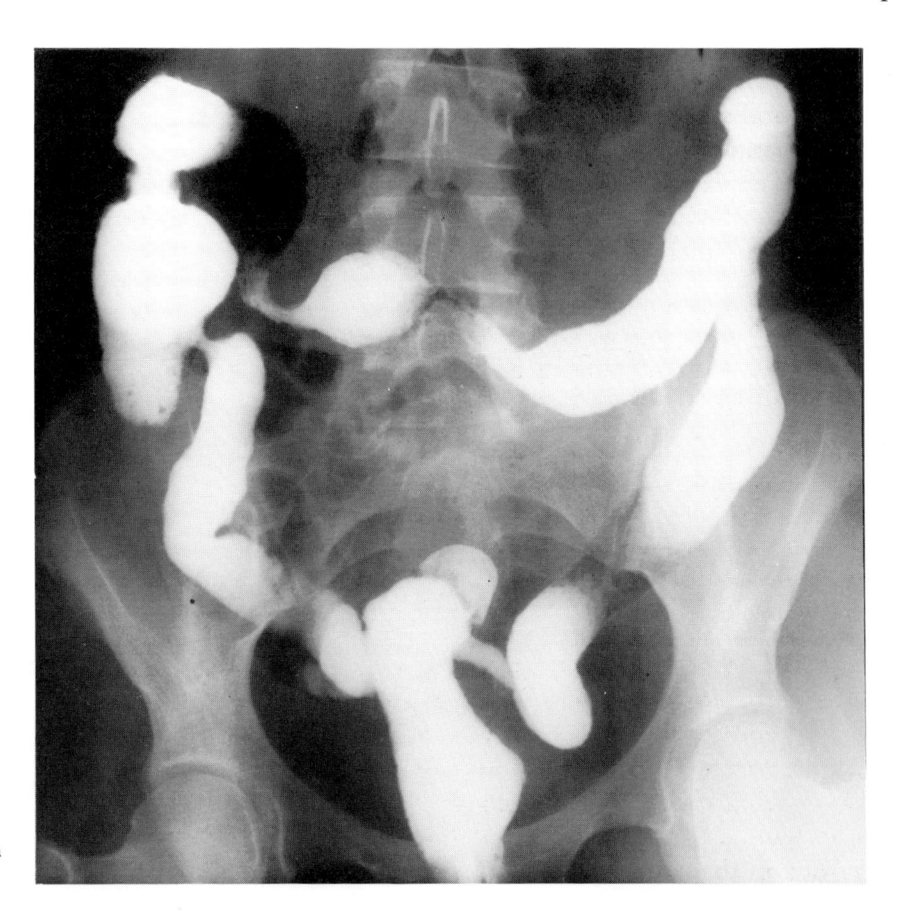

Figure 2.7 Radiograph of a colon with a barium enema, showing multiple strictures caused by total chronic ulcerative colitis. Total colectomy with an ileo-rectal anastomosis restored normal defaecation. Carcinoma can develop with this chronic disease in the colon or rectum.

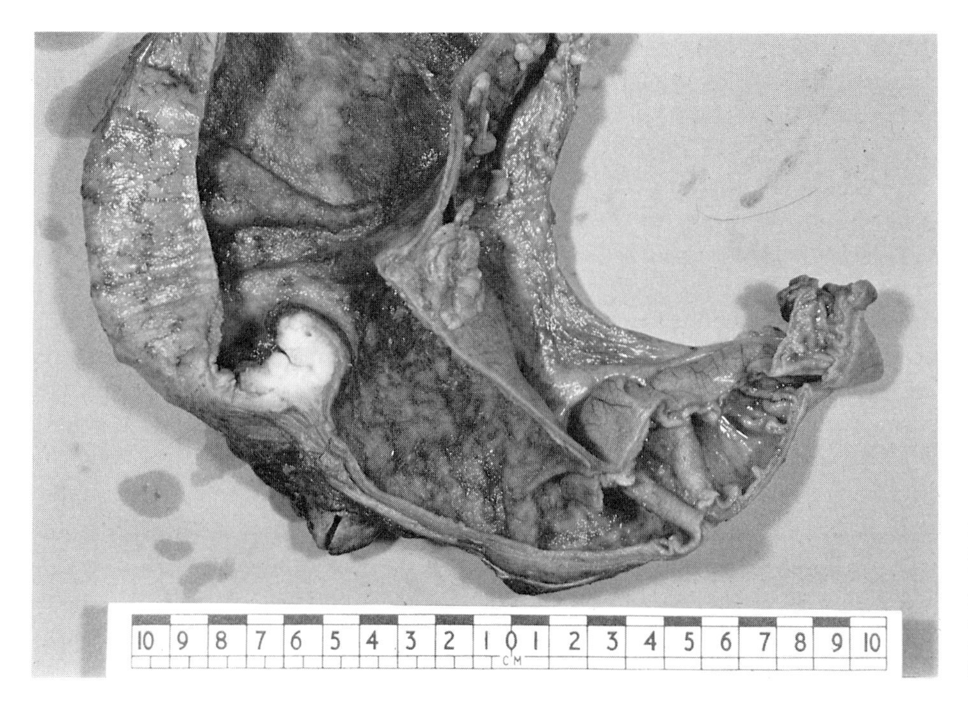

Figure 2.8 Carcinoma in a colon affected by chronic ulcerative colitis. The risk of carcinoma developing in the colon of patients with total chronic ulcerative colitis of 10 years' duration is 30 times greater than it is in the normal population.

changes in the gastric mucosa, characteristic of an autoimmune lesion. Chronic ulcerative colitis may possibly be an autoimmune disease causing ulceration and disintegration of the wall of the colon. Cancer occurring in autoimmune diseases is worthy of further study.

We admire the ideas and penetrative thoughts of our ancestors, whose questions here are of the greatest interest. The subject of immunology, however, had not then emerged and they knew little of the complicated immune system of the body and its role in the prevention and control of cancer. Several decades were to elapse before vaccines and sera were used in cancer treatment. There is every likelihood that further immunological research will explain why cancer develops in other lesions and diseases.

Question 4: Are there any proofs of cancer being a hereditary disease?

Answer: Whether cancer, or any other disease, be, strictly speaking, hereditary, has, like any other opinions, been positively asserted, or positively denied. Whether children born of cancerous parents be more liable to cancer than others, from any structure or organisation of the body, or other rooted principle of the constitution, may, by attentive observation, be discovered; and if it should be so proved, we might be led to the prevention of cancer by medicine, by well-regulated diet, or a circumspect manner of education, and of living. If it be proved, on the contrary, that cancer is not hereditary, the minds of many would be relieved from the distress of perpetual apprehension.

Comment: This is an important question, for in addition to the scientific problems involved, the subject is the cause of much apprehension. At the time the members of the committee asked this question there was no scientific answer, for genetics had not emerged. A considerable amount of research is being carried out on genetics and experimental tumours and a clear account was given by Koller *(1957)*. Inbred strains of mice were largely used in the experimental work and Koller states that no tumour

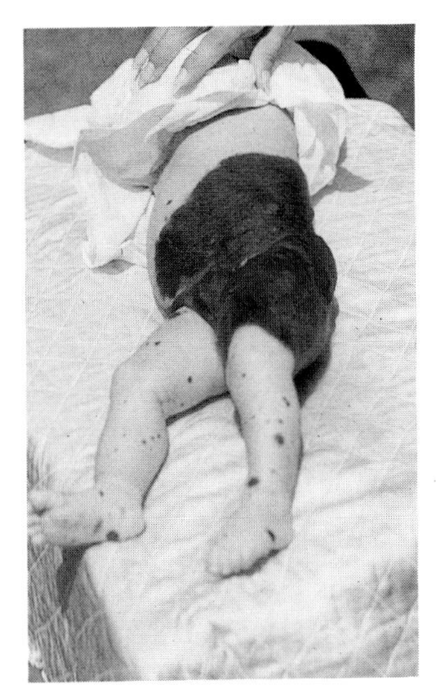

Figure 2.9 A child with the rare condition of "bathing trunks naevus", a congenital deformity.

determined by a single gene had been found; the studies indicate that many genes are involved in determining the animal's susceptibility and the genes have a cumulative effect. He points out that the problem is complicated, as shown in the studies of mammary cancer in mice, where three factors are concerned: genetic constitution, that is, genes which condition susceptibility; oestrogenic hormones; and a cytoplasmic factor.

The possibility that human cancer has a genetic basis is suggested by a number of family pedigrees showing the high incidence of particular cancers in members of one family, but there are many factors to consider which affect their value. However, Koller states that the evidence indicates, at least in certain families, the presence of a genetic factor in breast cancer causation. Thus daughters of women with breast carcinoma are in a higher risk group for this disease than others.

He also points out that leukaemia shows a tendency to appear in relatives, and familial studies of gastric cancer show a higher incidence of cancer in the relatives of patients with the disease than in the controls. The high incidence of the same cancer in some families is suggestive of a genetic factor; and this applies especially to gastrointestinal cancer, including cancer of the stomach, colon and rectum. The familial incidence of retinoblastoma, neurofibromatosis and multiple exostoses of bone is well known. Familial adenosis of the colon and the rectum is a disease where the risk of developing carcinoma is extremely high. Xeroderma pigmentosum is another familial disease with a high cancer risk when the skin is exposed to strong sunlight.

Cancer has been studied in twins and their family pedigrees; the results increase the evidence that stomach cancer has a hereditary basis, but the genetic factor in breast cancer is secondary.

There are practical connotations of all this evidence and it is advisable that persons in the high risk group for cancer should have routine health check-ups; those with premalignant lesions should undergo preventive cancer treatment and genetic counselling is now done for prospective parents in high risk cancer families. Patients with malignant diseases which

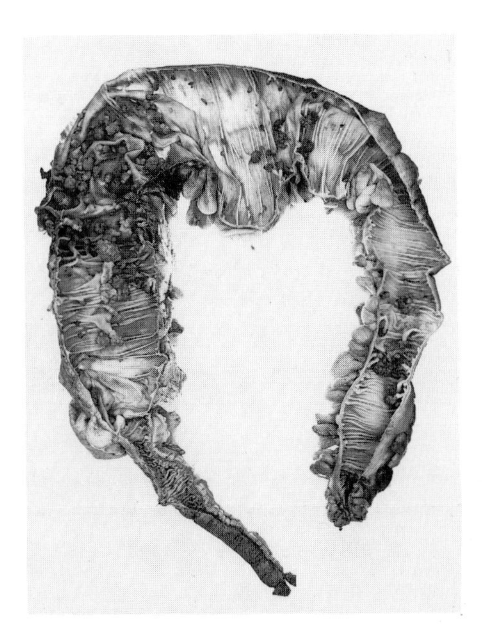

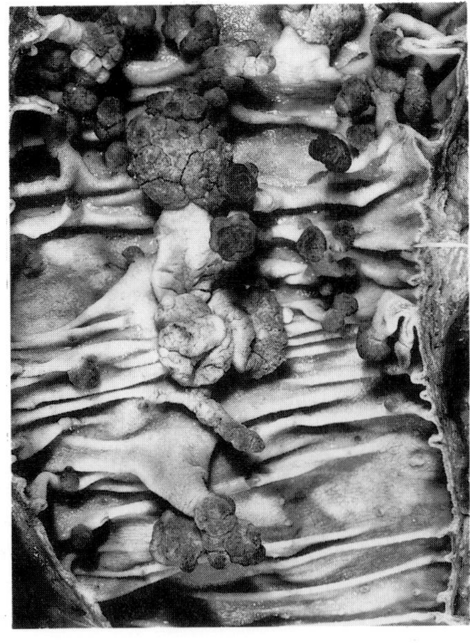

Figure 2.10 *Left:* A colon with familial polyposis and a carcinoma. *Right:* The carcinoma in the ascending colon.

are treated with chemotherapy are being followed-up to determine whether their children are more likely to develop cancer.

Question 5: Are there any proofs of cancer being a contagious disease?

Answer: This query constantly requires some explanation and the Committee was endeavouring to collect all the facts, even the most trifling, as they may direct us to the knowledge of things of great importance.

Comment: There is no evidence that cancer is contagious; the incidence of cancer in doctors and nurses who care for patients with cancer is no higher than in others. Relatives of cancer patients need not fear close proximity with them. It seems that the committee were wondering if cancer had an infective aetiology, but they had no knowledge of oncogenic viruses, or viral carcinogenesis. The newer aspects of carcinogenesis, including aspects of viral carcinogenesis, were discussed by Warwick *(1973)*. Warwick quotes Huebner and Todaro, who put forward the oncogenic hypothesis to explain various facets of oncogenesis, including the fact that while cancer does not appear to result from an infective process, it nevertheless has a viral aetiology in animals, in some cases. It is postulated that mammalian cells contain genes which when expressed release the particular cells from constraints regulating their normal growth pattern, so the cells become malignant. These genes are termed "oncogenes"; there are others called "virogenes", which contain the information to code an RNA virus, which can function alone or concomitantly. Activation of both genes would cause malignant transformation and the release of virus; activation of the oncogene alone would lead to transformation without the release of virus. Almost all tumour-inducing viruses in animals so far investigated cause sarcomas or leukaemias, while, as pointed out by Warwick, the majority of human cancers are carcinomas. Up to the present no human malignant tumour has been proved to be of viral aetiology, although there is evidence associating the Epstein–Barr virus (EBV) with Burkitt's lymphoma.

A detailed and comprehensive account of the part played by viruses in the origin of tumours was given by Dmochowski *(1957)*, who also gave an extensive list of references to the literature up to that date.

Question 6: Is there any well-marked relation between cancer and other diseases? If there be, what are those diseases to which it bears the nearest resemblance, in its origin, progress and termination?

Answer: Some have affirmed and others deny.

Comment: The development of cancer in other diseases has been described in the comment under question 3.

Regarding any resemblance in origin, progress and termination between the cancerous diseases and other diseases, there is none for they are in a class by themselves.

Question 7: May cancer be regarded at any period, or under any circumstances, merely as a local disease? Or, does the existence of cancer in one part afford a presumption that there is a tendency to a similar morbid alteration in other parts of the animal system?

Answer: An answer could be highly important. A surgeon who is said to have great skill in removing cancerous breasts has said that, in many truly cancerous affections of that part, he has found on examination that the uterus exhibited the marks of the same disease, and that the state of the uterus was his guide in determining him to extirpate or avoid operating upon diseased breasts. If the uterus was discovered to be affected, he refused to perform the operation, having constantly found it unsuccessful under such circumstances, yet it does not follow that all extirpations of the breast will be successful, if the uterus be free from disease. When operations fail to remove the whole disease which in some cases is impracticable, the sufferings of the patients are aggravated and their lives shortened by operation; of course they should not then be performed. In practice we must distinguish between the extirpation of a diseased part and the cure of the disease. It is worthy of observation whether external injuries ever give rise to cancer, or merely aggravate and put in action a disease which before existed.

Comment: This question is very important both from the academic and practical viewpoints and it indicates considerable perspicuity on the part of the committee members at that time. It is generally considered that cancer is initially a local disease which later becomes a generalised disease with the formation of micrometastases at first, and later macrometastases in other organs and tissues. The time scale for these developments in the disease process remains unknown, but we recognise that the primary tumour can be small and give rise to multiple metastases. The treatment of the patient with primary cancer is different from that of the patient with disseminated disease, so assessment and staging of the disease are essential when the treatment programme is arranged. With our sophisticated techniques of investigation an accurate assessment can usually be made.

Research continues to elucidate the properties of cancer to invade contiguous tissues, lymphatic and blood vessels and to form metastases in the regional lymph nodes and in distant organs.

In the answer to this vital question the members of the committee concentrated on breast cancer, which causes us considerable concern today, for it is the commonest cancer in women. It is an unfortunate fact that many patients already have disseminated carcinoma of the breast when they are first seen for treatment, although initially the disease is localised in the breast. When metastases are present in the axillary nodes the survival rate after treatment is markedly diminished. Mastectomy is contra-indicated for patients with disseminated carcinoma, unless it is confined to the axillary nodes. Every patient must therefore be thoroughly investigated to determine the stage of the disease. In contrast to the treatment available in the early 19th century, in addition to surgery we now have radiotherapy and chemotherapy, which includes hormonal therapy, to be used according to the stage of breast carcinoma.

The surgical opinion given to the members of the committee, that mastectomy is contra-indicated if there is uterine carcinoma, was very sound. It is not stated whether the surgeon considered the uterine carcinoma was primary or metastatic. (In the present author's experience, primary or metastatic carcinoma is uncommon with breast carcinoma.) He was wise in pointing out that surgical treatment, unless performed for the correct indications, might place the patient in a worse position than before the operation. When generalised disease is present, treatment with hormonal therapy and/or chemotherapy is indicated. If there is localised pain, especially with osseous metastases, radiotherapy can give good relief. Surgical treatment may be necessary to relieve obstructions; for endocrine ablation procedures; for pain relief by various neurectomies and cordotomy; and as debulking operations before chemotherapy and radiotherapy are instituted.

Question 8: Has climate, or local situation, any influence in rendering the human constitution more or less liable to cancer, under any form, or in any part?

Answer: Regarding cancer it is not only necessary to observe the effects of climate and local situation, but to extend our views to different employments, as those in various metals and manufactures; in mines and collieries; in the army and navy; in those who lead sedentary, or active lives; in the married and single; in the different sexes, and in many other circumstances. The cancer to which chimney-sweepers are subject is known, but not accurately understood, and more but fruitless observations have yet been made upon it, except such as relate to operations.

Comment: This is a comprehensive and enlightened answer to an important question. Could the question have been sparked off by the observation made 27 years previously by Percivall Pott about chimney-sweepers' scrotal cancer? The committee also pointed out that more work, other than surgical operations, was required to understand the reason for the development of this disease. About 130 years were to elapse before the synthesis, by Kennaway, Cook and their colleagues, of benzpyrene from coal-tar. In the meantime, Butlin in 1892 examined the subject in detail (see Chapter 4).

It is very likely that Percivall Pott's observation stimulated the members of the committee to consider newer aspects of the cancer problem, although the complete cancer panorama was hidden from their eyes. Nevertheless, they were moving into the areas of environmental, occupational and geographical cancer, in addition to hinting that life-styles might be implicated. Epidemiology has provided us with important scientific data and all these subjects embracing cancer have had a remarkable development, which is described in other chapters of this book.

Here, only brief comments will be made on various matters which were raised in the committee's answer.

Geographical studies concerning the distribution of cancer have shown wide variations in continents, countries and nations. For example, breast carcinoma is very common in women in the UK and the USA, but very uncommon in Japanese women living in Japan. The study of the incidence of cancer in emigrant populations has provided important information. Gastric carcinoma is common in Japan, but is declining in the UK; and hepatocellular carcinoma is common in Bantu natives, but is rare in the UK. These and many other facts are now the object of intensive epidemiological research in order to define the different influences which are in operation.

The sex incidence of various forms of cancer is a matter of constant study but many of the questions involved still remain unanswered. For example, why is carcinoma of the breast the commonest cancer in women and one of the rarest in men? The age incidence of cancer likewise always attracts considerable attention. Here we can enquire why malignant tumours in children commonly arise in mesoblastic tissues, whilst those in adults usually arise in ectodermal tissues. Why does breast carcinoma attain its maximum incidence at the age when women are undergoing important hormonal changes? The influence of the marital status and childbearing are also important, for example, in carcinoma of the breast and uterus.

The problems associated with the prevention of occupational cancer, and its treatment, are now matters of great concern. This subject is dealt with in Chapter 4. The members of the committee raised the question of cancer and various metals and manufactures, but this was before the introduction of carcinogens such as asbestos and vinyl chloride.

The importance of working in mines and collieries was not overlooked, for doubtless the committee members were aware of the reports that had been made of specific miners' sickness in workers in the mines at Schneebey and Joachimsthal from the 16th century onwards. About a century was to elapse, however, before it was recognised that many of the sick miners were dying of lung cancer. The subject was considered in detail by Glucksmann *et al. (1957)*, who stated that these mines contained a lot of dust, in which there were possibly traces of arsenic, cobalt and other metals, and that this was thought to cause the high incidence of lung cancer, but when a high level of radioactivity was observed in the air of the mines, that also was considered a possible cause of the disease.

The committee members had no knowledge of radiation and its carcinogenic action; the growth of that subject has really been enormous and we now have to consider the atmospheric and global effects of radiation.

The committee gave a hint that life-style might be important where cancer development is concerned, by mentioning "sedentary and active" lives. We now recognise the importance of stress and strain and of habits and customs. The serious tobacco cancers were not recognised at that time, nor was the connection of cancer with alcohol; however, the committee's answer did include the words "many other circumstances".

Question 9: Is there a particular temperament of body more liable to be affected with cancer than others, and if there be what is that temperament?

Answer: The normal temperament has been often used by medical writers without any precise meaning. It is here meant to signify any nature or acquired habit of body, which may dispose to or resist the influence of cancer.

Comment: In the previous comment mention was made of stress and strain; there is experimental evidence that the incidence of tumours in small animals is higher in those that have been subjected to various stresses and strains than in controls. Some cancer patients are seen who report that a period of stress and strain preceded their symptoms, but more research is necessary here. It is possible that changes occur in the endocrine system, especially in the adrenal glands. The association between smoking tobacco and cancer in the lungs and other organs is one of the biggest problems we need to solve today and some attention is being given to the personalities of inveterate smokers, since both factors might be concerned with the development of cancer.

Question 10: Are brute creatures subject to any disease resembling cancer in the human subject?

Answer: It is not known at present whether brute creatures are subject to cancer, though some of their diseases have a very suspicious appearance. When this question is decided we may enquire what class of animals is chiefly subject to cancer; the wild or domesticated; the carnivorous or the grainivorous; those which do and those which do not chew cud. This investigation may lead to much philosophical amusement and useful information; particularly it may teach us how the prevalence or frequency of cancer may depend upon the mannerisms and habits of life.

Comment: It is interesting to see the way the members of the committee were seeking new information about cancer by turning to cancer in animals under different conditions, including the possible influences of the human domestic environment. It appears that at that time there was very little information about cancer in animals. The subject was considered in great detail by Innes *(1958)*, who stated that Bashford and Murray in 1904 were amongst the first to call attention to the universal occurrence of cancer throughout vertebrates, and he gave valuable references to the literature. He points out that if all domesticated animals were allowed to survive for their natural span of life, the morbidity and mortality from cancer might approximate those in humans. The immunity of apes and monkeys to cancer is an interesting observation. The important work of Cotchin must be acknowledged here, and references to his publications are given by Innes. Attention is called to the conclusions reached by Innes from a study of his personal data and wide experience. He states that there are differences in cancer between humans and animals, but they are not fundamental, being related to the different susceptibilities of animal species to different varieties of cancer and to the higher and lower incidence in the various organs and tissues. Important differences are the low incidence of cancer in the mammary glands of the cow and in the stomach of all animals, in marked contrast to their frequency in humans. The reasons for these differences are not apparent; does the continual milking of cows confer immunity? Cancers occur quite often in the mammary glands and testes of dogs. Innes describes cancers which are peculiar to certain species of animals. Thus eye cancer occurs in Hereford cattle, osteosarcoma in long-legged dogs, osteogenic tumours in the canine mammae and leukaemia in Scottish terriers. Research in comparative oncology should continue, for it might yield important results.

Question 11: Is there any period of life absolutely exempt from the attack of this disease?

Answer: It seems to be generally admitted that cancer is most frequent in old or advanced age; but this is not satisfactorily proved. Nor is it certainly known what is the earliest period of life at which cancer has been observed to take place; though no case of that disease has yet been noticed before

20 years of age; at least not before the time of puberty when the parts most frequently affected with cancer undergo a great and conspicuous change; so that some connection may possibly be observed between puberty and this disease. The same may perhaps be observed at the time of the final cessation of the menses.

Comment: The relationship between the age of people and the incidence of cancer in various organs is a subject of great interest and importance. Since the above answer was written in 1802 there has been a considerable growth in our knowledge. For example, we now recognise intrauterine carcinogenesis and know that cancer has been seen in new-born babies; and increasing numbers of cancer patients under the age of 20 years are being seen today. The emergence of paediatric oncology is an important, fairly recent development. The committee members were right to call attention to the changes that occur at the times of puberty and the cessation of menstruation. We do not yet understand their influence, which is chiefly of an endocrine nature, on the development of cancer.

In general, the incidence of cancer increases as age advances, but the age curves differ somewhat according to the organ or tissue which is affected. This subject and many others, including marriage and childbearing, were dealt with by Stocks *(1958)*. That author pointed out that the death rate from cancer of some internal organs, for example, the lung, kidney and brain, appears to be lower for people aged over 70 years, but this might be due to less complete recognition of the disease in advanced age. In some countries death rates from uterine cancer reach a peak at about 50 years of age, but this is not so in England and Wales, where in 1945–1949 the rates per million aged over 35, 45, 55, 65 and 75 were 92, 314, 513, 628 and 696. Stocks explains the method of calculating cohort rates and its importance in attempting to find reasons why cancer inception in an organ becomes more frequent as age advances.

The fact that the incidence of cancer increases with age has practical national connotations, for treatment and continuing care facilities have to be increased for an ageing population, as in the UK and other countries.

The committee members had no knowledge of transplacental and intrauterine carcinogenesis, which are of considerable interest and practical importance today. The subject has been dealt with by Tomatis *(1973)*, who states that the first reports were published by Larsen (1947), Smith and Rous (1948) and Klein (1952), and he gives a long list of references to the extensive literature which has been built up about the subject. He reviews the experimental evidence which indicates that a chemical carcinogen given to a pregnant woman can reach the foetus, interact with the foetal cells and induce tumours in the offspring. He also calls attention to the human evidence, including the reports of the development of vaginal adenocarcinoma in the daughters of women who received stilboestrol therapy during pregnancy. The daughters were diagnosed with this disease at ages between 14 and 22 years. There is obviously great practical importance in preventing the exposure of pregnant women to any carcinogen; for example, to chemicals, hormones and X-irradiation. It is now advised that no pregnant woman should smoke tobacco, to safeguard the foetus from its likely ill-effects.

In children aged from 1–14 years cancer is the major cause of death, apart

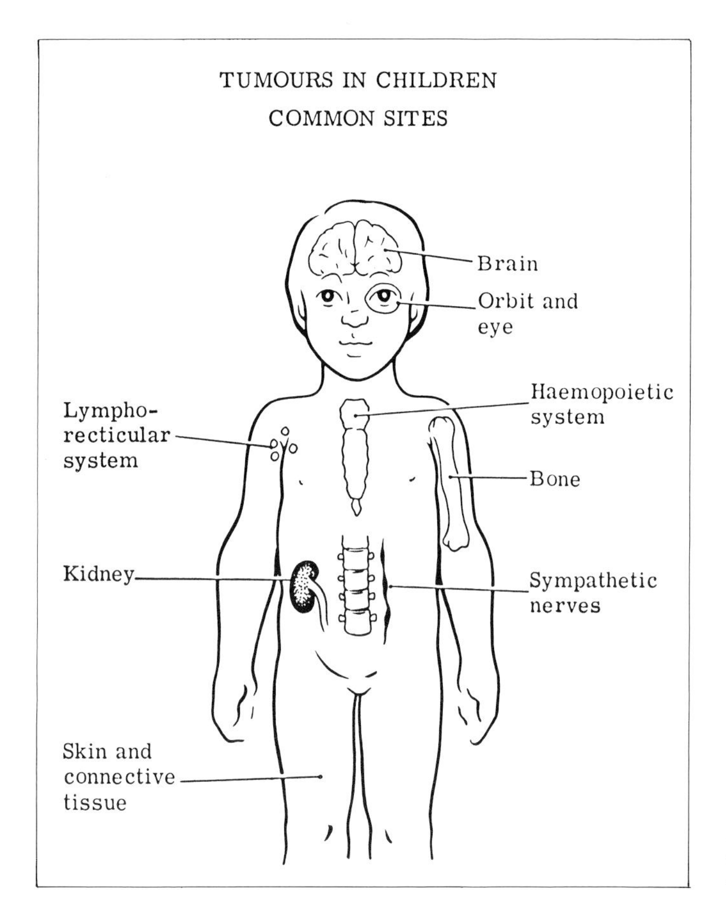

Figure 2.11 The organs and tissues which are the most common sites of tumours in children.

from accidents. As stated previously, the spectrum of cancer in children is different from that in adults; in the former the leukaemias, embryonal tumours and sarcomas are the common types. The differences in the anatomical distribution in the two groups are very striking; in children, after the leukaemias, tumours of the central nervous system, lymphomas, tumours of the sympathetic nervous system, soft tissues, kidney and bone are prominent. Modern treatment, including the development of chemotherapy and combined modalities, has considerably improved the prognosis in childhood cancer.

Question 12: Are the lymph glands ever affected primarily in cancer?

Answer: This query goes to the very root of the inquiry with respect to cancer, which has been hitherto said always to originate in the glandular system, without distinguishing, however, the particular set of glands. In cases of the breast, the lymphatic glands appear to be affected only in a secondary way, when the disease is making progress. It is probable that careful attention to the objects of this query would lead to many new observations respecting the first seat, cause, and effect of cancer.

Comment: It is apparent from the answer given to this easy question that the committee members were unaware of the group of lymphomas, including Hodgkin's disease, which are well known today. Doubtless, attention was being given to affections of the lymph glands (now termed "nodes") at that time, for in 1832 Hodgkin, of Guy's Hospital in London, recorded a series of patients with enlarged lymph nodes and splenomegaly, which became known first of all as lymphadenoma and then as Hodgkin's lymphoma. Much work has been done on lymphomas and patients can now be cured.

Investigations concerning the aetiology of the lymphomas have not yet given us an answer, although research into Burkitt's lymphoma, a lymphomatous tumour first reported by Burkitt *(1958)*, suggests that it has a viral aetiology. Considerable attention has been paid to this disease, which affects boys more than girls, and epidemiological findings, virus isolation and serological studies support the postulated viral aetiology. This may therefore be the first human tumour to be proved of viral aetiology and will vindicate the answer of the committee that "this query goes to the very root of the inquiry with respect to cancer", although it seems they had no idea of such a development.

That they were familiar with the spread of carcinoma through the lymphatic vessels to the regional lymph nodes is clear from their observation on the progress of breast cancer.

Question 13: Is cancer under any circumstances susceptible of a natural cure?

Answer: Many diseases and accidents, to which the human body is liable, are cured, or repaired by some process of the constitution peculiarly and admirably adapted to the kind of disease and accident. No instance has ever occurred, or been recorded, of cancer being cured by any natural process of the constitution. When an indurated and enlarged part of a truly cancerous disposition begins to inflame and to be disturbed, the morbid principle may be considered as having overpowered the shield or barrier formed around it for the defence of the constitution.

Comment: There are authentic reports of the spontaneous regression of malignant human tumours. This subject was considered by Everson and Cole *(1966)*. Neuroblastoma in children has a well-known propensity for spontaneous regression. This is a very interesting tumour, with a tissue-type specific antigen against which cell-mediated immunity might be directed. Spontaneous regression occurs particularly in infants under 6 months of age, even with widely disseminated disease *(Schwartz and colleagues, 1974)*. Malignant melanoma is another interesting tumour where spontaneous regression can occur. Currie *(1973)* states that the evidence that such regressions are immunological is not wholly convincing and that other factors may be at work, including spontaneous differentiation, as is commonly seen in tumours such as neuroblastomas, which may have little or no immunological basis. He also points out that tumour regression can take place after viral and bacterial infections, due to their direct effects.

The reference of the committee members to "constitutional" responses to disease or accident is extremely interesting and was far-seeing at that time when immunology had not emerged and they could not explain their ideas in scientific terminology. Even now we cannot predict the future developments in cancer immunotherapy and immunoprophylaxis, although immunodiagnosis is being used and is developing in an interesting way.

This series of 13 questions and answers published early in the 19th century has real relevance to cancer at the present time, towards the end of the 20th century. The committee members' insight regarding the cancer problem, evident from the way they formulated their questions, is quite remarkable. They certainly asked the right questions considering the state of knowledge about cancer that existed at that time. The answers they were able to obtain from the medical profession are illuminating and demonstrate the grasp of the subject of those who gave the information, in addition to the way they looked into the future.

Whilst the answers to the questions asked in 1802 require further elaboration, which is now possible because of the development of scientific methodology, research, study of the basic oncology sciences and our present understanding of the whole subject of cancer, in closing this chapter it is appropriate to ask some additional questions, the answers to which would illuminate the problem. These questions are as follows: How do cancer cells differ from normal cells? What is the mechanism of carcinogenesis? What are the mechanisms of the hormonal control of neoplasms?

REFERENCES

Burkitt, D. (1958). A sarcoma involving the jaws in African children. *Br. J. Surg.*, **46**, 218–23

Currie, G. A. (1973). Human cancer and immunology. In Raven, R. W. (ed.) *Modern Trends in Oncology*, Part 1: Research Progress, pp 127–43. Butterworth & Co., London

Dmochowski, L. (1957). The part played by viruses in the origin of tumours. In Raven, R. W. (ed.) *Cancer*, Vol. 1, pp 214–305. Butterworth & Co., London

Everson, T. C. and Cole, W. H. (1966). *Spontaneous Regression of Cancer*, W. B. Saunders, Philadelphia and London

Glucksmann, A., Lamerton, L. F. and Mayneord, W. V. (1957). Carcinogenic effects of radiation. In Raven, R. W. (ed.) *Cancer*, Vol. 1, pp 497–539. Butterworth & Co., London

Innes, J. R. M. (1958). Malignant diseases of domesticated animals. In Raven, R. W. (ed.) *Cancer*, Vol. 3, pp 73–115. Butterworth & Co., London

Koller, P. C. (1957). The genetic component of cancer. In Raven, R. W. (ed.) *Cancer*, Vol. 1, pp 335–403. Butterworth & Co., London

Schwartz, A. D., Dadash-Zadeh, M., Lee, H. and Swaney, J. J. (1974). Spontaneous regression of disseminated neuroblastoma. *J. Paediatr.*, **85**, 760–3

Stocks, P. (1958). Statistical investigations concerning the causation of various forms of human cancer. In Raven, R. W. (ed.) *Cancer*, Vol. 3, pp 116–72. Butterworth & Co., London

Tomatis, L. (1973). Transplacental carcinogenesis. In Raven, R. W. (ed.) *Modern Trends in Oncology*, Part 1: Research Progress, pp 99–126. Butterworth & Co., London

Warwick, G. P. (1973). Newer aspects of carcinogenesis. In Raven, R. W. (ed.) *Modern Trends in Oncology*, Part 1: Research Progress, pp 61–97. Butterworth & Co., London

CHAPTER THREE

The Establishment of Cancer Hospitals

The first hospital to be devoted exclusively to the care of patients with cancer was opened in Rheims in 1740, through the generous benefaction of Jean Godinot (1661–1739), who bequeathed to the city a considerable sum of money for the erection and maintenance of a cancer hospital. He was a Canon of Rheims Cathedral and described as "a charitable and pious man who had devoted his whole life to caring for poor patients and to relieving their misfortunes" *(Ledoux-Lebard, 1906)*. It was a small hospital, directed by the staff of the Hôtel Dieu, with a bed complement of 12, but that number was always found to be too small to meet demands and it was increased as funds became available.

At that time the popular belief that cancer was contagious was particularly strong in the Rheims region and patients with cancer were avoided as though they had leprosy. The fear of infection was so great that in 1779 the inhabitants of Rheims succeeded in having the cancer patients transferred outside the city, where a new hospital building had been constructed and named the Hôpital Saint Louis. This hospital was used entirely for patients with cancer until 1846, when the fear of cancer contagion was much less.

THE CANCER HOSPITAL IN LONDON

The present author is able to write with affection and knowledge about this famous hospital, having spent the greater part of his professional life on the surgical staff. His first appointment was as Surgical Registrar (1934–1939) and this was followed by appointments as Assistant Surgeon (1939–1946), Surgeon (1946–1961), Senior Surgeon (1961–1969), and Consulting Surgeon (1969 to the present date).

The Cancer Hospital was opened in 1851 and was the first hospital in the UK to be used exclusively for patients with cancer. It was founded by the generosity of William Marsden, who was a great philanthropist of the 19th

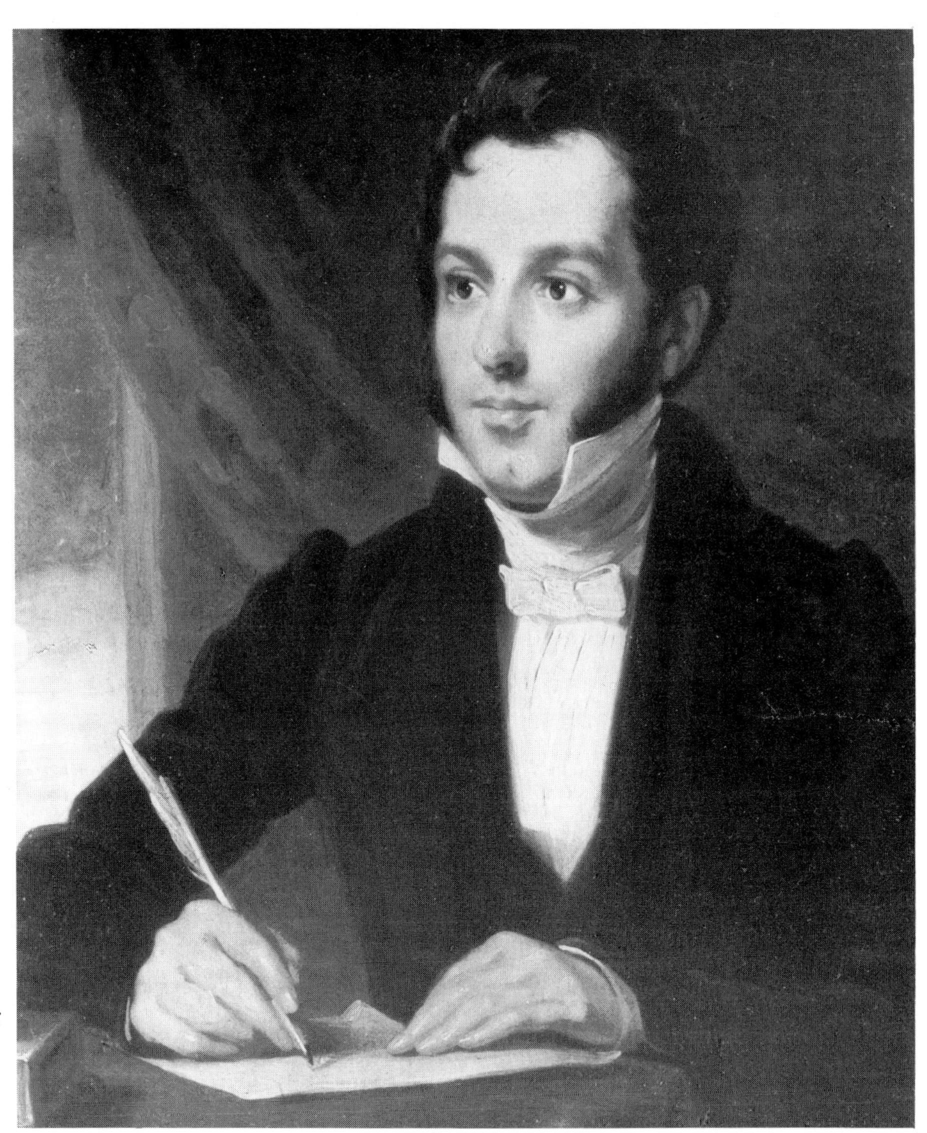

Figure 3.1 William Marsden, founder of the Royal Free Hospital (1828) and the Cancer Hospital (1851). The latter was renamed The Royal Marsden Hospital in 1954.

century. The title was changed from the initial Cancer Hospital to The Royal Cancer Hospital (Free) in 1936. Subsequently it was thought that the word "Cancer" in the title might cause concern to patients attending the hospital and also diminish the number of referrals, so the title was again changed, to The Royal Marsden Hospital, in memory of the founder.

William Marsden, a Yorkshireman, was born in 1796 and was later apprenticed to a druggist in Sheffield. He showed considerable ability within a few years and was therefore offered a partnership, which he refused because he was determined to become a surgeon. Consequently, he left the home farm for London, meeting his future wife on the coach. He soon became an assistant to a surgeon called Dale, who practised in Holborn near St Bartholomew's Hospital, so he was able to carry out his duties as an assistant surgeon and also work as a medical student at St Bartholomew's. Here he was taught by the famous John Abernethy, an inspired teacher of surgery at that time.

The admission of patients to hospitals was not easy, because they had to produce a Governor's letter of authorisation. William Marsden disagreed with this system and eliminated the difficulty by establishing The Royal Free Hospital in 1828 and later the Cancer Hospital in 1851. This important development was recorded at a meeting arranged by him and held on 10 February 1851 at his residence in Lincoln's Inn Fields, as follows: "Cancer, a malady that has hitherto been incurable and one that exists to a far greater extent than is generally supposed, has never been sufficiently provided for, it is therefore the opinion of this meeting that a specific and separate asylum be established for the treatment of all persons, male and female, afflicted with cancerous affections and that the establishment be called the Free Cancer Hospital." The provision of free treatment and ease of admission without a letter of recommendation were always stressed at the hospital, for it was to be "a special refuge for poor persons afflicted with the fearful disease".

Following this inaugural meeting, a dispensary for out-patients was opened in Cannon Row, Westminster, in May 1851, the medicines being purchased from a local chemist. Case-records were compiled which embodied the history, treatment and progress of each patient. The number of patients who were seen increased rapidly by referrals from all over the country, which justified the belief that such a special hospital was needed. This was an important observation, because there were people, even in high places, who not only doubted the wisdom of the development but were actually opposed to it. Queen Victoria, probably acting on advice, declared that she could not contribute to a "hospital for the exclusive treatment of one disorder".

History records other occasions when new and visionary enterprises have received scanty encouragement to go ahead and even open opposition. However, William Marsden was not deterred from bringing his scheme to fruition and made a great success of the Cancer Hospital. Within 2 years he had the satisfaction of having the support of 700 subscribers and an annual income of over £2000. The contribution of a Mrs Wolridge is recorded, for she offered a sum of 50 guineas on condition that 19 similar donations be given to the funds. A sum of 1000 guineas was thereby subscribed and Mrs Wolridge is commemorated today by the Wolridge Ward in the hospital.

The marked increase in cancer mortality in the London area at that time is stressed in the *First Surgeons' Report* by William Marsden and Weeden Cooke. In 1839 the number of deaths registered was 483, but in 1850 there were 889. The medical profession, however, failed to see the need for a special cancer hospital and the antagonism of the medical press to all special hospitals is shown by the following criticism, amongst others: "against the serious abuse afflicting the profession, namely the rampant tendency to multiply specialist institutions"! In their first report the surgeons acknowledged "with deep gratitude and reverence the manifest favour of Divine Providence which has attended their first efforts in the establishment of your charity". They believed that they had been "permitted to be the means of adding somewhat to the extension of knowledge of this malignant malady". Their dual objectives of caring for cancer patients and studying cancer diseases are highly commendable and this splendid work has been continued to the present time.

Facilities were urgently needed for in-patients; these were lacking in the dispensary in Cannon Row. Therefore, in October 1852, Hollywood House was rented for the sum of £60 per annum. These premises were situated "abutting the high road from London to Putney at New Brompton about three quarters of a mile beyond the Consumption Hospital on the same side of the way". Accommodation was for 20–25 patients, who were first admitted on 1 November 1852. It is interesting to find that in females the most frequent sites for cancer were the breast and uterus, and in males the face and tongue. The average age for cancer was 43 years and five times more women were affected than men.

In the early years of the hospital there were difficult financial problems, which were exacerbated by the Crimean War, but the useful sum of £5000 was bequeathed by a Mrs Wilson, whose benefaction is commemorated by the Wilson Ward in the present hospital. This money made it possible for the Secretary's office and the boardroom to be removed from Cannon Row to 5 Waterloo Place, Pall Mall. In 1855 they were moved again, with the Out-patients' Department, to 167 Piccadilly. The work load of the hospital continued to increase, so that it became apparent that the hospital must provide more accommodation for patients. Fortunately, a site was found in Fulham Road, Brompton, opposite the hospital for patients with "consumption", and was purchased for the sum of £4500. A building with a capacity of between 60 and 70 beds was planned and an appeal was opened for the necessary funds. The building site was "nearly an acre in extent with a frontage of one hundred and thirty-five feet having two houses erected on it". It was possible to buy it largely because of the benevolence of Angela Burdett Coutts, who loaned the sum of £3000. The new building was designed by David Mocatta so that it could be extended later to accommodate 300 beds. On 30 May 1859, the foundation stone of the present hospital was laid by Angela Burdett Coutts. The Bishop of London presided at the ceremony, the music was played by the band of the Grenadier Guards, and the bells of St Luke's Church, Chelsea, were rung from 2pm to 5pm. In the evening a foundation dinner was held at the Thatched House Tavern in St James' Street, London W1.

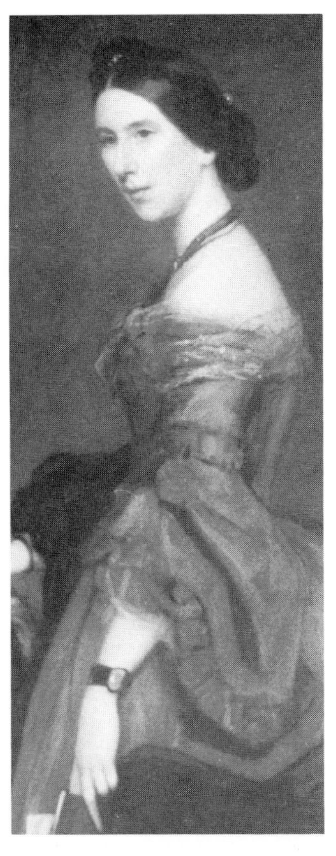

Figure 3.2 Angela Burdett Coutts (1814–1906).

At the next annual meeting of the Governors a warm tribute was paid to William Marsden in the following terms: "It was resolved, that the cordial thanks of this meeting are pre-eminently due, and are hereby tendered to William Marsden, Esq., M.D., Principle Surgeon of this Charity, for his zealous and unremitting exertions on behalf of the afflicted patients brought under his charge. That this anniversary specially recognises, under the Divine blessing, Dr Marsden's singularly successful treatment of the distressing disease of cancer, his liberal devotion of so much valuable time and attention in intercepting, arresting and more or less relieving the large number of cases annually admitted into the Hospital, or treated as out-patients, his careful tabulation of the origin, symptoms and pathological development of the cases open at any time to the inspection of medical practitioners, the experience derived from which materially influences the treatment of wealthier patients suffering from the same painful malady. That the above resolution be engrossed and presented in a suitable form to Dr Marsden, and that it be inserted in the leading morning papers."

The strength of the continuous professional antagonism to setting up special hospitals in London can be measured by considering the leading article in the *British Medical Journal* issued on 1 September 1860. Here it is written: "We are afraid the public are not yet in any way indoctrinated with the present professional feeling against the evils of special hospitals. One of the most unjustifiable of these institutions is the Cancer Hospital founded by Dr William Marsden, and now rebuilding in the Brompton Road." This stern opposition did not deter Marsden and his supporters from pursuing their objective. He was fortunate that members of the general public persisted in their refusal to be so indoctrinated as was advocated in the *British Medical Journal*. In fact, their support increased and the funds were provided to complete the first stage of the building in 1861 at a cost of over £8000. The valuable help given by Angela Burdett Coutts is commemorated by her portrait, which hangs in the hospital today. In addition, an anonymous benefactor, described in the report as "a benevolent lady in the country", gave a handsome donation of £1000.

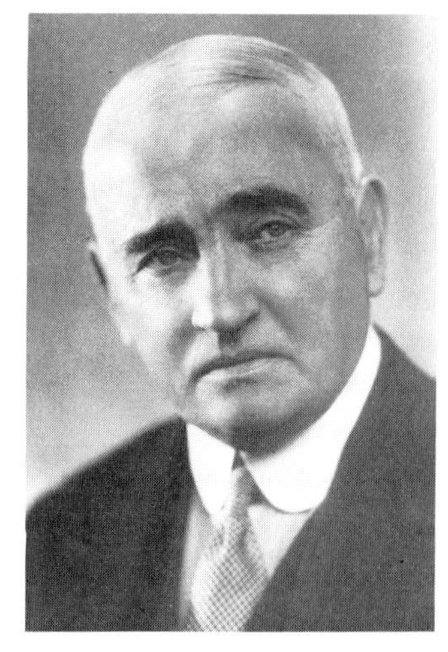

Figure 3.3 William Ernest Miles (1869–1947).

On 1 January 1862 the patients were moved from Hollywood House to the new hospital built on its present site, with a possible bed complement of 300. Marsden's dream had now come true. His work had begun in a small dispensary for cancer out-patients and culminated in a hospital for in-patient treatment and care.

Marsden died in 1867 aged 70 years, having served his hospital as Senior Surgeon for 15 years. He was succeeded in that post by his son, Alexander Marsden. It was a happy occasion when in 1954 the hospital was renamed The Royal Marsden Hospital after its illustrious founder, for he was a great doctor with vision and courage and full of sympathy for all in distress.

He would have been gratified by the continuous growth of the hospital, including the ever-increasing number of patients treated, as by the end of the 19th century it was firmly established. At that time the treatment of cancer was largely surgical, so the professional staff consisted of six Surgeons, including Alexander Marsden and the outstanding surgeon Charles Ryall (later Sir Charles Ryall). There were two Assistant Surgeons, one being the illustrious Ernest Miles.

Special mention is made here of the work of Ernest Miles, the great British surgeon who conferred enormous distinction and lustre on the hospital he served so faithfully and well. The present author enjoyed his

THE CANCER HOSPITAL
THE CANCER HOSPITAL (FREE)
SUPPORTED ENTIRELY BY
VOLUNTARY CONTRIBUTIONS

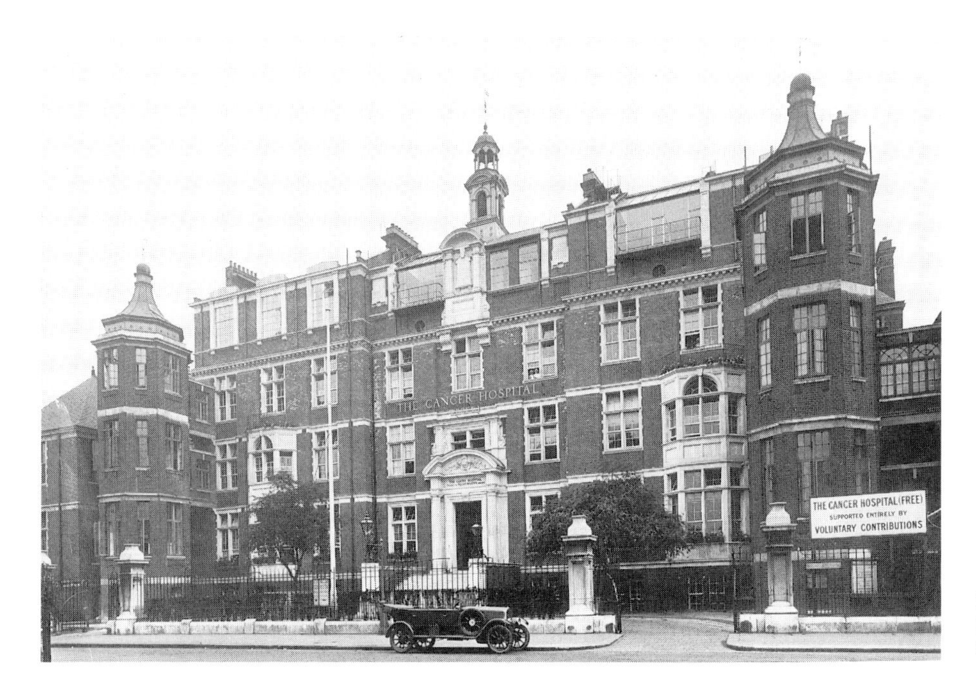

Figure 3.4 The Cancer Hospital (Free) in Fulham Road, London, about 1925.

friendship for many years and was his junior colleague when he was Senior Surgeon at the Gordon Hospital in London. Miles originally studied the pathology of carcinoma of the rectum, including the local and lymphatic spread of this tumour, on which he based and designed his operation of abdomino-perineal excision of the rectum, which he performed in a most dexterous manner. The present author was privileged to assist that master-surgeon when he performed the operation for a group of distinguished surgeons towards the end of his career. Surgeons from all over the world visited Miles at his hospitals to observe him perform this major operation and other surgical procedures. Miles not only demonstrated with beautiful clarity every step of the operation (the Miles operation), but also invited the visiting surgeons to spend time with him in the surgeons' room, where he discussed different surgical problems with them with the aid of his diagrams on the blackboard he had installed in the room so that he could illustrate his work. The visitors' book kept in the room bears witness to the large number of eminent surgeons who came to the Cancer Hospital to see and talk with Miles.

Other members of the staff at that time included two anaesthetists and two pathologists. It is salutary to remember the simple techniques of anaesthesia which were available at that time and the respiratory system affections which often complicated major operations; there were no antibiotics. Enormous advances have been made in anaesthetic agents and in methods of administration, with peroperative monitoring of patients. There has also been a spectacular growth in pathology, so that we now have important specialties such as histopathology, biochemistry, haematology, bacteriology, cytology and virology. These disciplines are essential for the investigation, treatment and monitoring of patients with oncological diseases.

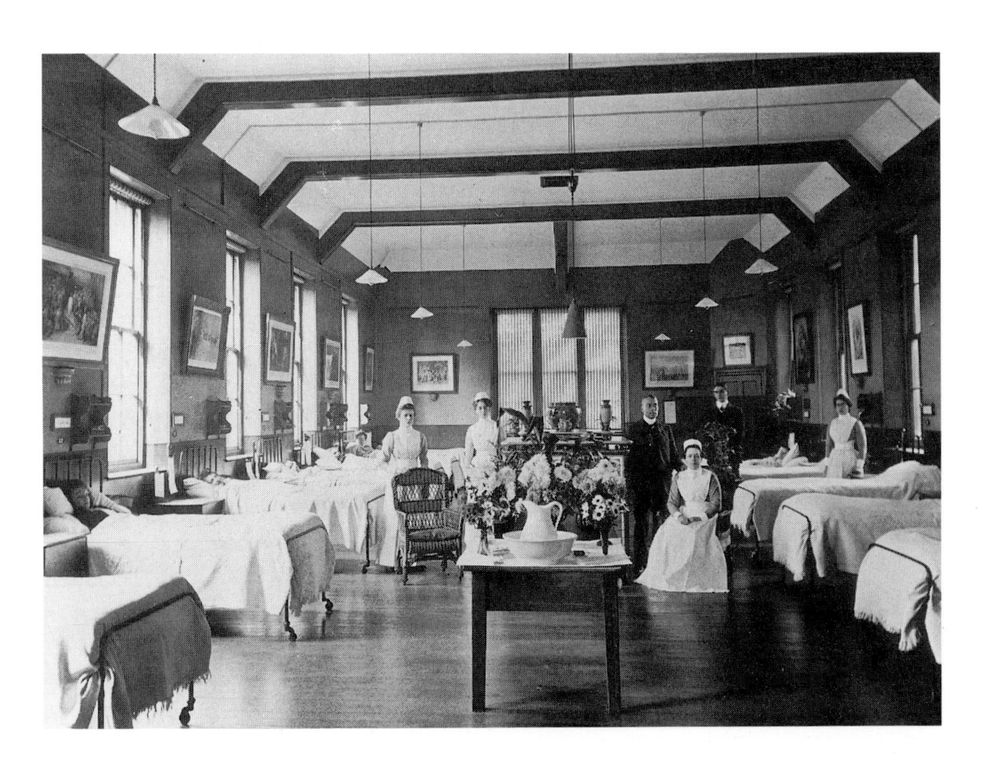

Figure 3.5 A ward in the Cancer Hospital (Free) in Fulham Road, London, in the early 1900s.

Other developments at the Cancer Hospital

In 1874 the surgeons used a new instrument, called the Galvanic cautery, "for the relief of pain by electricity and the destruction of tumours by the same means". In subsequent years the electric cautery was used to treat tumours in selected patients.

Great discoveries were imminent. Thus X-rays were discovered by Roentgen in 1895 and radium by Pierre and Marie Curie in 1898. It is not possible to measure the value of these discoveries in medicine and the countless number of patients who have benefited from them.

The staff of the Cancer Hospital responded quickly, and at once recognised the enormous value of radiation in the management of their patients. Thus, in 1901, X-rays were being "extensively used in intractable cases which seem appropriate for its employment". Radium was used in the treatment of malignant tumours in 1903 and it is believed that the Cancer Hospital was the first hospital in the UK to use this method of treatment.

It is interesting to note that a quantity of radium was placed at the disposal of G. H. Plummer, who was Director of the Department of Pathology and who wisely journeyed to Vienna to see the results of radium treatment in cancer patients by Professor Exner. Naturally, the general public showed enormous interest in this new cancer treatment, but the surgeons at the Cancer Hospital remained very critical about it and the present author recalls his discussions about the use of radium many years later with Ernest Miles, who still remained critical.

The surgeons warned the public about "the reputed cures which so frequently appear in the Daily Press". They pointed out that the most reliable treatment was "early surgical interference" and that if patients came for treatment in the early stage of the development of cancer they might "be freed from their disease by thorough removal of the affected part".

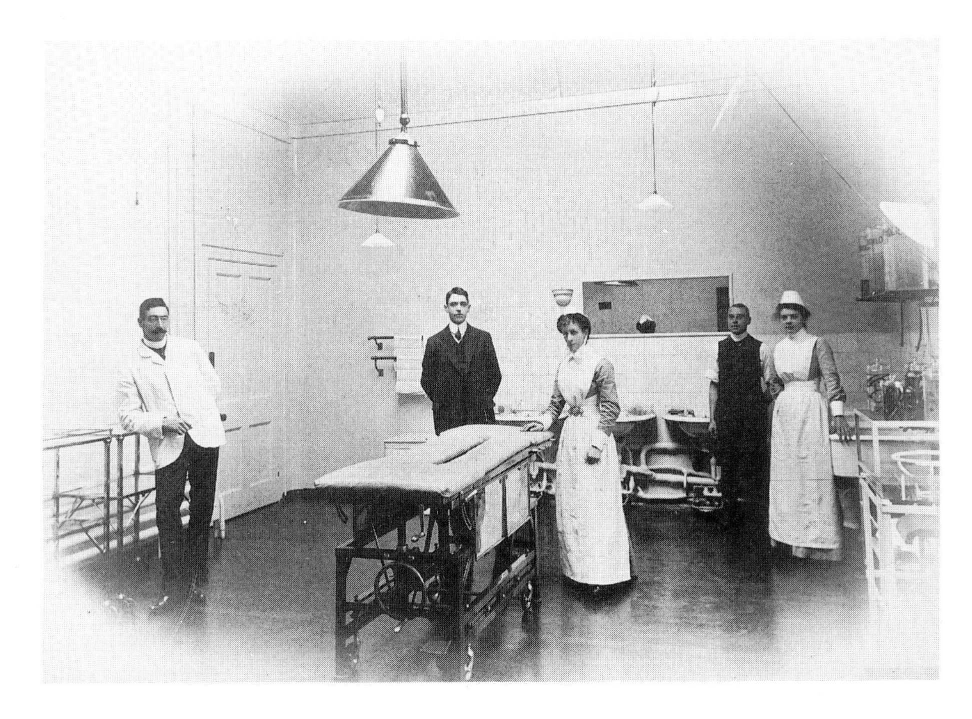

Figure 3.6 An operating theatre in the Cancer Hospital (Free) in the early 1900s.

The present author can detect the influence here of Ernest Miles, as he remembers Miles' dictum for cancer treatment: "the biggest possible operation for the earliest possible case".

In 1984 there was a swing away from radical cancer operations to more conservative procedures and the more frequent use of combined treatments — surgery, radiation and chemotherapy. However, the lessons taught by the master-surgeons of the past should not be forgotten.

The growth of knowledge

During this century and especially during recent decades enormous strides have been made in our knowledge of the causation, prevention, diagnosis and treatment, including rehabilitation, of the oncological diseases. The Cancer Hospital has made a big contribution to these advances and its facilities and staff have been considerably expanded. It was soon realised that the skill of a physician was necessary in the care of patients and a physician was therefore appointed to the staff. This was the beginning of the important Medical Department. Who could have foreseen the advent of medical oncology and modern chemotherapy?

The establishment of the Radiotherapy Department

In 1903 an Electrical Department with an X-ray machine and a quantity of radium for clinical use was formed under the direction of J. D. Pollock. As stated earlier, Dr Plummer was interested in the effects of radium. The Electrical and Radiotherapy Department was instituted in 1910 under the directorship of Robert Knox, who retained that post until his death in 1928. Knox was a famous pioneer in radiotherapy, and had an international reputation.

The necessity of having a physicist in the department was realised in 1910, so the position of Honorary Physicist was given to C. E. S. Phillips, who retained it until he resigned in 1926.

The Physics Department was then established as an independent department of the hospital under the direction of W. V. Mayneord, who became Professor of Physics as Applied to Medicine, and he held this dual appointment until his retirement in 1965.

In 1929 the Radiotherapy Department received academic recognition when the University of London created a Chair of Radiology (the first in the UK) tenable at the Cancer Hospital and appointed J. Woodburn Morison to it. The work and importance of the department grew under his direction and the present author recalls his association with Morison and numerous discussions about radiotherapy in cancer when he was Surgical Registrar at the hospital. At that time Chaoul in Germany introduced a new technique using low-voltage X-rays for treating superficial cancers, especially those in the skin. Morison was impressed with the method and arranged to have a Chaoul Apparatus installed in his department. He died in 1938 and was succeeded by David Smithers (later Sir David Smithers).

Department of Pathology

The necessity for a Pathology Department was recognised early in the hospital's history, for in 1856 the pathology-anatomist and resurrectionist

Robert Knox (1791–1862), was given a post on the staff, which he held until he died 6 years later. The post was then not filled for several years, the work being undertaken by a surgeon.

It was realised later that research into cancer causation was an important function of the hospital and should be done in parallel with patient care. Furthermore, it was decided that this research should be carried out in the Pathology Department. In 1893 G. H. Plummer was therefore appointed to the staff. Initially Plummer supported the protozoal theory of cancer aetiology, for in 1892 he had described cellular inclusions known as Plummer's bodies. Later he considered the aetiological agent to be a vegetable parasite of the yeast group of fungi and published his article on "The parasitic theory of cancer" (1903).

He was a distinguished pathologist and was elected a Fellow of the Royal Society. He left the Cancer Hospital in 1904 to take up an appointment at the Lister Institute, and was succeeded by two pathologists, Alexander Paine and D. Morgan, but the dual appointment was not a success, so the latter resigned in 1908.

It was decided to change the name of the department to "The Cancer Research and Pathological Department" under the direction of Paine. The increasing importance of cancer research was well recognised, so in 1909 a decision was made to erect a new building, with the title "The Cancer Hospital Research Institute". It was opened formally by H.R.H. The Duke of Connaught on 23 May 1911. This historic event marks the inauguration of many decades of cancer research, which has continued to the present day and has been conducted by outstanding scientists who have made impressive contributions to our knowledge.

The first Director of the Institute was Alexander Paine (1866–1933), who held the appointment from 1909–1921. He had supervised the planning and

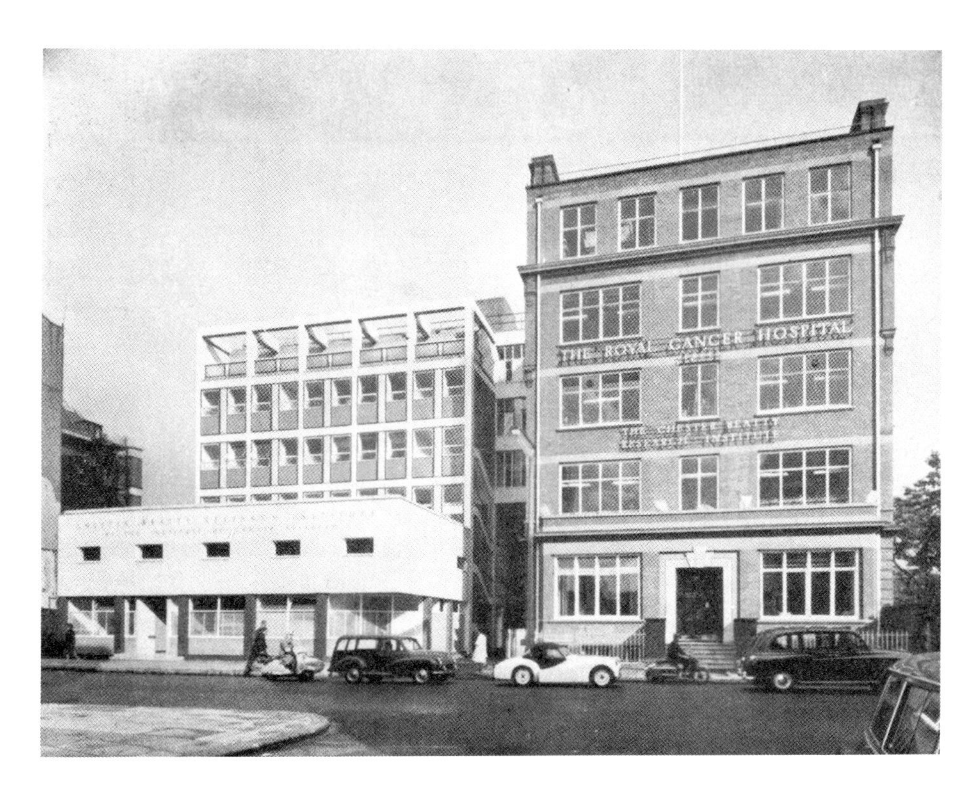

Figure 3.7 In 1939 the Royal Cancer Hospital Research Institute was transferred to new quarters, through the benevolence of Sir Chester Beatty, and renamed the Chester Beatty Research Institute in his honour.

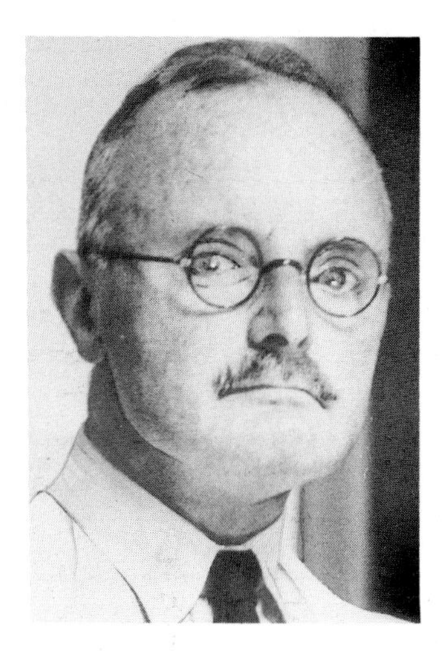

Figure 3.8 Sir Ernest Kennaway (1881–1958).

the provision of its equipment. He then built up his staff of workers, who subsequently distinguished themselves in the world of science.

The second Director was Archibald Leitch (1878–1931), who immediately commenced to carry out experimental research on carcinogenic tars and oils and made a considerable contribution to our knowledge of chemical carcinogenesis. As pointed out by Brunning and Dukes *(1965)*, he was one of the first to call attention to the long delay that occurs between the application of tar to the skin of mice and the appearance of the cancer. He also demonstrated in 1922 that shale oil and lubricants derived from it are carcinogenic, thus explaining the cause of mule-spinners' cancer. This "delay period" described by Leitch, which is a feature of carcinogenesis, was an observation of profound importance and was elucidated later in considerable detail by Kennaway *(1957)*.

In 1928 Leitch was appointed by the University of London to be its first Professor of Experimental Pathology, in recognition of his outstanding scientific work. It was tragic that his successful career was cut short by ill health, for he died at the early age of 53.

The third Director was Ernest Kennaway (1881–1958) (later Sir Ernest Kennaway), who succeeded Archibald Leitch in 1931 and retained his post until 1946. During that period of 15 years, which included the Second World War years 1939–1945, scientific discoveries of great importance (described in some detail in Chapter 17) were made by Kennaway and his colleagues. These discoveries of chemical carcinogens and their synthesis have illuminated the problem of cancer aetiology.

The present author had the privilege of knowing Kennaway and his colleagues when he worked as Surgical Registrar at the hospital. He had innumerable opportunities to hear about their discoveries and to take part in discussions.

Lady Kennaway, a voluntary worker in the Institute, for many years gave her husband immense support and valuable help in biological and statistical research, which Kennaway proudly acknowledged. All his colleagues and friends admired and cannot forget his magnificent fortitude in overcoming the physical handicap of his distressing chronic illness and they marvelled at his great accomplishments in such adverse circumstances.

Sir Ernest Kennaway was succeeded as Director of the Research Institute by Alexander Haddow (later Sir Alexander Haddow), who, with his gifted staff, added considerable lustre and international fame to the Institute through outstanding scientific achievements.

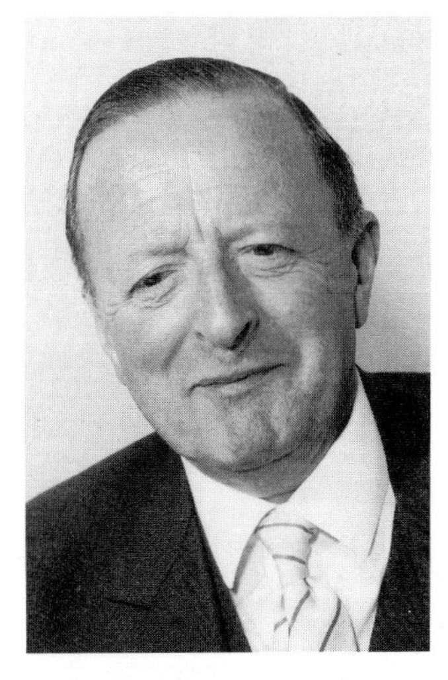

Figure 3.9 Sir Alexander Haddow (1907–1976).

Retrospect and prospect

The author, who has served on the surgical staff of the Cancer Hospital in London for 50 years and has witnessed with considerable pride its development and close association with the Institute of Cancer Research, has given its history in detail here, as the account is valuable not only for its description of the formation and growth of the hospital, but also because it shows how the management of patients with oncological diseases, including prevention, diagnosis and the multi-modal treatment, has progressed over nearly 150 years. The hospital has played a leading role in this progress.

The value of collaborative work by those who are engaged in clinical and research oncology, including the constant interchange of ideas and problems between doctors and scientists, and the essential feedback from the laboratory to the clinic, is clearly demonstrated here.

The Royal Marsden Hospital and Institute of Cancer Research, Royal Cancer Hospital, which is its present title, is a living monument to these ideals and a splendid model on which future developments of this nature can profitably be based.

The modern features of the hospital were described by Banks *(1959)*, who was formerly House Governor and Secretary to the Board of Governors. The development of the various departments and refurbishing of the wards during recent decades are very impressive and have contributed much to the treatment, care and comfort of the patients.

Under the National Health Service Act (1948) the hospital was incorporated in the new Service and designated as a teaching hospital, a designation which recognises its association with the Institute of Cancer Research, which is a constituent of the British Postgraduate Medical Federation and is therefore under the aegis of the University of London. This notable achievement would have gladdened the heart of the founder of the Cancer Hospital, William Marsden.

THE CHRISTIE HOSPITAL AND HOLT RADIUM INSTITUTE IN MANCHESTER

The Christie Hospital and Holt Radium Institute, which is concerned mainly with the treatment of patients with cancer and associated diseases, was opened on its present site in Manchester on 5 November, 1932, and was the result of the amalgamation of the Cancer Pavilion and Home in Stanley House, Withington, with the Holt Radium Institute, which was established originally at the Manchester Royal Infirmary.

The history of these components is very interesting. The Cancer Pavilion was founded in 1895 with a legacy from Sir Joseph Whitworth. It was renamed the Christie Hospital in recognition of the support of Richard Copley Christie, one of the executors of Joseph Whitworth's will. The work of the hospital expanded rapidly from its original number of 100 patients per year to more than 400 patients by the late 1920s. It was the first hospital in the North of England to treat cancer patients with radium.

The Holt Radium Institute was established in 1914 with a monetary subscription from Edward Holt, who was a former Lord Mayor of Manchester and the owner of a brewery. The institute was sited first at the Manchester Royal Infirmary, then in 1920 it was moved to premises in Nelson Street, Manchester.

Although the hospital and the institute were housed in separate buildings, they worked together daily in close cooperation which was so successful that it was decided to unite them in a specially constructed building. This was completed in 1932 in Withington, a suburb of Manchester, and named the Christie Hospital and Holt Radium Institute.

At this time the Director of the hospital was Ralston Paterson, the well-known radiotherapist. He wished to establish a research unit and accomplished his aim with the assistance of his wife, Edith Paterson, who was a radiotherapist and radiobiologist, and Walter Dale, a biochemist specialising in radiation chemistry.

After the end of the Second World War temporary accommodation was provided for the sections of Radiation Chemistry, Experimental Chemotherapy, Radiobiology and Cytogenetics. The Physics Department and Edith Paterson's Department of Experimental Haematology were both on different sites, the latter being housed over the archway entrance to the private wing of the Christie Hospital. This unit was the nucleus for the three successive phases by which the laboratories expanded, beginning when Ralston and Edith Paterson retired in 1962 and their name was given to the laboratories. They were succeeded by Professor Laszlo Lajtha, who was appointed the first full-time Director of Research. His previous appointment was Head of the Radiobiology Laboratory of the Churchill Hospital, Oxford, where his speciality was experimental haematology. He continued to maintain this subject as his main research interest when he moved to Manchester. In 1970 he was appointed to the newly created Chair of Experimental Oncology at the University of Manchester.

The expansion of the laboratories in three phases, which was initiated in 1962, involved the creation of new sections of Carcinogenesis, Epithelial Kinetics, Cellular Biophysics, and Immunology. The laboratory building also houses Professor Crowther's Department of Medical Oncology and separate units of Paediatric Oncology, Pharmacokinetics and Endocrinology. In a basement area the linear accelerator is housed.

It will be obvious that the laboratories are a disciplinary establishment for many aspects of cancer research with participation in clinical research, which is primarily carried out by Professor Crowther in the Department of Medical Oncology housed in the same building, with the collaboration of the hospital complex.

Commensurate with the development of the laboratories and the increasing number of research projects, the staff has grown considerably, including postdoctoral staff, postgraduate students and visiting fellows from many countries. In addition, there are technical and clerical staff to support all the work.

Financial support is provided jointly by the Cancer Research Campaign, the Medical Research Council and the National Health Service. Finance for new buildings has been provided by the local Women's Trust Fund. In addition to this valuable donation, substantial funds are received for the Paterson Laboratories from industry and the general public.

This is the largest cancer research institute in the UK and it has gained an international reputation for its work. The institute works in close collaboration with the Christie Hospital, which has continued to expand with recent developments to extend the Radiotherapy and Diagnostic Radiology Departments and to provide a new Treatment Planning Suite. The pharmacy is also being extended to provide an aseptic suite for the preparation of drugs.

Another major building project for the Christie Hospital is the construction of a new Adult Leukaemia Unit containing a ward of 10 beds and facilities for the care of patients who are being treated with bone marrow transplants and intensive chemotherapy for acute leukaemia.

The author expresses his appreciation of the assistance of P. K. Shields, Unit General Manager of the Christie Hospital and Holt Radium Institute, who provided him with valuable sources of information.

ROYAL BEATSON MEMORIAL HOSPITAL IN GLASGOW

This cancer hospital, the first in Scotland, was established in 1886 and during the next century it gained an important international reputation. The history of the development of the Royal Beatson Memorial Hospital is of great interest and the author is very indebted to Derek A. Dow, Archivist to the Greater Glasgow Health Board, for kindly providing him with valuable information and a copy of *A Short History of the Glasgow Royal Cancer Hospital, since its Inception in 1890 with a Statement of What it has done in Scotland for Cancer Patients and Cancer Research* (issued by the Board of Directors and written at their request by Sir George Thos Beatson, M.D., K.C.B., D.L.). The present author has drawn all his information about this hospital from these sources and expresses his gratitude to Derek Dow for his valuable help.

The initial Glasgow Cancer Hospital resulted directly from the efforts of Hugh Murray, who founded the Glasgow Cancer and Skin Institution at 409 St Vincent Street in 1886. The first general meeting of those associated with its work was held on 1 December 1889, and on 3 December 1889 a committee was formed to liaise with Dr Murray to establish the Cancer Hospital proper. They acquired premises at 163 Hill Street, formerly Cowcaddens Free Church Manse, and the hospital was opened by the Duchess of Montrose, free of debt, on 13 October 1890.

There were 10 beds for in-patient care and the objective was to treat patients with cancer in all its stages by medicine because it was felt that surgical treatment was not only useless but could actually be harmful. This attitude to the treatment of cancer was contrary to the general opinion of the medical profession at the time, for it was believed that cancer began as a limited local disease and no drug could affect its progress. The only practical use of medicine was to relieve the pain and only wide surgical excision at an early stage could provide hope of a cure.

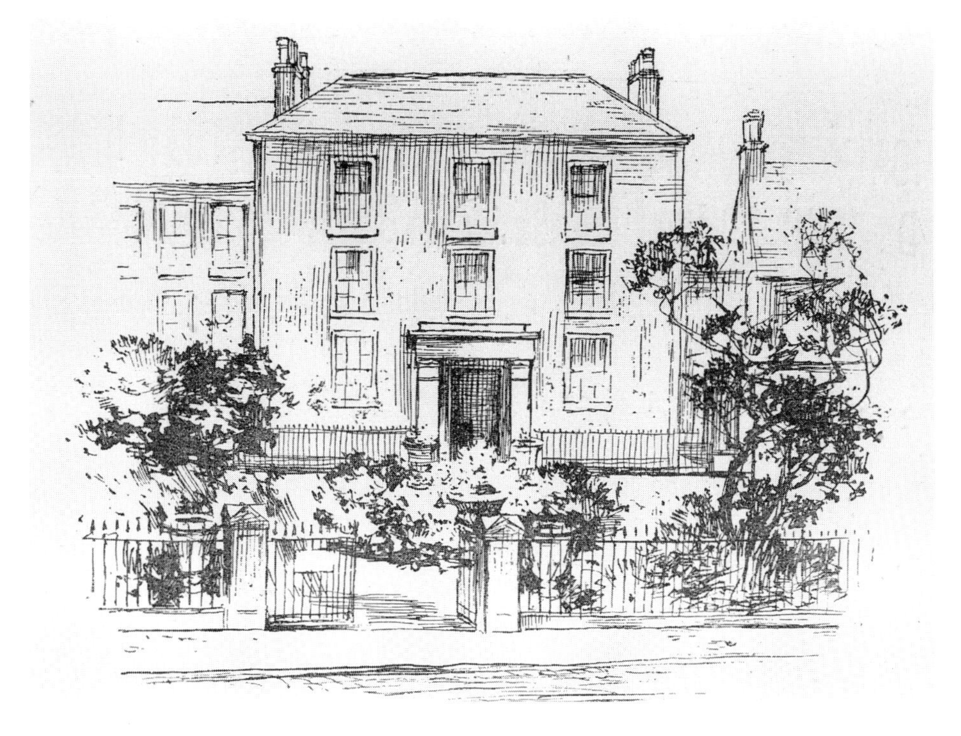

Figure 3.10 The original Glasgow Cancer Hospital opened in 1890.

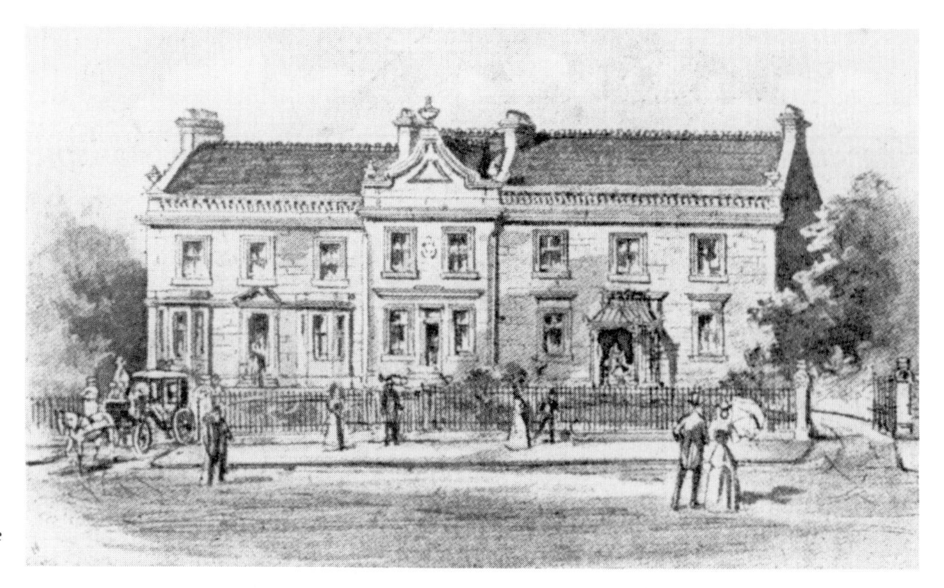

Figure 3.11 The 1896 extension to the Glasgow Cancer Hospital.

It is of interest to note that the hospital established a system of home nursing for patients who were terminally ill. The importance of domiciliary nursing care for patients with cancer and in support of their families was recognised by the Marie Curie Memorial Foundation in the 1950s, when it established its National Day and Night Cancer Nursing Service.

The directors of the hospital declared their intention to carry out research in cancer and to establish teaching programmes. It appears that the success and development of Scotland's first cancer hospital were hindered by its directors' belief in the medical treatment of cancer, which caused the medical profession to withdraw its approval, and the support and confidence of the public declined.

It is not surprising, therefore, that the Glasgow Cancer Hospital severed its connection with the Glasgow Cancer and Skin Institution in 1894, and it is important to note that Sir George Beatson had joined the staff in 1893. The hospital then took up a recognised position amongst the charitable institutes of Glasgow. It was decided to limit its work to cancer patients only, a full staff of medical officers was appointed, which included a pathologist, and an out-patient department was established at 22 West Graham Street.

The original building in Hill Street soon proved to be too small so the houses situated at 132–138 Hill Street were purchased to provide sufficient accommodation. As a result many serious and distressing cases no longer had to be refused admission. It was also felt that the accommodation for the nursing staff was unsatisfactory. These buildings, one of them the old manse of St George's-in-the-Fields with a stone in one of its walls bearing the inscription in Latin "Glory to God Alone", were converted into a suitable hospital with 30 beds and a pathology laboratory. The new hospital buildings were opened on 22 October 1896 by Her Grace the Duchess of Montrose, who announced that most of the beds had been named after and furnished by individual persons.

The hospital, now providing better facilities for the treatment and comfort of patients, increased its scope of work not only in Glasgow but also over a large part of Scotland. Advances were occurring in medical science which necessitated new treatment methods, so that further accommodation was required, including separate rooms for patients who could not be suitably treated in the general wards.

The directors had constantly desired to establish and equip a research department for the scientific investigation of cancer. This was an added reason for reconstructing and extending the existing hospital on the present site, which was quite adequate for the purpose. An appeal for funds was made to carry out the new plans for extension. Work was completed by the end of 1911 and the new hospital was opened on 30 May 1912, by H.R.H. Princess Louise, who made the important announcement that King George V had agreed that the institution should henceforth be known as the Royal Cancer Hospital. The new hospital contained 50 beds and seven small rooms for special cases, an X-ray Department, Pathology Department and Dispensary. There was accommodation for the Research Department and separate quarters for the nurses.

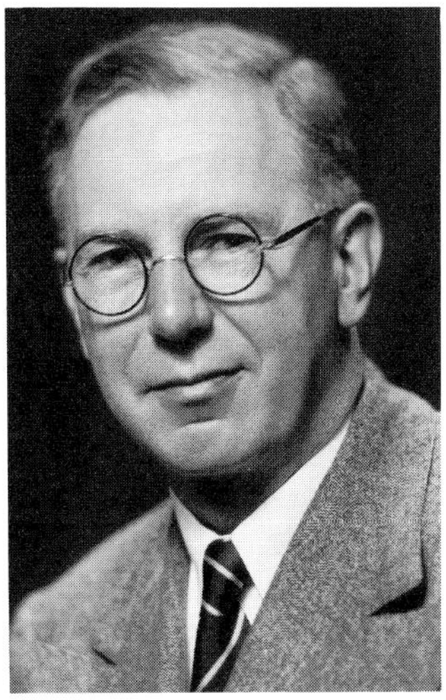

Figure 3.12 Philip R. Peacock (1901–), Director of Research at the Glasgow Royal Cancer Hospital 1928–1966, made important contributions to our knowledge of carcinogenesis.

The first Director of Research was appointed in 1912 but little progress was made until after the end of the disruption caused by World War I. An important development occurred in November 1928, when Beatson persuaded Lady Burrell to donate radium worth £10 000 to the hospital. On 10 June, 1930, a new Nurses' Home was opened by the Duchess of Montrose and the Glasgow and the West of Scotland Radium Institute, housed in the former Home, was inaugurated by Principal Rait of Glasgow University. Dr P. R. Peacock was appointed Director of Research in 1928 and he held this post until his retirement in 1966.

In the post World War II Scottish Hospitals Survey there was a gloomy account of the 72-bed hospital and institute which were not large enough to form the basis of a Regional Cancer Centre for the West of Scotland. It was considered that the hospital's name was unfortunate and would have an adverse effect.

It is noted that during those years it was inappropriate to speak of cancer in public and the name of another cancer hospital in London was altered from the Cancer Hospital to The Royal Cancer Hospital and finally The Royal Marsden Hospital.

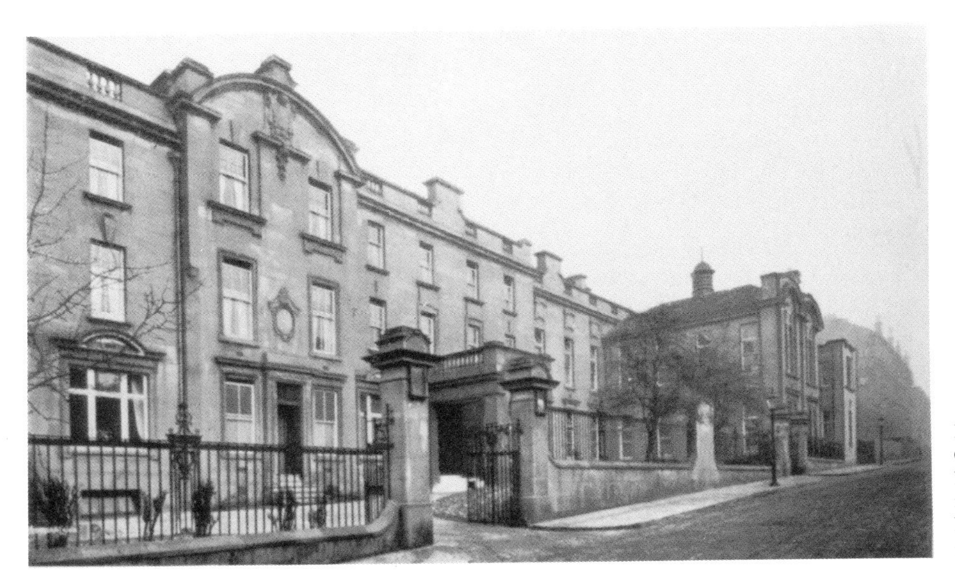

Figure 3.13 The new Glasgow Cancer Hospital opened in 1912 as the Royal Cancer Hospital. It was renamed the Royal Beatson Memorial Hospital in 1952. This photograph was taken in the mid-1920s.

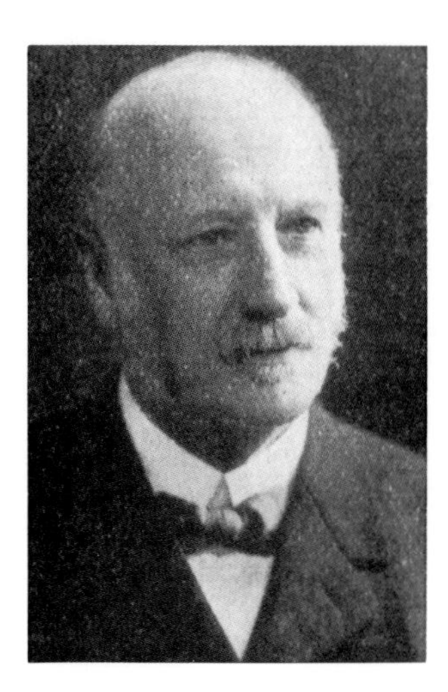

Figure 3.14 Sir George Beatson (1848–1933).

The hospital managers were undaunted by criticisms and they provided new accommodation for laboratory research, which was opened in April 1951. They also altered the title of the hospital in 1952 to the Royal Beatson Memorial Hospital, in memory of its greatest supporter. A further expansion occurred in November 1956, when 13 more beds for radiotherapy were made available; and in 1963 the first phase to re-equip the Pathology Department was completed.

The hospital and oncology scenes are continually changing and the subsequent history of the Royal Beatson Memorial Hospital is a good illustration of this. The Glasgow Hospitals Survey in 1965 was very critical of this hospital with its 44 beds for general surgery and urology and 37 beds for radiotherapy and described it as old, isolated and difficult for access since it was built on more than one level. The Survey concluded that the hospital should be abandoned, the beds for radiotherapy transferred to the Western Infirmary and the Cancer Research Unit placed in a major teaching hospital. This assessment influenced all subsequent decisions. In 1966 the Glasgow Institute for Radiotherapy had units at Belvedere, the Western Infirmary and the Beatson. In 1967 a new name was adopted, the Beatson Institute for Cancer Research, and in 1971 it was decided to seek a new location, with the result that in 1976 the institute moved to its present home in Garscube. Finally, the previously independent Royal and Western Infirmary Schools of Radiography were amalgamated in 1971, and later rehoused in the Beatson as the Glasgow School of Radiography.

Sir George Beatson died on 16 February, 1933, at the age of 85. His name is enshrined in the Beatson Institute for Cancer Research and he will be remembered for ever for his work in the development of hospital facilities for patients with all stages of cancer and for his memorable observations on the effects of oophorectomy in patients with advanced carcinoma of the breast.

THE FIRST CANCER SERVICE IN A GENERAL HOSPITAL

The special management, including treatment, of patients with oncological diseases has been recognised for decades by the medical profession and especially by those who are responsible for their care. The complexity increased with the introduction of new treatment modalities, rehabilitation and continuing care. This concern for cancer patients stimulated the formation of cancer departments and services in our general hospitals.

The first cancer service was established in 1791 at the Middlesex Hospital in London.

John Howard, a surgeon and pupil of Percivall Pott, who had probably stimulated his interest in cancer, proposed to the Board of Governors that since "the deplorable situation of cancerous paupers was casually the topic of conversation" and "the Middlesex Hospital having at this time several wards unoccupied", an airy ward be appropriated for this specific disease where patients with cancer might remain "until either relieved by art, or released by death". Howard was given an endowment of £3000 for the new service by Samuel Whitebread. The plan was agreed and a ward with 12 beds was opened to receive patients on 19 June 1792.

This historic event occurred when the Middlesex Hospital was a small general hospital; it had been founded in 1745 with only one special service, for midwifery. The cancer service steadily grew so that by 1893 it occupied the upper floor of the main hospital building. There was considerable financial support for it, which made it possible to erect a separate hospital wing with a complement of 49 beds and this was opened in 1900. It was realised that clinical work in cancer should be linked with pathology and research and this linkage was achieved later by creating the Cancer Research Laboratories and the Bland-Sutton Institute of Pathology. The Middlesex Hospital Cancer Charity thereby achieved an international reputation for this work, which was carried out by many distinguished surgeons, including Charles H. Moore and Sir John Bland-Sutton. These were followed by others who have brought great distinction to their hospital, including Lord Webb-Johnson, Sir Gordon Gordon-Taylor and W. Sampson-Handley.

Like the ideas of many other visionary pioneers, those of John Howard regarding cancer care were far ahead of his time, for he fully realised the necessity of specialisation in this discipline. His book was published posthumously and entitled "*Practical Observations on Cancer* by the late John Howard, Fellow of The Royal College of Surgeons and Surgeon Extraordinary to the Cancer Ward in the Middlesex Hospital, London. Printed for J. Hatchard 1811; 144 pages". On page 126 he stated: "I am almost led to believe that if external and internal means of relief are applied with due discrimination of judgement sufficiently early, the knife even may be superseded."

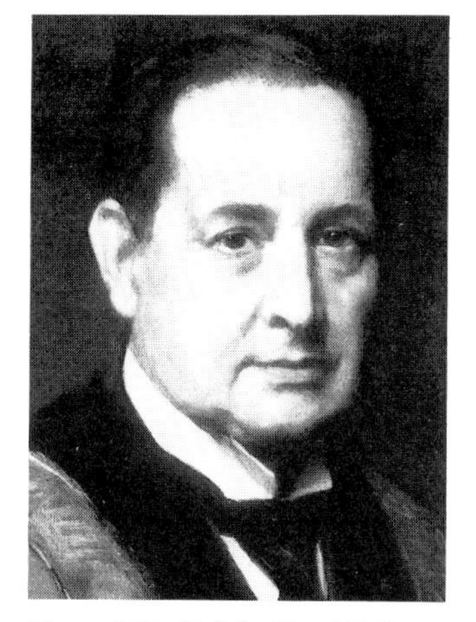

Figure 3.15 Sir John Bland-Sutton, President of the Royal College of Surgeons of England.

OTHER GENERAL HOSPITALS

It is noteworthy that a number of other general hospitals have followed the example of the Middlesex Hospital in establishing cancer departments and services for the management of patients with cancer. Follow-up departments have been organised so that patients can be periodically reviewed and assessed following definitive treatment and the necessary continuation treatment given. The development of radiotherapy for cancer patients necessitated the installation of elaborate and expensive machines and equipment housed in specially constructed departments. The basic staff requirements were for radiotherapists, nurses, radiographers, physicists and technicians. The oncology services in a number of general hospitals are based on the Radiotherapy Department and more recently they have been designated as the Department of Radiotherapy and Oncology.

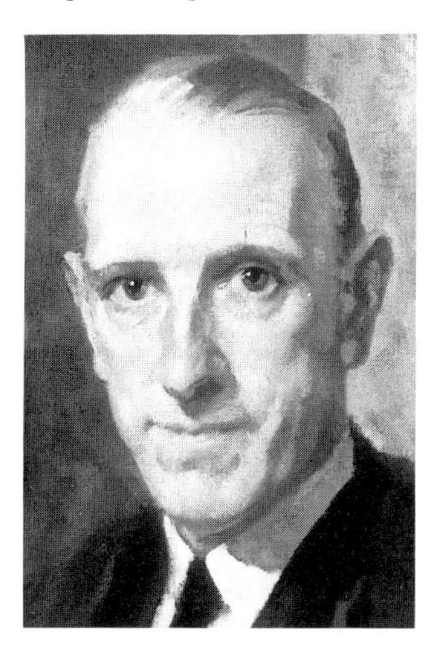

Figure 3.16 Lord Webb-Johnson, President of the Royal College of Surgeons of England. He gave the 1940 Bradshaw Lecture: "Pride and prejudice in the treatment of cancer".

THE INSTITUTION OF FOLLOW-UP DEPARTMENTS

The follow-up of the majority of patients who have received definitive treatment in hospital for many different diseases is now an organised routine service. It is difficult, therefore, to understand the situation when this vital work was not done and there was no follow-up department in our hospitals. Since all the patients were lost sight of, there was no record of their subsequent condition and fate and all the valuable data concerning the end-results of treatment were lost. Specialists had no scientific evidence of the value of different methods of treatment, due to the lack of data on subsequent patient morbidity and mortality. The provision of all follow-up services for patients with cancer is axiomatic, so that survival rates and

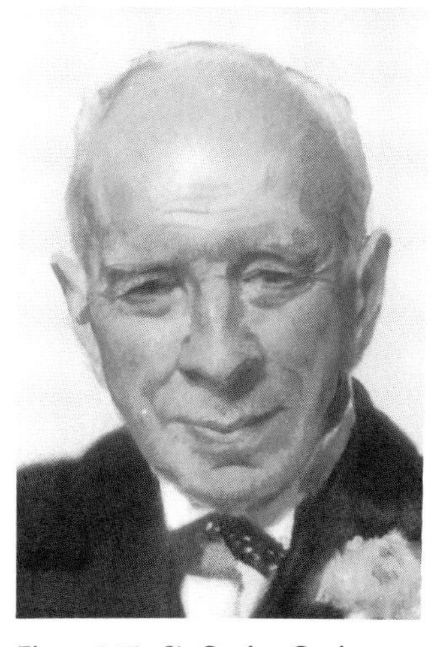

Figure 3.17 Sir Gordon Gordon-Taylor (1878–1960). In 1935 he and Philip Wiles published *Interinnominoabdominal (Hindquarter) Amputation.*

other measurements of the value of different methods of treatment can be obtained. Individual clinicians with a special interest in certain groups of patients enquired into the end-results of their treatment but there was no organised follow-up department to cover all the patients with cancer.

The present author played a key role in the development of follow-up departments when he was appointed to the new post of Medical Officer in charge of the Follow-up Department at St Bartholomew's Hospital, London, in 1932. Later he used this experience to organise the follow-up scheme at the Royal Cancer Hospital, when he was appointed Surgical Registrar there in 1934.

At St Bartholomew's Hospital the Follow-up Department had been formed in 1922 with the objective of ascertaining the ultimate value of the treatment of in-patients. Previously certain patients were seen periodically following their discharge from the wards, but no systematic survey was made of large groups of patients. The present author produced evidence of the value of follow-up studies for all patients with cancer in two reports from his department. These were (1) "An investigation into the end-results of the treatment of cancer of the breast", and (2) "A study of cancer of the buccal cavity with the end-results of treatment" *(see Raven, 1933).* The author made a number of observations, including the dearth in the literature of careful reports of series of cases of breast cancer with reference to the late results of treatment. He pointed out that the immediate results are so good, with only a small operative mortality, that we are prone to regard our treatments too favourably in the light of longer-term end-results. It was shown that the prognosis in breast carcinoma is very unfavourable and "it is time we regarded the position in its true character". After the implantation of interstitial radium needles had been introduced as treatment for breast carcinoma it was necessary to compare the survival rate with that from excisional surgery. It is interesting to read the following statement which the author made 56 years ago (1932): "A study of survival rates in carcinoma of the breast shows that involvement or otherwise of the regional lymph nodes is the touchstone by which the prognosis must be assessed. Other factors must also be considered, namely the resistance of the patient and the relative malignancy of the carcinoma. Carcinoma of the breast is a much more widespread disease than it has hitherto been thought to be."

Enormous advances have been made during the last 50 years; today when patients are first seen we can use imaging techniques and other sophisticated diagnostic methods to see whether they have generalised disease, and we now have systematic treatment modalities with which to treat them.

INTERNATIONAL CENTRES FOR CANCER RESEARCH AND TREATMENT

There are important cancer societies and centres for cancer research and treatment in many countries, an overall picture and account of whose activities is of great interest and value, and is provided in the *International Directory of Specialized Cancer Research and Treatment Establishments, (1978)*, published by the International Union Against Cancer under the auspices of the Committee on International Collaborative Activities (CICA).

A subcommittee under Dr R. Lee Clark (Houston, Texas, USA) and Dr S. Eckhardt (Budapest, Hungary) was appointed to supervise the preparation and collection of data and the publication of definitive editions. A preliminary edition of limited coverage had been published in 1974. The preparation of the first definitive edition, which contained information on about 490 establishments, was begun in June 1975 and that of the second edition, which contained data on about 680 establishments in 82 countries, in January 1978.

The latter edition describes the immense amount of research and clinical cancer work which is being carried out throughout the world in four major types of institute:

(1) Comprehensive cancer centres. These are autonomous and are concerned with the care of patients with cancer, clinical and basic cancer research, and the training of personnel. Most have a cancer registry, a social welfare service and an education programme.
(2) Cancer research institutes. These, also autonomous, are concerned with a wide spectrum of basic and clinical cancer research, which is carried out by medical and scientific staffs and technicians, and they usually have the facilities for training research workers.
(3) University departments or biomedical research centres which are engaged in an integrated programme of cancer research.
(4) Special cancer hospitals or other hospitals with a separate department or unit for the diagnosis and comprehensive multidisciplinary treatment of all types of cancer or of cancer of a specific site or sites. Such a department or unit usually has a Director who coordinates cancer treatment and also carries out clinical research.

This valuable book is recommended for careful reference and study of the international effort in cancer research and treatment.

Roswell Park Memorial Institute

Roswell Park Memorial Institute was founded in 1898 at the University of Buffalo Medical School and its university status continues to the present day. In its 90 years of existence it has made outstanding achievements in cancer research and treatment, which are recognised world-wide. The author gratefully acknowledges his indebtedness to Dr Edwin A. Mirand, Associate Institute Director from 1951 to the present, who kindly supplied him with all the information on which the following account is based.

Roswell Park Memorial Institute is a division of the New York State Health Department and has a staff of more than 2600, including approximately 325 physicians and scientists. It maintains a 277-bed hospital, which admits approximately 7000 patients annually, and out-patient clinics which handle more than 65 000 patient visits each year. The linkage thus established between cancer research and the care of cancer patients is very valuable, as is also the professional and public education the institute gives on all aspects of oncological diseases.

The founder of the institute, Dr Roswell Park, clearly recognised the importance of organised research in an institution embodying all the necessary resources. His original concept attracted leading authorities in medicine and science in the USA and other countries to visit him and to set up other cancer centres. Born in 1852 at Pomfret, Connecticut, in the 30 years following his appointment as Professor of Surgery at the University of Buffalo School of Medicine he became a leader in the field of surgery and cancer and gained an international reputation. He was amongst the first to call attention to the contested fact that cancer was steadily increasing. How very true this observation remains today. In his impressive account of the life and achievements of Dr Park, Dr Mirand *(1988)* describes him as a man with boundless determination and energy. He was a superb teacher and he built up an outstanding record as a professor and researcher. He was also widely read in many other subjects and wrote extensively, was a skilled musician and a brilliant conversationalist.

Dr Park realised he required financial help to establish his cancer research laboratory, and this was provided by Edward H. Butler, Sr, publisher of the *Buffalo Evening News*, who had many prominent and influential friends. The latter were successful in obtaining New York State funding for Dr Park's project, which has now developed into a complex of more than 30 buildings.

Dr Park died in 1914 at the age of 62, after a life full of rich accomplishments which is an outstanding example of dedicated work in the field of cancer. In 1946 the institute he had founded, the New York State Institute for the Study of Malignant Diseases, was renamed the Roswell Park Memorial Institute in his honour.

Early research carried out there included the study of transplantable rodent tumours, the parasitic theory of the causation of cancer, and antibodies in mice recovering from experimental tumours. By 1911, the staff had realised the need for a hospital where the results of research could be applied clinically, for their research now included the study of the preparation and action of vaccines, the search for parasites in cancer, the transplantation of mouse and fish tumours and the investigation of immune

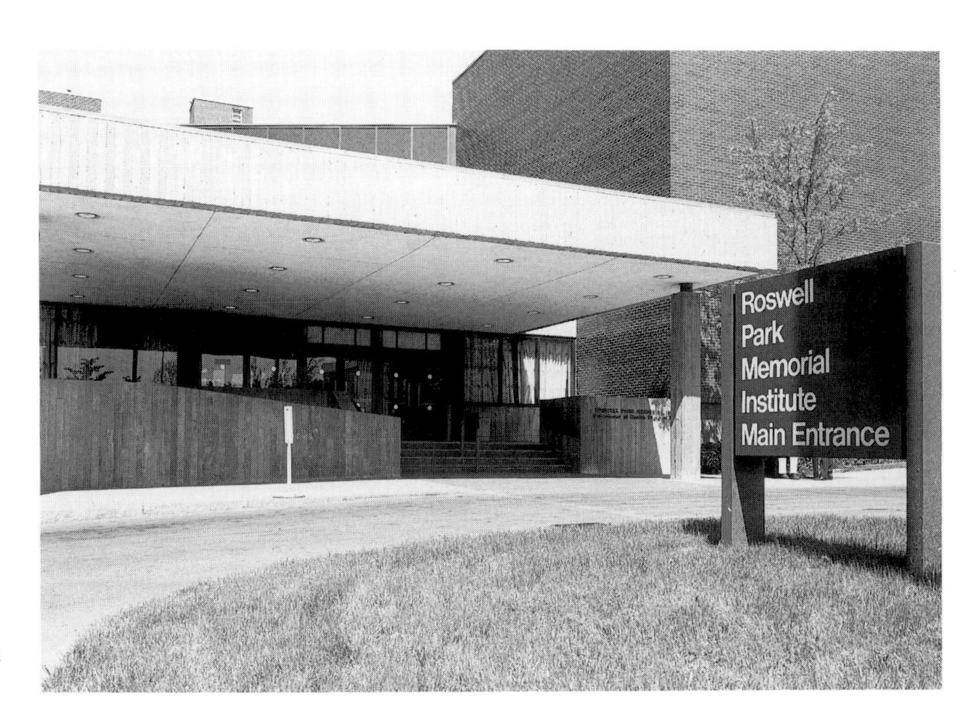

Figure 3.18 Roswell Park Memorial Institute.

reactions in cancer. The first hospital building was a 30-bed facility and this was followed in 1940 by a hospital with 100 beds. Since then, the size and work of the hospital have continued to expand to their present imposing dimensions. The research scientists are concerned with the basic subjects relating to cancer, including biology, chemistry and physics, and the feed-back system between the laboratory and the clinics ensures the application of all new research findings in the prevention and treatment of cancer.

The broad-based cancer education programme developed by Dr Mirand is an important division of the centre's work. The institute provides opportunities for medical students from the State University of New York at Buffalo to work in the out-patient clinics and to attend seminars. Resident physicians from many different countries receive training. Postgraduate research training is given in basic and clinical sciences and intensive courses in nursing oncology are organised.

Permanent institute Directors since Dr Park have been Dr H. R. Gaylord (1904–1923), Dr B. T. Simpson (1924–1943), Dr L. Kress (1945–1952), Dr G. E. Moore (1952–1967), Dr J. T. Grace (1967–1970), Dr G. P. Murphy (1970–1985) and currently Dr T. Tomasi.

The constant contribution which is being made there to our knowledge of cancer aetiology, prevention and treatment is an outstanding record of progress and achievement in the control of cancer.

The University of Texas M. D. Anderson Tumor Institute and Hospital

This well-known comprehensive cancer centre was established on 30 June 1941 by the 47th Legislature of the State of Texas. In addition to the State government support it received, private philanthropy was an important factor in its creation. On 10 March 1942 an agreement was made between the M. D. Anderson Foundation, which had been established as a trust in 1936, and the University of Texas Board of Regents, that the institute would be the first unit of the proposed University of Texas Medical Center. In 1964 the institute moved to its permanent quarters in the centre.

Dr Ernest A. Bertino was appointed the first (Acting) Director and he was succeeded by Dr Randolph Lee Clark, who as Surgeon-in-Chief and Director made an important and valuable contribution to the progressive growth and development of the organisation. Since his retirement he has continued to serve the centre as President Emeritus. The current President is Dr Charles H. LeMaistre.

The extent of the growth and expansion of the centre is shown by the wide range of its present fields of activity: experimental cancer research, cancer treatment and rehabilitation, clinical cancer research, cancer control and professional education. All this work is carried out at the M. D. Anderson Hospital and Lutheran Pavilion, the Tumor Institute and a new clinic building. There is also a rehabilitation hospital situated 6 miles from the main campus. A research division and a veterinary division are located in Science Park, about 120 miles away.

Experimental research is carried out on a wide spectrum of fundamental problems in the aetiology of cancer, and there is an extensive programme of clinical research on many aspects of human cancer.

The large hospital, which provides care for both in- and out-patients, has facilities and staff for the diagnosis and treatment of all varieties of cancer and allied diseases. The treatment modalities available include surgery, radiotherapy, chemotherapy, immunotherapy and patient rehabilitation.

Professional education forms an important part of the centre's work. There are postgraduate training positions for both nationals and non-nationals; training facilities for clinical fellows, postdoctoral fellows, project investigators, residents and graduate trainees; and rotation facilities for undergraduate medical, nursing, dental and paramedical students.

The development of the University of Texas M. D. Anderson Tumor Institute and Hospital has been most impressive and the work it carries out is of great international interest and importance.

Memorial Sloan–Kettering Cancer Center

This famous cancer centre in New York, USA, was promoted by Dr J. Marion Sims, the father of modern gynaecology, who stated: "A cancer hospital is one of the greatest needs of the day, and it must be built. We want a cancer hospital on its own foundation — wholly independent of all other hospitals. Let me beg you to take steps at once to inaugurate a movement which must culminate in a great work so much needed here and now. The subject is too large and its interest too great to be lodged in a pavilion subsidiary to any other hospital." His statement encouraged others to found the New York Cancer Hospital; he himself unfortunately died before his dream materialised. The hospital was incorporated on 31 May 1884 and opened in December 1887, its name being changed in 1899 to General Memorial Hospital for the Treatment of Cancer and Allied Diseases. The hospital's design was noteworthy for the circular wards and special system of ventilation. The advantages of circular wards were considered to be that they increased the amount of natural light, promoted cleanliness by impeding dust accumulation, provided the nurses with better means to observe the patients, and helped to create a more cheerful atmosphere.

An important development occurred when Dr James Ewing, who joined the staff in 1913, succeeded in converting the hospital's role as a general hospital into that of an institution devoted entirely to the study and treatment of cancer, the original objective of the founders. Dr Ewing was later joined by Dr James Douglas, a mining engineer and metallurgist, whose gifts of radium, funds and scientific knowledge were governed by the Douglas Deeds, which stipulated that Dr Ewing should become President of the General Memorial's Medical Board and the hospital's pathologist and that the hospital should be exclusively for cancer care and affiliated with Cornell University Medical College. The agreement was formalised in 1914, and in 1916, as stipulated in the Douglas Deeds, the word "General" was eliminated from the hospital's name.

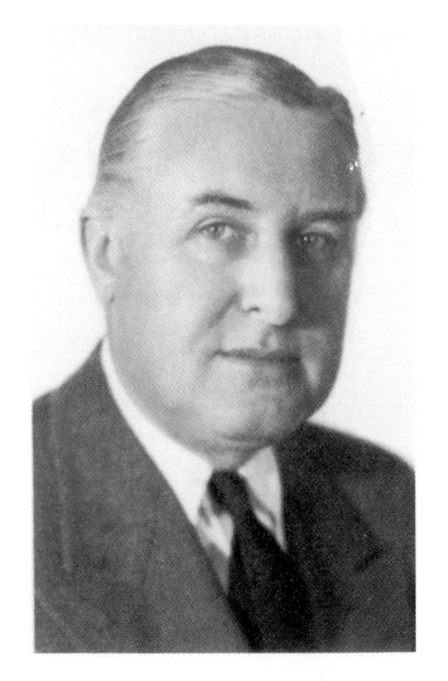

Figure 3.19 Frank E. Adair.

Marie Curie visited the hospital in 1921 and inspected the apparatus used for collecting radium emanation. The radon was enclosed in gold seeds or tubes for the treatment of cancer patients.

The work of the hospital continued to grow under distinguished professional staff. In 1938, for example, the attending staff included such well-known surgeons as Hayes E. Martin, Bradley L. Coley, Frank E. Adair and George T. Pack, and many others. There were 125 nurses on the staff and educational courses were arranged to standardise nursing care and to provide special cancer nursing.

The educational and training programmes for residents and other doctors are an important feature of the work of the hospital aimed at improving the care of cancer patients. In 1927 a fellowship programme was established through the generosity of John D. Rockefeller, Jr, and by 1938 fellows had come from about 30 states and 20 countries. During the years 1939–1944 new programmes in nursing, clinical and laboratory research were created though Rockefeller's generosity and concern.

An outstanding development was the construction of a new, modern hospital on land given by the same benefactor, with funds contributed by the General Education Board and Edward S. Harkness. Scientific and clinical work expanded. In 1939 Dr Cornelius P. Rhoads became Director of the Memorial Hospital and played an essential role in its evolution into a modern medical centre. He initiated and developed the discipline of cancer chemotherapy and Dr Kanematsu Sugiura conducted work on transplanted animal tumours as a tool for testing chemotherapeutic agents. In the chemistry laboratory Dr Helen Q. Woodard tested blood serum for phosphatase and her work contributed greatly to the understanding of bone disease. Radiotherapy was developed by the installation of a 1 000 000 volt X-ray machine, then the largest of its kind for treating cancer.

Another outstanding development took place in 1945 when Alfred P. Sloan, Jr, and Charles F. Kettering established the Sloan–Kettering Institute. Their research experiences at General Motors encouraged them to believe that similar research techniques could be implemented to elucidate cancer problems. The institute was opened in 1948. It is most important to note that although the Sloan–Kettering Institute was organised as a separate corporation, its members worked in conjunction with the staff of the Memorial Hospital and Dr Rhoads was the Director of both organisations. In 1950 the institute became affiliated with Cornell Graduate School of Medical Sciences, thus providing PhD programmes for young scientists during training.

In 1950 the James Ewing Hospital opened as a result of a cooperative effort between the City of New York and the Memorial Hospital, and it enabled patients in New York City to receive the same care that Memorial Hospital patients received. In 1968 Ewing Hospital was absorbed by the Memorial Hospital and renamed the Ewing Pavilion. In 1975 it was converted into a research facility and its name was changed again, to Arnold and Marie Schwartz International Hall of Science for Cancer Research.

Many outstanding people continued to support the development of this great enterprise. Laurence S. Rockefeller has devoted more than half his life to it, and numerous others have given liberally of their skills and funds, serving the institution in different positions. Edward J. Beattie, Jr, joined the staff in 1965 as Attending Surgeon and Chief of the Thoracic Service and in 1966 he was appointed Chairman of the Department of Surgery. Later that year he became Chief Medical Officer of the Memorial Hospital and he held this post until his retirement in 1983. He is well known for his surgical skills and his development and support of the multidisciplinary work on cancer. Dr Samuel Hellman, first Chairman of the Department of Radiation Therapy, established the joint Center for Radiation Therapy. He was appointed Physician-in-Chief of Memorial Hospital in 1983. When the

Sloan–Kettering Institute was reorganised in 1982, Dr Richard A. Rifkind was appointed its Chairman. In the meantime a new hospital had been planned and built, a 19-storey building containing 565 beds, which opened in 1973 for the clinical investigation and comprehensive care of patients suffering from cancer.

The first Directors of the Memorial Hospital, Dr Ewing and Dr Rhoads, were followed by several other illustrious physician administrators: Dr John R. Heller, Dr Frank Horsfall, Dr Lewis Thomas and Dr Paul Marks.

The author is greatly indebted to Patricia Turi, Administrative Coordinator, Public Affairs Department of the Memorial Sloan–Kettering Cancer Center, for the brochure entitled *A Century of Commitment*, which provided him with all the information for this section.

The American Cancer Society

This is the world's largest private health organisation concerned with cancer. It was established in 1913 by only 15 men, as the American Society for the Control of Cancer. In its first year of activity about 10 000 dollars were raised to finance the project and a pamphlet was published entitled *Facts About Cancer* to educate the public. In those days both professional and public attitudes with regard to cancer were entirely different from those prevalent today. In fact it was difficult even to mention the word "cancer" to the public, who regarded the disease's development with fear and despondency, for the results of treatment were very poor. Cancer research lacked the scientific equipment, methodology and knowledge we possess nowadays and aroused but little interest and enthusiasm in scientists and clinicians. This was the background against which the Society was formed with the grand objective of the total control of cancer in the human race. Since then it has grown enormously, has organised and activated enlightened programmes of work and provided an infinite amount of help and influence throughout the whole world. The present author gratefully acknowledges the information about the Society kindly supplied to him by Gerry S. de Haven, Vice President for International Activities, and also that taken from the book *Crusade*, the official history of the Society by Walter Ross, formerly Director of Special Publications at the American Cancer Society. This book gives a complete account of the inauguration and development of the Society into the enormous present-day institution, with its impressive research programmes and policies. In addition, it gives valuable information about medical statistics, cancer aetiology and the results of research into cancer detection and prevention, and is strongly recommended for detailed study by all who are concerned with cancer control. It is only possible here to give the briefest glimpse of the work and accomplishments of the American Cancer Society, which is carried out by more than two million volunteers, American men, women and children who implement programmes in public and professional education, provide various services for patients and their families and support the enormous research programme of the Society.

Its national headquarters are in Atlanta, Georgia, and it has 58 incorporated chartered Divisions, one in each State, in Puerto Rico, the District of Columbia and six metropolitan areas. All Divisions are represented on a

National Board which plans the programmes of research, education and service to cancer patients, in addition to formulating policies. Members are drawn from every discipline relative to the work of the Society.

The Society works closely with other professional societies, including the American Medical Association, the American College of Surgeons, the United States Public Health Service, medical societies and health departments. Its influence is shown by its annual expert testimony to Congress on the specific needs for government funds for the National Cancer Institute's (NCI) various cancer control activities. The Society collaborates with the NCI in many public and professional education and service projects.

Educating the public about cancer is an important part of the Society's work. It stresses the value of a medical check-up for all adults and defines seven cancer warning signals which require immediate medical attention. Whilst regular clinical examination is an important safeguard against cancer, other safeguards are publicised which concern the six most frequent cancer sites: the lungs, colon and rectum, breast, uterus, skin and mouth. Tumours in these sites can be prevented, detected, diagnosed and cured.

The Society has a comprehensive professional education programme which is designed to continue and supplement the education started in medical, dental and nursing schools and to complement the work of professional societies, health departments and other health agencies. National conferences are organised and Clinical Fellowship Programmes are financed so that hospital residents can improve the management of cancer patients. Support is also given to post-resident clinicians and professors of clinical oncology.

Cancer patients and their families are assisted through the Society's Service and Rehabilitation Programmes, which provide information and counselling services, various amenities, including equipment and the application of surgical dressings in the homes of patients, and transportation facilities. The rehabilitation of patients is carried out very extensively and includes ostomy care, laryngectomy care and the Reach to Recovery to enable mastectomy patients to live normally. Rehabilitation is also provided for patients with disabilities related to cancer.

An important part of the Society's work is research into all aspects of cancer, including its prevention, development, incidence and treatment. All varieties of fundamental scientific research are supported, but special emphasis is placed on epidemiological and statistical research. Notable work has been done on cancer of the lung. For example, in 1951 a large statistical investigation was made of the smoking habits of 188 000 men in nine States, which necessitated 22000 American Cancer Society volunteers carrying out interviews over a period of 4 years. This survey showed a marked relationship between smoking and lung cancer and heart disease.

In 1982 the Society launched a long-term epidemiological study of one million men and women aged 30 or more to determine whether environment and life-styles are related to the onset of cancer and other diseases. A search will be made for clues of cancer causation and factors that might prevent cancer.

At the time of writing (January 1989), the Society is due to soon move to splendid new headquarters in Atlanta, built on 4 acres of land provided by Emory University and adjacent to its medical campus. The three new national officers of the Society are: William M. Tipping, Executive Vice-

President; Gerald P. Murphy, Senior Vice-President for Medical Affairs; and John Laszlo, Senior Vice-President for Research.

1988 was the 75th anniversary of this Society, which goes from strength to strength, its future prosperity assured. It is impossible to measure the enormous contribution to cancer control that it has made during the past 75 years and that it will doubtless continue to make in years to come.

Institut Curie in Paris

This famous institute was established in 1909 in honour of Marie Curie and it has expanded considerably and continuously since then. Scientific research on the aetiology, environmental factors, prevention, early diagnosis and treatment, including surgery, radiation, chemotherapy, hormonal therapy and immunotherapy, of all varieties of cancer is carried out in the research department and hospital by its distinguished staff of scientists and clinicians.

Pierre and Marie Curie discovered radium in 1898 and were awarded the Nobel Prize in 1903. In 1909, in order to provide Marie Curie with the best possible research facilities, the University of Paris created the Institut du Radium, where she directed the Laboratory of General Physics and Radioactivity. Claudius Regaud, Professor of the Faculty of Medicine at Lyon and already well-known for his research, was appointed by the Institut Pasteur to direct the Laboratory of Radiophysiology, with the specific objective of studying the biological effects and the medical applications of ionising radiation.

The Institut Curie was founded to apply the effects of radium in the treatment of various cancers, and it continued to develop in this domain in which it was the precursor. In 1920 the necessity of creating a department for the medical application of radiation became apparent and this led to the birth of the Foundation Curie. The results obtained in 1921 in the treatment of cancer placed the Foundation's methods in the first rank world-wide, and the faith in their work which the founders were able to instil in important benefactors allowed the Institut to serve as a model for establishing cancer centres both in other parts of France and in other countries. Due to the knowledge and energy of Claudius Regaud, novel and revolutionary ideas for that period were born at this institute which are now fundamental in hospital medicine.

Towards the end of the 19th century scientists were aware of the still mysterious Röntgen rays discovered in 1895, the products of electricity, and of Becquerel rays, which are emitted spontaneously by certain natural elements, including radium, which was discovered by Pierre and Marie Curie and isolated in 1898 by Marie Curie. In the Faculty of Medicine at Lyon, Claudius Regaud, a still little known scientist, passionately concentrated his efforts on the study of the radiobiological effects of radium. In 1909 Emile Roux, Director of the Institut Pasteur in Paris, speaking of the importance for humanity of the development of radioactivity, and the Rector of the University of Paris, Louis Liard, conscious of the role which the University must assume, together recognised the necessity of uniting the physicians, chemists and biologists to study radioactivity and the biological effects of ionising radiation as a corporate effort.

An Institut du Radium of the University of Paris was therefore created, composed of twin laboratories, namely, the Pavilion Curie (physical and chemical laboratories), directed by Marie Curie, and the Pavilion Pasteur (biological laboratory), which was entrusted to Dr Regaud.

Construction work began in 1911, but it had scarcely been completed in 1914 when the First World War broke out, and it was not until 1919 that the Laboratoire Curie, which had been used for defense purposes during the war, and the Laboratoire Pasteur, which had remained closed, took any part in the work for which they had been built. In 1920 the project became a reality and the creation of an organisation in the form of a foundation was decided upon. Dr Henri de Rothschild, a generous benefactor who had already made a gift of half a gramme of radium to the Institut, provided the initial donation, and Dr Roux obtained an official grant for the creation of "a radium therapy establishment for the treatment of all illnesses by radium, in particular cancer".

Finally, the University made a 10-year grant to the Institut du Radium of a strip of land situated behind the Institut du Chimie, a few metres from the Laboratoire Pasteur in the Rue d'Ulm. The statutes of the "Foundation Curie" were laid down on 27 May 1921. It has earned universal renown for its work in many aspects of cancer and particularly in the medical application of radiation.

From 1919 Regaud was surrounded by physicians and biologists each of whom was chosen for his competence in his own speciality, but also, and perhaps above all, for his character, enthusiasm and team spirit. Regaud did not come alone from Lyon to Paris, but brought with him his pupil, Dr Antoine Lacassagne, licentiate in sciences and hospital intern, who was the son of the Professor of Legal Medicine in the Faculty and assured of a fine career in Lyon. Against the advice of his friends, however, the pupil chose to follow his patron and took up an appointment at the Institut Pasteur to concentrate on research. It was a decision he did not regret, for he later became chief assistant of Regaud and succeeded him as Director of the Foundation in 1937. He became a master of radiobiology and cancerology and his achievements earned him an international reputation.

Many notable scientists and clinicians have made important contributions to cancer problems at the Institut Curie. In 1935 Dr Francois Baclesse did his work on techniques of radiotherapy which has had a big influence on the development of this treatment modality. In subsequent years the volume of work has continued to increase, both in cancer research and in clinical aspects, and it is clearly recognised that these main divisions are closely interlinked and progress conjointly.

In 1988 the building of a new hospital was commenced to amplify still further both cancer research and the treatment of patients with cancer at the Institut Curie. The facilities for the care of in-patients and out-patients in the hospital will be greatly increased by this necessary expansion of its work in surgery, radiotherapy, hormone therapy and immunotherapy. In addition, emphasis will continue to be placed on environmental cancer, and on prevention and early diagnosis of malignant diseases.

The author gratefully acknowledges the assistance of Mireille Vitry, Unité de Communication, who supplied him with a leaflet of presentation of the Institut and a brochure giving the most important historical features and detailed information on the cancer research and treatment carried out at the Institut Curie.

Institut Gustave-Roussy

The Institut Gustave-Roussy is well known internationally for its work in cancer research and the treatment of cancer patients. As is the case in many cancer centres in different countries, the research and clinical disciplines in cancer are linked together and the work proceeds concurrently, thus ensuring a constant feedback of new knowledge between the laboratory and clinic for the benefit of patients, and establishing an environment for the interchange of ideas and for mutual discussions between researchers and clinicians.

The Institut Gustave-Roussy, directed for many years by Professor Pierre Denoix, is one of 20 French anti-cancer centres. It is the direct descendant of the hospital section of the Institut du Cancer which was conceived in 1930 by Professor Gustave Roussy, who wished to create a combined clinical and research establishment under a single management charged to maintain its cohesion.

The centre comprised the Institut de Recherches Scientifiques sur le Cancer directed by Professor Roger Monier, the progeny of the laboratory section of the Institut du Cancer, and three research units of the Institut National de la Santé et de la Recherche Médical. These three units were: the Unit of Statistical Research, under Professor Daniel Schwartz, which was directly associated with the Institut Gustave-Roussy; the Institute of Radiobiological Clinical Research, directed by Professor Maurice Tubiana, which was situated in the same building as the Institut Gustave-Roussy; and the Institute of Cancerology and Immunogenetics, directed by Professor Georges Mathe.

In addition, in 1962 an association was formed for the development of cancer research, presided over by Jacques Crozemarie. This constituted a meeting point for discussion by the members of the five entities.

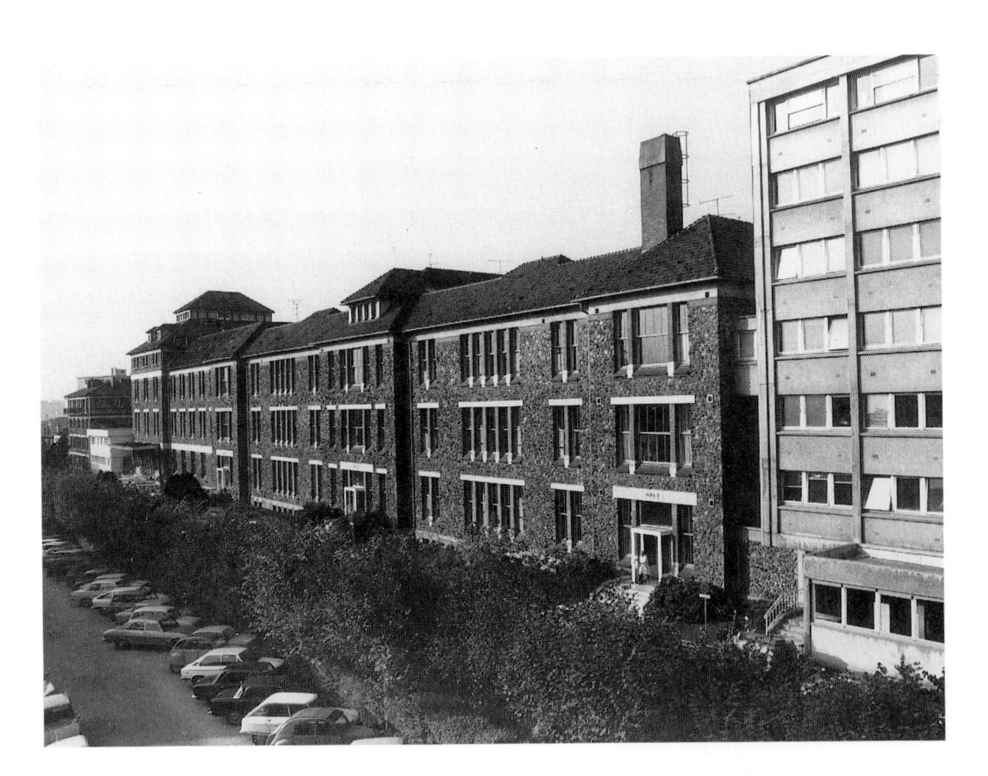

Figure 3.20 The original Institut Gustave-Roussy.

The history of the development in stages of the anti-cancer complex at Villejuif then proceeded as now briefly described according to the year of inauguration.

1921. Creation at the Hôpital Paul-Brousse of the first centre which was designed specially for cancer patients by L'hermite and Gustave Roussy. A regional centre for the fight against cancer was created in Paris in 1925 with Professor Roussy as its Director.

1926. Creation of the Institut du Cancer de la Faculté de Médecin de Paris at Villejuif, situated 3 kilometres to the south of Paris. When the hospital section was opened in 1934, Professor Roussy was appointed the Medical Director.

The Institut du Cancer, like the Hospice Paul-Brousse, was built on the highest area of the region and similarly with an outlook facing towards the south; the research laboratories and the morgue faced the north. Situated far from the smoke of factories, it enjoyed the pure air of the region of Arcueil-Cachan and of Bourg-la-Reine, the heights of Chevilly and the Valley of the Seine.

1930–1934. Creation of the Foundation for the Development of the Institut du Cancer under the presidency of Gustave Roussy, at that time Doyen of the Faculty of Medicine and Rector of the University of Paris.

1950. The Institut du Cancer was renamed "Institut Gustave-Roussy".

The Institut Gustave-Roussy has developed in an impressive way so that it now includes the complex of Hautes-Brugères at Villejuif which was completed in 1980 with 440 beds, and a complex at Le Grange et Savigny-le-Temple, opened in 1961 with 164 beds and designed to care for patients for whom the method of treatment or their distant domicile necessitates prolonged hospitalisation but does not require the use of sophisticated equipment. If radiotherapy is necessary this is carried out at Haut-Brugères.

Since the inauguration of the Institut Gustave-Roussy in 1921, its distinguished scientific and clinical staff have made important contributions to our knowledge of cancer and large numbers of cancer patients have been treated and helped in many ways.

The author is indebted to Nicole Guery, Director of the Institut Gustave-Roussy, who supplied him with a copy of *I.G.R. Soixante Ans Après Inauguration — Institut Gustave-Roussy 1921–1981*, from which all the information in this section has been taken.

Istituto Nazionale per lo Studio e la Cura dei Tumori, Milan, Italy

The first divisions of this institute, the Victor Emanuel III National Institute for the Study and Cure of Cancer, founded in 1925, were opened in March 1928 by its principal animator, Prof. Luigi Mangiagalli, a gynaecologist and active politician. Initial capacity was for about 200 in-patients, in two wards: clinical/surgical and gynaecological. Three essential service units were included: anatomical pathology, radiology and biology.

Several additions have been made to the original nucleus. In 1969 the first comprehensive mono-unit was inaugurated, which houses most of the divisions for the in-patients. A second unit, opened in 1984, with further divisions for both patients and diagnosis, brought total in-patient capacity to 500. A new building under construction on the remaining space on the site will potentiate and enlarge the areas for research and laboratories. The hospital now has 15 divisions for in-patients, is supported by 15 divisions devoted to diagnosis and special therapy and has almost 1500 employees.

The first Head of the institute, Prof. Gaetano Fichera (1928–1935), has been followed by Prof. Pietro Rondoni (till 1956), Prof. Pietro Bucalossi (till 1975) and finally the present Director, Prof. Umberto Veronesi.

The institute includes a highly rated nursing school specialising in the care of cancer patients. It also supports the European School of Oncology, founded in 1982, whose purpose is to propagate and inform medical personnel occupied chiefly in the field of oncology.

It has always taken part in scientific exchange and discussion on an international basis and has made some very valuable contributions, including results with the drugs Adriamycin and Daunomycin, which are among the best known scientific products introduced for some time past for cancer treatment throughout the world. Of primary importance was the development of adjuvant chemotherapy after mastectomy; in the same field the achievement of conservative surgery for breast cancer made it possible for a large number of women to undergo less mutilating surgery. Important research has also been done on the role of human papillomavirus in cervical lesions.

Today research is divided among five divisions: molecular biology, cell kinetics, carcinogenesis, immunology and experimental chemotherapy. Major studies are being carried out on new monoclonal antibodies and their clinical applications.

The author is grateful to Dr Edoardo Majno for the above information.

REFERENCES

Association of American Cancer Institutes (June 1985). *ACCI Newsletter* (Mirand, E. A., ed.), p. 12

Banks, J. D. (1959). Features of a cancer hospital. In Raven, R. W. (ed.) *Cancer*, Vol. 6, pp 453–63. Butterworth & Co., London

Brunning, D. A. and Dukes, C. E. (1965). The origin and early history of the Institute of Cancer Research of the Royal Cancer Hospital. *Proc. Roy. Soc. Med.*, **58**, 33–6

International Union Against Cancer (1978). *International Directory of Specialised Cancer Research and Treatment Establishments*, 2nd edn. UICC Technical Report Series, Vol. 33, Geneva

Kennaway, E. L. (1957). The incubation period of cancer in man. In Raven, R. W. (ed.) *Cancer*, Vol. 1, pp 6–23. Butterworth & Co., London

Ledoux-Lebard, R. (1906). *La Lutte Contre le Cancer*, p 9. Masson et Cie, Paris. Quoted by Haagensen, C. D. (1933) in "An exhibit of important books, papers and memorabilia illustrating the evolution of the knowledge of cancer", *Am. J. Cancer*, **18**, 56–7

Mirand, E. A. (1988). Dr Roswell Park and our 90th Anniversary. *Buffalo Physician and Biomedical Scientist*, 26–8

Raven, R. W. (1933). Report from the Follow-up Department of St Bartholomew's Hospital. In *Saint Bartholomew's Hospital Reports*, Vol. 66, pp 45–124.

Ross, W. *Crusade*. Arbor House Publishing Company, New York

CHAPTER FOUR

Voluntary Cancer Organisations

Voluntary cancer associations, which have been established in many countries throughout the world, have for many decades carried out an immense amount of work that is of the utmost importance and value in all aspects of the cancer field. The members of these associations continue to give freely of their time and expertise to different aspects of the work. In broad terms, their main objectives are to support and develop cancer research and to help patients with cancer in every possible way. To attain these objectives an enormous amount of money is required, so voluntary associations are engaged in fund-raising on a massive scale.

Patients with cancer at any stage of the disease and their families have many needs which must be supplied and serious problems that must be solved. This important subject was dealt with most helpfully by Joan Gough-Thomas *(1959)*. She stated that the first building in Europe for the care of patients suffering from cancer was erected in Rheims in 1740 at the instigation of Canon Godinot. In 1796 the first Committee of the Boston Dispensary considered organised home-care for cancer patients on a long-term basis and they established a public dispensary "so that the sick might be attended and relieved in their own homes at less expense to the public than in hospital and that those who had seen better days might be comforted without being humiliated".

Joan Gough-Thomas called attention to the address which Sir Charles Loch, Secretary to the London Charity Organisation Society, delivered in 1885 to the Metropolitan Provident Medical Association, in which he stated that a means was needed for investigating medical care recipients and enabling patients to continue with medical treatment after their discharge from hospital.

In connection with this early work for the care of cancer patients in the community it is extremely interesting to interpolate the modern concept of rehabilitation and continuing care in cancer and the practical ways in which it is being implemented with great benefits for patients and their families. Such work is attracting international interest today, in addition to other developments in the UK, where, for example, the Marie Curie Memorial Foundation is establishing special rehabilitation and continuing care units.

In her detailed and informative article Joan Gough-Thomas has traced the development of social services in different countries where the special needs of patients with cancer were recognised. Charitable organisations have been established to provide hospitals and clinics, treatment facilities, including radiotherapy, home-care and financial help for patients who require it. Other activities of these organisations include cancer research and community education about cancer. The author gives specific examples of the organisations and appropriate references to the literature.

THE MARIE CURIE MEMORIAL FOUNDATION

This Foundation is an outstanding example of a composite cancer voluntary organisation which is working on a national scale throughout the UK. A detailed account is given here of the work it has carried out since its foundation in 1948. The present author has had a very close connection with the Foundation and has helped in its development from its inception to the present day.

Attention is called to the historic document *Report of the Marie Curie Memorial Foundation 1948–1953. Incorporating the First Annual Report 1952–1953*, which contains a description of the inauguration of the Foundation and details of its Council and Committees and their membership. The account given here is based upon this document, from which various passages are quoted.

After preliminary discussions the inaugural Committee met in London on 7 July 1948, "under the chairmanship of Mrs Warren Pearl with Squadron-Leader T. B. Robinson as secretary and at this meeting the Memorial was brought into being. The Founder Members included Lord Moynihan, Lady Waddilove and Dame Louise McIlroy. By the end of 1948 formalities were completed with the Charity Commissioners, the Public Control Department of the London County Council and the Inland Revenue Authorities, and a limited test appeal for funds had produced £11 000. About this time unofficial approaches were made to other organisations to ensure that no duplication of effort should occur and in order not to transgress the work of other Charities.

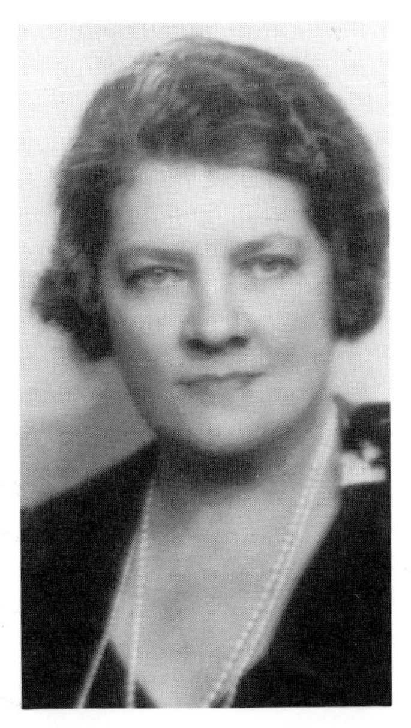

Figure 4.1 Mrs. A. L. Warren Pearl, a founder member of the Foundation. Nursing Home in Birmingham named in her honour.

On 22 May 1949 the Trust Deed, prepared by the Honorary Solicitor, was signed by Mrs Warren Pearl, Lady Waddilove and Lord Moynihan as Trustees and at the end of the summer months the appeal for funds was reintroduced. Despite the fact that external conditions had worsened, the income for this period of 4 months exceeded £10 000. The results of the two short appeals convinced the Committee "that it would be possible to raise a large sum of money which could be devoted to the welfare and assistance of patients suffering from cancer, and, in order that it could discharge its obligations to the donors fully and wisely it was considered essential to seek the advice and cooperation of a larger body of people, who, through their knowledge of public affairs and health problems, could assist in the administration of these funds judiciously."

Accordingly, a meeting of the first Council was called and took place on Wednesday, 1 March 1950, with Mrs A. L. Warren Pearl in the Chair. The other 19 members of this first Council are named in the Report.

At this meeting the present author outlined a programme which he had devised for the work of the Foundation. This was to be based on the findings of the Joint National Survey Committee which had already started work under his chairmanship in January 1950. This Committee composed of members of the Inaugural Committee of the Marie Curie Memorial Foundation and of the Committee of the Queen's Institute of District Nursing had been set up "to enquire into the conditions of patients with cancer being nursed at home throughout the country, in order that their needs could be assessed and methods sought for the alleviation of their problems."

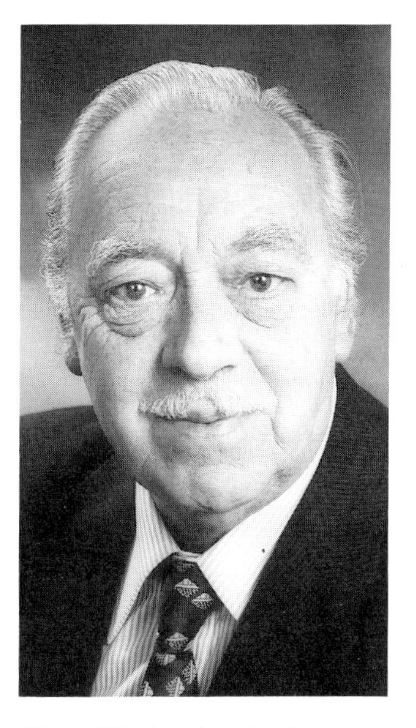

Figure 4.2 Squadron-Leader T. B. Robinson, Secretary of the Marie Curie Memorial Foundation from 1948 to 1977.

The Council took the following actions as described in the Report: "The Council appointed an Executive Committee under the chairmanship of Mr Raven, and the original Inaugural Committee became the Appeals Committee of the Council. There have been several changes in the composition of the Council and of the Executive Committee since that time, and we are pleased to record the acceptance of the chairmanship of the Council by Lord Kershaw in April 1951. Mr R. W. Raven, who was already Chairman of the Executive Committee and of the Joint National Survey Committee, was invited to become Deputy Chairman of the Council in April 1951 and Lord Amherst of Hackney kindly consented to become Honorary Treasurer in April 1950." He was succeeded in December 1981 by Sir Malby Crofton.

On the retirement of Lord Kershaw in 1961 the present author was appointed Chairman of the Council and the Earl of Wemyss and March Deputy Chairman.

In 1956 Her Majesty Queen Elizabeth, the Queen Mother, graciously granted her patronage to the Foundation and in the succeeding years her continued interest has provided profound encouragement and inspiration.

Squadron-Leader T. B. Robinson, who had been intimately connected with the work from its inception, including carrying out the two test appeals for funds, was the Secretary of the Council until he retired in 1977, when he was succeeded as Executive Secretary by Paul A. Sturgess. In 1985 the latter retired and Major-General M. E. Carleton-Smith was appointed Director-General.

A Charity is greatly dependent on the support of voluntary helpers, and special mention is made here of the important work of Lady Heald and her colleages, who raised considerable funds to enable the Foundation's work to proceed.

The rapid expansion of this work necessitated the formation of other committees of the Council, which are listed in the Report. An important development was the establishment of the Committee for Scotland, composed of a distinguished membership from all parts of the country, in June 1952 under the chairmanship of the Earl of Wemyss and March, with headquarters in Edinburgh. Before details are given about the growth of the Foundation's work, attention is drawn to the findings of the Joint

National Survey, because the needs of patients with cancer being nursed at home 36 years ago, soon after the inauguration of the National Health Service in 1948, are clearly shown there.

Joint National Survey Committee

The Joint National Survey Committee was formed in January 1950 at the present author's suggestion, with representation from the Foundation's Inaugural Committee and the Queen's Institute of District Nursing. The author was appointed its Chairman and Miss E. Elliott the Organising Secretary. It was the first time a survey had been made concerning the "conditions and circumstances of cancer patients being nursed in their own homes. In view of the frequent cases of hardship encountered in this connection, the Foundation had taken as one of its principal objects the provision of a welfare service to help domiciliary cancer cases, as an ancillary to those services already provided by the National Health Service, and it was thought that such a Survey would indicate where help was most needed."

The work began in January 1950 and culminated in April 1952, when the Committee published its *Report on a National Survey Concerning Patients with Cancer Nursed at Home*. The Committee met finally on 9 June 1952 to receive the published report, which proved to be a valuable guide for the activities of the Foundation.

Since this is a historic document a detailed account of the research is given here. The Committee was greatly indebted to many individual experts and organisations for advice and help concerning the form of questionnaire used in the investigation (a facsimile is shown in the report), and the procedure adopted, for practical help with the Survey, and for information about voluntary welfare services. The questionnaire includes 50 questions, with a number of subdivisions, covering the condition of the patient, amenities of the home, nursing and welfare services available and needs as not yet met. Space was allowed for comments of the nurses who were responsible for filling up the questionnaires.

The questionnaires were distributed to all home nurses attending the sick, by the Medical Officer of Health responsible for domiciliary nursing under Section 25 of the National Health Service Act. In the metropolitan area the distribution was undertaken by the Central Council for District Nursing in London and in a few areas questionnaires were sent direct to voluntary nursing associations at the request of the Medical Officer of Health concerned. The cooperation of 179 Medical Officers of Health was secured, so the report is based on a total number of 7050 patients with cancer being nursed at home. A punch card system (a facsimile of which is shown in the report) was used for the analysis of the data received, which covered patients in England, Scotland, Wales and Northern Ireland. The Committee recorded its gratitude to Miss Elliott M.A., A.M.I.A., for all her competent work in organisation and analysis.

The special needs of patients with cancer nursed at home were considered in detail in the report. The provision of domiciliary nurses, especially to nurse patients during the night, was stressed, for it was found that there were many patients who required such help urgently at short notice and lack of it could cause much additional suffering for the patient and con-

FACSIMILE OF QUESTIONNAIRE (original size 13in. by 8in.)

CONFIDENTIAL

JOINT NATIONAL SURVEY COMMITTEE

Chairman R. W. RAVEN, Esq. O.B.E. F.R.C.S. Hon. Secretary S/Ldr BERNARD ROBINSON, F.C.C.S.
Organising Secretary Miss ELIZABETH ELLIOTT, M.A., A.M.I.A.

MARIE CURIE MEMORIAL & QUEEN'S INSTITUTE OF DISTRICT NURSING

Tel. Sloane 1095 124, SLOANE STREET, LONDON, S.W.1

SECTION I

(a) Age of patient: (b) Male/Female (c) Married/Single/Widowed/Separated.
(d) (Former) Occupation:
(e) Home run by: Patient/Husband or Wife/Daughter/Son/Other relative/ Friend/Housekeeper or Landlady.
(f) Is patient receiving medical attention? Yes/No.
(g) What caused patient to seek medical advice?

SECTION II

(a) Present general condition of patient: Active/Convalescent/Bedridden
(b) " local " " Improving/Static/Deteriorating.
(c) Is one of the following present?
Tracheotomy/Gastrostomy/Jejunostomy/Colostomy/Cystotomy.
(d) Can patient attend to above?
(e) If not what is done?
(f) Degree of suffering: Slight/Moderate/Severe.
(g) Equipment or appliances required:
(h) " " " available:

SECTION III

(a) Nature of Locality: Town/Village/Country.
(b) Residence: House/Bungalow/(......Floor) Flat.
(c) Number in household: Adults .... Children ....
(d) Number of rooms: Living .... Bedrooms ....
(e) Has patient own room? Yes/No.
(f) Is a bathroom available? Yes/No.
(g) What lavatory accommodation is available? Indoor/Outdoor.
(h) Is above easily accessible to patient? Yes/No.
(i) Is patient on a special diet? Yes/No.
(j) Are there reasonable cooking facilities? Yes/No.
(k) Is a Meals on Wheels service available? Yes/No.
(l) If so, who runs it? Local Authority/B.R.C.S./W.V.S./Other voluntary body.
(m) Does above provide invalid diets? Yes/No.
(n) Is above used by patient? Yes/No.
(o) Has dwelling: Running Hot Water/Main Water/Main Drainage/Gas/Electricity.
(p) Is Home Help service available? Yes/No.
(q) " " " " used by patient? Yes/No.

SECTION IV

(a) 1. Frequency of District Nurse's visits:
2. Is another nurse in attendance? Yes/No.
3. Is night nursing necessary? Yes/No.
4. If so is it done by Nurse/Relative/Friend/Others/Not available.
5. Are reasonable washing facilities available ? Yes/No.
6. Is laundry done by: Commercial laundry/Relative/Friend/Home Help/Patient/Others.
7. Are dressings necessary? Yes/No.
8. Quantities used: Large/Medium/Small
9. Are these obtained under National Health Scheme? Yes/No.
10. How are these dressings disposed of?

(b) 1. Does hospital follow up the case? Yes/No.
2. Is patient likely to need: Convalescent treatment/(Re)admission to hospital.
3. Is there an urgent unfilled need of any of the following:
Additional nourishment/Special Foods/Clothing/
Bedlinen/Nursing furniture/Nursing appliances/Home Help/
Night Sitter/Facilities for recreation/
4. Is there any need not listed above?
5. Is patient in touch with his or her Religious Denomination? Yes/No.
6. If not does he or she wish to be? Yes/No.
7. Is patient in touch with any welfare organisation? Yes/No.
8. If so which one?

Nurse's signature...............Town or district................Date............

Any additional information or other comments may be written on the back of the questionnaire.

51

Figure 4.3 The questionnaire used by the Joint National Survey Committee of the Marie Curie Foundation and the Queen's Institute of District Nursing.

siderable anxiety for the family. The Foundation solved the problem by organising its Day and Night Nursing Service for cancer patients at home on a national scale (see later in this chapter).

The need for residential nursing homes was clearly shown in the Survey, for there was evidence of considerable hardship in many families with one member with cancer at home and there were some patients who required in-patient medical and nursing care. It was found that some older patients were reluctant to leave their homes in spite of poor conditions and it was felt that they would be prepared to enter a nursing home rather than a public institution. In addition to providing skilled medical and nursing care for the patients, nursing homes would relieve much stress and strain for their relatives. Accommodation would be provided not only for the continuing care of seriously ill patients, but also, for short periods, for other cancer patients in order to give their families a much needed rest or help during domestic emergencies.

The nursing homes would not be regarded as homes for incurable patients, since groups of patients could be admitted for convalescent care and when they were undergoing radiotherapy as out-patients at hospitals. It was pointed out that if more facilities were available for convalescent care, patients could leave hospital sooner after surgical and other forms of treatment. This was the forerunner of our present-day concept of rehabilitation and continuing care for cancer patients, which is being developed practically by the Marie Curie Memorial Foundation by the establishment of Rehabilitation and Continuing Care Units.

The Foundation proceeded to establish 11 Nursing Homes for patients with cancer in different parts of the UK, with a total number of 380 beds (see later in this chapter).

The need for community education about cancer and for information on various aspects of cancer and all the facilities which are available for the needs of cancer patients is highlighted in the report, where it is stated: "The question of the education of the public regarding the early symptoms of

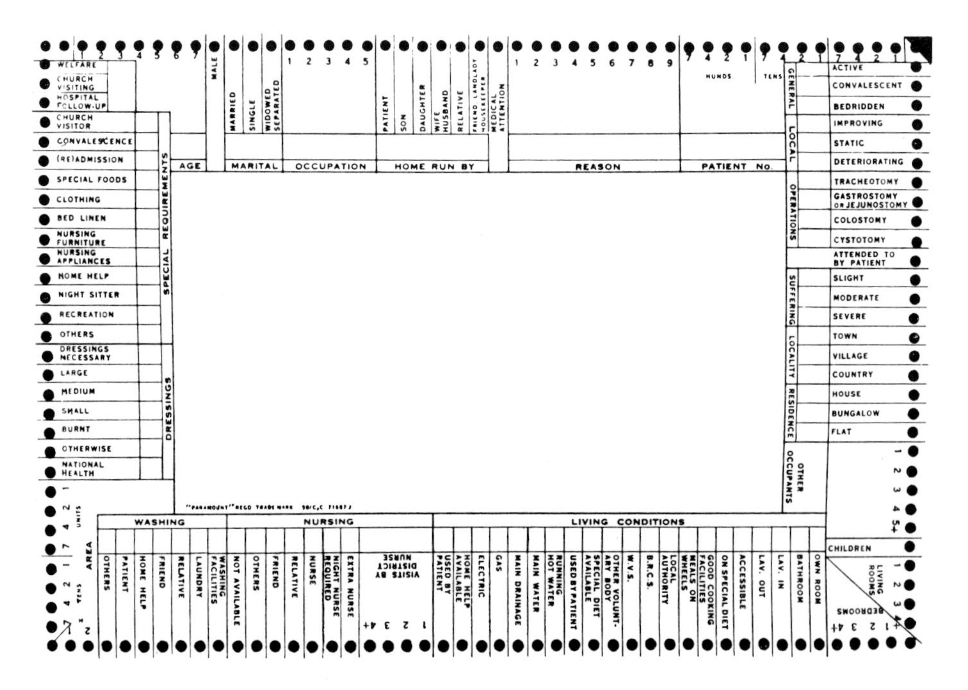

Figure 4.4 The punch card system used for the analysis of the data collected in the national survey.

cancer, the benefits of obtaining early treatment, and certain other aspects of the disease is most important. Valuable pioneer work is being done by voluntary bodies, such as the Chelsea Cancer Education Committee, and should be extended. The facts already quoted in this Report show the suffering which is caused by ignorance leading to delay in seeking treatment. Certain other information concerning cancer, such as the non-infectious nature of the disease, if known to the families of these patients would allay considerable anxiety."

In consequence of this particular conclusion, the Foundation established its Education and Welfare Department, whose work is described later in this chapter.

The report also describes other needs of cancer patients, including an extension of the home help service; the provision of special nursing and other equipment; recreational facilities, including occupational therapy and congenial company for elderly patients; individual case-work and the organisation of voluntary helpers. It is interesting to note that some of these needs brought to light so many years ago are now being satisfied through the provision of Day Centres for cancer patients.

In the total management of cancer patients, the care of the "whole" patient is of paramount importance. This means treatment of their physical condition and satisfying their spiritual needs. The report showed that nearly 75% of the patients investigated were receiving pastoral care from their religious denominations. The mental suffering of patients can be considerable, for it is often caused by the prospect of an incurable and sometimes a lengthy illness. It is very salutary for us to read the phrases "sent home from hospital to die" and "discharged as incurable", which appear very frequently in the questionnaires. Today increasing care and attention are being given to the spiritual needs of patients by developing pastoral care and counselling services for both patients and their families, and help is also being provided for the bereaved.

The report contains 22 tables, which summarise important data relative to the 7050 patients investigated, of whom 2685 were males and 4365 were females. Nearly 70% of the patients were aged 60 or over and more than 24% were aged 75 or over. It was amongst the elderly patients that some of the most serious problems were found. For instance, some patients depended upon an equally aged wife or husband; others had outlived all their friends and relatives and suffered acutely from neglect and loneliness. A noticeable number of patients were blind, either as the result of cancer or from other causes, and 55% of all patients were bedridden. It was clear that the degree of activity of the patients depended to a great extent on the character and temperament of the patient. The hope of recovery helped many patients to postpone invalidism, which is so important for the family as well as the patient. Many serious problems can be avoided so long as the patient remains independent and self-supporting.

The *Report on a National Survey Concerning Patients with Cancer Nursed at Home* was compiled 36 years ago, soon after the National Health Service was established, and it gives a clear account of the conditions and needs of cancer patients in the UK at that time. A comparison with the circumstances of domiciliary cancer patients today demonstrates the impressive advances in general care and management which have taken place since then. Important developments have also occurred in specific treatments

TABLE 8

JOINT NATIONAL CANCER SURVEY

GENERAL CONDITION OF PATIENTS

General Condition	*Total*	*% of 7,050*
Active	1,456	21
Convalescent	1,455	21
Bedridden	3,916	55
Unknown	223	3
TOTAL ..	7,050	100

TABLE 9

JOINT NATIONAL CANCER SURVEY

LOCAL CONDITION OF PATIENTS

Local Condition	*Total*	*% of 7,050*
Improving	812	12
Static	1,862	26
Deteriorating	4,129	58
Unknown	247	4
TOTAL ..	7,050	100

Figure 4.5 Tables 8 and 9 from the *Report on a National Survey Concerning Patients with Cancer Nursed at Home.*

for all varieties of cancer and in symptom control, including pain relief. The voluntary charity associations have also made very valuable contributions to this work.

Development of the work of the Marie Curie Memorial Foundation

It should be remembered that the Foundation's pioneer and comprehensive service for patients with cancer was planned and started 40 years ago and that during the ensuing years our knowledge of cancer, including its prevention, diagnosis and treatment, and of methods of rehabilitation and continuing care has increased enormously. For example, medical oncology was in its infancy then as compared with today and there has been impressive growth in all the other divisions of oncology.

The following description of the work and main activities of the Foundation is based on the details given in the First Annual Report.

Nursing Homes for cancer patients

One of the first objectives of the Foundation was to set up special Nursing Homes for all categories of patients suffering, or having suffered, from cancer to give them "nursing care and attention, a balanced diet, peaceful surroundings, physiotherapy and occupational therapy". "All categories" include patients needing hostel accommodation while attending hospital for radiotherapy as out-patients, patients who are convalescent after surgical treatment or radiotherapy and patients with persistent cancer. It was decided "that no Home should be entirely devoted to caring for patients in the third category, but should take a percentage of convalescents as well, in order to bring an atmosphere of hope to the Home, which is necessary as much for the staff as for the patients themselves". At that time there were unfortunately very few Homes available for patients with advanced cancer and many of them were known as "Homes for the Dying".

During the year 1950 visits were made to various parts of the UK to find properties which could be used, and converted if necessary, for patients

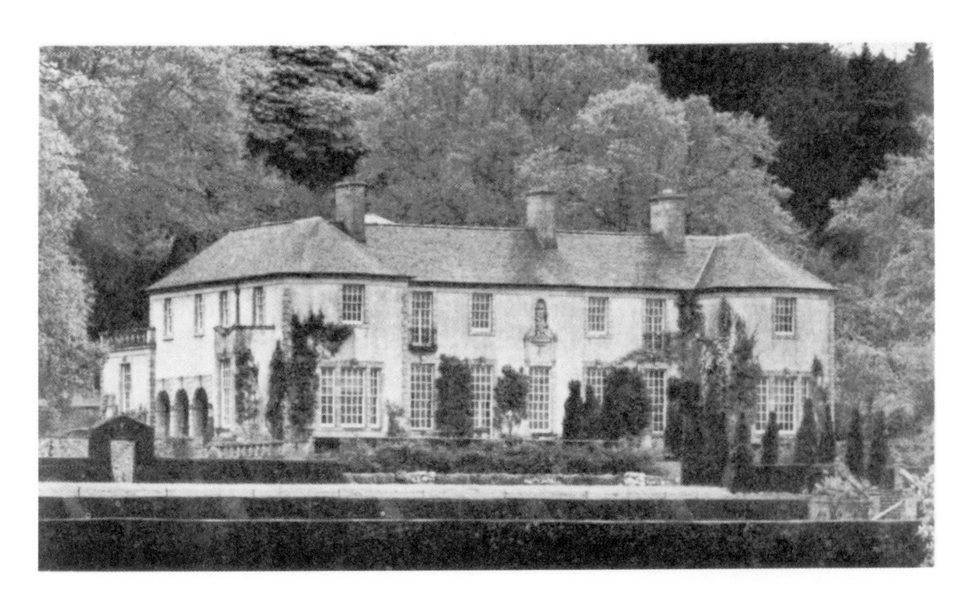

Figure 4.6 Hill of Tarvit Nursing Home at Cupar, Fife, which was opened in December 1952.

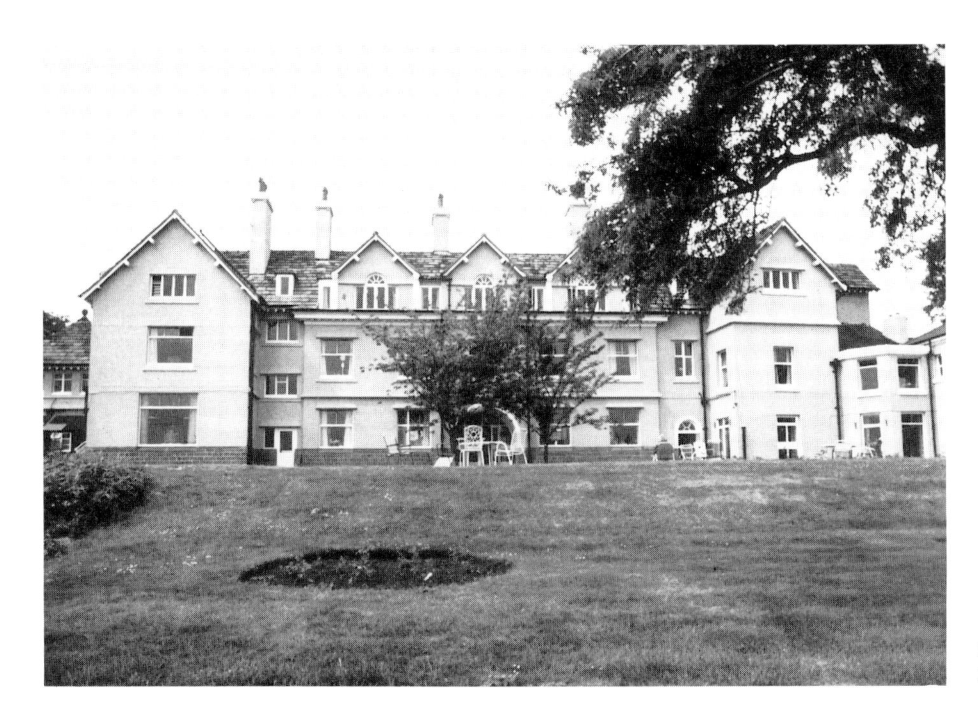

Figure 4.7 Sunnybank Nursing Home, Liverpool.

with cancer. An approach to the National Trust resulted in securing the property known as Sprydencote, situated at Broadclyst, Devon, at a nominal annual rental. This was followed by the offer from the National Trust for Scotland of the property known as Hill of Tarvit, situated at Cupar, Fife, at a peppercorn rent of one shilling per annum. In January 1953 arrangements were made to purchase Tidcombe Hall, Tiverton, Devon, which was already equipped as a Nursing Home, and Sprydencote was closed. In March 1953 the lease was secured of another Nursing Home, called Edenhall, situated at Lyndhurst Gardens, Hampstead, London, for the care of cancer patients in the London area.

The value of the work carried out in these Nursing Homes was apparent and it was recognised that there was a need for similar services in other parts of the country. Consequently, properties were acquired and converted into Nursing Homes in Newcastle upon Tyne (Conrad House), Solihull (Warren Pearl House), Liverpool (Sunnybank), Caterham, Surrey (Harestone), Glasgow (Strathclyde House), Penarth, Wales (Holme Tower) and Ilkley, Yorkshire (Ardenlea).

The developments which were occurring in cancer care and the need for modern accommodation with all the appropriate facilities and equipment made it necessary to acquire new and purpose-built Nursing Homes. Consequently, well-planned buildings were established in Edinburgh (Fairmile) — Hill of Tarvit was closed; Glasgow (Hunter's Hill) — Strathclyde House was closed; Belfast (Beaconfield); and Penarth (Holme Tower) — the original Home was closed. In Hampstead, London, Edenhall was demolished and a new Home with the same name was built in its place.

At all these Nursing Homes the patients are under the care of visiting doctors; there is a full establishment of a Matron and nursing staff and a domestic staff. Each Nursing Home has a House Committee whose members give valuable voluntary help in its administration, visiting patients and providing certain amenities and in many other useful ways.

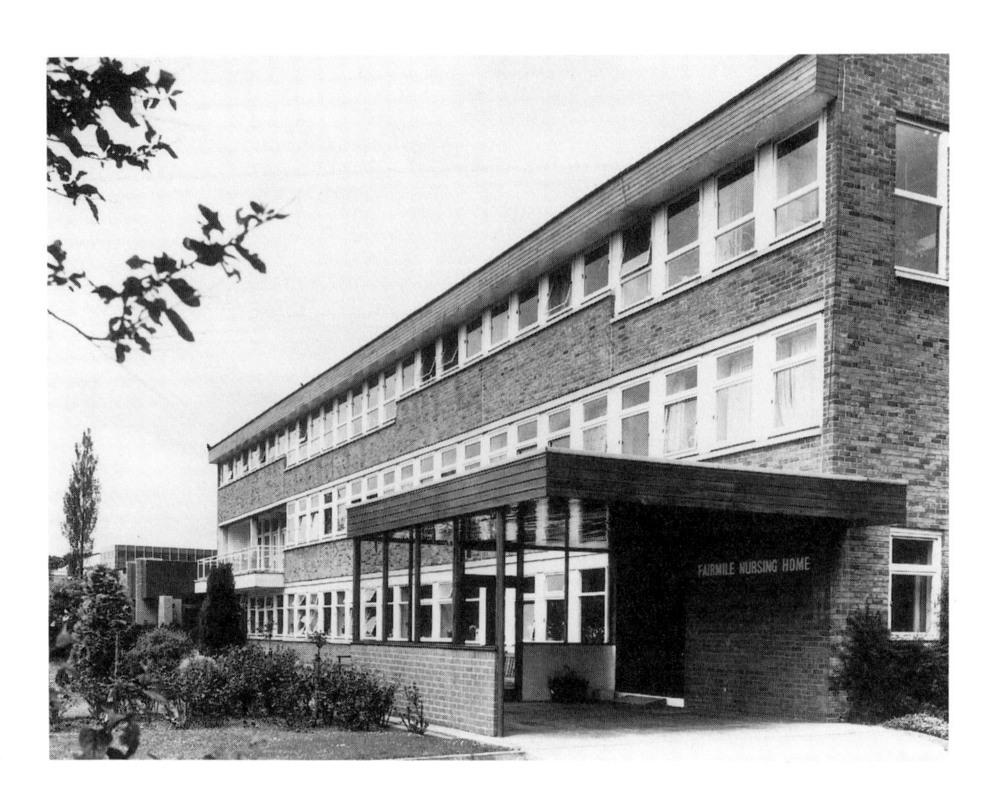

Figure 4.8 Fairmile, the purpose-built Nursing Home in Edinburgh.

The Foundation's Domiciliary Day and Night Nursing Service

In the report of the Joint National Survey Committee in 1952 detailed consideration was given to the special and numerous needs of patients with cancer who were being cared for in their own homes. The outstanding need was for home nurses to look after such patients throughout the day and especially during the night. The responsibility was too much for the families of the patients to undertake, however willing they were to endeavour to meet the requirements. Furthermore, it was found that families and patients frequently required nursing care urgently at short notice. The Foundation solved this important problem of suffering and anxiety by organising its Domiciliary Day and Night Nursing Service on a national scale. During subsequent decades the scope of the work has increased enormously and the Service has succoured and supported many thousands of cancer patients and their families.

There is now an ever-increasing need for the care of cancer patients in the community. For example, during the past 5 years the expenditure of the Foundation on the Day and Night Nursing Service has increased by no less than 492%. The Service is generally jointly funded with the National Health Service and it provides the help of about 4000 part-time local nurses who give treatment, care and support to seriously ill cancer patients and their families in the patients' own homes. It is quite unique to the Foundation and provides nursing care which is not normally available through the National Health Service. There is still a need to expand it, however, for the need is great.

For efficient administration the country has been divided into definite areas and regional nurse coordinators have been appointed — experienced nurses with administrative skills, who are also developing in-service training and education in cancer nursing for the community nurses.

Recently the Foundation has initiated complementary schemes linking community services to the Marie Curie Homes and to home-care teams and hospices. These partnerships have proved their worth in terms of giving a community dimension to the Homes and hospices, better in-service training facilities, improved support for nurses and good patient care integrated at primary health care level.

A home-care team has been established at the Marie Curie Home "Sunnybank", where the service is fulfilling a real need in the city of Liverpool. A similar team will be established at the new "Holme Tower" at Penarth in Wales, and a team of nurses is being trained who will provide the service in Newcastle upon Tyne and its environs.

Welfare work

There are many patients with cancer uncontrolled by definitive treatment who wish to remain at home with their families in their own familiar environment and whose relatives are willing and anxious to take care of them in this stage of their illness. Nevertheless, the members of the family usually require considerable practical support and assistance. The chief requirements which were elicited by the Survey are day and night nurses, nursing equipment, extra comforts, laundry help and recreational facilities.

During the initial years of its work the Foundation received many requests for advice and information of various kinds which were promptly answered, but there were many patients who required more than this. As a first step towards satisfying some of their needs, funds were allocated to the Central Council for District Nursing in London for distribution amongst the District Nursing Associations, and also to the Committee for Scotland. It was stated that the money should be used to pay for night nurses and provide other needs, and a report on how the money was spent should be made to the Executive Committee so that future allocations of funds for specific purposes could be considered. The pilot scheme was very successful in demonstrating the different ways in which patients and relatives can be helped to overcome the difficulties and anxieties caused by a long and distressing illness.

Educating the public about cancer

Educating the public to recognise the early warning symptoms and signs of cancer was an aspect of the Foundation's work which was discussed at the first meeting of the Council in March 1950. At that time it was not advocated, professionally and officially, that the public be educated about aspects of cancer; in fact there was opposition to it being done, largely because those who opposed it thought it might cause cancerphobia. How things have changed today, for this work is now encouraged and supported internationally and being done throughout the world.

The Foundation has regarded education of the public about cancer as an important part of its welfare programme, as knowledge alleviates fear, and education about cancer not only embraces the facts concerning cancer itself but is also concerned with the way it is treated and with giving people information about all the available facilities to mitigate their anxiety and distress.

The first step forward by the Foundation in active cancer education for the public was taken in November 1951, when the Chelsea Cancer Education Committee (whose Honorary Secretary was Joan Gough-Thomas), which had already received a grant from the Foundation for its pioneer work, became one of the Foundation's affiliated Committees. It was felt that this would benefit both organisations.

Special reference is made here to the Chelsea Cancer Education Committee, which carried out much of the early work in this subject in the UK. It started its work in April 1949 at the instigation of the present author and with the enthusiastic support of Alderman G. L. Tunbridge, who was the Mayor of Chelsea, and Joan Gough-Thomas. Public meetings were organised and were attended by large audiences. Many people were obviously keenly interested and desirous of learning more about cancer. Educational leaflets were carefully written and distributed to give useful information to the public.

In December 1951 the Foundation's Executive Committee appointed an Education Sub-Committee to consider the preparation, publication and distribution to the public of educational material about cancer; Joan Gough-Thomas became its Chairman and the present author its Vice-Chairman. Suitable leaflets were then designed to give the lay person as much information as possible about cancer in a simple form. This included the way in which a cancer starts, the early warning symptoms, its methods of treatment, and how people can protect themselves against it.

It is interesting to notice here the beginning of the concept of cancer prevention and its practical application to the habits, customs and general life-style of people.

This most important subject attracted very little attention at that time, in the early 1950s, but 35 years later cancer prevention has assumed a major role in cancer control. In fact, it is now agreed that it provides the brightest hope for the world where cancer is concerned, and it is believed that more than 75% of cancers could be prevented if people took the right actions according to our present knowledge.

The method by which the leaflets were to be distributed was carefully studied by the Committee, who thought it was unwise at that time to distribute them indiscriminately. They therefore decided to write in the first instance to all Medical Officers of Health, enclosing a specimen of Leaflet Number 1 entitled "What is cancer?" and asking if a supply of the leaflets could be sent to Public Health Departments for distribution to the public as they became available. The response was encouraging, so the leaflets were distributed by this method; requests were also made for posters.

Many requests were received for lectures to be given about various subjects connected with cancer, including early diagnosis, treatment and research, and also about the work of the Foundation. Lectures were delivered in many different parts of the UK to audiences representing the medical and nursing professions and the lay public.

Special mention is made of the lecture delivered at the request of the Central Council for Health Education on the occasion of the meeting of representatives of the World Health Organisation at their London conference in April 1953. The members were impressed with the work carried out by the Foundation in the field of cancer education and asked to be kept informed of future developments.

The account which is given here of the inauguration and development of cancer education for the public in the UK is of historic interest and importance, so many details have been included. The results that were obtained over succeeding decades show what can be achieved, in spite of opposition, when such an object is pursued with careful planning and enthusiasm.

Great credit is due to the Chelsea Cancer Education Committee and the Foundation; much encouragement for the pioneer work was given by the interest which was taken by the Ministry of Health and by the Central Council for Health Education.

Growth of the Foundation's work

Reference to the Marie Curie Memorial Foundation's Annual Report 1984–1985, which is headed "The nation's most comprehensive cancer charity", shows the impressive growth which has taken place since the Foundation was formed in 1948. Demand for the in-patient facilities in the 11 Nursing Homes situated in England, Scotland, Wales and Northern Ireland continues to increase. The Foundation's guiding philosophy is the rehabilitation and continuing care of cancer patients through the provision of special units for that purpose. The nationwide Domiciliary Nursing Service, generally jointly funded with the National Health Service, provides the help of about 4000 part-time nurses, for the treatment, nursing care and support of patients with cancer and their families in their own homes. The nurses stay with the patients during the whole day and night, as necessary. The Domiciliary Day and Night Cancer Nursing Service is unique in the world.

The Research Institute

The Research Institute was commissioned in 1961 and for many years carried out laboratory cancer research which was concentrated mainly on carcinoma of the human breast and prostate, which are hormone-related neoplasms and common varieties of human cancer. It was hoped that valuable contributions would be made to their control. The programme of work continued under the direction of D. C. Williams. On his death, new research projects were introduced by the new Director, G. Currie. One of the main functions of the Research Institute is to bridge the gap between clinicians and scientists.

The Education and Training Department of the Foundation was established to improve the care and treatment of patients with cancer through the continuing education of doctors, nurses and the other members of the caring professions. Emphasis is placed on interdisciplinary education, for it is recognised that the care of patients with cancer is carried out by team-work. The teaching consists of short courses for doctors and nurses, seminars, workshops, conferences and symposia. The need to increase the cancer constituent of the medical curriculum for medical students is well recognised. This work is being usefully expanded. The annual

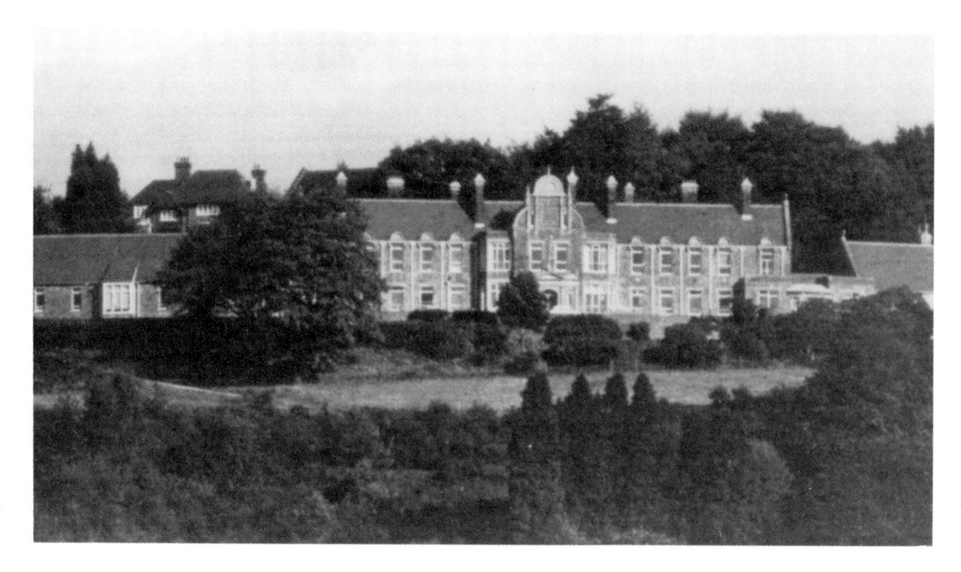

Figure 4.9 The Marie Curie Memorial Foundation's Cancer Research Institute at Limpsfield, Surrey. It includes well-equipped laboratories and some residential accommodation for research scientists.

symposium on cancer, held for 19 years at the Royal College of Surgeons of England, attracted many nurses, doctors and members of the paramedical professions.

Rehabilitation and continuing care in cancer

The Marie Curie Memorial Foundation clearly recognises the importance of this concept, which has been developed and described by its Chairman *(Raven, 1986)*, and is establishing special R.C.C. Units with the necessary professional knowledge, skills and facilities in the major Homes in different regions of the UK. This subject is integrated with the educational and training programme of the Foundation. There is considerable interest in the concept, both nationally and internationally, and in its practical application to meet the needs of patients with cancer. Work in this area is bound to grow in the years to come.

Closely connected with the R.C.C. Units is the need for whole-time clinical oncologists to take care of all the patients attending the units, with their different requirements and problems. Some of these patients are residents in the Homes but many are visitors to the Day Centres.

THE NATIONAL SOCIETY FOR CANCER RELIEF

The National Society for Cancer Relief (Cancer Relief Macmillan fund) was founded by Douglas Macmillan in 1911, following the death of his father from cancer. At first it was known as the Society for the Prevention and Relief of Cancer but this name was changed to the National Society for Cancer Relief in 1924 when it was registered as a Benevolent Society. Although the registered title still remains, the Society is known today as the Cancer Relief Macmillan fund, because it is through the Society's Macmillan fund, which is named after the founder, that services are funded.

The Society's activities were initially entirely voluntary and were concerned with promoting a better understanding of cancer by gathering and disseminating information about its prevention and relief.

Work was seriously interrupted by World War I, but after the war the Society continued its cancer education campaign, using booklets, letters to the press, lectures and the quarterly *Journal of Cancer*.

As the work developed emphasis was placed increasingly on cancer relief, beginning with the provision of grants to cancer patients who were in financial need. The first full-time paid member of the staff was appointed in 1930 and the activities of the Society then increased rapidly, so that by 1939 grants to patients had risen to £9000, and by 1950 to more than £23 000.

During the 1950s the foundations of today's national charity were laid. Countess Mountbatten of Burma became President, and by 1959 grants to patients had risen to £101 514.

Early in the Society's history Douglas Macmillan had envisaged other forms of cancer relief and in the 1930s he had expressed his objectives for the Society in the following words: "I want even the poorest people to be provided with the latest and best advice both for avoiding cancer and for recognising and dealing with it when it exists. I want to see 'homes' for cancer patients throughout the land, where attention will be provided freely or at low cost, as circumstances dictate. I want also to see panels of voluntary nurses, who can be detailed off to attend to necessitous patients in their own homes." The Macmillan home-care nursing teams and in-patient facilities which Cancer Relief subsequently set up are now two of the most important aspects of its work.

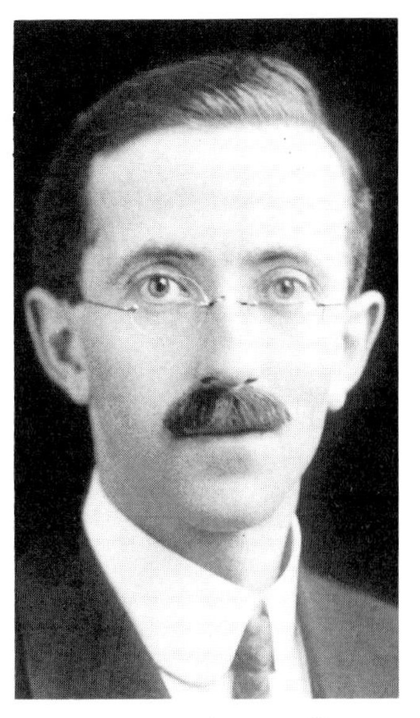

Figure 4.10 Douglas Macmillan, M.B.E.

In 1964 Douglas Macmillan resigned as Chairman of the Society. His place was taken by Her Grace the Duchess of Roxburgh. In 1966 Her Royal Highness the Duchess of Kent became the Society's Patron, and Michael Sobell became its President.

Cancer Relief began to give financial support to in-patient care in 1969. Grants were given towards the building of St Ann's Hospice, Cheadle; the Douglas Macmillan Home, Stoke-on-Trent; and St Luke's Nursing Home in Sheffield. Another development occurred when the Colostomy Welfare Group became the first associated charity of Cancer Relief.

In 1973 Major Henry Garnett became Deputy Chairman and Chief Executive of the Society. In 1975 the Society extended the in-patient aspect of its work by building the first Macmillan in-patient unit, which is run by the National Health Service, at Christchurch Hospital, Christchurch, Dorset. This marked the beginning of its programme of building to provide in-patient facilities for cancer patients. Since that time it has built 12 continuing care homes in England, Scotland and Wales and during 1976 and 1977 it built and equipped eight Macmillan "mini-units", two-bedded wards with a visitors' room, attached to community hospitals in Wales.

1975 was also the year in which Cancer Relief set up its first team of Macmillan nurses trained to care for cancer patients in their own homes. Both in its in-patient units and through its domiciliary nursing services Cancer Relief has sought to make more widely available to cancer patients skills for the control of pain and their overall care. The first grants for Macmillan home-care nursing services were made to St Joseph's Hospice in Hackney, London; St Columba's Hospice in Edinburgh; and the Dorothy House Foundation in Bath.

In 1980 the development of the highly successful Macmillan nursing teams was accelerated by the investment of £2½ million in 3-year grants, to establish them nationwide. The immediate emphasis was on placing services in areas where few facilities already existed. There are now more than 330 Macmillan nurses, working in more than 120 teams throughout the country.

In order to extend the skills of cancer care even further, in 1980 Cancer Relief became involved in medical and nursing education, at first mainly within its own Macmillan services. It is now directing substantial funds towards the establishment of a series of Macmillan lectureships in university medical schools and departments of nursing throughout the country, with the objective of extending knowledge of the skills of cancer care to the widest possible medical audience.

In 1981 the Mastectomy Association became the third associated Charity of Cancer Relief, and in 1984 the Countess of Westmorland succeeded Sir Michael Sobell as President of the Society. The Macmillan Education Unit was established as part of the Society's education programme at that time and its charitable income had reached £5 million. Financial help for patients, which is given through the Patient Grants Department, continues to be a vital aspect of its work. In 1985 the sum of £1.8 million was paid out to patients in order to alleviate many kinds of practical hardships. Also in 1985 Major Henry Garnett became Chairman of the Society in succession to Sir Charles Davis.

The author is most grateful to Miss Sue Childs for providing this account of the history of the Cancer Relief Macmillan fund.

THE IMPERIAL CANCER RESEARCH FUND

The foundation of the Imperial Cancer Research Fund on 4 July 1902 was an event of outstanding importance in the history of oncology, for this world-famous cancer research institute was the first to be formed in the UK whose work was primarily concerned with the basic problems in the aetiology of cancer. An account of the origin and early history of the Fund was given by Cuthbert Dukes in a lecture to the staff of the Fund on 27 November 1964 *(Dukes, 1965)*. Dukes was a friend of the present author, who is indebted to the published version of this lecture for much of the information in this section.

At the time of the Fund's foundation in 1902 it was known as the Cancer Research Fund. The title "Imperial" was added at the second general committee meeting on 8 July 1904, when the chair was taken by H.R.H. the Prince of Wales (later King George V), who was the first President. At the close of this meeting His Royal Highness stated that with the consent of His Majesty King Edward VII the Cancer Research Fund would in future be called the Imperial Cancer Research Fund.

The original concept and organisation

Dukes states that the idea to found a cancer research fund seems to have originated in a conversation between Henry Morris, who was a member of the Council of the Royal College of Surgeons of England, and a prospective donor of money to the Fund. A preliminary meeting was arranged by Henry Morris early in 1901 to discuss the proposal. It was decided that the object should be "the investigation of the cause, nature and treatment of cancer" and that the Royal College of Physicians and the Royal College of Surgeons should be requested to take control of the investigations. The Royal Colleges agreed, provided that the necessary money was supplied without any appeal being made by them. Official approval of the Royal Colleges was given on 4 July 1902 and it was soon apparent that sufficient financial support would be made available from charitable sources.

Attention was given to the early organisation necessary for the development of the Fund and an Executive Committee was formed, of which Sir William Church was elected Chairman, Henry Morris Treasurer and Frederick Hallett Secretary. It is of interest to note that Sir William Church, who at that time was President of the Royal College of Physicians, continued as Chairman for 22 years, and, as Dukes stated, seldom missed a meeting throughout the whole of that period. Henry Morris (later Sir Henry Morris) was elected President of the Royal College of Surgeons in 1906. He was the surgeon who was in charge of the Cancer Department of the Middlesex Hospital in London for more than 20 years and therefore greatly involved in cancer work. Frederick Hallett (later Sir Frederick Hallett), retained his post as Secretary for the long period of 31 years and on his resignation in 1933, due to ill health, the Executive Committee expressed "their deep appreciation of the way he had guided the Fund and of his far-sighted ability in drafting its constitution" *(Dukes, 1965)*.

Laboratory accommodation

The provision of laboratories for the research work of the Fund was an important initial problem needing to be solved. It presented no difficulties, however, as rooms were provided behind the Conjoint Examination Hall on Victoria Embankment (Sir Frederick Hallett had been Secretary to the Conjoint Examination Board since 1887).

The appointment of Superintendent of Research was advertised and E. F. Bashford was chosen out of 12 candidates. The selection committee were impressed by his scheme of research work to be undertaken if he were successful, entitled "A draft of scheme for enquiring into the nature, cause, prevention and treatment of cancer". As Dukes points out, it was a comprehensive survey of the cancer problem as seen at the turn of the 20th century, and served as the plan for most of the research work done by Bashford and his colleagues during the first 6 years of the Fund's existence.

Bashford is remembered as the originator of the Bashford needle and for his publications on the zoological distribution of cancer, the transplantability of animal tumours and induced resistance to them. He also prepared the first series of Scientific Reports of the Fund, which were the most important contribution to the literature of cancer research in this country during the first decade of the 20th century. He resigned from his post after 12 years because of ill health and died at the early age of 49 years, from heart failure.

Soon after his appointment Bashford was joined by several distinguished research assistants. Special mention is made of J. A. Murray (1873–1950), who had already published several papers on histopathology. An important contribution was made to cancer research by his discovery that in female

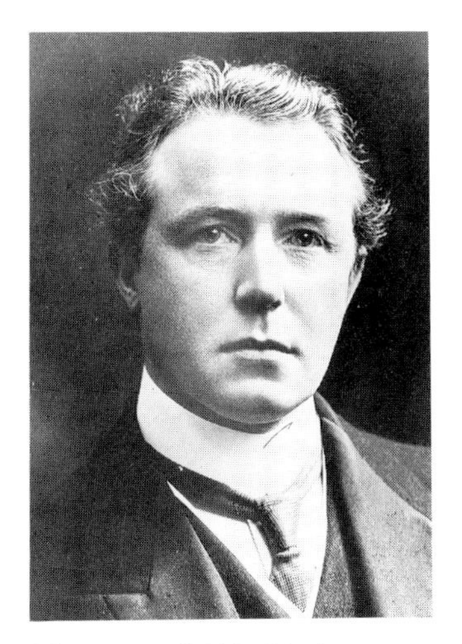

Figure 4.11 E. F. Bashford.

mice with an immediate cancer ancestry breast carcinoma is more than twice as frequent as in mice without this ancestry. This led to more research on mouse genetics, which continued in future years.

Developments continued

In 1908 the Royal Colleges were making new arrangements for holding their examinations. They sold the examination hall on the Embankment and began negotiations to build a new one in Queen Square, Bloomsbury. This was completed in 1912. Accommodation for research laboratories for the Fund was provided on the 4th and 5th floors of the new building and the Fund carried out most valuable work there during the long period from 1912 to 1938.

The Director for most of this time was J. A. Murray, with W. Cramer, an esteemed research scientist who retired from the Fund in 1939. Murray was succeeded by W. E. Gye in 1935. It is not the author's purpose here to even summarise an account of all the valuable cancer research carried out by the Fund during those and subsequent years by its very distinguished scientific staff, which has greatly increased our knowledge of many aspects of cancer.

Laboratories situated at Mill Hill

New buildings for the laboratories were completed at Burtonhole, Hole Lane, Mill Hill, London. These comprised the main laboratory block,

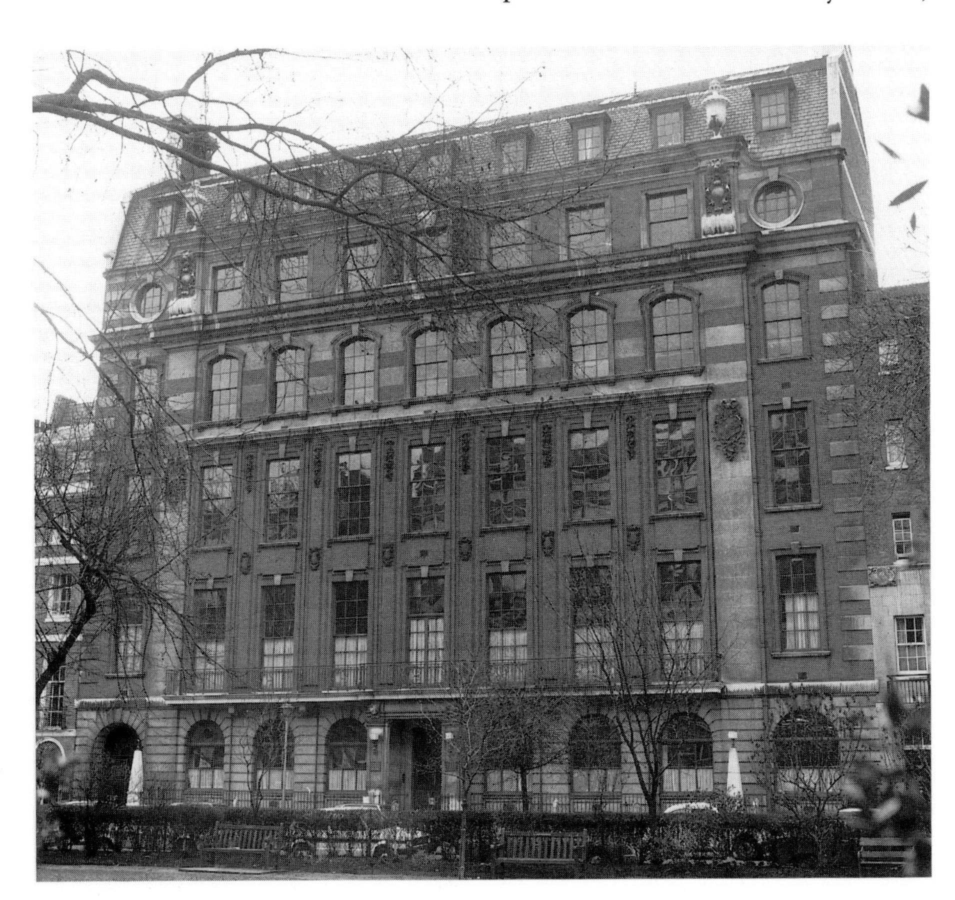

Figure 4.12 The Examination Hall of thè Royal College of Surgeons of England in Queen Square, Bloomsbury, London, the 4th and 5th floors of which accommodated the Research Laboratories of the I.C.R.F. from 1912 to 1938.

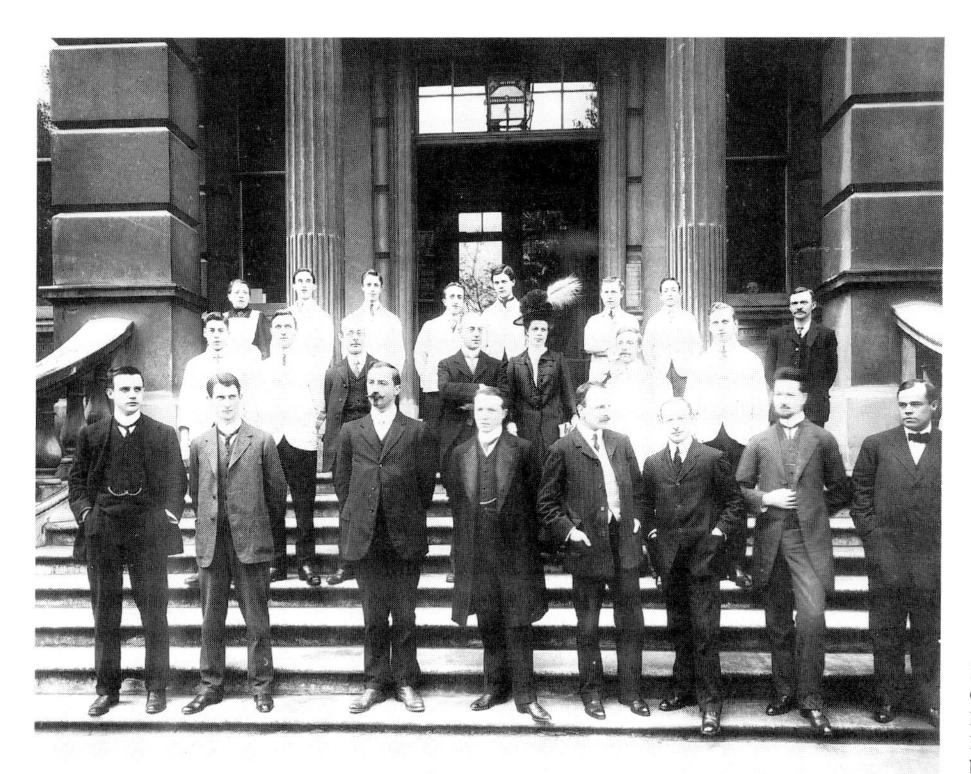

Figure 4.13 The staff of the Imperial Cancer Research Fund in 1909. On the left of the Superintendent, E. F. Bashford, is J. A. Murray, who later became Director.

animal houses, stables and two cottages for staff members. Removal of the laboratories from Queen Square was carried out in July 1938 and arrangements were made to set up a central office at the Royal College of Surgeons in Lincoln's Inn Fields (see *Thirty-Sixth Annual Report for the Year 1937–1938)*. The new laboratories were formally declared open on 27 June 1939 (see *Thirty-Seventh Annual Report for the Year 1939–1940)*.

It is interesting to read in the latter publication the report of the Director, Dr Gye, on the scope of the cancer research carried out by the Fund. The research subjects included carcinogenesis, hormones in relation to breast cancer, comparative reactions of normal and malignant cells in tissue cultures to some chemotherapeutic compounds, and tumours caused by filtrable viruses.

The Mill Hill laboratories, where so much of the early research work of the Fund was carried out, were closed in December 1985 on the expiry of the lease of 50 years. The research work was taken over and expanded in a new Developmental Unit in Oxford and at the Clare Hall Laboratories at South Mimms.

The new laboratories at Lincoln's Inn Fields, London

The Fund's new laboratories, which had been planned for a number of years, occupy a site adjacent to the Royal College of Surgeons of England. The development was outlined in 1954 and illustrations of the splendid new building are shown in the *Sixtieth Annual Report and Accounts 1961–1962*, which also contains a detailed description of them. There are excellent laboratories and ancillary rooms, accommodation for the administrative staff and for meetings, and a library. The building makes impressive and fitting headquarters for the Fund, the staff having moved there in August

1962. The final phase of the development was marked by the visit of Her Majesty the Queen and His Royal Highness the Duke of Edinburgh on 11 June 1963.

The large growth of the Imperial Cancer Research Fund and the great scope of its cancer research programme are clearly portrayed in the report of the Director of Research, Sir Walter Bodmer, who was appointed on 1 July 1979 in succession to Sir Michael Stoker, who was Director from 1968 to 1979.

Plans are being considered for further expansion of the research programme at Lincoln's Inn Fields, at the Clare Hall Laboratories and at other important units. With the outstanding staff new approaches are developing for the solution of cancer problems in the visionary interrelated research programme.

CANCER RESEARCH CAMPAIGN

The establishment of The British Cancer Campaign in 1923 was an event of outstanding importance and great value in the cancer world. The Certificate of Incorporation was issued on 23 May 1923 with the name The British Empire Cancer Campaign; subsequently "Empire" was omitted from the title. It is very interesting to read about the people who were concerned with its formation and the events which led to its development.

During the early years of the 20th century increasing attention was focused on cancer research projects. In 1902 the Imperial Cancer Research Fund (see earlier in this chapter) was established under the joint auspices of the Royal College of Physicians and the Royal College of Surgeons of England. In 1913 the government set up the Medical Research Committee, which later became the Medical Research Council, to sponsor serious medical research. Research in cancer was actively developing in a number of hospitals and universities in the UK and was supported financially from a number of sources, including the Medical Research Council, funds from universities and hospitals and funds from private donors. All the creative effort required coordination so that the results of research could be properly assessed, information exchanged and advice given. Furthermore, no central organisation was in existence to which research scientists could apply for funds for their research projects.

Several people clearly appreciated the need to establish such a central organisation — The British Cancer Campaign — whose work would consist mainly in giving grants for cancer work in laboratories and institutions other than its own. This facet distinguishes the work of the Campaign from that of the Imperial Cancer Research Fund, which in the main carries out cancer research in its own laboratories.

Founders of the Campaign

Special mention is made here of the people who were responsible for setting up the Campaign and for the early development of its work. Much of the credit is due to J. P. Lockhart-Mummery, who was then Senior Surgeon at St Mark's Hospital in the City of London and who was offered a personal gift of £20 000 in gratitude for his skilful care by a patient, Sir Richard Garton, whom he had convinced of the need for a new cancer organisation.

He declined the gift and Sir Richard then gave £20 000 anonymously to establish the Campaign and became its first Treasurer; however, many years elapsed before the donor's name became known.

Amongst other associates of Lockhart-Mummery was a member of Parliament, Godfrey Locker-Lampson, and the early meetings were held in the House of Commons. An important meeting was convened there on the night of the budget debate in 1923 and amongst those present were Lord Dawson of Penn (the King's Physician), Sir Thomas Horder (later Lord Horder), Sir Bernard Spilsbury and Sir Edward Marshall-Hall. Captain E. J. C. Chapman was appointed Secretary and he carried out the early correspondence from his offices situated off Southampton Row in London.

Launching the Campaign

The Campaign owes a great debt of gratitude to the British Red Cross Society for the help given in its launching. The Red Cross provided the office accommodation in their premises at 19 Berkeley Street, London, and also helped in the appeal for funds so that it could be carried out more cheaply and quickly.

At the first full meeting of the Executive Council, held at 19 Berkeley Street, Captain Chapman was appointed General Secretary and he held this post with great distinction for 23 years.

An original structure of 16 committees was envisaged, but the number was reduced to six during the first year, with meetings in most cases at monthly intervals and never less than quarterly.

From its early days the Campaign has had important associations with the Royal Society and the Medical Research Council; each nominated a member of Council and they jointly nominated five members to what is now the Scientific Committee. This arrangement remains unchanged and has proved to be of continuing benefit.

Early grant awards

The earliest grant awards were made during the first year of the Campaign's existence, to the Middlesex Hospital and the Cancer Hospital (now the Royal Marsden Hospital), each of which received £2500. A third award of £330 was made to Dr Louis Sambon to investigate the possible link between vermin and the spread of cancer.

The major part of the money raised in the first year — nearly £60 000 — was carried forward to the next year, thus commencing the tradition of awarding grants in any one year from the funds raised in the previous year. This system was modified for the first time in the accounts for the year 1982.

Recipients of early grants

Malcolm Donaldson, gynaecologist at the Royal Hospital of St Bartholomew in London, was closely associated with the Campaign for 48 years and carried out splendid work in cancer. He was a pioneer in cancer education for the community and founded the Cancer Information Association in

Oxford. He received a grant from the Campaign in 1924 for his valuable work and for the last few years of its existence his Association was funded largely by the Campaign. He resigned from the Grand Council of the Campaign in 1972, owing to ill health.

An early grant (1924) was made to Dr E. C. Dodds (later Sir Charles Dodds), who was appointed to the Chair of Biochemistry at the Middlesex Hospital in 1925 at the early age of 25 and was the first Director of the Courtauld Institute on its opening in 1928. He was associated with the Campaign until his death in 1973, being a member of its Scientific Committee for 21 years and then its Chairman for the next 15. His outstanding work, which included the introduction of stilboestrol, the first synthetic oestrogen, earned him international acclaim and he was given a unique series of honours and distinctions.

Developments

In 1930 the Campaign moved its headquarters to 12 Grosvenor Crescent, London, still as a tenant of the British Red Cross Society, then again to No. 11 next door. It stayed there until 1970, when it moved to the present premises in Carlton House Terrace. The great generosity of Sir Michael Sobell enabled it and the Royal College of Pathologists to obtain a 99-year lease of these premises, which they share on most reasonable terms.

Fund-raising

A fund-raising organisation was carefully developed with the establishment of county organisations and a network of local committees. Many of the early area Councils were autonomous and those in Yorkshire and in the North of England continue their work in this way, supporting research in their respective areas.

The public image of the Campaign was greatly enhanced in 1924 when H.R.H. the Duke of York accepted the invitation to become its President and 3 years later His Majesty King George V graciously consented to become Patron. When the Duke of York became King George VI in 1937 the Duke of Gloucester became President and held this office until 1973, when he was succeeded by Prince Richard of Gloucester.

The Campaign continued to grow in the late 1930s but on the outbreak of the Second World War in 1939 a deliberate decision was made to cease fund-raising so that all resources could be devoted to the war effort.

Further development

In the period of post-war reconstruction changes were made in the Campaign. In 1946 Lockhart-Mummery resigned from his post as Honorary Secretary, having edited the *Annual Report* for 23 years, and in 1947 he relinquished the chairmanship of the Executive Committee.

The original General Secretary, Captain Chapman, handed over his post to Captain F. B. Tours, O.B.E., R.N., after 23 years' service. In 1948 the National Health Service was created and it is interesting to note that the Campaign's income was growing, and thereby its research activities. 1955 saw the establishment of the Research Unit in Radiobiology at Mount

Vernon Hospital, and its new building was opened in 1957 by the Duke of Devonshire, who had succeeded Lord Horder as Chairman of the Campaign in 1956.

Income continued to grow, so that by the time the Duke of Devonshire retired in 1981 it had increased 25-fold since he had commenced his chairmanship 25 years earlier. The Duke had made a remarkable contribution to the entire work of the Campaign in many other ways and he was liked and respected by everyone concerned with it. His sister, Lady Elizabeth Cavendish, kindly agreed to succeed him as Chairman.

In 1970 several changes occurred, in addition to the move to 2 Carlton House Terrace, London. The Committee structure was revised and a new integrated one was adopted. Also, Brigadier K. D. Gribbon succeeded Captain Tours, who retired after 24 years' service as General Secretary.

Apart from making grant awards for research projects, the Campaign undertook other activities. A significant development was the establishment of a professorial Department of Cancer Medicine at the Institute of Cancer Research and the decision was made to follow this by setting up five Chairs. The first incumbent at the Institute was Professor P. K. Bondy from the University of Yale, who held the post until 1977, when he returned to the USA. The post was then vacant until 1982, when Professor T. J. McElwain was appointed.

A second Chair was established at the University of Manchester, to which Professor D. Crowther was appointed in 1972. There followed a Chair at Cambridge University in 1973 — Professor N. M. Bleehen; Glasgow University in 1974 — Professor K. C. Calman; and Southampton University in 1976 — Professor J. M. A. Whitehouse.

Another important development was the establishment of a Chair in Cancer Epidemiology at the Institute of Cancer Research in 1975. This was held by Professor M. R. Alderson until 1981, when he left for another appointment and Professor Julian Peto was appointed to succeed him. In 1982 a Chair of Radiation Oncology was set up at Liverpool University and based at Clatterbridge Hospital, Professor H. M. Warenius being appointed to it. These Chairs have linked laboratory research with the treatment of cancer patients and have had outstanding success. In addition, they have given training to young doctors specialising in medical oncology and have fostered the recognition of medical oncology as a medical speciality.

The policy of the Campaign has always been to invest in people rather than in buildings or equipment, but there have been notable exceptions when important assistance has been given. This has included laboratory extensions and the provision of apparatus and equipment which have been needed urgently.

The title of the Campaign was changed in 1981 to Cancer Research Campaign. There is a continuing, notable expansion of the scope and scale of its work, which is made possible by the corresponding growth in its income. The work which has been accomplished by all the staff and numerous supporters throughout many decades has been truly remarkable, for it has enabled a large number of researchers and clinicians to carry out valuable work in all aspects of the cancer problem.

The Cancer Research Campaign's *Annual Report 1986. Handbook 1987* gives a most impressive account of the wide spectrum of its present activities and clearly illustrates the enormous progress of its work in the UK.

The Campaign's programme in cancer research is being coordinated to exploit the opportunities to develop it for the direct benefit of patients suffering from cancer. An important part of the clinical research programme is the investigation of the psychological and social problems experienced by patients with cancer and finding methods of relief. The Campaign is also funding cancer education for the public, professionals, patients and their relatives, provides financial support for an impressive list of institutes, laboratories, and departments whose staffs are engaged in cancer work in the UK and allocates many individual fellowships and awards.

The author thanks Dr Joan Austaker of the Wellcome Unit for the *History of Medicine*, University of Oxford for the article entitled "The Campaign 1923–1983" in *Cancer Research Campaign Annual Report 1982.*

THE INTERNATIONAL UNION AGAINST CANCER (UICC)

The International Union Against Cancer is a world-wide federation of non-governmental agencies and organisations which are concerned with all aspects of cancer. It was inaugurated in October 1933 at a Cancer Congress held in Madrid, when prior to the closing ceremony Dr Jacques Bandeline of France spoke as follows: "I wish to move a motion calling for the creation of an international organisation to promote the fight against cancer through research, therapy and the development of social activities." This proposition was agreed unanimously with enthusiasm. For several years the need had been felt for an international organisation to deal with some of the international problems caused by cancer and to try to control the malignant diseases and coordinate research programmes.

The UICC is constituted of members who are voluntary anti-cancer organisations, such as leagues, societies and associations, foundations, comprehensive cancer institutions and cancer research and treatment centres, specialised hospitals, and, in certain countries, Ministries of Health. The Union derives its income from dues which are paid by leagues, societies, foundations, private donors and other institutions.

Following the passing of Dr Bandeline's motion in Madrid in 1933, preparatory meetings were held in Paris in 1934 and 1935 to determine the statutes of the future Union. The first meeting of the General Assembly was held on 4 May 1935 in Paris, with representatives from 43 countries and 67 national cancer organisations. A Latin name was given to the Union: "Unio Internationalis Contra Cancrum". Since that time the Union has been internationally known as the UICC. The General Assembly elected Justin Godart, a former French Minister of Public Health, as President and designated Dr Bandeline as its Secretary-General and Paris as the headquarters.

Programme of work

The programme of work for the UICC was considered at the first meeting and it was decided to establish an international quarterly publication called *Acta, Unio Internationalis Contra Cancrum* to be devoted to international cancer problems. It was the first publication of this kind. Other projects included work on an illustrated tumour nomenclature, the collection of reliable statistics using an international standardised procedure, and the organisation of the Second International Cancer Congress. This was held in Brussels in September 1936 and attended by representatives from 43 countries. The Third International Congress was held in Atlantic City in September 1939 but was somewhat disrupted by the world events which culminated in the outbreak of World War II.

After the end of the war, the activities of the UICC were reviewed by Justin Godart, and Professor J. H. Maisin of Belgium became the new Secretary-General. With the generous assistance of the American Association for Cancer Research, the Fourth International Congress took place in St Louis in September 1947. The present author recalls this stimulating and successful congress which was the first UICC congress he attended and at which he presented a contribution on malignant melanoma, a subject which at that time did not receive the great attention that is given it today, for its incidence is markedly increasing.

It is interesting to record the subsequent congresses which were organised by the UICC and to note the special cancer problems discussed. In 1950 the Fifth International Congress was held in Paris and new topics were discussed, which included the morphology and biochemistry of cancer cells and the important subject of carcinogenesis.

The Sixth International Congress took place in Sâo Paulo, Brazil, in July 1954. Public and professional cancer education now created growing interest and the prevention of cancer became a subject for study. The role of voluntary organisations in cancer control was recognised and this stimulated their growth and importance. It was decided that international congresses should be held every 4 years and this practice has continued to the present time.

The Seventh International Congress took place in London in July 1958 and important papers of great interest were presented. The subjects dealt with included research in virology, biochemistry, carcinogenesis, chemotherapy and observations made possible by electron microscopy.

The Eighth International Cancer Congress opened on 22 July 1962 in Moscow, with 5000 participants from 70 countries, and more than 1000 papers were presented. The Proceedings, which were published in Russian, English and French, summed up the state of knowledge at that time. Specialists all over the world were able to see clearly the advances taking place in the medical field and particularly in oncology in the USSR.

In the meantime new headquarters of the UICC, with a full-time staff, were established in Geneva. The decision was taken to set up an International Agency for Research on Cancer (IARC) in Lyons, France, to be administered by WHO, with Dr J. Higginson as its first Director. The publication *Acta*, the Union's official organ since 1935, was replaced by the *International Journal of Cancer*, with Dr E. A. Saxen of Helsinki, Finland, as its Editor-in-Chief, and this became one of the world's leading publications in this field.

The Ninth International Cancer Congress was held in October 1966 in Tokyo. Environmental factors as a cause of many varieties of cancer attracted considerable attention and for the first time the subject of the molecular basis of translation of the genetic message was examined.

The Tenth International Cancer Congress took place in Houston, USA, in May 1970. Here the multidisciplinary team approach in the treatment of cancer was strongly advocated. Such team-work has now been adopted almost universally and is essential with the important developments in cancer therapy.

The Eleventh International Cancer Congress was held in October 1974 in Florence, where considerable attention was focused on immunotherapy. The importance of cancer prevention was stressed, and also that of public and professional education. A significant result of this congress was a marked increase in international collaboration between the voluntary cancer organisations.

It is of historic interest to record the various themes and subjects of these congresses for they give an indication of the growth of oncology. The Twelfth International Cancer Congress took place in October 1978 in Buenos Aires and it is interesting to note that caution was expressed regarding the value of cancer immunotherapy, especially in the treatment of solid tumours. This waning of the initial enthusiasm was opportune, for even today immunotherapy has very limited clinical application; much more knowledge of the immunology of cancer is required. There were many discussions about the importance of cell membranes in cancer and the interaction between genetics and environmental factors.

The Thirteenth International Cancer Congress, at which the number of participants exceeded 9000, was held in September 1982 in Seattle, USA. Increased emphasis was given to the work of voluntary cancer organisations. Reviews were presented of advances made in the clarification of the mechanisms of chemical carcinogenesis and of the genetic and environmental factors which condition the development of cancer.

The Fourteenth International Cancer Congress was held in August 1986 in Budapest, Hungary, and was attended by a very large number of international delegates. A broad spectrum of important and growing subjects relating to cancer was considered and discussed in plenary lectures, sessional meetings and poster sessions. A special session was devoted to rehabilitation and continuing care in cancer. The new programme of Treatment and Rehabilitation and Continuing Care was set up at the congress in Seattle under the chairmanship of Dr I. Elsebai and the new project of Rehabilitation and Continuing Care under the chairmanship of the present author.

Programmes of the UICC

An important development in the work of the UICC was the establishment of individual programmes to increase our knowledge and expertise in certain defined subjects. These programmes are executed by individuals and committees composed of voluntary experts in different cancer fields. The subjects covered are: Detection and Diagnosis; Tumour Biology; Epidemiology and Prevention; Professional Education; Campaign, Organisation and Public Education; International Collaborative Activities; Fellowships and Personnel Exchange; Smoking and Cancer; Treatment and Rehabilitation, and the Multidisciplinary Project on Oral Cancer.

The classification and staging of cancer

The classification and staging of cancer in different organs and tissues are subjects of great clinical importance. The classification involves an assessment of the disease when the patient applies for treatment and the recording of the facts and physical signs by a system of symbols. When the disease has been thus recorded, the stage it has reached can be assessed and the prognosis determined. The classification can be correlated with a particular method of treatment. Patients with the same classification and treated by the same method can be compared as regards survival rates and the results of different treatments can be evaluated.

This subject is considered in this section about the UICC because in 1958 the Union published a book of great importance which describes a classification of breast cancer by clinical stages on the basis of the TNM system, which was developed by Professor Pierre Denoix of France. The adoption of this system internationally has enabled oncologists to group their patients according to their classification for specific methods of treatment and to assess and compare the results.

The precursor of the TNM classification

In 1939 the present author *(Raven, 1939)* published a new classification based on clinicopathological findings, for carinoma of the breast. Reference was made to this article by M. Harmer in an editorial in *Clinical Oncology* entitled "The case for TNM", in which he stated: "Raven published an article in which he described, with the aid of symbols, the extent of the disease as determined surgically, radiologically and pathologically but with emphasis on the three components: tumour, nodes and metastases. In this sense it was a forerunner of TNM."

In his article the present author had stated that there was a real need for a uniform classification for breast carcinoma with the continued evolution of treatment and the development of radiation methods, either alone, or in conjunction with excisional procedures, so that the end-results from each method could be compared for further advances to be made. For an appraisal of these methods groups of comparable cases according to the extent of the disease should be considered. He called attention to the classification of carcinoma of the cervix uteri whereby the results of each treatment method could be compared in the same stage of the disease (see *League of Nations Health Organisation Atlas* (1938) — Cancer of the Cervix. Stockholm).

Requirements for a satisfactory classification

In his article published in 1939 the present author stated that a satisfactory classification of breast carcinoma must embrace the following clinicopathological findings:

(1) The local condition: (a) skin involvement, (b) pectoralis fascia involvement, (c) pectoralis major muscle involvement, and (d) costal cartilage, rib or sternum involvement.

(2) The regional lymph nodes: (a) axillary lymph node involvement according to the group, (b) axillary perinodal connective tissue involvement, (c) supraclavicular lymph node involvement, and (d) mediastinal lymph node involvement.

(3) Distant structures: (a) visceral involvement, and (b) bone involvement.

He called attention to previous classifications of breast carcinoma where patients were classified into groups according to certain gross clinical findings and no account was taken of the detailed spread of carcinoma in its various phases which markedly affect the prognosis.

The classification proposed by Raven in 1939

The proposed classification based on clinicopathological findings correlates the condition in the breast itself with the contents of the axilla and other more distant regions which may be the site of metastases.

The stage of the disease in the breast is indicated by a number (for example, I); the stage of the disease in the regional lymph nodes is indicated by a letter (for example, a), and if the disease has spread to the perinodal connective tissue, a dash (′) is placed after the letter (for example, a′); if the disease has spread to other organs of the body, then the first two letters of the organ or organs involved are added (for example, lu — lung; li — liver). The final stage of the disease is clear when these various regions have been assessed and the symbols have been combined, for example, I a′ lu.

It is necessary to assess the stage of the disease both in the breast and in the regional lymph nodes. In the proposed classification the following assessments were defined.

The disease in the breast. Stage I. The carcinoma is strictly confined to the breast. Stage II. The carcinoma infiltrates the skin (Stage II skin). The carcinoma infiltrates the pectoralis fascia (Stage II fascia). Stage III. The carcinoma infiltrates the pectoralis muscle (Stage III muscle). The carcinoma ulcerates through the skin (Stage III ulcer). Stage IV. The carcinoma infiltrates the ribs or costal cartilage or sternum (Stage IV bone). The carcinoma infiltrates the whole breast with peau d'orange of the skin and/or infiltration of the underlying pectoralis fascia or muscle (Stage IV whole breast).

The disease in the regional lymph nodes and perinodal connective tissue. Stage a. The carcinoma involves the lymph nodes under the lower border of the pectoralis major muscle. Stage b. The carcinoma involves the lymph nodes under the tendon of insertion of the pectoralis major muscle. Stage c. The carcinoma involves the lymph nodes under the tendon of the pectoralis minor muscle. Stage d. The carcinoma involves the supraclavicular lymph nodes. Stage e. The carcinoma involves the mediastinal lymph nodes.

If the carcinoma has transgressed into the perinodal connective tissue the symbol ′ is placed opposite the appropriate group of lymph nodes affected, for example, a′ or d′ etc.

Examples of the classification were given as follows:

Case. Carcinoma of the breast which infiltrates the pectoralis major muscle. There are metastases in the lymph nodes under the lower border of the pectoralis major muscle and the carcinoma has spread to the perinodal connective tissue. Classification = III (muscle) a′.

Case. Carcinoma infiltrates the whole breast with peau d'orange of the skin and infiltration of the pectoralis major muscle. The lymph nodes under the lower border of the pectoralis major muscle and the lymph nodes under the tendon of the pectoralis minor muscle are involved. There are metastases in the lungs. Classification is IV (whole breast) a, c, lu.

This classification of breast carcinoma which was described originally by the present author in 1939 is given detailed consideration here because it has historic importance and interest as the precursor of the international TNM classification of malignant tumours in many sites of the body, published by the UICC.

TNM classification of malignant tumours

In 1944 P. F. Denoix of the Institut Gustave-Roussy in France conceived the TNM system of classification *(Harmer, 1977)* and proposed that it should be a "pure clinical description of the extent of the disease based on the clinical examination, simple radiology and endoscopic findings". This approach was criticised because of the impossibility of assessing many visceral tumours by this method alone, a good example being ovarian tumours. Thus it was accepted that laparotomy was necessary to establish ovarian malignancy. Other specialists argued that for other particular tumours additional investigations were required for a correct classification and histopathologists claimed that it would be foolish to ignore their findings. It was agreed, therefore, to define, for tumours in each specific site, the investigations which are permissible to identify the several degrees within each of the three categories, T, N, and M.

A detailed account of the discussions and publications by the UICC during these early years is given by Harmer *(1977)*, who is an Honorary Consulting Surgeon to the Royal Marsden Hospital in London. He became a member of the UICC Committee on TNM classification in 1958 and was Chairman from 1968 to 1974, when he became the secretary of the committee.

A booklet entitled *TNM Classification of Malignant Tumours of Breast, Larynx, Stomach, Cervix Uteri, Corpus Uteri* was published by the UICC and AJC (American Joint Committee on Cancer Staging and End Results Reporting) in Geneva in 1972. In the Introduction, Harmer stated that discussions on this form of classification began in 1953, and that the UICC published the first of its brochures, *Cancer of the Breast and Larynx*, in 1958, this being followed by *Cancer of the Buccal Cavity and Pharynx* in 1963. Eight other brochures, with a total number of 22 sites of cancer classified by TNM, were combined in a single booklet called *Livre de Poche*, which was published in 1968. During approximately the same period the American Joint Committee published 10 fascicles dealing with about a dozen sites of cancer. Large numbers of the *Livre de Poche*, translated into nine languages in addition to English, and of the American fascicles have been circulated throughout the world. The TNM classification is known and accepted internationally as the best method for recording the extent of cancer in different sites of the body and for comparing the end-results of treatment. Harmer stated that the classification has failings, so that a continuing effort is necessary to refine it when new facts and figures become available.

The 4th fully revised edition of the *TNM Classification of Malignant Tumours* was published in 1987. It contains an up-to-date site classification and eliminates all variations, and chapters are added on tumours which previously were not classified.

The general rules of the TNM system

A detailed account of the TNM system of classification of cancer in all sites and anatomical regions is given in the 4th edition *(1987)*, which includes the following general rules. To describe the anatomical extent of the cancer, an assessment is made of three components, as follows: T describes the extent of the primary tumour, N describes the absence or presence and extent of regional lymph node metastases and M describes the absence or presence of distant metastases. The addition of numbers to these three components indicates the extent of the cancer as follows: T0, T1, T2, T3, T4; N0, N1, N2, N3; and M0, M1.

All tumours should be confirmed by histopathology and any tumours not proved must be reported separately. There are two classifications for each site. Clinical classification before treatment is designated TNM (or cTNM) and is based on all the pretreatment clinical and investigatory evidence. Pathological classification is designated pTNM and is the post-surgical histopathological classification. This is based on the pretreatment evidence supplemented or modified by the evidence acquired from surgery and from pathological examination.

The pathological assessment of the primary tumour (pT) entails a resection of the primary tumour or a biopsy which is adequate to evaluate the highest pT category. The pathological assessment of regional lymph nodes (pN) entails the removal of nodes which is adequate to validate the absence of regional lymph node metastases (pN0) and sufficient to evaluate the highest pN category. The pathological assessment of distant metastases (pM) entails microscopic examination.

It is explained in the 4th edition that knowing the exact clinical stage is essential in order to select and evaluate therapy; the pathological stage gives the most precise data for estimating progress and calculating the end-results of treatment. When there is doubt about the correct TNM category of a particular tumour, the lower, less advanced category is chosen. This will also be reflected in the stage grouping. When there are multiple simultaneous tumours in one organ, the tumour with the highest T category is classified and the multiplicity or the number of tumours is indicated in parenthesis; for example, T2(m) or T2(5). With simultaneous bilateral cancers of paired organs, each tumour is classified independently. With tumours of the thyroid gland and liver, nephroblastoma and neuroblastoma, multiplicity is a criterion of T classification.

BRITISH ASSOCIATION OF SURGICAL ONCOLOGY

The emergence of oncology as a multidisciplinary subject of which surgical oncology is an important component had profound professional effects on different groups of specialists, including surgeons. The present author discussed the possible formation of the British Association of Surgical Oncology with Ian Burn and other surgical colleagues. As a result of his initiative and after detailed discussions about the project, including its administration, objectives, constitution and committee structure, the Association was established in 1972. The author was elected its first President and a National Committee was formed.

The Association attracted a large membership of general and specialist surgeons in the UK and radiation oncologists and medical oncologists were also welcomed. Regular meetings are organised and are held in different regions of the country, at which the members are encouraged to present accounts of their work and to take part in discussions.

In 1972, when the British Association of Surgical Oncology was established, it was foreseen that in the future surgery would continue to play a major role in the diagnosis, staging, definitive treatment, rehabilitation and continuing care of patients with neoplastic diseases. For many patients it would be combined with medical and radiation treatment, both for the local control of primary tumours and for metastatic tumours.

It was realised quite clearly that general and specialist surgeons would continue to be responsible for the management of many patients with cancer affecting the organs and tissues of the body. In addition to this heavy responsibility, many general and specialist surgeons have to deal with other non-malignant conditions. A number of surgeons have a very special interest and role in surgical oncology and academic units were established for surgeons with a total commitment to it. The need for these special academic units was clearly seen.

Provision should be made for surgical oncology in the education and training programme of surgeons when they will have to carry a heavy workload of patients with neoplastic diseases, for every help should be given them in their responsible work. The surgical oncologist must be well trained in surgery and must have a sound knowledge of the basic oncological sciences. The subject of training in surgical oncology has been studied in detail by the British Association of Surgical Oncology.

Since its formation in 1972 *(Raven, 1973)* the Association has continued to expand in many directions. The membership has grown, and the following surgeons have held the office of President: R. W. Raven, 1972–1977; Lord Smith, 1977–1980; I. J. Burn, 1980–1983; Professor A. Cuschieri, 1983–1986, and Professor H. Ellis, 1986 to date. A notable achievement of the Association was the publication of the *Journal of Clinical Oncology*, with an international circulation, by Academic Press. With the subsequent establishment of the European Society of Surgical Oncology, constituted in 1981, this journal was merged with the *European Journal of Surgical Oncology* under the auspices of the European Society and the British Association, with Harvey White as Editor. The new journal has a large international circulation and is also published by Academic Press.

An important landmark in the history of the British Association of Surgical Oncology was the Joint Annual Meeting held in London in 1987 with the Association of Head and Neck Oncologists of Great Britain, the Society of Head and Neck Surgeons (USA), and the Society of Surgical Oncology Inc. (USA). There was a large number of participants from many countries, which indicated the importance of surgical oncology and the great interest in this discipline throughout the world.

THE ASSOCIATION OF HEAD AND NECK ONCOLOGISTS OF GREAT BRITAIN

The Association of Head and Neck Oncologists of Great Britain was formed in 1968 through the initiative of the present author, who consulted colleagues who were responsible for the management of patients with neoplastic diseases of the head and neck. New surgical techniques were being developed and combination treatments of surgery, radiotherapy and chemotherapy were being used for an increasing number of patients. There was therefore a need for joint discussion and joint consultation between surgical, radiation and medical oncologists concerning the problems associated with malignant diseases of the head and neck. The proposal that an Association of Head and Neck Oncologists of Great Britain be formed was welcomed with enthusiasm by the different specialists who were working in this field. The Association was therefore established and the present author was elected the first President (1968–1971). The executive officers were chosen and a National Committee was formed. The membership consists of surgical, radiation and medical oncologists. Regular meetings of the Association have been organised in subsequent years and a historic landmark was its participation in the Joint Annual Meeting held in London in 1987, described above.

Past Presidents of the Association have been as follows: R. W. Raven, 1968–1971; M. Lederman, 1971–1974; Sir Douglas Ranger, 1974–1977; R. Morrison, 1977–1980; Professor D. N. F. Harrison, 1980–1983; and I. A. McGregor, 1983–1986. The present President is Professor P. M. Stell, 1986 to date.

In the years that have followed the establishment of the Association, the team-work envisaged between surgical, radiation and medical oncologists and plastic surgeons and other specialists has grown considerably, for the diagnosis, treatment, rehabilitation and general management of patients with complex and serious neoplastic diseases of the head and neck. All the facilities for this work should be concentrated in special oncology centres and there is an obvious need to train a limited number of head and neck oncologists to work at these centres.

The Association has given careful consideration to the education and training of head and neck oncologists. Surgical oncologists working in this special field should undergo the necessary training in general surgery before having specialist training in head and neck surgery. There must be continuing education in the basic oncology sciences, as for the other clinical oncologists.

REFERENCES

Cancer Research Campaign. *Annual Report 1986. Handbook 1987*

Dukes, C. E. (1965). The origin and early history of the Imperial Cancer Research Fund. *Ann. Roy. Coll. Surg. Engl.*, **36**, 325–38

Gough-Thomas, J. (1959). The social, economic and welfare problems of patients with cancer. In Raven, R. W. (ed.) *Cancer*, Vol. 6, pp 375–88. Butterworth & Co., London

Harmer, M. (1977). Editorial — The case for TNM. *Clin. Oncol.*, **3**, 131–5

Imperial Cancer Research Fund. *Thirty-Sixth Annual Report for the Year 1937–1938*. December 1938

Imperial Cancer Research Fund. *Thirty-Seventh Annual Report for the Year 1939–1940*

Imperial Cancer Research Fund. *Annual Report and Accounts 1985–1986*

Imperial Cancer Research Fund. *Sixtieth Annual Report and Accounts 1961–1962*. 9 April 1963

International Union Against Cancer (1987). Hermanek, P. and Sobin, L. H. (eds) *TNM Classification of Malignant Tumours*, 4th fully revised edn. Springer-Verlag, Berlin

Raven, R. W. (1939). A clinico-pathological classification of cancer of the breast. *Br. Med. J.*, **1**, 611–13

Raven, R. W. (1973). The British Association of Surgical Oncology. Address at the first meeting of the Association, 8 June 1973. *Ann. Roy. Coll. Surg. Engl.*, **53**, 305–10

Raven, R. W. (1986). *Rehabilitation and Continuing Care in Cancer*. Published on behalf of the International Union Against Cancer by Parthenon Publishing Group, Carnforth

CHAPTER FIVE

Historic Contributions to Cancer Literature

Major treatises on many aspects of cancer have been published in the 20th century, which clearly demonstrate the growth in our knowledge about malignant diseases. This growth has had an enormous influence on our conception of their nature and our attitudes to their prevention and the care of patients afflicted by them. An increasing number of patients can now be cured, a fact which has engendered a more optimistic attitude towards cancer throughout the world. The emergence of the basic oncological sciences and new methods of diagnosis and treatment was profoundly important. A study of the evolution of knowledge and the advances in the management of patients as portrayed in these treatises is of great interest.

THE TREATISE BY JACOB WOLFF

This massive work by Jacob Wolff consists of four volumes entitled *Die Lehre von der Krebskrankheit, von den altersten Zeiten bis zur Gegenwarte,* which were published by Gustav Fischer in Jena, Germany, in 1907, 1911, 1913 and 1928, respectively.

The first volume was reviewed by E. F. Bashford *(1907)*, who was the first Director of the Imperial Cancer Research Fund in London. His review gives a clear insight into the state of cancer research and the quantity and quality of cancer literature at the turn of the century. It is very favourable and is quoted here in detail. He wrote: "Dr Jacob Wolff's volume on the history of cancer from ancient times to the present is in reality a contribution to the history of medicine generally, and one of the most painstaking and valuable with which we are acquainted. Dr Wolff does not merely paraphrase the writing of those who have laboured at cancer. He does much more, for he is obviously learned in the history of medicine and possessed of special knowledge of cancer. Having himself no hypothesis to support, he has impartially reviewed and ably criticised the work of others, and has assigned to the workers of the past the position they seem to merit. Among their contemporaries Dr Wolff brings out very clearly how conceptions of cancer throughout the ages reflect the progress of medicine as a whole. The volume brings the progress of our knowledge of cancer up to modern experimental research of which no account could be taken. Within the space of 750 pages he has condensed an enormous amount of information never before contained in one volume; for this reason and because of its reliability it cannot fail to become a valuable book of reference.

Naturally it is not a book which is easy to read, but we have laboured through it with profit. At the present time such a volume meets a want, in that it covers the whole extent of the work which has been done on cancer. The investigation of cancer is one of the fashions of the hour. As the author points out in his preface, much printer's ink could have been spared had those engaged in the study of cancer been informed of what others had thought and written before them. Hypotheses long tested and found wanting crop up again and again in the pages of Dr Wolff's book, often supported by masses of evidence identical with that which had already proved insufficient to previous generations. He might have added that such repetition is occurring today.

Dr Wolff has gone to the primary sources for his information. We can only admire the industry which has enabled him to cover so vast a field as the literature of cancer, and to consult and quote his authorities at first hand. The book has the added value of being excellently arranged, supplied with a full table of contents facilitating consultation and provided with a good index. We heartily recommend it to the medical profession generally, and particularly to all who contemplate adding to the literature of cancer. The perusal will save 'cancer researchers' much useless labour; perhaps it may restrain some of them from re-inflicting the exploded hypotheses of the past upon the readers of the present. The volume is printed and illustrated in accordance with the traditions of Gustav Fischer's well-known house."

Following such a favourable reception of the first volume as given by Bashford's review, the succeeding volumes were doubtless successful too. The second volume deals mainly with the aetiology of cancer; the third is concerned with statistics and cancer occurring in animals and plants, and the fourth gives a systematic presentation of the surgical treatment of specific varieties of cancer. It is to be noted that surgical treatment was the conventional treatment for cancer at that time, for the modalities of radiotherapy and modern chemotherapy had still not emerged.

RADIUM TREATMENT OF CANCER, BY STANFORD CADE

This book by Stanford Cade (later Sir Stanford Cade) was published by J. and A. Churchill, London, in 1929. Cade was a leading British surgeon who specialised in the treatment of cancer at the Westminster Hospital in London. In the Preface he wrote: "I am primarily a surgeon, and radium therapy is only an effective weapon in the armamentarium available for the treatment of the patient afflicted with cancer. Patients are entitled to expect the selection and use of the most effective form of treatment for their special needs. If the choice of treatment in a given case of cancer depends upon a surgeon not conversant with the possibilities of radium, the choice will inevitably be that of surgery; the converse is true and is applicable to the radiologist."

Since these words were written great progress has been made in the treatment and general management of patients with cancer. A clinical oncologist can no longer work in isolation but must be a member of an oncology team which works in joint consultation regarding the diagnosis and the formation of the treatment programme. Members of the team must be familiar with modern treatment modalities, including their indications, side-effects, complications and end-results.

When Cade's book was published radium therapy for cancer was still in its infancy. The author gave descriptions of the different radium techniques used at that time and commented: "In a science so young and of such rapid development they may be of historic interest only before many years, or even months, have passed." He described the radium technique applicable for the treatment of cancer in various anatomical sites and illustrated the end-results of treatment by quoted case-records.

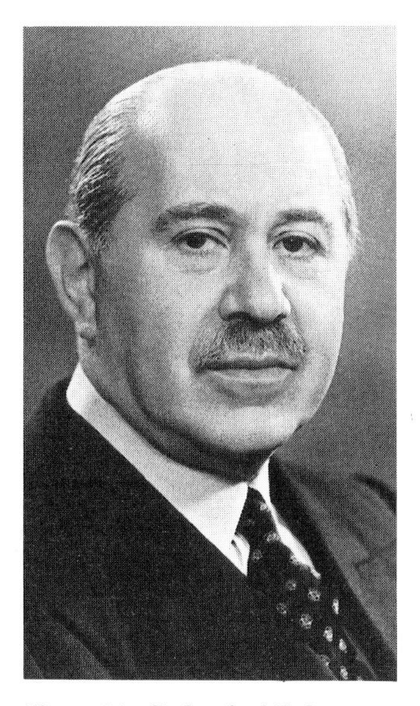

Figure 5.1 Sir Stanford Cade.

This pioneer work carried out by Cade and his colleagues at Westminster Hospital more than 50 years ago is of important historical interest and fully merits its detailed inclusion in this chapter.

Cade explained that the rapid advances which had occurred during the preceding 10 years in the radiation treatment of cancer had changed the conception of tumour operability and that surgical excision was no longer the only means of making a cancer disappear. Nevertheless, the new modality had a limited use, but wider than that of surgery alone. In certain cases radium was the treatment of choice and in others combination treatment was a possible means of prolonging life, but no patient should be untreated, however inoperable the cancer. He pointed out that all the surgeons at the Westminster Hospital appreciated the possible value of radium treatment, and that cancers of the tongue, lip, palate and brain were treated entirely by radium. He also stated that radium treatment abolishes, or at least minimises, operative mortality and mutilation.

Methods of irradiation

Cade described four methods, which are discussed in detail here because they are of historic interest and importance. The objective is to give the whole tumour a homogeneous dose which is sufficient to cause its disintegration while having only minimal effects on the surrounding healthy tissues. The four methods are the cavitary method; interstitial irradiation; surface application; and distance irradiation.

Cade considered that distance irradiation had great future possibilities and reported that it was being used in the Radium Institutes of Brussels and Paris. Large quantities of radium were applied at distances of 10 cm or more from the skin, which meant that much larger doses of irradiation could be given without causing skin damage. The treatment was given in special rooms and required 4 g or more of radium, which was placed in a box suspended above the patient, with a window in it to allow the rays to be beamed on the tumour. The method had been used with good results for patients with cancers of the breast and uterus.

An outstanding feature of Cade's book is the inclusion of beautiful coloured drawings, which were executed with exquisite skill by Sewell, an extremely good medical artist of the time. He was based at the Royal College of Surgeons of England, and his excellent work illustrated many medical books and articles in journals. He was well known to the present author, for whom he executed many coloured drawings illustrating the techniques of operative surgery, the pathology of tumours and anatomical dissections.

In Cade's book the coloured drawings show the type and situation of the primary cancer before radium treatment and appearances of the tumour at various times after treatment. They are specially impressive in showing the results achieved by radium in the treatment of carcinomas situated in the lip, tongue, floor of the mouth, palate and oropharynx.

Treatment of cervical lymph nodes

In one chapter of his book Cade gave a valuable review of the management of the cervical lymph nodes in patients with carcinoma of the mouth. He wrote: "The marked failures of incomplete operations for the removal of cervical glands, the hopelessness of cases where the glands are irremovable and the death of patients from cervical deposits although the oral cavity is normal, are convincing proofs of the importance of early treatment."

He cited the collective experience of all the Westminster Hospital surgeons and made the following important conclusions, which are worthy of study by clinical oncologists today.

(1) Incomplete operation which does not conform with Crile's dissection is by itself not recommended because of the great risk of local recurrent disease.
(2) Incomplete operation with postoperative interstitial radium has been abandoned because of the risk to large blood vessels and unsatisfactory end-results.
(3) Incomplete operation followed by surface irradiation with Columbia Paste collars has given better results, but is not the ideal treatment.
(4) Surface irradiation using Columbia Paste collars alone has been successful in some cases, but there was no proof that node metastases were present; in other cases postradiation recurrences occurred.
(5) Crile's operation has given good results, but is by itself considered insufficient if malignant glands are present, and is not indicated if malignant glands are not present.

Cade recommended block dissection of the cervical nodes followed by postoperative radiotherapy, when the presence of metastases was proved microscopically. It is of historic interest that radiotherapy was given by the application of a Columbia Paste collar, with an average of 70 mg of radium, giving a total dose of 10 000 mg hours.

Cade gives accounts of the radium treatment of cancer in all parts of the body for which radiation techniques had been developed. It is fascinating to study the care and ingenuity shown by cancer specialists in applying the new treatment modality. Reference is made here to certain procedures which have much historic interest.

Cancer of the larynx

The old classification of intrinsic and extrinsic cancers is supplanted here by "endolaryngeal, epilaryngeal, lateral pharyngeal and hypopharyngeal tumours". Today this classification has been replaced by laryngeal (old term "endolaryngeal") and hypopharyngeal (old terms "epilaryngeal", "lateral pharyngeal" and "hypopharyngeal") cancers.

Cade stated that laryngeal cancer treated by laryngofissure had a good prognosis, but radium treatment was superior because it permitted better voice production. He cited the fenestration method based on the technique of Ledoux *(1923)* and practised by Finzi and Harmer *(1928)* with outstanding success and gave a detailed account of the procedure as described by Harmer *(1927)*. A window was cut in the lateral ala of the thyroid cartilage to provide access for the insertion of radium needles in the larynx. Usually seven needles, each containing 1.3 mg of radium, were used and left in position for 7 days.

The treatment of "epilaryngeal" cancer described here illustrates the use of interstitial platinum radon seeds of 1.8–2 mCi strength. These were implanted in and around the tumour and left in position for 10–14 days.

Cancer of the hypopharynx

Cade used the classification of "lateral pharyngeal" and "hypopharyngeal" tumours. The former are tumours of the pyriform fossa; the latter include postcricoid and posterior wall tumours. The modern classification of carcinoma of the hypopharynx includes all the tumours arising in the epiglottis, down to the pharyngo-oesophageal junction. Cade described surface irradiation with a Columbia Paste collar for the treatment of lateral pharyngeal tumours and stated that it gave good palliative results. He considered hypopharyngeal cancer to be "rapidly fatal and lends itself badly to surgical removal" and an inoperable disease as a rule. The first stage of treatment consisted of a tracheostomy and a lateral pharyngotomy on the "sound side" so that platinum radon seeds could be introduced in and around the tumour, and the pharynx closed. The second stage was done 4 weeks later, when the whole neck was irradiated by applying a Columbia Paste collar. In discussing the management of these tumours, Cade quoted the classical work of Wilfred Trotter *(1913)*, the London surgeon who performed pioneer surgical operations for cancer of the mouth and pharynx.

Since that time notable advances have been made in the management of carcinoma of the larynx and pharynx, which are based on a precise understanding of the pathology of these tumours which occur in defined sites. Developments have occurred in radiotherapy, which is now given from external sources such as a linear accelerator. The surgical operations of laryngo-pharyngectomy and laryngo-oesophago-pharyngectomy have been developed, to give restoration of normal deglutition. The operative mortality of these major operations is low and the end-results, which include some patients being alive without recurrence after 10 years, are encouraging *(Raven, 1958)*.

Carcinoma of the breast

The treatment of this disease which occurs so frequently in women has rightly attracted enormous attention for many decades and the subject still continues to be debated. The introduction of treatment by radium was an important landmark in the long history; the work of Sir Geoffrey Keynes in this connection is described in Chapter 12.

Stanford Cade devoted a chapter to this subject. He stated: "Modern surgical teaching lays stress on the importance of an extensive operation, wide removal of fascia and careful dissection of the axilla." He pointed out that there could be recurrences long after the primary treatment had been given and that it must be assumed that inactive disease had been present all the time, but not recognisable clinically. We now speak of micrometastases and realise their importance.

Regarding the treatment of primary breast carcinoma, Cade considered that the great advantage of radium therapy was that its therapeutic action extended beyond the field covered by surgical excision. The technique of radium therapy used at Westminster Hospital had progressed from surface application of radium to the insertion of interstitial radium needles, and finally a combination of these techniques was used. The combined technique was suitable for treating the majority of operable and inoperable breast carcinomas and based on the "Radium Halsted" method, which covered a much wider area of tissues than the most extensive excisional operation.

Cancer of the uterus

There was initial enthusiasm for using radium to treat cancer in certain organs, but this has waned with greater experience of the end-results, the recognition of radioresistant tumours and the development of modern radiation techniques. The treatment of carcinoma of the cervix uteri, in marked contrast, has certainly stood the test of time, for irradiation techniques are still of prime importance for these tumours.

Stanford Cade quoted Sir George Newman *(1927)*, Chief Medical Officer of Health, who wrote concerning radiation therapy for uterine cancer: "Broadly speaking, the results obtained are the equal of those obtained by operation, viz, survival to 5 years of about 40 per cent of patients suitable for operation. In addition, survival to a similar period of about 12 per cent of patients who are inoperable is secured. ... Further, radiological treatment supplies an efficient palliative in many cases in which cure cannot be hoped for ... It is clear that one of the most serious deterrents to patients needing early advice and treatment for cancer is the dislike of operation. If this fear can be removed by substituting another method of treatment, a great impulse might be expected in the movement for securing the attendance of patients at hospital in an earlier stage of their malady."

Cade described the methods of radiation treatment which had been devised by different authorities for use in their clinics: (1) intrauterine and vaginal radiation applications; (2) treating the tumour by means of radium needles; and (3) intra-abdominal application of radiation, which was supplementary to (1) and (2).

An important contribution to the development of radiotherapy for carcinoma of the cervix uteri was made by Malcolm Donaldson at the Royal Hospital of St Bartholomew, London. The present author had many fruitful discussions about many cancer problems with this distinguished gynaecologist, including ways and means of achieving the early detection of cancer in different parts of the body and developing community education about different aspects of cancer.

Carcinoma of the rectum

The position regarding the surgical treatment of carcinoma of the rectum over 50 years ago was summarised in the Report on cancer of the rectum *(Ministry of Health, 1927)* concerning nearly 6000 cases operated on in 10 different countries, which was briefly quoted by Stanford Cade. There was an average period of 12 months between the first symptom of the disease and its surgical treatment, and rather less than 50% of the patients were considered operable. About one-sixth of the patients who underwent radical surgery died from the operation or causes connected with it, and two out of every five patients submitted to the radical operation were alive 3 years later.

The early method of radium treatment was to introduce a sound carrying radium tubes into the lumen of the rectum, but this caused serious complications. It was followed by the technique of surgical exposure of the carcinoma and the interstitial insertion of radium needles, the results of which were encouraging. This method was used by Sir Charles Gordon-Watson *(1928)*, who was Surgeon at the Royal Hospital of St Bartholomew in London and well known to the present author, who had the privilege of seeing him perform the operation. His work was quoted by Cade, in addition to that of Neuman and Coryn *(1928)*, which includes diagrams showing the technique of the operation.

The treatment of carcinoma of the rectum with radium has not proved satisfactory and we have recognised that adenocarcinoma of the rectum has radioresistance. With modern methods of external radiotherapy there is renewed interest in combined radiation and surgical treatment of carcinoma of the rectum and radiation alone as palliative for advanced local tumours.

Other sites

In his book Stanford Cade discussed the treatment by radium of cancer in other important sites in the body, including the prostate, urinary bladder, penis and vulva. He demonstrated that many of the carcinomas in these sites are radiosensitive. With the development of modern external techniques, radiotherapy has an important place in their management today.

Cade gave an interesting account of radium treatment for *carcinoma of the oesophagus*, which failed because of the great difficulties of obtaining access to the tumour and delivering to it an adequate dose of radiation. He pointed out that the failure was not due to radioresistance of the carcinoma. Whilst radium treatment is not used today for the treatment of oesophageal carcinoma, the great value of external radiotherapy has been clearly proved when it is used either alone or in combination with oesophagectomy operations.

Regarding the common and dangerous *carcinoma of the stomach*, Cade called attention to the poor prognosis which often followed surgical treatment. He felt that radium therapy might prove useful, but that its future was speculative. Though in subsequent experience tumour regression has occurred in isolated cases, radiotherapy of gastric carcinoma has not developed either alone or combined with surgical treatment.

The increasing incidence of *cancer of the lung* was causing Cade and others considerable concern. He felt that it was necessary to call attention to the possible value of radium treatment for lung cancer as the initial results were encouraging and the development of distance therapy from a "radium bomb", permitting more accurate radiation beaming of the tumour, might give better results. It is interesting to observe that external radiotherapy from modern equipment now plays an important role in the management of various forms of lung cancer.

The treatment of *tumours of the cerebrum and cerebellum* by radium presented difficulties and the results were adversely affected by secondary vascular changes in the surrounding normal tissues and the presence of oedema. The insertion of interstitial radium needles had been attempted but this technique was found to be unsatisfactory. Another method used was preliminary cerebral decompression followed by a course of surface irradiation of the tumour with a Columbia Paste helmet for a period of 2–3 weeks, but the results failed to impress.

Cade divided *epithelioma of the skin* into fungating and ulcerative varieties. He states that the former is more radiosensitive and responds to surface irradiation, while the latter variety requires a bigger radiation dosage with interstitial irradiation alone or followed by surface irradiation to promote healing. He points out that some rodent ulcers are radioresistant but that unless they are invading bone the majority of these tumours respond well to irradiation treatment.

Cade concluded his book with a short chapter on the protection of those who work with radium and stressed that adequate precautions against radiation effects must be taken by everyone who handled or used radium needles or radium tubes. This was important advice in those early days of the development of radiotherapy.

CANCER, EDITED BY R. W. RAVEN

This work, which covers all aspects of cancer, was conceived, planned, contributed to, edited and brought to fruition by the present author. It consists of six volumes plus an index volume, which were published by Butterworth and Co., London, during the years 1957–1959. It was subsequently updated by new material in the volumes entitled *Cancer Progress*, which were also edited by the present author and published by Butterworth & Co. in 1960 and 1963.

It was perhaps the first occasion that such a comprehensive treatise on cancer had been published. A perusal of the extensive coverage of the subjects, which include all aspects of cancer research, laboratory, epidemiological, statistical and clinical; cancer prevention; pathology; treatment modalities of surgery, radiation and chemotherapy, and a number of general subjects concerning public health and nursing aspects of cancer, including rehabilitation of patients; patients with persistent cancer; social, economic and welfare problems of patients with cancer and cancer registration, etc, must lead to the conclusion that such a synthesis of knowledge was really the first presentation of oncology. In these volumes it is shown that "cancer" has become "oncology".

It is apposite here to refer to the Preface, from which the following quotation is taken. "The control of cancer is one of the important problems requiring urgent solution for it is a major threat to life of all nations and none is excluded from its effects. The mortality from the disease rises annually and a concerted effort is required to attain our object. There is need for a close partnership of all who are engaged in different aspects of the work and the facilities for quick access to information concerning advances being made in fields other than their own. These volumes will help to fill this need, for they are planned with the object of including many of the relevant aspects of the subject. 'He alone can conceive and compose who sees the whole at once before him.' (Fuseli, quoted by John Ruskin in *Modern Painters*, 1896).

In planning this synthesis of knowledge care was taken in the choice of subjects and to show each in its right perspective. 'To try to approach truth on one side and another, not to strive or try, nor to persist in pressing forward on any one side with violence and self-will — it is only thus, it seems to me, that mortals may hope to gain any vision of the mysterious goddess... He who will do nothing but fight impetuously towards her on his own, one, favourite, particular line, is inevitably destined to run his head into the folds of the black robe in which she is wrapped.' (Matthew Arnold in *Essays in Criticism*, 1865).

It is recognised that some of the subject matter in these volumes is in a state of flux, that knowledge is still imperfect and further progress will occur."

Volume titles

Volume 1, entitled "Research into causation", contains chapters dealing with carcinogenesis; chemical mechanisms of normal and abnormal cell division; biochemistry of cancer induction; hormones and neoplasia; viruses and tumours; nutrition and the genesis of tumours; genetics and cancer; environmental factors in the production of human cancer; carcinogenic effects of radiation; and the incubation period of cancer in man.

Volume 2 is concerned with the pathology of malignant tumours, including general pathology; biological characteristics of neoplasms; and modes of spread of malignant tumours. There are separate chapters dealing with the pathology of malignant tumours of different organs and tissues of the body.

Volume 3 contains sections and chapters dealing with additional aspects of pathology, including immunology and cancer; cancer cells in tissue culture; malignant diseases in domestic animals; and statistical investigations concerning the causation of human cancer. There are sections which deal with the geography of cancer; occupational cancer; cancer education; and cancer detection.

Volume 4 is devoted to the clinical aspects of malignant tumours which affect the different organs and tissues of the body.

Volume 5 deals with radiotherapy of cancer and includes chapters on the general aspects, including the physical properties of radiation; the biological basis of radiotherapy; dosage; methodology; radioisotopes; protection from radiation; and radiation reactions. There are chapters which describe the radiotherapy of cancer in all the organs and tissues of the body.

In Volume 6 cancer chemotherapy and hormonal therapy are considered in detail. The final section, dealing with the public health and nursing aspects of cancer, contains chapters on cancer rehabilitation; the treatment of patients with persistent cancer; the social, economic and welfare problems created by cancer; psychological aspects; cancer registration; and the prevention of cancer.

A simple perusal of the contents of this treatise written more than 25 years ago will give the reader information concerning the broad spectrum of activities in research and clinical work which was carried out at that time.

THE SURGICAL TREATMENT OF MALIGNANT DISEASE, BY SIR HOLBURT J. WARING

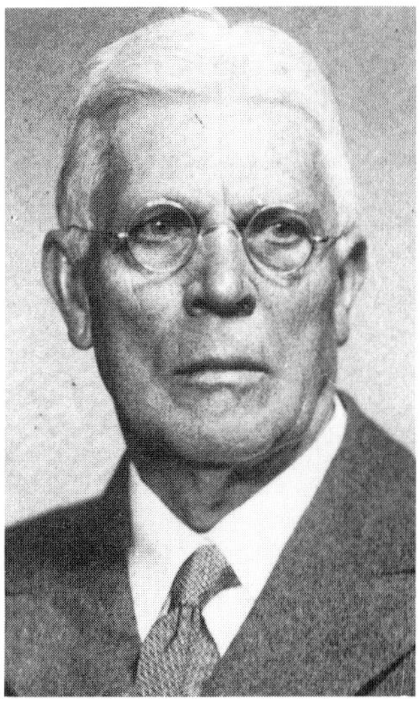

Figure 5.2 Sir Holburt J. Waring.

This notable book by Sir Holburt J. Waring, who was Surgeon to the Royal Hospital of St Bartholomew, London, and became President of the Royal College of Surgeons of England, was published in 1928 by Humphrey Milford, Oxford University Press. The present author was his house-surgeon at St Bartholomew's Hospital and greatly values a copy of this book which Sir Holburt inscribed and presented to him.

In the Preface we read: "The subject, in the main, has been treated from a clinical and surgical point of view; but to a limited extent, the pathological aspect of malignant disease, in so far as it has bearing on clinical diagnosis or surgical treatment, has been dwelt upon." In the 49 chapters of the book there is detailed coverage of malignant disease of all the organs and tissues of the body with splendid descriptions of the surgical operations for their treatment. Reference is made also to treatment by radiological methods where this is indicated. There are 19 beautiful colour plates and the book is profusely illustrated also with black and white drawings. These were largely carried out by the well-known illustrator Mr Kirkpatrick Maxwell.

When this book was written 60 years ago the treatment of malignant diseases was predominantly by surgery. Cancer operations were based on a sound and detailed knowledge of tumour pathology, especially the spread of cancer by local infiltration and by the lymphatic system. A detailed knowledge of the lymphatics of the body was therefore essential, as the operations were designed to extirpate the local tumour and the regional lymph nodes. This principle is clearly presented in Waring's book, which was a definite milestone along the road which has led to the establishment of surgical oncology as a recognised discipline.

PATHOLOGY OF TUMOURS, BY R. A. WILLIS

This classical book on the pathology of tumours was written by Professor R. A. Willis, who was Sir William H. Collins Professor of Human and Comparative Pathology at the Royal College of Surgeons, London. It was published in 1948 by Butterworth & Co., London.

In the Preface the author states that the book is the outcome of his special interest in tumours during his 20 years as a hospital pathologist. Most of the material on which the book is based was studied in the pathology laboratories of the Alfred Hospital in Melbourne, Australia; the author also held a research appointment in the Pathology Department of the University of Melbourne. The book was published while he held his appointment at the Royal College of Surgeons of England, where his work included restoring the museum and teaching.

His book, which extends to 992 pages plus an index, is the record of his personal observations and conclusions. Throughout he has used his own material as much as possible, making frequent references to articles he had already published and to his earlier book entitled *The Spread of Tumours in the Human Body*. A feature of the book is the inclusion of many brief reports of cases illustrative of the subjects under discussion.

The book also contains many illustrations, all from material the author had studied and in most cases previously unpublished. With few exceptions they are microphotographs. Emphasis is laid on less common tumours and showing less familiar and special features. References to the literature are given at the end of each chapter.

No attempt is made here to review the contents of the book, but special features should be mentioned. In the chapter on carcinoma of the stomach Willis discusses possible causative factors. He states that he had examined hundreds of gastric ulcers and carcinomas but had seen only three examples of unequivocal ulcer-cancer. Other causative factors are dealt with, including gastritis, benign epithelial neoplasms, and pernicious anaemia. With regard to the latter he states that in his opinion the evidence is inconclusive that true pernicious anaemia or achlorhydria predisposes to gastric carcinoma and that further data must be carefully evaluated to reach a final decision. He also discusses the ingestion of possible carcinogenic substances, the physical state of ingested food and the influence of heredity, which he considers is not a very important causative factor. In the chapter devoted to epithelial tumours of the breast, he gives a historical introduction in which he states that whilst Hippocrates and his contemporaries knew of breast cancer, an earlier still, and perhaps the first specifically reported, case of breast tumour was recorded by Herodotus as having occurred in Atossa, the daughter of Cyrus and the wife of Darius I, about 520 BC. The author calls attention to the fact that John Hunter *(1837)* recognised the surgical importance of the multicentric origin of some cancers of the breast and their association with cystic changes in the breast, and quotes the following passage: "It (cancer) often arises in distinct points of the same breast, but seldom at the same period; and some of these may be so much in their infancy when the operation is performed as not to be observable, but afterwards increase and require a second operation. The surrounding substance of the breast has often little tumours, sometimes containing a blackish fluid; these may be called cancerous hydatids. It is therefore best to extirpate the breast completely at once, to remove the whole complaint."

It is of profound interest to ponder on these words of Hunter at the present time and to remember that in a significant percentage of women with carcinoma of the breast the disease is multicentric in origin. Today the operation of excision of the carcinoma — the so-called "lumpectomy" procedure — is frequently performed; Hunter advised mastectomy.

Regarding the aetiology of carcinoma of the lung, our knowledge of the important role of tobacco and our attempts to curtail its use have increased enormously since Willis wrote his book in 1947. He states, "It is quite possible that the inhalation of carcinogenic hydrocarbons, or other substances in soots, smokes and dusts, including tobacco smoke, is an important causative factor, but proof of this will entail much more pathological and experimental research."

It is interesting to note that Willis considered that melanoma is a relatively rare disease and that almost all melanomas arise in moles. He does not mention the important factor of exposure of the skin to excess sunshine, but calls for closer study of melanosis and melanomas in animals to help in the solution of some of the problems of histogenesis. Melanomas are well known in horses, dogs and other animals.

The book is divided into two parts: Part 1 contains 12 chapters on general tumour pathology; Part 2 contains 50 chapters on the pathology of tumours of special organs and tissues.

In Chapter 6, dealing with tumours in animals, Willis gives a brief outline of the main tumours which occur spontaneously in different classes of animals and states that much information of value for human pathology remains to be learnt from the study of animal tumours. The occurrence of particular kinds of these tumours is also referred to in the appropriate chapters in Part 2.

The close of Part 1 deals with the subject of neoplasia. Willis states: "Histopathologists and experimentalists have been building up a secure foundation of knowledge of tumour causation and behaviour; and — healthiest omen — pathologists are beginning to pay attention to biologists, and biologists to pathologists. All are coming slowly to realise that progress in embryology, in genetics, in cytology, in biochemistry, in endocrinology and in pathology are all inextricably linked; that pathology is extended physiology; and that disturbances of growth studied by one specialist are of interest to all."

The present author is in complete agreement with this opinion and finds it to be a perfect description of the multidisciplinary subject of oncology.

TREATMENT OF CANCER AND ALLIED DISEASES (2nd EDITION), EDITED BY GEORGE T. PACK AND IRVING M. ARIEL

The nine volumes in this work — copyright 1940 and 1958 by Paul B. Hoeber, Inc., Medical Book Department of Harper and Brothers — were printed in the USA and published in the UK by Pitman Medical Publishing Co., Ltd.

They are devoted to the clinical aspects of cancer management and make a notable contribution to the literature on cancer. The editors are known internationally for their outstanding work in the cancer field while holding appointments at important hospitals in New York. Dr Pack and the present author enjoyed a very happy friendship which extended over many years.

The series is jointly dedicated to James Ewing, who carried out valuable cancer research work and made an enormous contribution to the whole subject of neoplastic diseases, and to John D. Rockefeller, Jr., in recognition of his outstanding devotion to the cause of medical research and education. The latter will always be remembered for establishing the Rockefeller Fellowships to give physicians training in clinical cancer therapy at the Memorial Hospital.

The nine volumes, which deal with the treatment procedures for tumours in the different organs and tissues of the body, were written by recognised authorities on neoplastic diseases from prominent cancer centres in many parts of the world. In several chapters there are introductions giving a broad perspective of cancer treatment in the speciality discussed. The text was entirely rewritten and reorganised for the 2nd edition, to take account of the great advances which had been made in the previous two decades in the treatment of cancer.

In Volume 1 the principles of treatment are dealt with by 55 authors and there are 505 illustrations. There is a wide coverage of this subject, with sections on organisation; diagnosis and pathology; surgery; radiation, including radioactive isotopes; hormone therapy; chemotherapy; and the general care of the patient with cancer. The final chapters are concerned with the methods of reporting the end-results of cancer treatment and specific methods of calculating survival rates. This particular volume is doubtless unique in concentrating solely on the treatment of cancer in all its different aspects and is a magnificent precursor of the outstanding volumes which follow.

The whole work constituted another historic landmark in the evolution of oncology as we understand it today.

THE AMERICAN CANCER SOCIETY CANCER BOOK, EDITED BY ARTHUR I. HOLLEB

This book published in 1986 makes an impressive addition to the cancer literature. The editor, who is Senior Vice-President for Medical Affairs of the American Cancer Society, has been a close friend of the present author for many years and is an active member of the Rehabilitation and Continuing Care for Cancer Committee of the International Union Against Cancer, in addition to being a member of the Council.

The extensive text is concerned with the main subjects of prevention, detection, diagnosis, treatment, rehabilitation and care, and these are covered in 650 pages which also include a Directory of Resources, Glossary and Index. The book is divided into two main parts, plus an introduction by the editor, entitled "An overview of cancer today". Part 1 is devoted to "Where we stand in the battle against cancer". It contains 14 chapters on fundamental general subjects such as modern cancer therapy, principles of cancer chemotherapy, radiation therapy, rehabilitation of the cancer patient, cancer and pain, genetics and cancer, and cancer prevention.

Part 2 is concerned with specific cancers and their treatment and these important subjects are covered in 20 chapters written by well-known experts on each subject. The book is usefully illustrated with clear line drawings.

It was written for the general public and is the most comprehensive and authoritative ever published for this particular readership. The detailed information given will doubtless greatly help individuals and families to understand the needs of their loved ones in their suffering and also give them valuable knowledge about cancer prevention.

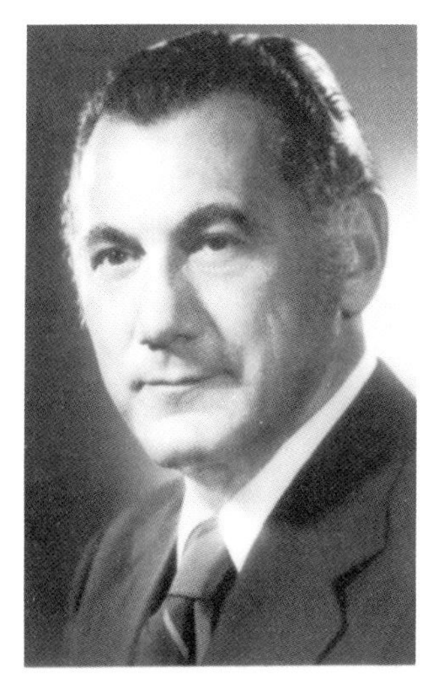

Figure 5.3 Arthur I. Holleb, Chief Medical Officer of the American Cancer Society from 1968 to 1988.

This book was published for the American Cancer Society by Doubleday & Company, Inc., New York. The present author wishes to pay a special tribute here to the American Cancer Society for its dedicated work in the control of cancer. The Society was founded in 1913 as the American Society for the Control of Cancer and has made many valuable contributions in research, education and service. It is the largest voluntary health agency in the world to be funded entirely by contributions from the public. It has 58 divisions and relies on the efforts of more than 2 million devoted volunteers, who serve nationwide. The literature published by the Society covers many aspects of cancer and is widely read by both professional and lay people throughout the world. *The American Cancer Society Cancer Book* is an outstanding example of the high quality of the Society's extensive cancer literature.

The important historic contributions to the literature on cancer which are described in this chapter are by no means the only ones that have been made. In fact, it would be a herculean task to even list the many valuable and major works written by numerous authorities throughout the world.

REFERENCES

Bashford, E. F. (1907). Review. "A history of cancer". *Br. Med. J.*, **1**, 1061

Finzi, N. S. and Harmer, D. (1928). Radium treatment of intrinsic carcinoma of the larynx. *Br. Med. J.*, **2**, 886

Gordon-Watson, Sir Charles (1928). Radiation in the treatment of cancer of the rectum. *Rep. Int. Conf. Cancer, London*, pp 100–6

Harmer, D. (1927). Radium treatment of carcinoma of larynx and tongue. *St Bartholomew's Hospital Reports*, Vol. 60, pp 113–26

Hunter, J. (1837). In Palmer, F. (ed.) *Lectures on the Principles of Surgery*, Vol. 1

Ledoux, L. (1923). La radio et radium therapie en oto-rhino-laryngologie. *J. Belge de Radiologie*, **12** (2), 60

Ministry of Health (1927). Report on cancer of the rectum. *Reports on Public Health Subjects*, No. 46, pp 1–70. H.M. Stationery Office, London

Neuman, F. and Coryn, G. (1928). The radio-surgical treatment of cancer of the rectum. *Rep. Int. Conf. Cancer, London*, pp 128–30

Newman, Sir George (1927). Prefatory note to "Report on cancer of the uterus" by J. E. Lane-Clayton. *Reports on Public Health and Medical Subjects*, No. 40, p 5. H.M. Stationery Office, London

Raven, R. W. (1958). *Cancer of the Pharynx, Larynx and Oesophagus and Its Surgical Treatment.* Butterworth & Co., London

Raven, R. W. (ed.) (1957–1959). *Cancer.* Butterworth & Co. London

Raven, R. W. (ed.) (1960 and 1963). *Cancer Progress.* Butterworth & Co., London

Trotter, W. (1913). Operative treatment of malignant disease of the mouth and pharynx. *Lancet*, **1**, 1075

CHAPTER SIX

The Broad Image of Oncology

Oncology is defined as the multidisciplinary subject compounded of arts and sciences which is concerned with the nature, aetiology, prevention, diagnosis and definitive treatment of the group of diseases known traditionally as cancer (but now proposed to be called "oncological diseases") and with the rehabilitation and continuing care of patients suffering from them.

The component of arts comprises the treatment modalities of surgery, medicine and radiation, and rehabilitation and continuing care. The component of sciences comprises a large group of basic sciences which is making fundamental academic and clinical contributions to our knowledge of the nature, aetiology and behaviour of oncological diseases.

The broad image of oncology should be clearly seen in this way by all oncologists, both research and clinical, because their work is closely interrelated. Oncologists cannot work in isolation; team-work is essential and members of the team must have the ability to communicate and have some general knowledge of the main aspects of the subject.

Oncology is divided into a system of subdivisions which are clearly defined to show the broad spectrum of research and clinical work which it embraces. They are listed in Table 1.

RESEARCH ONCOLOGY

Many individuals have increased our knowledge of cancer, through their observations and research work, over a long period of several centuries. During recent decades, with the development of laboratory sciences, scientific methodology and new equipment, the volume of research work has expanded considerably, resulting in important discoveries being made, including advances in patient care and management, and an increase in our knowledge of the nature and aetiology of the oncological diseases.

Table 1 The subdivisions of oncology

Research oncology
Laboratory and experimental research
Epidemiology research
Clinical research
Clinical oncology
Rehabilitation and continuing care
Surgical oncology
Medical oncology
Radiation oncology
Nursing oncology
Gynaecological oncology
Paediatric oncology
General practice oncology
Social oncology
Prevention and screening programmes
Community education
Resettlement of patients
Oncology philosophy
Recognition and solution of major problems

In past years an enormous expenditure of research effort and time was spent in the study of tumours induced in small animals. Whilst important discoveries were made and many scientific data accumulated, they made only a limited contribution towards the solution of the problems of human cancer. Increasing attention is now focused on the spontaneous malignant tumours occurring in humans and on the development of laboratory sciences, including molecular biology, without the need for experiments on animals. The key subject where illumination is essential is the mechanism of carcinogenesis; already a wide range of physical and chemical carcinogens is recognised. Considerable research is being done, therefore, on cellular chemistry, including nucleic acid and protein metabolism; on genetics and oncogenes; on immunology; and on virology. There is further discussion about these basic sciences later in this book.

Epidemiological and statistical research continues to develop and valuable aetiological clues have been provided which have resulted in prevention programmes being formulated. Studies are proceeding concerning the life-style of people, including their environment, occupations, habits and customs. More information is being gathered about the geographical distribution of the oncological diseases and about their incidence in emigrant populations, and reasons are being found for differences in incidence. Already we have sufficient data from epidemiological results to believe that about 75% of oncological diseases could be prevented if the right actions were taken.

It should be remembered that clinicians have made valuable contributions to the knowledge of oncology through their research, which has often been of an observational nature. Particular mention is made here of the historical observations made by Percivall Pott in 1775 about the high incidence of cancer of the skin of the scrotum in chimney-sweeps. These eventually led to the isolation and synthesis of dibenzpyrene, the carcinogen present in coal-tar, by Kennaway and his colleagues around the year 1930 (see Chapter 17).

CLINICAL ONCOLOGY

The basis of clinical oncology is rehabilitation and continuing care of patients with cancer. Rehabilitation begins with diagnosis and this is followed by definitive treatment with the objective of restoring the patient to a life of good quality. Clinical oncology includes the specialities of surgical, medical, radiation and nursing oncology, in addition to the recognised modalities of gynaecological oncology and paediatric oncology. The clinical oncologist in each discipline requires a sound knowledge of the theory of oncology described in Chapter 7, which is acquired by a continuing learning process throughout professional life. Before specialising in clinical oncology he or she must have a complete basic medical training so as to develop clinical knowledge and technical skills in the chosen art of surgery, medicine or radiation disciplines. He or she should understand the indications, results and complications of the different oncology treatments, which may be given singly or in combination. The "treatment triad", comprising surgery, medicine and radiation, is used increasingly for cancer patients, especially now that more effective chemotherapy is available.

The practice of oncology is described in Chapter 8, but certain observations are made here in this context.

The surgical oncologist must be a well-trained technical surgeon with a good background of operative experience in general surgery, or a surgical speciality, who concentrates either wholly or part-time on surgical oncology. Whilst there are some surgeons who have a total or major interest in oncology, it is recognised that there are many general and specialist surgeons who carry a heavy oncological work-load in addition to their other responsibilities. Education and training in oncology will enable all to acquire new knowledge and skills to help them in their work.

The medical oncologist is basically a well-trained skilful physician who acquires special knowledge and experience in the care and management of patients with oncological diseases, including leukaemias and lymphomas. Special expertise is required to carry out modern methods of diagnosis, including endoscopy techniques of all types. The medical oncologist has special knowledge of the expanding disciplines of chemotherapy and hormonal therapy, in addition to responsibilities for the general treatment and care of the patient.

The radiation oncologist is basically a well-trained clinician who then acquires special experience and expertise in treating patients with oncological diseases by different methods of radiation. He or she is also concerned with the general management and care of the patients and many also undertake chemotherapy and hormonal therapy.

The gynaecological oncologist is a well-trained general gynaecologist who develops special knowledge of the oncological diseases of the female pelvic organs and genitalia, and of the diagnosis and treatment of such diseases. He or she may be totally committed to oncology or practise it as a special interest in addition to general gynaecological work.

The paediatric oncologist may be a physician or surgeon with the appropriate basic education and training in paediatrics who is devoted to the care of children with oncological diseases, including leukaemias, lymphomas and various solid tumours. These sick children are usually investigated, diagnosed, treated and cared for in special paediatric clinics and hospitals.

Nurse oncologists are fully trained and experienced nurses who have subsequently acquired special knowledge in oncology and skills in the treatment, management and nursing care of patients with oncological diseases. They are taking an increasing and important part in chemotherapy, including administering carcinostatic drugs and monitoring the patients undergoing different treatment regimens. They play a vital role in the rehabilitation and continuing care units and are skilled in methods of symptom control and the management of patients with chronic pain. Patients may be treated in hospital, special homes or hospices; there are also many patients in the community who require special care in their own homes. Some nurses specialise in pain control management and are accordingly designated "pain nurses".

It is emphasised that all clinical oncologists are educated in the basic oncological sciences to a different extent according to the modality of treatment with which they are concerned — surgery, medicine, radiation or nursing. For example, the medical oncologist must have an in-depth knowledge of clinical pharmacology, whilst the radiation oncologist must be well versed in radiobiology and radiation physics. The surgical oncologist needs to have a sound knowledge of pathology, including histopathology, cytology, biochemistry, haematology and the modes of dissemination of malignant tumours.

Oncology in general practice

The doctor in general practice has a big responsibility in many aspects of oncology, so this subject should occupy an important place in the medical curriculum of medical undergraduates so that they are properly prepared for their work.

The general practitioner should play an important role in cancer prevention and screening programmes, including making the early diagnosis of oncological diseases. After the definitive treatment of patients in hospital he or she must undertake the responsible work of rehabilitation and continuing care as a member of the oncology team, so close liaison with the other team members must be established. Many patients with oncological diseases wish to be treated and cared for in their own homes for the remaining period of their lives. Consequently, they and their families need to be given much support and help by the home-care team, of which the family doctor and the nurse are important members.

SOCIAL ONCOLOGY

This important subdivision of oncology is concerned with the community in relation to the general and widespread incidence of oncological diseases and with solutions to the problems which they cause.

Prevention

The prevention of oncological diseases means the avoidance of any form of these diseases in any stage of their development, whether this is early or late. From the historical viewpoint the recognition of prevention is a relatively recent event, which is of fundamental importance for people throughout the world because of its enormous practical value today and in the future. In fact, prevention offers the brightest hope for the future, where these diseases are concerned, for it could save countless lives in all nations and preclude much suffering.

The following quotation is taken from the Preface to *The Prevention of Cancer (Raven and Roe, 1967)*: "In recent years knowledge of causes and causative mechanisms has been accumulating rapidly; numerous chemical, physical and viral agents are now known to be capable of causing cancer in experimental animals. In some cases it has been shown beyond reasonable doubt that exposure to the same or similar agents leads to the induction of cancer in man. This newly acquired knowledge makes possible a new approach to the problem of human cancer, namely cancer prevention."

The prevention of oncological diseases is one of the most outstanding medical challenges today in view of their occurrence world-wide and the high mortality they cause. Its importance is stressed by the realisation that about 75% of oncological diseases could be prevented if people responded to our present knowledge about their causation and protected themselves. This would mean alterations in the life-style of many people. For example, in the Western world the tobacco cancers cause the majority of deaths from malignant diseases. Lung cancer is an epidemic of huge magnitude and is spreading throughout many nations. Consequently, if tobacco could be totally abolished from human use, very many lives could be saved. In the meantime a great effort is being made to dissuade young people from commencing the dangerous habit of smoking and to advise and help those who already do so to stop. Thus prevention is closely linked with community education whereby people are taught salient facts about cancer and the actions they should take, including making changes in their life-style, in order to avoid incurring a malignant disease.

Figure 6.1 *Below:* After smoking a clay pipe for many years this male patient developed a squamous cell carcinoma in the floor of the mouth where the stem of the pipe impinged. *Bottom left:* The squamous cell carcinoma involving the lower mandible. The affected floor of the mouth and the horizontal ramus of the left mandible were widely excised. *Bottom centre:* Photograph taken after the excision wound had completely healed. *Bottom right:* The patient 2 years and 2 months after excision of the carcinoma.

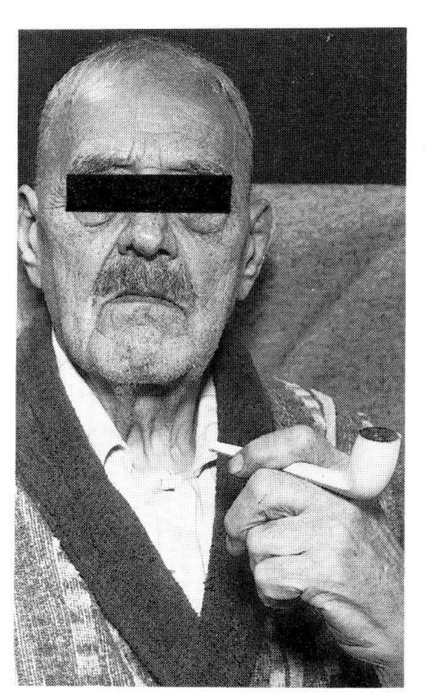

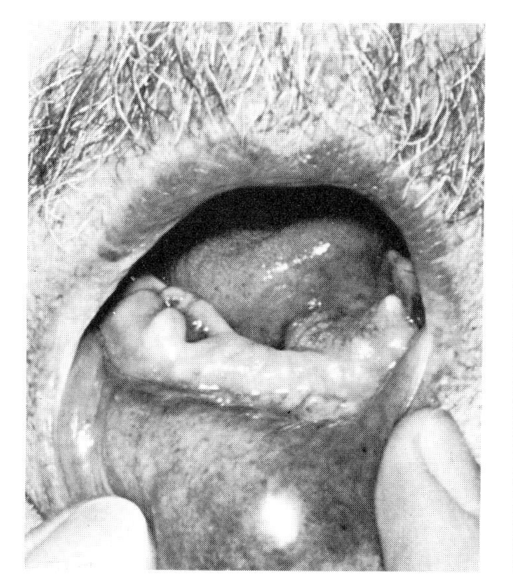

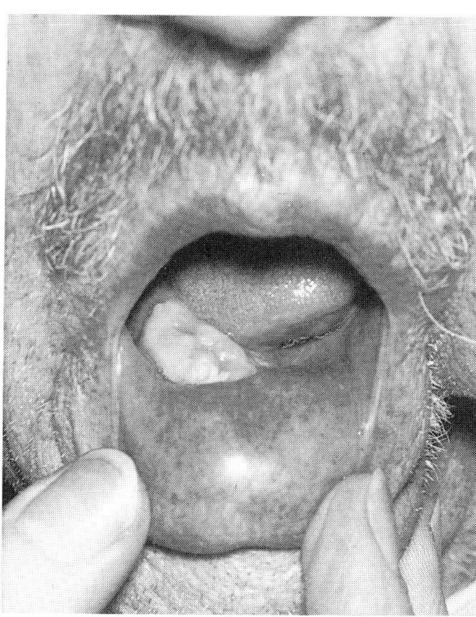

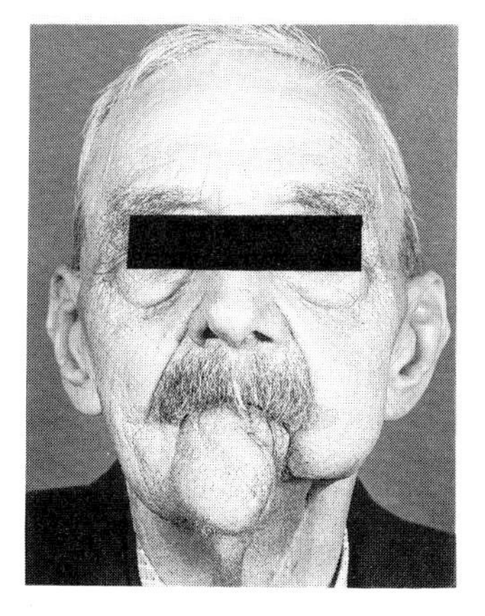

Community education

In order to be able to control and prevent oncological diseases the medical profession must take the public into their confidence and provide the relevant information about the diseases, so that they can gain collaboration and compliance in their work, in addition to engendering optimism and hope in place of much of the fear now experienced.

It is encouraging and noteworthy to see how much community education has increased in scope and content during recent years. Several decades ago it was considered inappropriate to even mention the word "cancer" because of its dismal connotations. Since then attitudes have changed completely and useful information and advice are now freely given. These important changes and developments have occurred through the efforts of governments, voluntary organisations and individuals.

The information for the community concerns the general nature and effects of the oncological diseases, including the known aetiological factors. The latter are combined with advice to people on how to protect themselves and avoid oncological diseases by appropriately changing their life-style, habits and customs.

Members of the community are taught about the early symptoms and signs of the diseases and given helpful advice on how to act under different conditions, including seeking a medical examination. All the information is suitably presented so that it does not cause fear and apprehension.

The value of periodic health examinations, including screening tests such as cervical cytology for carcinoma of the uterus and premalignant lesions, sputum cytology for lung carcinoma, and mammography to detect early breast carcinoma, is now appreciated.

"Well women" clinics can be attended by women who want to have clinical examinations and special investigations. There is also a need for "well men clinics", for clinics of this type are of real value to people who are in high-risk groups with regard to cancer.

Different methods of communication are used to educate the public and provide information. These include the media: the press, television and radio. Lecture and discussion meetings are arranged, and printed leaflets and booklets are available which give useful information on particular subjects, including the care of patients. Voluntary associations are also carrying out valuable work in community education, giving advice and support to well people, cancer patients and their families.

Resettlement of patients

The objective of rehabilitation and continuing care in cancer is to restore patients to a long, good quality life that is normal or near normal, depending upon the prognosis following definitive treatment (see Chapter 9).

Patients are finally resettled at home with their families and can resume their employment, in addition to engaging again in their recreational pursuits.

The work of resettlement is undertaken by different members of the oncology team, including the family doctor, community physician, community nurse and social worker. Consultation with the specialist oncologist is likely to be necessary.

Changes and readjustments to the patients' life-style and alterations in the home may also be necessary. After rehabilitation many patients can carry the same work-load as the normal population. Others may require adjustments to be made in their particular work or new work to be found for them. Thus their employers may need to be consulted; they are usually helpful and sympathetic in their response.

Following their rehabilitation, the patients are assessed for their resettlement programme, so that any defects can be corrected and any residual deformities measured and dealt with. The assessment also enables the patient to receive appropriate guidance concerning the need for adjustments to be made in his or her home conditions, life-style, employment and recreations.

ONCOLOGY PHILOSOPHY

Oncology philosophy is an important subdivision of oncology and is well worthy of attention, though it is dealt with only briefly here.

It embraces important questions which are designed to enlarge our conception of what is possible, it enriches our imagination, and it diminishes the dogmatic assurance which can close the mind to profitable speculation.

There are major and difficult problems in oncology which still await solution; much hard work remains to be done. The major problems are set out in Table 2.

Table 2 Major problems in oncology philosophy

1. Cell division and carcinogenesis mechanisms
2. Tumour invasion and metastatic mechanisms
3. Hormonal control mechanisms
4. Immunological mechanisms:
   Immunodiagnosis, immunotherapy, immunoprophylaxis
5. Cell chemistry, basic components and disturbance

PROGRESS IN ONCOLOGY

The broad image of oncology which has been portrayed in this chapter demonstrates the enormous progress which has been made throughout many centuries and especially during recent decades. This progress is clearly apparent when oncology is viewed against the historical background of "cancer", which stretches out over several millennia. The notable advances made during the last half century owe much to the developments in scientific education, training and methodology which have now culminated in the emergence and establishment of the multidisciplinary subject of oncology. This is our modern vehicle to ensure rapid progress in the future.

Basic contributions to modern knowledge have been made by different scientific disciplines using new scientific and clinical methodology, instruments and apparatus. The establishment of team-work between scientists and clinicians is a noteworthy achievement which should ensure there is a constant feedback of new knowledge between clinics and laboratories. It is fascinating to speculate about the nature and direction of the advances in oncology which will inevitably occur during the next half century. The study of the evolution of oncology from the era of antiquity to the present day is an absorbing intellectual exercise. It gives us a clear picture of the present position and provides indications for future progress in research and clinical oncology.

REFERENCE

Raven, R. W. and Roe, F. J. C. (eds) (1967). *The Prevention of Cancer*. Butterworth & Co., London

CHAPTER SEVEN

The Theory of Oncology

In the elaborate and extensive theory of oncology which is now established, the continuing and fundamental contributions which are being made by a number of different basic sciences can be clearly recognised. The close relevance of these sciences to oncology merits their title of basic oncological sciences. The practice of surgery is traditionally based on a sound background knowledge of surgical anatomy, surgical physiology and surgical pathology. By the same token the theory of oncology is translated into the practice of oncology for the benefit of patient care.

All oncologists need to study the basic oncological sciences, to which they will constantly refer throughout their professional lives, and clinicians will select for special study those sciences which are most relevant for their particular practice. It is, of course, impossible to acquire an in-depth knowledge of all the basic oncological sciences, but every oncologist should at least understand their terminology and general relevance to the work.

BIOLOGY OF CANCER

Attention must be focused on the individual cancer cell which becomes conglomerated to form the malignant tumour. The outstanding property of cancer cells is their destructiveness. They can invade contiguous tissues, including blood and lymphatic vessels; they can detach themselves from the parent tumour and multiply in other parts of the body, forming metastases in lymph nodes and organs. This process of invasion, metaplasia and multiplication can continue without restraint by the host.

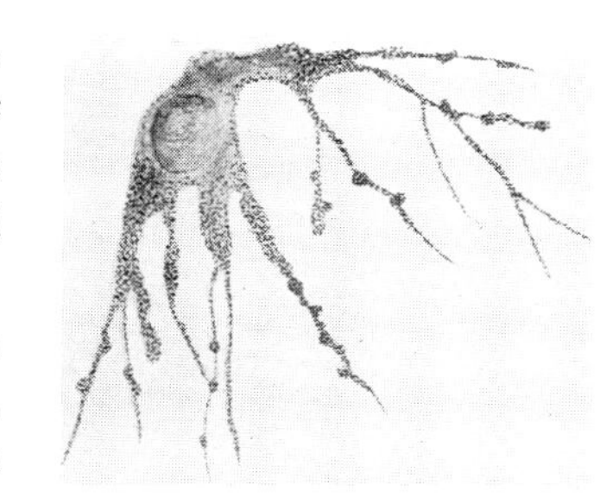

Figure 7.1 Photograph of a single melanoblast, the type cell of malignant melanoma, showing its pseudopodia processes containing melanin.

The cancer cell is a complex entity; it is larger than normal, has a division time-scale faster than normal and its energy requirements are increased. The cell membrane itself is a complex structure containing receptors which monitor the cell's environment, including the normal hormones and the abnormal cytotoxic chemicals. The membrane relays any relevant observations on its environment to the intracellular systems of genes and enzymes. In fact, the cell membrane is the "eyes and ears of the genes".

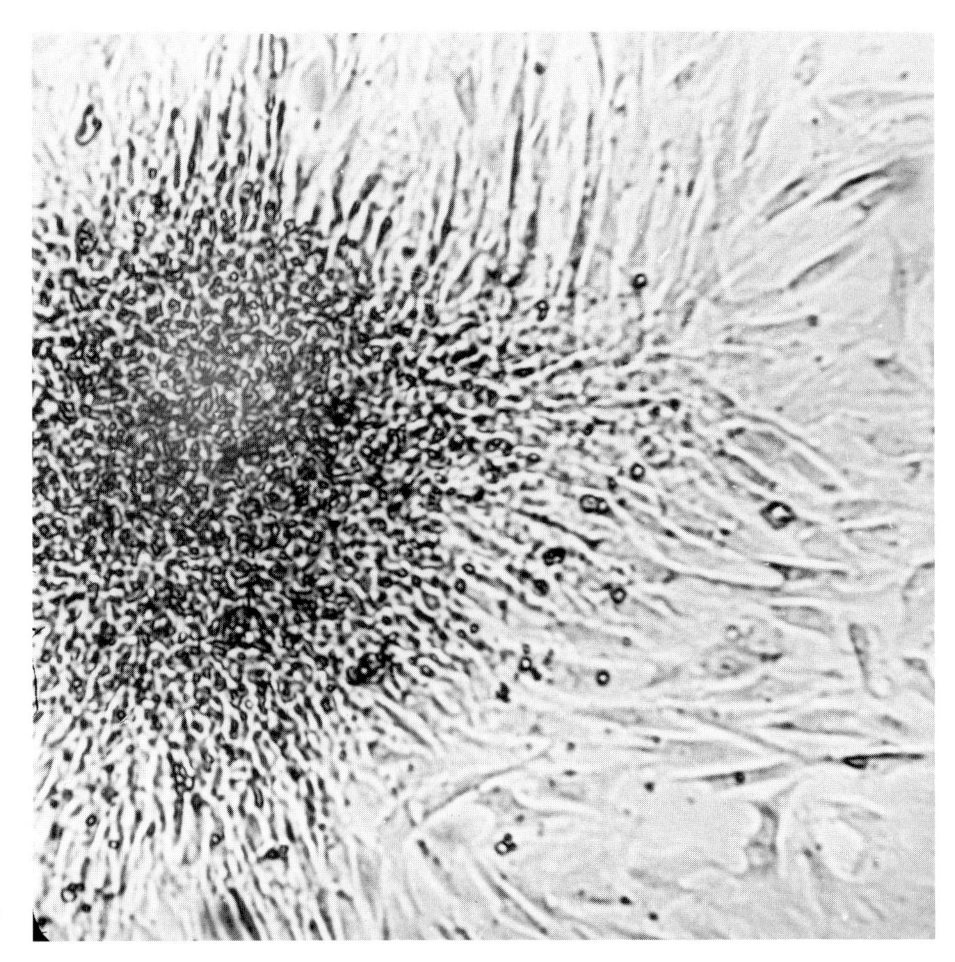

Figure 7.2 A fragment of a human breast carcinoma growing in tissue culture, showing the migration of cells from its periphery (X 135). Note the mound of epithelial cells.

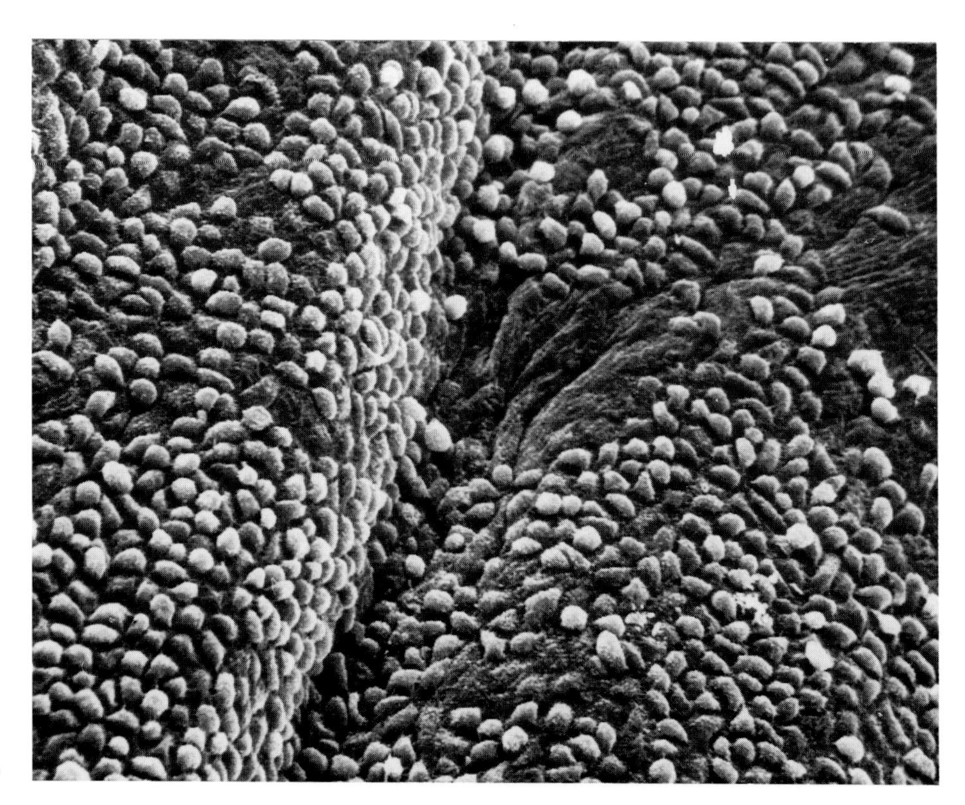

Figure 7.3 Ascitic tumour cells adhering to the peritoneum lining the abdominal cavity as viewed in a scanning electron microscope (X 800).

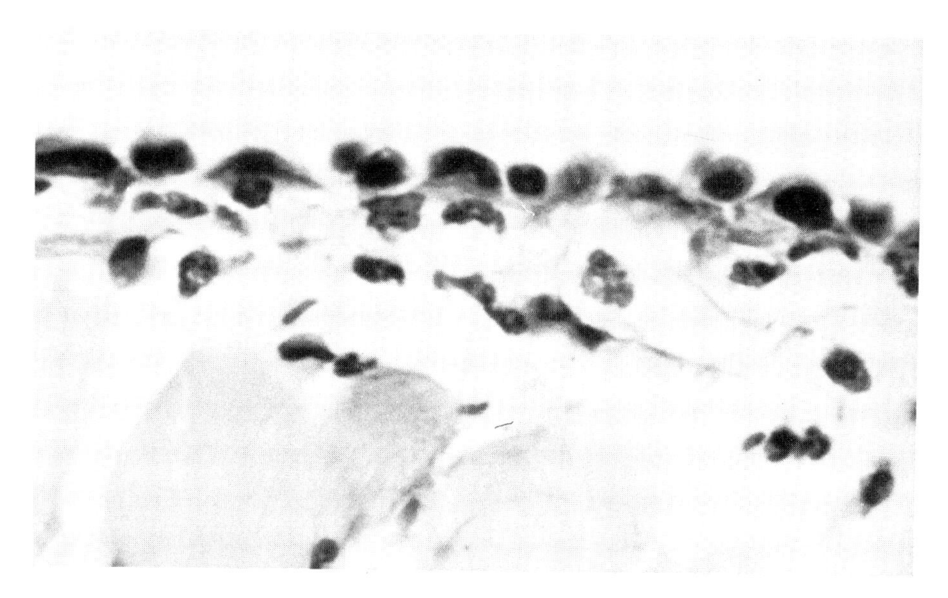

Figure 7.4 Ascitic tumour cells adhering to the peritoneum lining the abdominal cavity as viewed in a light microscope (X 200). The cells form a single layer on the surface and invasion has not yet occurred. A cellular response is taking place against the tumour, demonstrated by cells of the host, including polymorphonuclear leucocytes, which have migrated into the subjacent tissue.

The mechanism whereby a normal cell is changed into a cancer cell is known as carcinogenesis. Knowledge of how this process occurs still eludes us, although we recognise a wide range of carcinogens, both physical and chemical, in nature. The chemistry of the cell is the object of continuous research and much attention has been given to the changes in the chemistry of the cell nucleus which cause its malignant behaviour. Computer analysis is being increasingly used in this work, with the mathematical modelling of cell processes.

Growth control systems, including cytoplasmic and intercellular systems, are being investigated. Hormonal control systems are of fundamental importance in the development and treatment of breast and prostate carcinoma, and it is likely that other malignant neoplasms are under hormonal influences. An interesting beginning has been made to the understanding of these systems by the recognition of oestrogen, androgen and progesterone receptors in the cell membrane (see also Chapter 19).

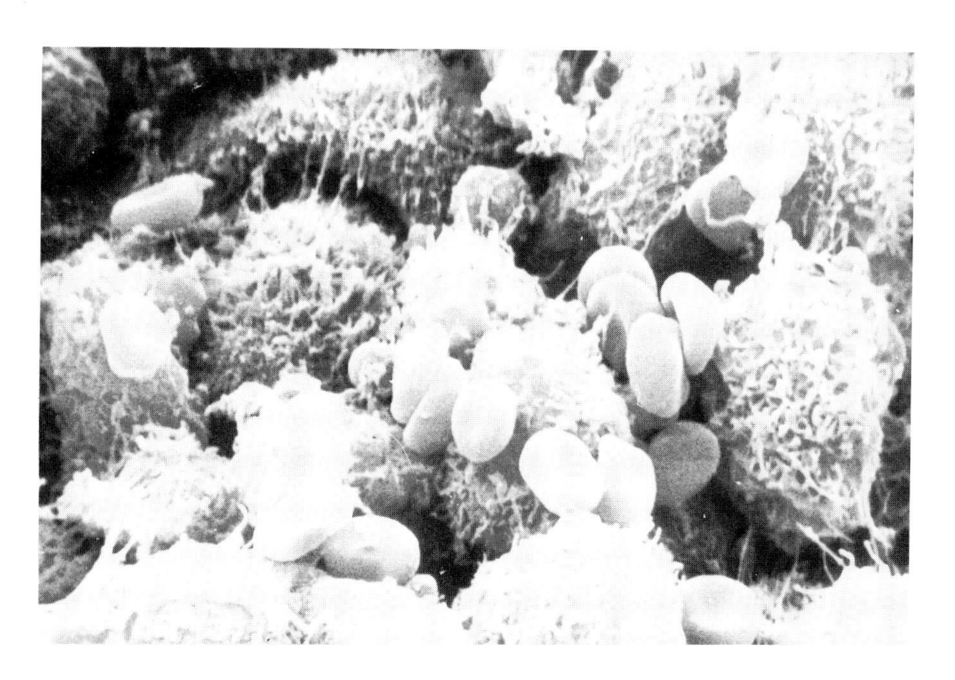

Figure 7.5 Ascitic tumour cells invading the peritoneum of the host as viewed in an electron microscope (X 11 000). The tumour has caused haemorrhage which is evidenced by the red blood corpuscles adhering to the sides of the tumour cells.

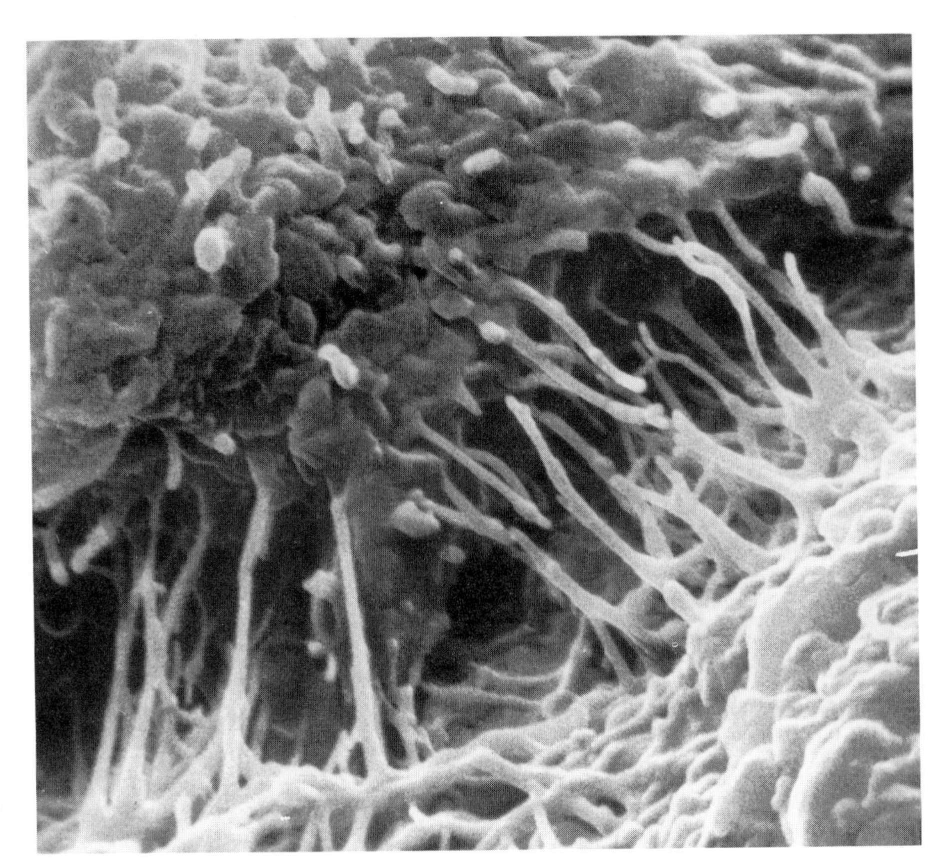

Figure 7.6 The interaction between an ascitic tumour cell and a host cell as viewed in an electron microscope (X 27 500). The alignment of the processes from each cell suggests that some sort of message, possibly a chemotactic one, is involved.

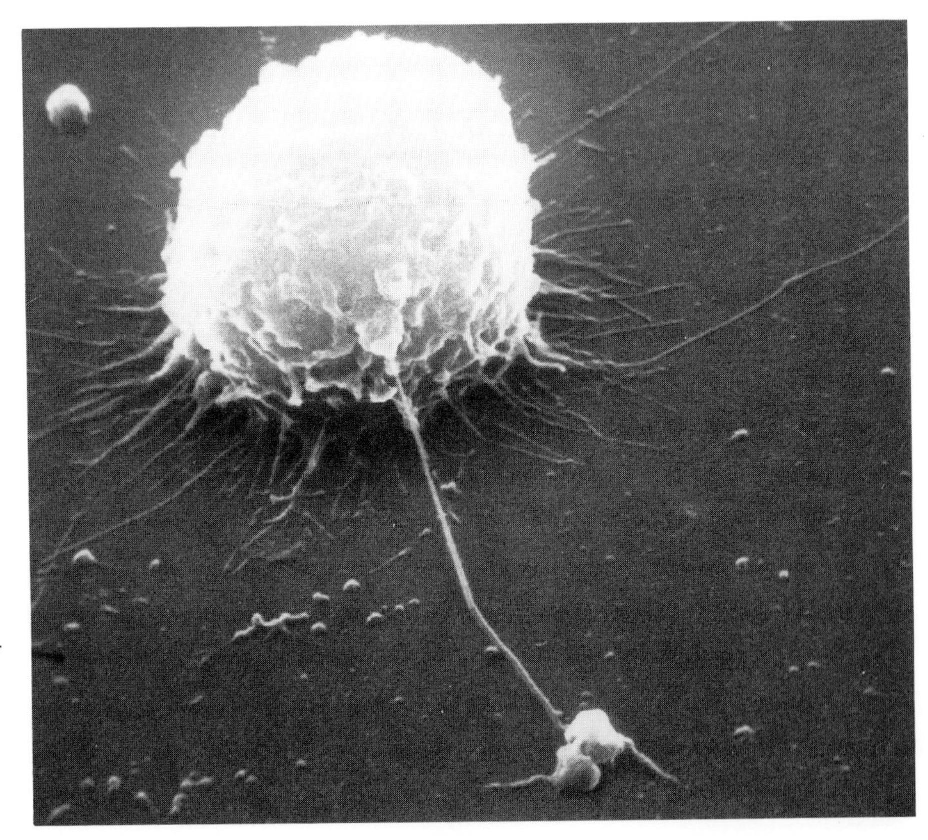

Figure 7.7 By subjecting tumour cells in tissue culture to proteolytic enzymes it is possible to observe their attachment to the substrate in an electron microscope. The large process seen here in the foreground with the bleb of cytoplasm at its end is the remnant of the ruffled membrane and indicates the direction of cell movement (X 10 500).

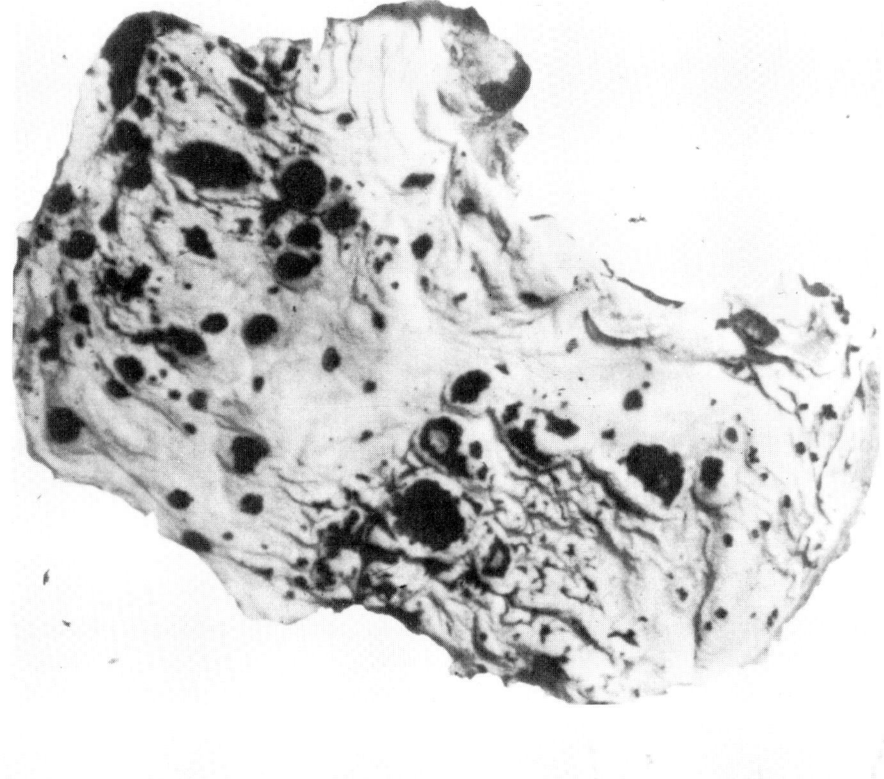

Figure 7.8 A stomach with multiple metastases of malignant melanoma — a rare condition.

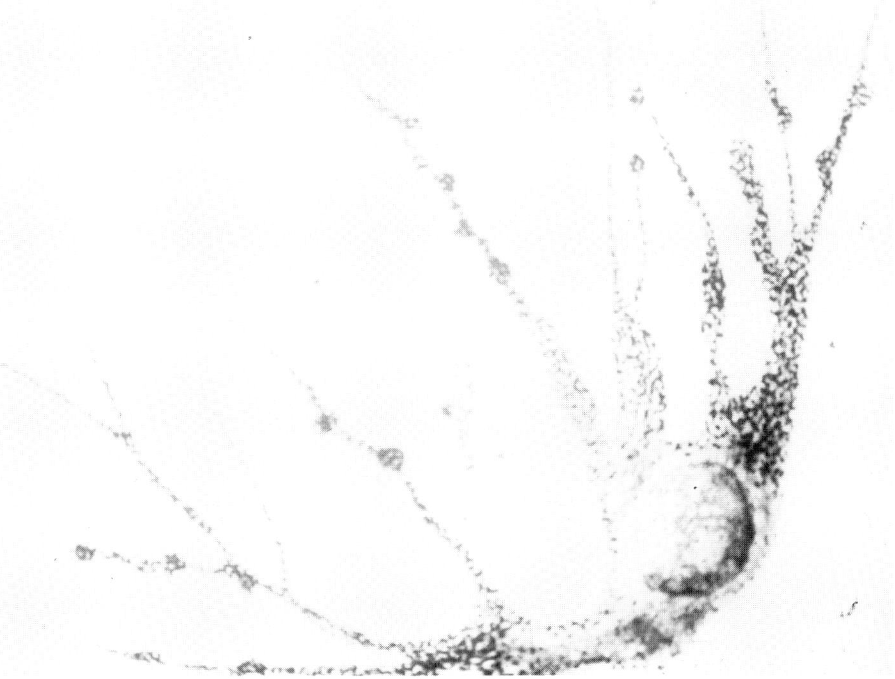

Figure 7.9 Histological specimen of a malignant melanoma of the oesophagus, showing irregular polymorphic cells without any pattern. Tumour giant cells are present and there are cells containing melanin.

PATHOLOGY

A sound knowledge of general pathology is essential in order to understand the natural history of the numerous and different oncological diseases and their effective treatment. Their effects, which are so serious for the host, must be clearly recognised, so that they can be rectified or minimised by appropriate management. Certain tumours can secrete chemical substances which can prove lethal for the patient unless their effects are neutralised at once.

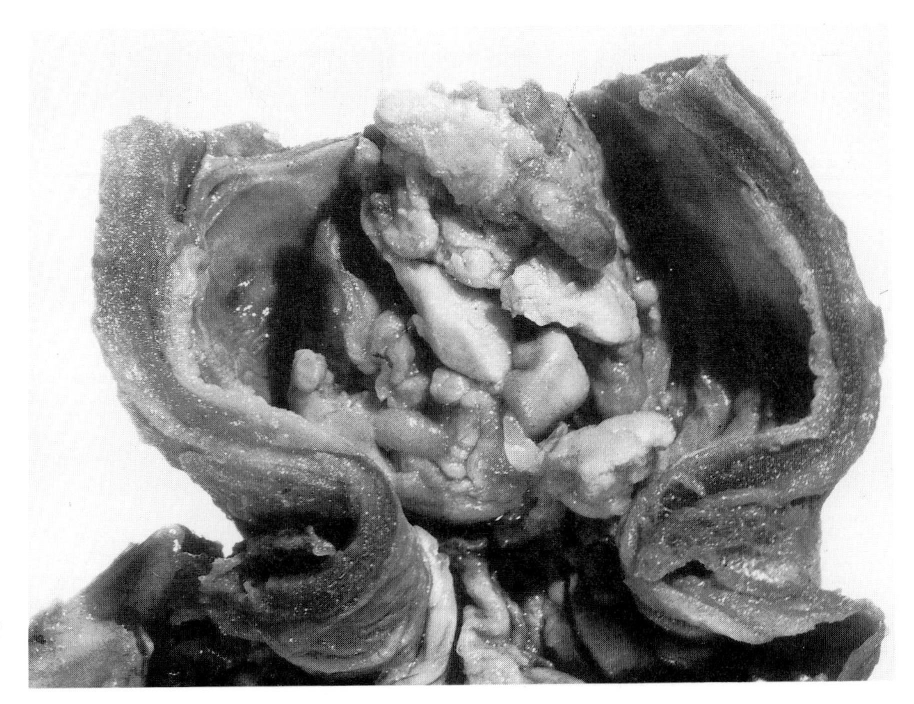

Figure 7.10 A specimen removed by a partial oesophago-gastrectomy with an oesophago-gastric anastomosis showing a primary malignant melanoma of the oesophagus of a female patient aged 52. This variety of melanoma is protuberant, polypoid and pedunculated.

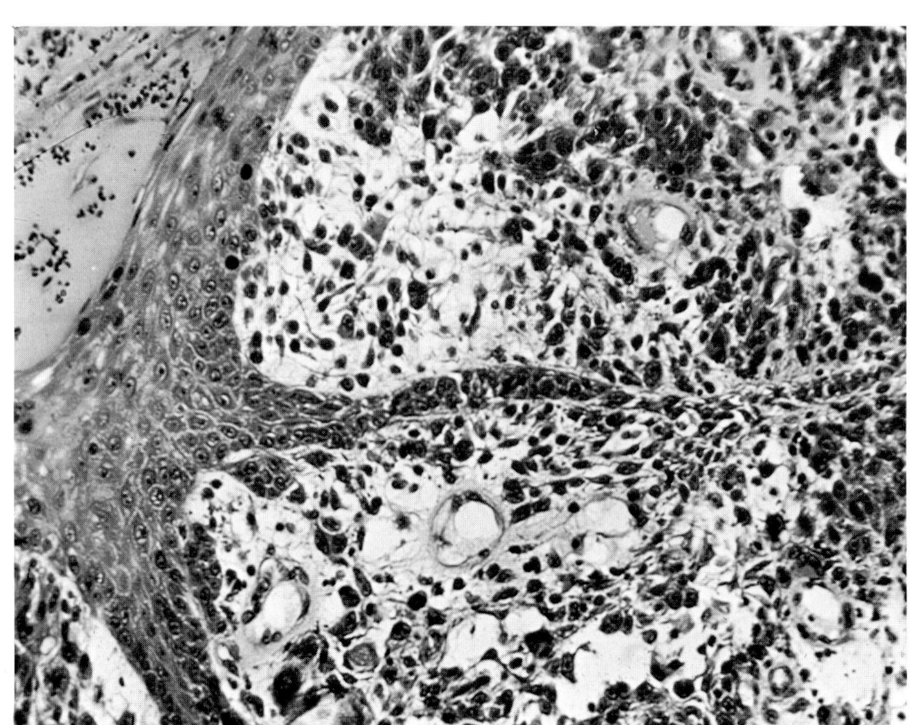

Figure 7.11 Malignant melanoma of the skin.

The subject of pathology includes several laboratory sciences: haematology, biochemistry, histopathology, cytology, microbiology and virology.

Haematology monitoring is routinely done in clinical practice, especially for patients who are undergoing chemotherapy. Supportive treatment with cell component therapy is frequently required, and allogenic marrow grafting, which needs knowledge of histocompatibility, is increasing in importance in the treatment of certain patients.

The academic and clinical importance of biochemistry is fully recognised and an increasing number of investigations are now available for diagnosis, treatment and patient monitoring. The oncologist must understand the alterations in the general body metabolism and the profound biochemical disturbances which are caused by the secretions from certain tumours. Clinical syndromes can be recognised, including the argentaffinoma syndrome, hypercalcaemia and hyperuricaemia, which are good examples.

VIROLOGY

Virology has gained increasing importance now that research oncologists are identifying oncogenic viruses. Oncogenes which directly cause malig-

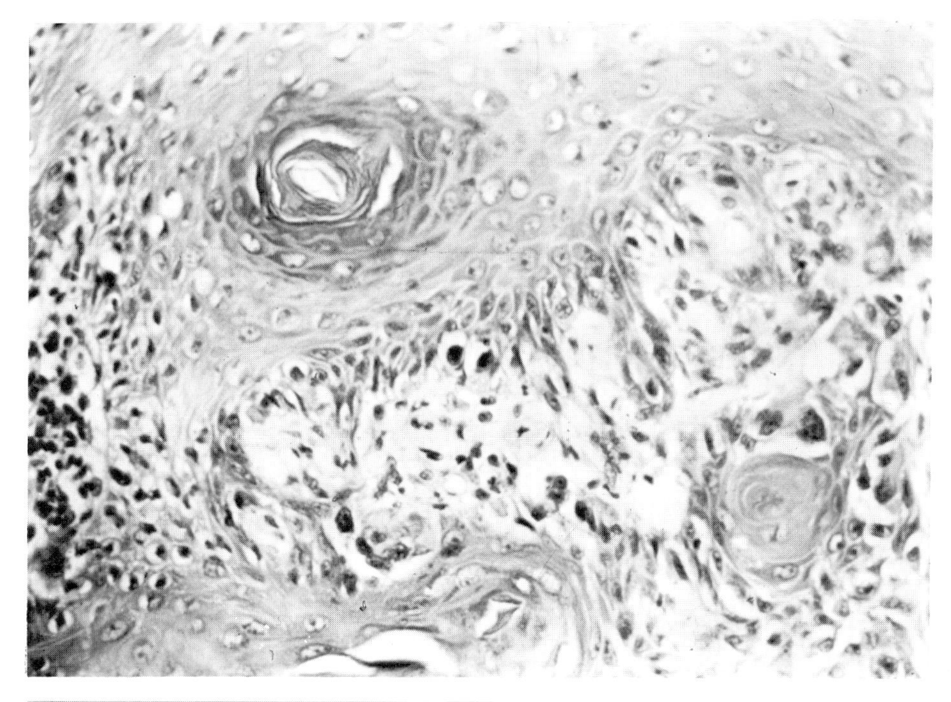

Figure 7.12 Junctional activity in malignant melanoma of the skin.

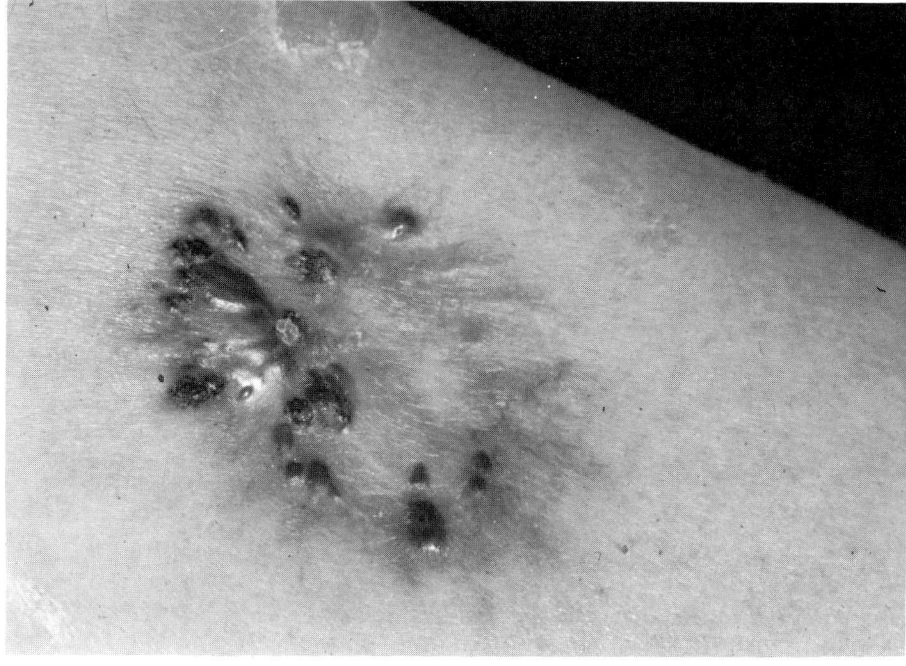

Figure 7.13 Malignant melanoma of the skin with satellite tumours.

nant transformation of cells growing in tissue culture have been found in human tumour cell lines and tumour tissues and isolated from them. These cellular genes are closely related to the viral genes which cause a number of animal tumours. There may be a viral genome in the neoplastic cell which could be inactivated by a monoclonal antibody, or dealt with through the DNA sequence.

Primary carcinoma of the liver is very common in African and some other countries and it is now thought that it supervenes in the liver of people who have had hepatitis B. This has led to the procedure of vaccinating young children against infection by the hepatitis B virus as a preventive treatment for carcinoma of the liver, a step which might represent the first immunoprophylactic measure against malignant diseases (see Chapter 22).

ENDOCRINOLOGY AND METABOLIC MEDICINE

The endocrine system plays a vital role in regulating the normal development of organs and systems in the body. It is therefore logical to assume that a close relationship exists with abnormal growth, a possibility which has been the object of clinical observations and research investigation for more than 100 years.

We now recognise the hormonal manifestations of a number of tumours and are learning more about ectopic hormone secretions which cause different clinical syndromes. Some of these are life-threatening, so immediate diagnosis and treatment are mandatory. Spectacular results are obtained in patients with carcinoma of the breast and prostate by manipulating hormonal control mechanisms through endocrine surgery, or by the administration of synthetic hormones. It is even possible to reverse breast carcinoma to benign tissue by hormonal treatment — bilateral oophorectomy and bilateral adrenalectomy — so that we can now visualise the possibility of healing early breast and prostate carcinoma by synthetic hormone administration when we understand the hormonal mechanisms of these diseases. Enormous progress has been made since 1896 when Beatson described the regression which occurred in advanced breast carcinoma after oophorectomy. A more recent advance in hormonal control is the measurement of the oestrogen receptor status of the primary breast carcinoma, which is a useful marker of its biological aggressiveness and hormonal responsiveness (see Chapter 19).

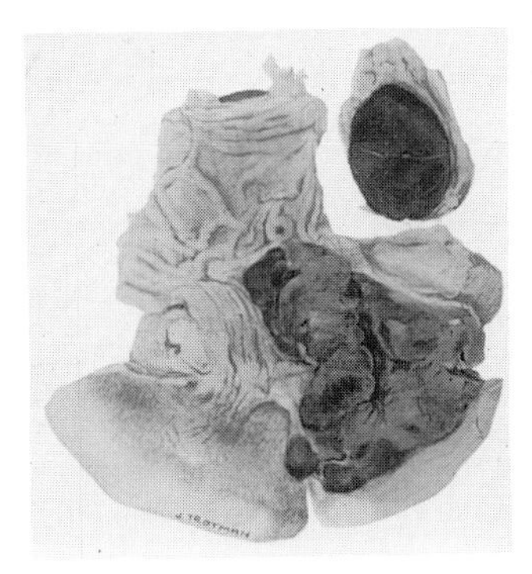

Figure 7.14 A rectum and anus excised because of a malignant melanoma of the anus with a lymph node metastasis.

CLINICAL PHARMACOLOGY

This is a rapidly expanding science of great potential value in treatment and we now have a wide range of different chemicals which are not only beneficial but also curative for patients with leukaemias and lymphomas. These chemicals are used alone, or in combination with surgery and radiation as the "treatment triad". Surgical techniques, such as arterial infusion and perfusion, have been developed to deliver the chemicals into the substance of the tumour. Complete tumour regression for many years has sometimes been achieved.

Inorganic chemicals, including arsenic, mercury and antimony, were first used to treat cancers many decades ago. For example, in 1922 Blair Bell introduced a treatment with lead, which was greeted with much initial enthusiasm, but it was later discarded. Current anticarcinogenic drugs and their analogues are complex organic chemicals, so it is essential to clearly understand the indications for their use, dosage schedules, metabolism and elimination from the body, together with their limitations, toxicity, chemical interactions and side-effects.

New chemicals are being constantly discovered which have exciting prospects, such as the prevention of neoplasia by retinoids; restoring and increasing immune reactions with thymic hormones and levamisole; and direct cytotoxic tumour effects with interferons or monoclonal antibodies (see Chapter 16).

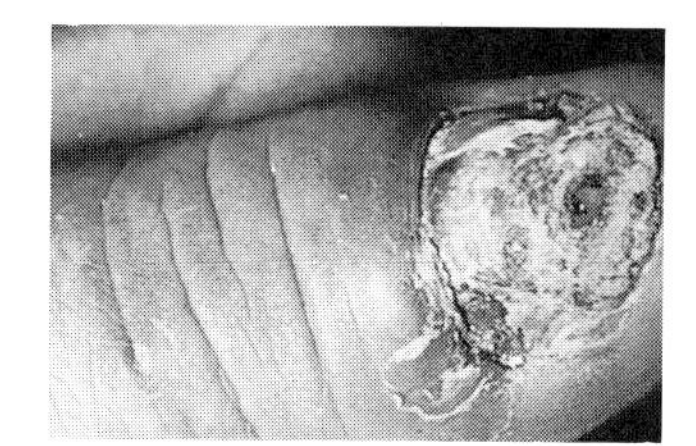

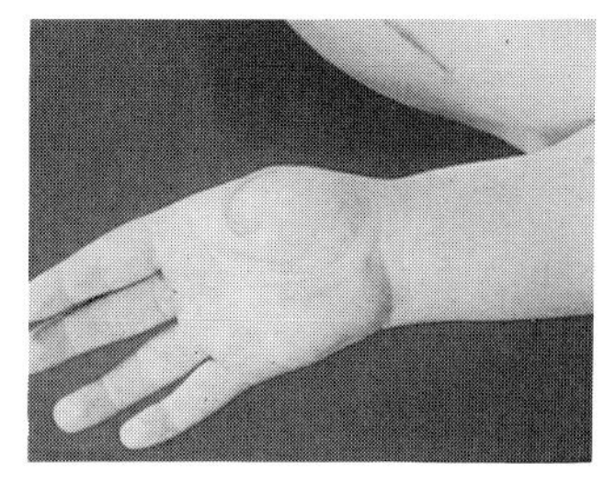

Figure 7.15 *Top:* This subungual malignant melanoma of a right thumb was treated by amputation of the thumb at the metacarpo-phalangeal joint. *Bottom:* The healed hand and axilla after amputation of the thumb and excision of the patient's right axillary lymph nodes.

IMMUNOLOGY

The role of immunological reactions in human cancers is being actively investigated, for it is postulated that they can modify or perhaps even control neoplastic diseases, which might explain the somewhat rare phenomenon of spontaneous regression of primary tumours and also metastases. Immune reactions might be responsible for dormant tumour cells becoming active after many years. The development of malignant diseases after periods of stress and strain might be attributable to depressed host immunity.

An increased incidence of certain malignant diseases, including non-Hodgkin's lymphomas and Kaposi sarcomas, has been observed in patients with immunodeficiency states. In such tumours where a virus might be implicated it might be that it is the virus and not the tumour which is under immune surveillance.

Considerable attention is being given to the possibility of carrying out cancer immunotherapy by manipulating in various ways the immunological reactions of patients. At the present time, however, there is no justification for this form of treatment, but it might develop in the future, in association with monoclonal antibodies.

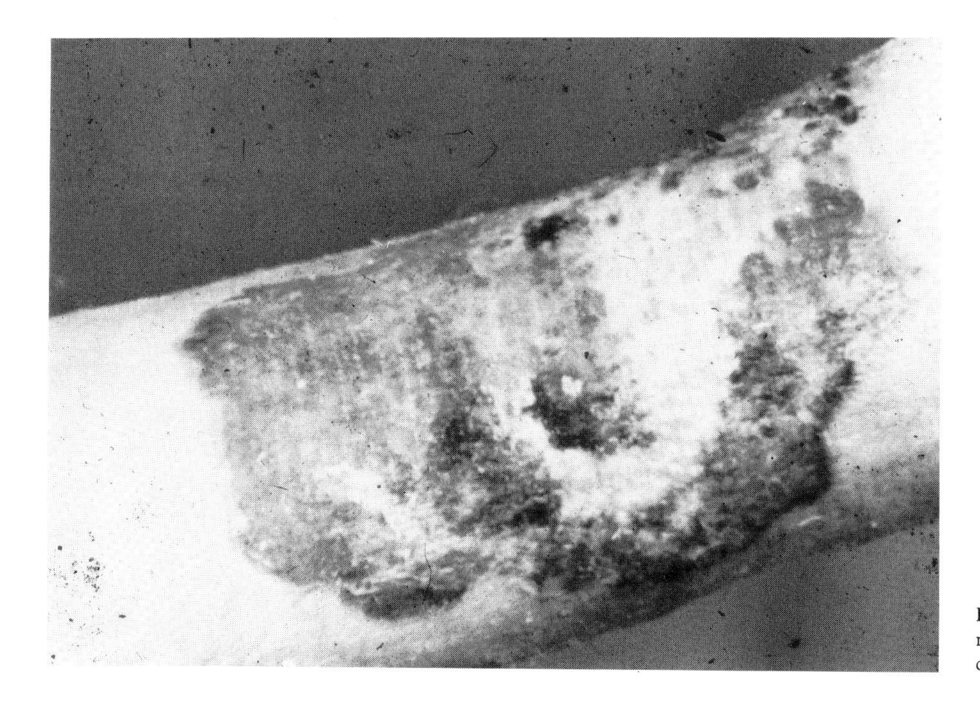

Figure 7.16 Extensive malignant melanoma of the skin of the leg, a condition with a poor prognosis.

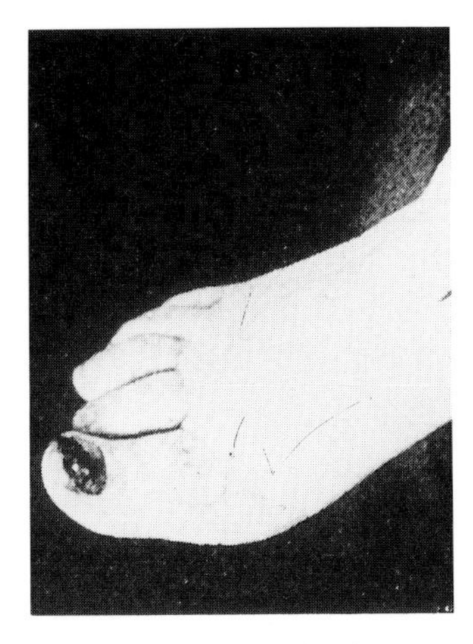

Figure 7.17 Subungual malignant melanoma of the great toe.

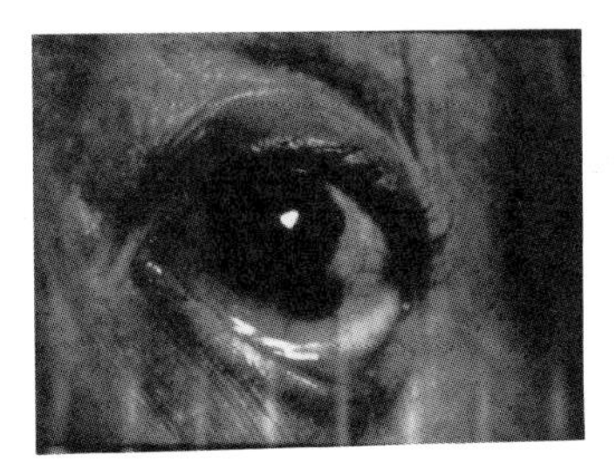

Figure 7.18 A subconjunctival melanoma.

Whilst cancer immunotherapy and cancer immunoprophylaxis are future possibilities, immunodiagnosis is already being used for certain neoplastic diseases. There is considerable interest in carcinoembryonic antigen (CEA) for monitoring the treatment of carcinoma of the colon and detecting recurrent and metastatic disease of this type. Another important test measures the alpha-fetoprotein in the serum of patients with primary hepatoma and the response of this tumour to treatment. It can also be positive in patients with testicular tumours. New tumour relationships and markers are being sought (see Chapter 20).

EPIDEMIOLOGY

This basic science is of great interest to all oncologists and it continues to give valuable information concerning the aetiology of malignant diseases. Important observations made by clinicians in the course of several centuries led to clues regarding the causation of cancer and in this work surgeons, too, played a part. Percivall Pott in 1775 described cancer of the skin of the scrotum in chimney-sweeps and Rehu in 1895 described the occurrence of tumours of the urinary bladder in workers in the aniline dye industry. In recent years an enormous amount of work has been done on the tobacco cancers, especially lung carcinoma, which are the major causes of death throughout the world and obviously the most preventable.

Epidemiology is now divided into three main disciplines. Descriptive epidemiology evaluates the cancer risks for large population groups and studies are carried out on the differences in the geographical incidence of oncological diseases. The incidence of different varieties of these diseases varies considerably in Western and Eastern nations.

Analytical epidemiology seeks to determine the causes of cancer in specific individuals who are affected and the reasons for the aggregation of malignant diseases in different groups of people.

Metabolic epidemiology studies the physical and chemical environ-

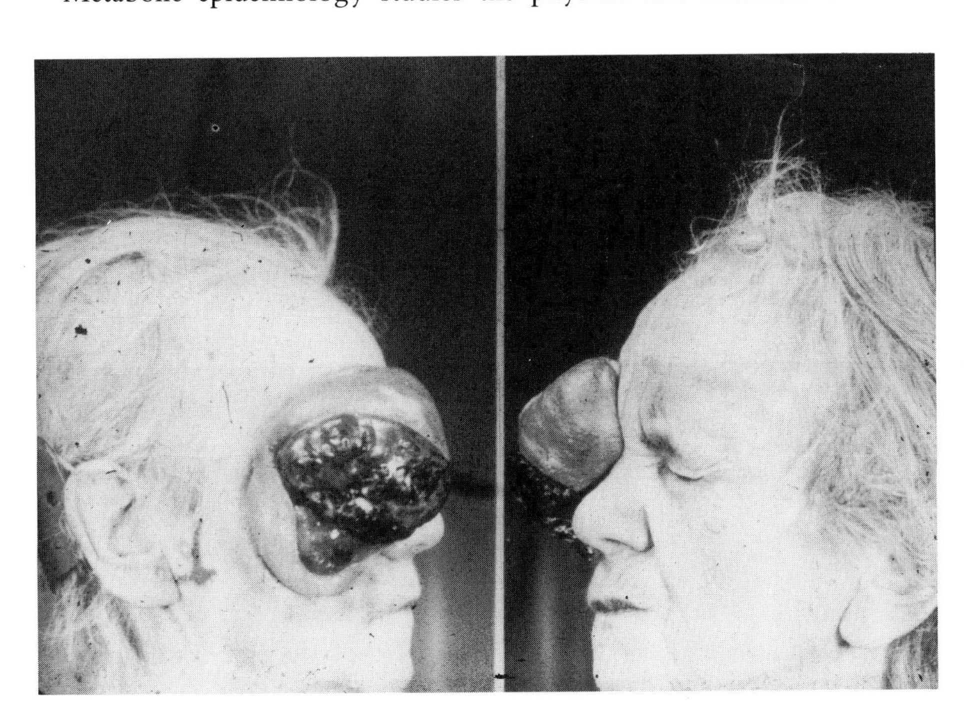

Figure 7.19 Advanced malignant melanoma of a patient's right orbit.

mental factors which are responsible for the causation of different cancers (see Chapter 18).

GENETICS

Increasing emphasis is nowadays being placed on this expanding science as it is recognised that genetic mechanisms are central to a clear understanding of the nature of the oncological diseases. Attempts are being made to find the causes for the loss of control of the regulation of growth, and also to understand the rôle of worn-out genetic material. Certain growth factors which are specific for the occurrence of T-cell lymphomas and small malignant neoplasms of the lung have been identified and analysed. Another more recent development is the discovery of biological control substances, including monoclonal antibodies and cloning suppression lymphocytes.

Immunogenetics and cytogenetics are now established disciplines which are contributing to the care of patients. The genetic inherited nature of some rare neoplastic diseases is recognised and has led to the present practice of genetic counselling (see Chapter 21).

COMPUTER SCIENCE AND MEDICAL STATISTICS

There is a constant and spectacular increase in the use of computers in research, clinical and administrative work in medicine. By their means countless amounts of information of all kinds can be stored and processed as required, and complex and repetitive mathematical operations can be carried out easily and accurately. When the present author was Registrar of Statistics to the National Radium Commission 50 years ago, his task of producing a detailed analysis of the results in the UK of the treatment of cancer with radium would have been accomplished far more quickly and easily had computers been available.

A computer is now essential in all aspects of oncological work: diagnosis, laboratory investigations, patient monitoring, the planning of radiotherapy, and records systems.

A sound knowledge of statistics and computers is essential for anyone who carries out clinical trials, for their design, data collection, analysis and interpretation of the results of treatment, and the presentation of the findings and their statistical significance.

RADIOBIOLOGY

This science should be specially studied by radiation oncologists and to a lesser extent by medical oncologists. The subject is concerned with cell kinetics and the characterisation of normal and neoplastic cells, the cell cycle, cellular division, cell loss and multiplication and the method of cell repair (see Chapter 15).

RADIATION PHYSICS

A sound basic knowledge of the physics of ionising radiations and their interactions with normal and neoplastic cells and tissues and with materials is necessary in order to provide safe and effective radiotherapy for patients with oncological diseases. All radiation oncologists must acquire a clear understanding of this science, and other clinical oncologists should be familiar with its principles.

ANTHROPOLOGY

Clinical oncologists must be concerned in the widest sense with the science of man, for throughout their professional lives they are studying man in the world environment. As humans we are all affected by group behaviour, relationships and methods of communication between doctors, colleagues, nurses and patients. An acquaintance with different cultures, the various beliefs people have about health, illnesses and their treatment in world health-care systems is helpful and desirable.

GERONTOLOGY

Gerontology is the science which is concerned with the process of aging. The possible connection between this natural process which affects all organs and tissues of the body and the development of neoplastic diseases has been contemplated for decades. Numerous studies have been made concerning the age-related incidence of malignant diseases. It is known that the process of carcinogenesis is proportional to the exposure time of the carcinogen and that carcinogenic effects occur as successive cellular mutations.

Tissue neoplasia incidence increases with age, but the incidence falls in the very old, although they are not immune. In the higher age-groups the multiple tumour synchronous rate is increased, premalignant conditions are more common, and carcinomatous transformation of benign tumours is increased.

The development of some of these basic sciences in relation to oncology is described in greater detail in specific chapters of this book. Increasing numbers of graduates are asking for guidance about the scientific education which is needed for a career in clinical oncology.

Special courses on the theory of oncology should be organised in order to satisfy the demands of trainees in oncology and also the needs of clinical oncologists. Sufficient time must be allowed for trainees to attend these courses at special centres and educational facilities should be provided in scientific departments which are easily accessible from oncology units.

CHAPTER EIGHT

The Practice of Oncology

The practice of oncology is concerned with the total care of patients with malignant diseases. This is epitomised in the concept of rehabilitation and continuing care. The rehabilitation of patients begins with diagnosis, when the treatment programme is designed by the oncology team with the objective of restoring them to a life of good quality and longevity. The prescription for recovery gives assurance and hope to the patients and their families. An accurate assessment is made of the patients' total requirements commensurate with the general and local conditions governing their prognosis. The programme is carefully explained to patients and their families so that their compliance is assured, together with their actual cooperation in the prescribed treatment and care.

CANCER DIAGNOSIS

It is essential that the diagnosis of cancer is correct, and when possible tissue pathology should be done. Enormous advances have been made, especially during the present decade, in developing sophisticated investigations for an accurate diagnosis and assessment of the extent of the disease. When the patient is first seen a detailed case-record is built up, which includes the history of the present illness, the past history and the family history. A description of the habits and life-style of the patient is also included.

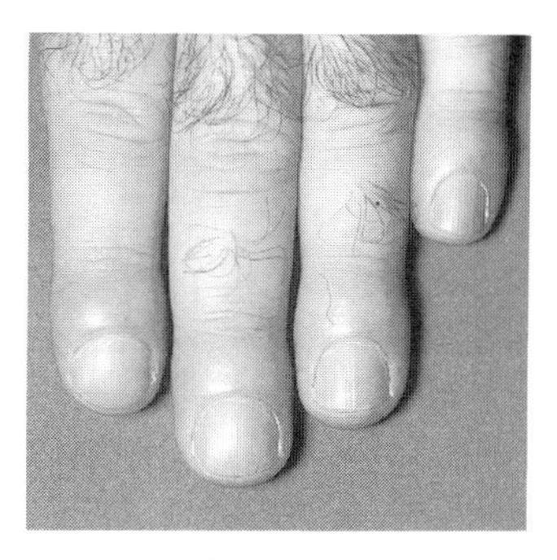

Figure 8.1 Clubbing of fingers of a patient with a primary bronchogenic carcinoma — an important diagnostic sign.

The clinical examination

Our predecessors had to establish the diagnosis largely on the results of clinical examination of the patient, as the present investigation facilities were not available. Even now, a clinical examination must still be meticulously carried out, as it will yield valuable information about the patient's general and local conditions.

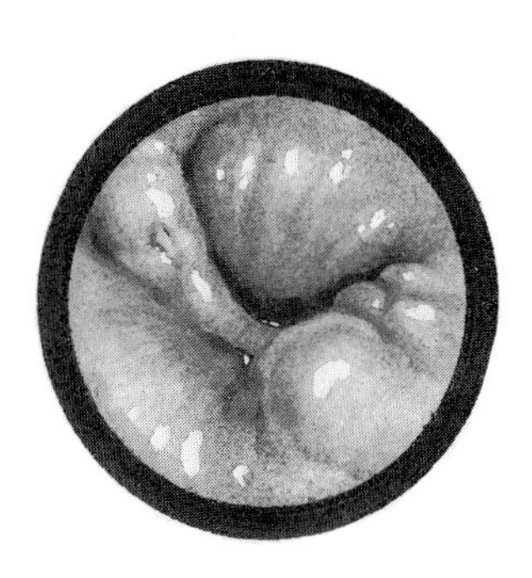

Figure 8.2 Oesophagoscopy showing a carcinoma of the oesophagus.

Methods of investigation

The appropriate investigations are made after the clinical examination and they provide important clues leading to a definitive diagnosis and a correct assessment of the malignant disease. They include haematology and biochemical profiles, urine examination, cytology of various kinds, tumour markers, and, when indicated, special tests (e.g. for thyroid function).

Routine radiological examinations are made of the chest and skeleton, together with barium meal and enema studies of the alimentary canal; intravenous pyelography; cholecystogram and visualisation of the extrahepatic bile ducts; and arteriograms, especially with renal neoplasms.

Endoscopy techniques of many varieties have been developed so that the interior of body cavities, viscera and ducts can be inspected and biopsies of lesions carried out.

Exfoliate cytology is a valuable method to reach a definitive diagnosis and relevant investigations have been perfected. They include cytology of sputum and urine, the contents of cysts, pleural and peritoneal effusions and gastric contents, and brush cytology of the oesophagus. The value of Papanicolaou's smear test for lesions of the cervix and corpus uteri is well known and this test has saved numerous lives in diagnosing premalignant and early carcinoma of this organ.

Histopathology of small biopsy specimens is of great value in the diagnosis of various tumours. It includes needle aspiration, Trucut biopsy and surgical biopsy. Marrow biopsy is necessary in certain malignant diseases.

A notable advance in the diagnosis of breast carcinoma and other breast conditions is the investigation by thermography, mammography and xerography. By these means small, early tumours which are not palpable can be identified and biopsied under direct vision.

Recently computerised axial tomography has been perfected and used routinely to identify the primary tumour and metastases. The whole body can be screened and the technique is valuable not only in diagnosis but also in monitoring the results of treatment.

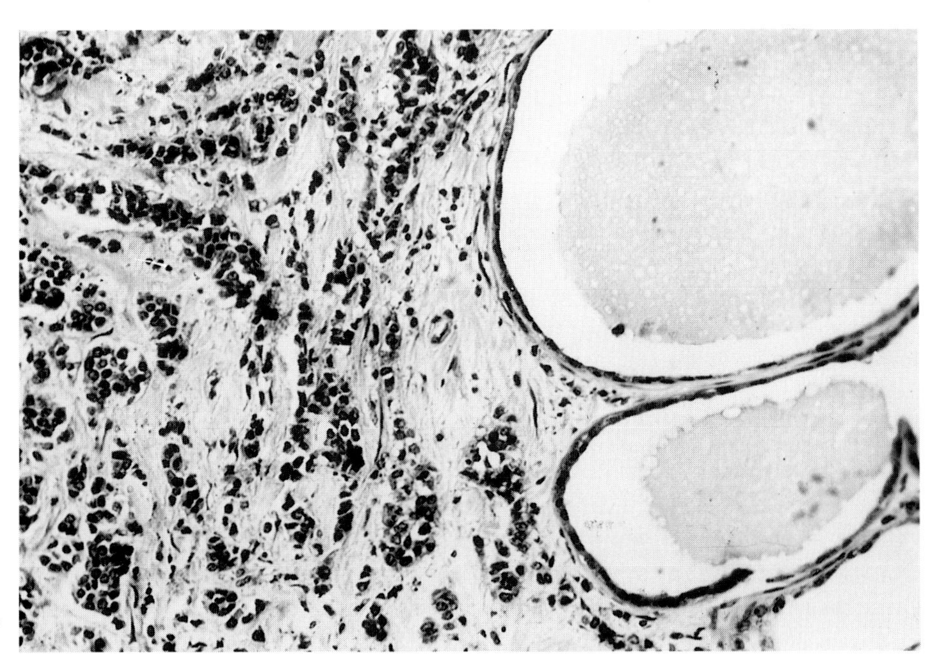

Figure 8.3 Histological specimen showing a breast carcinoma with large cysts.

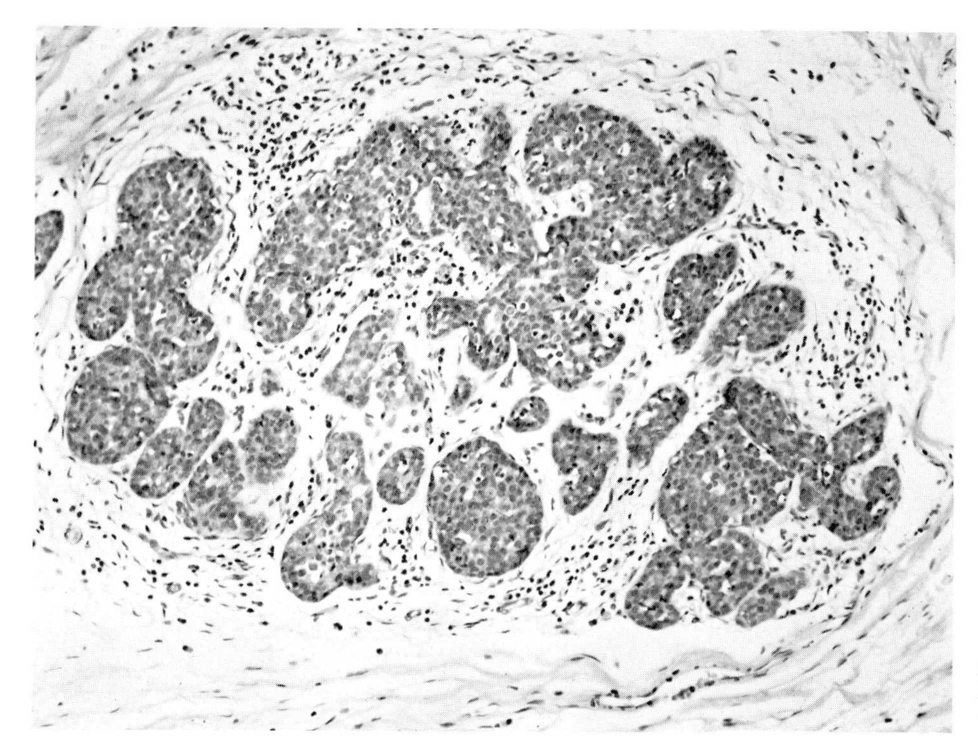

Figure 8.4 Histopathology specimen showing a lobular carcinoma *in situ* of the female breast.

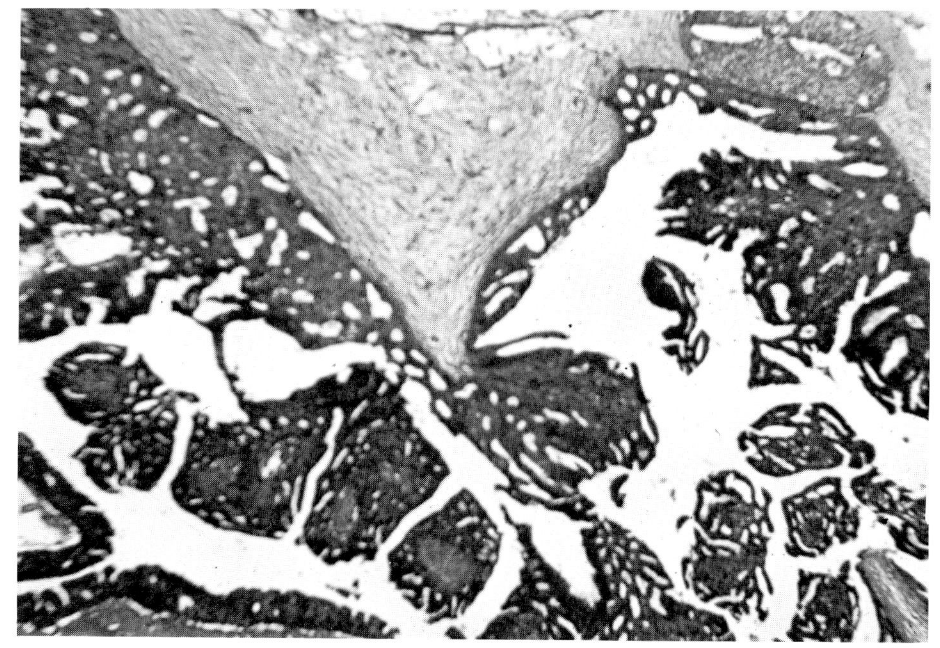

Figure 8.5 Histopathology specimen showing a cribriform intraduct carcinoma of the breast.

Bone scintiscans with isotopes are routinely used in primary and metastatic malignant disease of the osseous system. Lesions can be diagnosed in the presymptomatic phase of development.

Ultrasonography will differentiate solid and cystic tumours, especially those in the abdomen and pelvis, and is valuable in the diagnosis of tumours of the liver, gallbladder, extrahepatic biliary ducts, pancreas and kidney. The magnetic scanner, the latest type of scanner, can show the various parts of the human body in unprecedented detail. In addition to visualising the organs, this machine can also give information about the chemistry of the

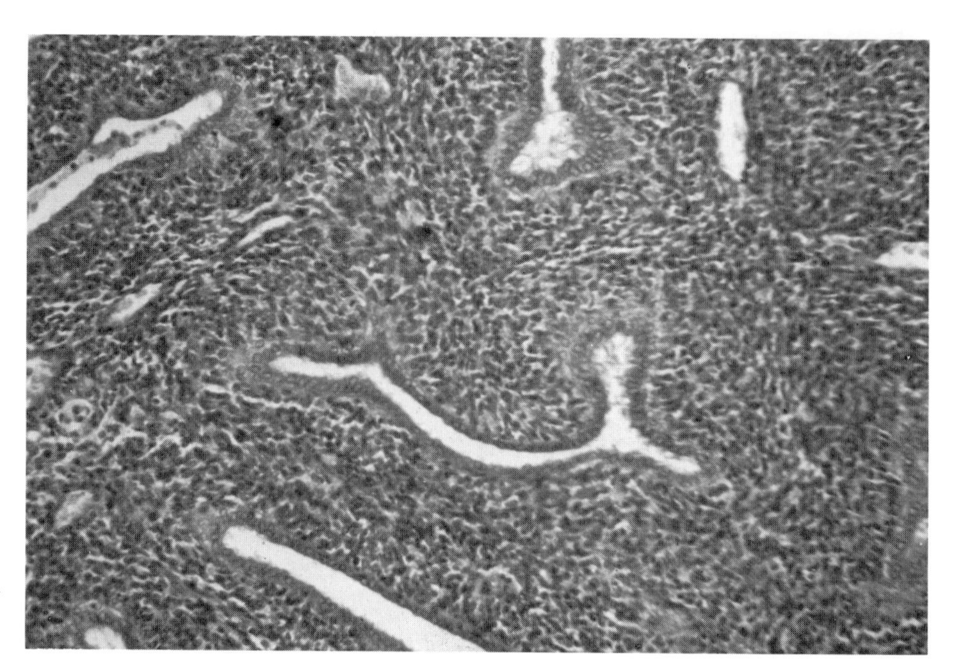

Figure 8.6 Histopathology specimen showing a fibrosarcoma arising in a fibroadenoma of the breast.

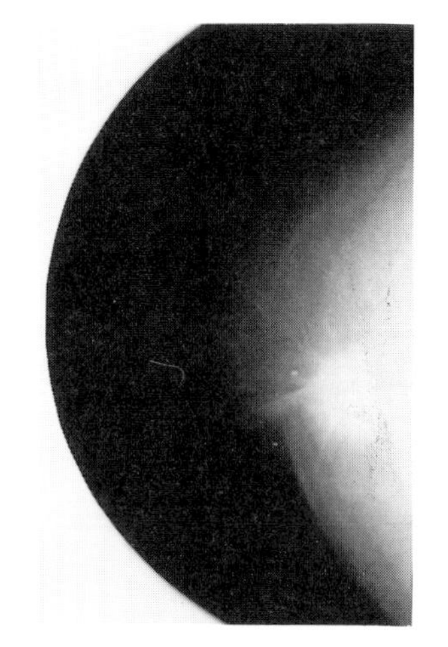

Figure 8.7 A mammogram showing a carcinoma of the left breast. Note the increased density and the spicules at the edge of the tumour.

body. It appears that a scanner will soon be available which can display both the structure and the function of different organs and tissues, whether normal or abnormal.

Immunodiagnosis

This method is a development of great potential value in the diagnosis of malignant diseases in individual patients and in screening populations and monitoring treatment *(Baldwin, 1977)*. In addition, the technique is already used to detect residual or recurrent tumours such as carcinoma of the colon.

The carcinoembryonic antigen (CEA) is associated specially with colonic

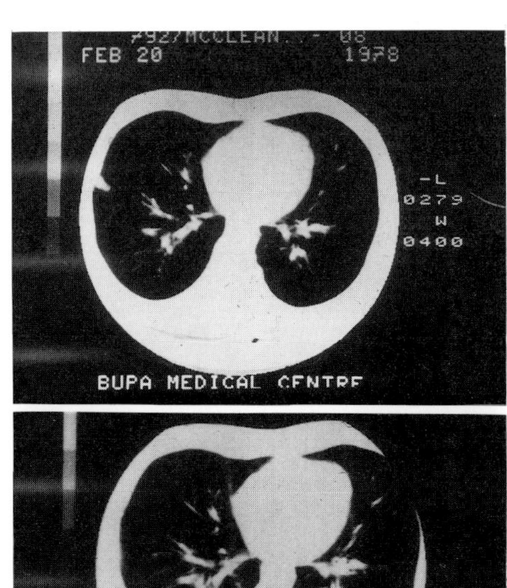

Figure 8.8 Computerised axial tomography showing metastases of a teratoma in the lungs. *Top:* Before treatment. *Bottom:* Regression of metastases and opening up of the bronchial tree after treatment.

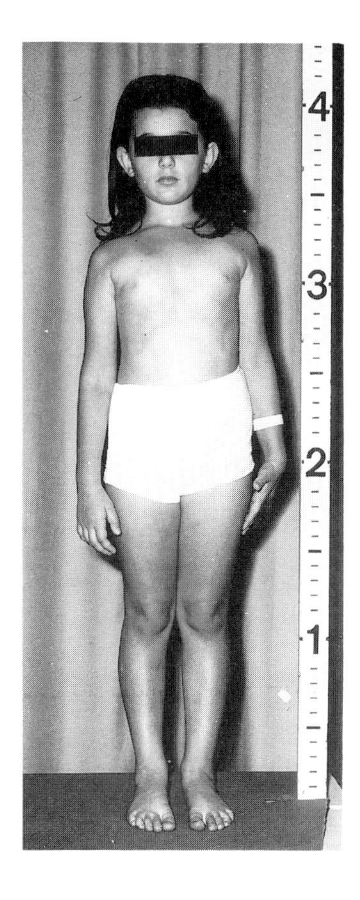

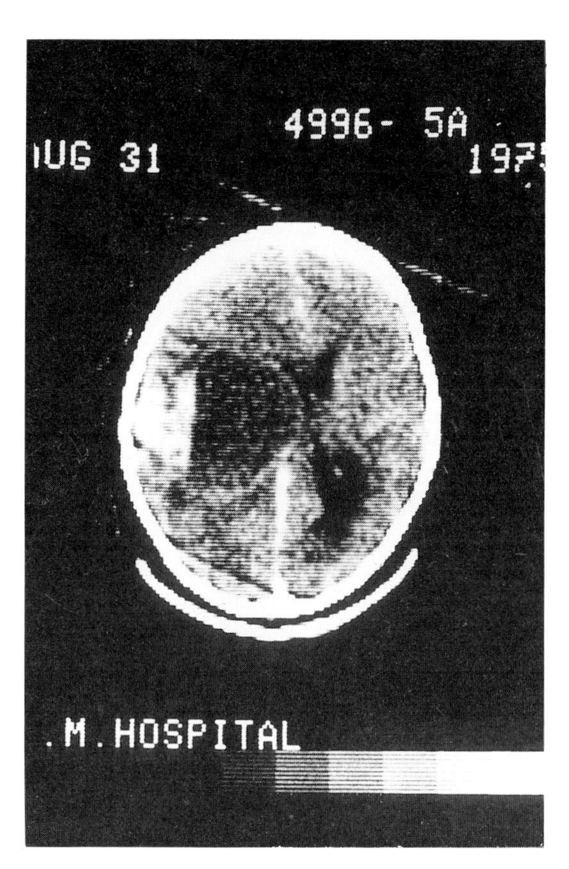

Figure 8.9 *Left:* A 9-year-old patient with a right spastic hemiparesis and right facial weakness caused by an oligochondroglioma of the brain. *Right:* The EMI brain scan of the patient, showing a large intracerebral tumour in the left parietal region, extending from the convexity to the midline. The outer third (light area) of the tumour is solid, whilst the inner two-thirds (dark area) is cystic. The right lateral ventricle is clearly outlined.

and rectal tumours and tumours of the stomach and pancreas. An association with other tumours may also be found.

The alpha-fetoprotein test is used in the diagnosis of hepatocellular carcinomas. Increased levels of the tumour-associated foetal protein are also found in patients with other liver diseases and in pregnancy.

The human chorionic gonadotrophin (hCG) test is valuable for diagnosing malignant tumours of the testicle, hydatidiform mole, and degenerative products of conception. It can detect occult malignant testicular diseases. The hCG levels increase considerably and rapidly when such tumours recur or spread and therefore guide the clinician in his choice of treatment. For a positive hCG test there must be syncytiotrophoblastic elements in the testicular tumour and not a pure seminoma *(Goldenberg* et al., *1981)*.

Ectopic hormone production

Considerable attention is now given to the production of ectopic hormones by tumours causing different clinical syndromes which lead to the identification of the primary tumour. The metabolic abnormalities caused can be lethal unless the primary tumour is excised or destroyed quickly and those such as hypercalcaemia, dilutional hyponatraemia and hypokalaemia are successfully treated.

Special mention is made of the dangerous hypercalcaemic syndrome associated with primary malignant tumours which produce parathyroid hormone, such as hepatoma, bronchogenic carcinoma, and kidney carcinoma, in addition to osteolytic osseous carcinoma metastases such as from breast carcinoma. In the argentaffinoma syndrome the pharmacological effects are seen from the excess production by the tumour of serotonin, killikrein and other proteolytic enzymes *(Raven, 1977)*.

Amongst the common tumours that produce ectopic hormones are those in the lung, thyroid gland, kidney, stomach and intestine. The effects of surgical removal or radiotherapy of the tumour can be monitored by measuring the decrease in the secretions of these polypeptides after treatment. This subject is dealt with in detail by Ellison and Neville *(1973)*.

It is apparent that the diagnosis of cancer is a continuous process in individual patients. The correct diagnosis must be made when the patient is first seen and an assessment of the extent of the disease is carried out. The presence of unrelated intercurrent diseases must also be diagnosed. After the patient has received definitive treatment for the cancer, the diagnosis of recurrent, spreading or metastatic disease must be made in the follow-up clinic.

ASSESSMENT OF PATIENTS

When a malignant disease has been diagnosed, an assessment is made of the conditions of the whole patient. This includes the psychological reactions to the diagnosis, which is carefully explained both to the patient and to his or her family in suitable terminology. At the same time the programme of treatment, designed, if possible, to restore the patient to a life of good quality, is explained so that patient-compliance can be obtained. The general physical state of the patient and the functions of the vital organs are studied. An exact assessment is made of the extent of the malignant disease locally and of the presence of macrometastases in the regional lymph nodes and other organs and tissues.

The oncology team will then decide whether the rehabilitation treatment programme should be designed to cure or to palliate the disease. Their decision determines the nature and scope of the definitive treatment by surgery, radiation, hormonal therapy, chemotherapy or combination treatment. There are special effects from these various treatments which have to be dealt with in postdefinitive rehabilitation and continuing care systems.

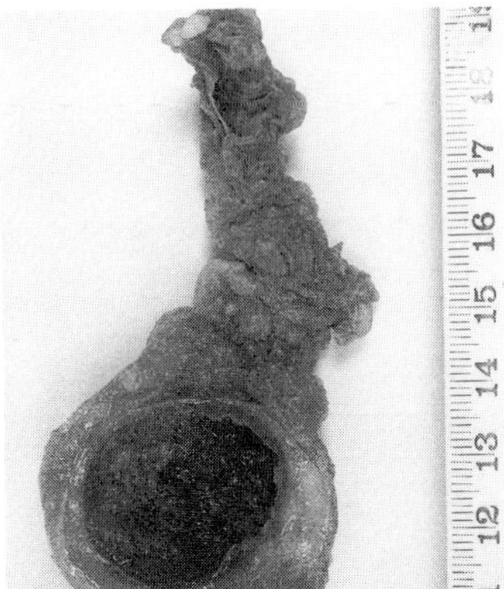

Figure 8.10 A seminoma in the undescended testicle of a 48-year-old patient. The testicle was placed in the scrotum when the patient was 11 and it was seen to be atrophic 6 years later. It enlarged for 9 months before orchidectomy was performed with ligation of the spermatic cord at the internal abdominal ring.

DEFINITIVE TREATMENT

The first phase of the rehabilitation of cancer patients after diagnosis and assessment is definitive treatment, which is given in hospital in most cases. The three methods of treatment employed are surgery, radiotherapy and chemotherapy, including hormonal therapy. For some patients combination treatment by all three modalities — the treatment triad — is indicated.

The main treatment modality for patients with cancer today and in the foreseeable future is surgery.

Oncological surgery

The scope of surgery in the management and treatment of patients with malignant diseases is shown in Table 3.

Table 3 Oncological surgery

Diagnostic biopsy
Staging surgery
Emergency surgery: perforations, obstructions, haemorrhage
Excisional surgery: curative or palliative
Debulking tumour surgery: less tumour bulk the better for the patient
Chemotherapy surgery: perfusion, infusion
Hormonal surgery: oophorectomy, adrenalectomy, hypophysectomy
Reconstructive and plastic surgery
Surgery to relieve cancer pain

The development of oncological surgery and the wide scope of its place in the treatment of patients with malignant diseases over a period of less than a century forms a large and brilliant part of the impressive history of surgery (Table 4).

Table 4 Major oncological operations

Surgeon	*Year performed*	*Operation*
Billroth	1881	Subtotal gastrectomy
Halsted	1890	Radical mastectomy
Schlatter	1897	Total gastrectomy
Von Mickulicz	1898	Oesophagogastrectomy
Wertheim	1900	Radical hysterectomy
Miles	1906	Abdominoperineal excision of rectum
Torek	1913	Oesophagectomy
Trotter	1913	Partial pharyngectomy
Graham and Singer	1933	Pneumonectomy

The master-surgeons of the past who designed and performed the major operations were guided by their knowledge of basic medical sciences, chiefly anatomy and pathology, and impressed by the need for radical procedures to remove the local malignant disease and thereby prevent local recurrences. They carried out their operations without the support of modern anaesthesia, blood transfusions and the nursing skills vital for patients today. Furthermore, there were no antibacterial chemicals, no rehabilitation techniques such as we have today and none of the facilities for patient care that we now have in our postoperative and intensive care units.

The role of surgery in the treatment of malignant diseases has expanded considerably, as shown in Table 3, and modifications have been made in the technique of many operations, as a result of clinical trials and an assessment of survival and recurrence rates. A notable example is the treatment of breast carcinoma, which is the subject of much investigation and discussion today (see Chapters 12, 13 and 19).

Radiation treatment

The study of the history of the development of the treatment of malignant diseases by different forms of radiation and the evolution of the impressive radiotherapy techniques which are used today is fascinating. The radiation treatment of cancer is a major discipline. It is used alone for certain diseases and combined with surgery and chemotherapy, including hormonal therapy, for others. This form of treatment developed in the space of less than a century: Roentgen discovered X-rays in 1895, Becquerel discovered

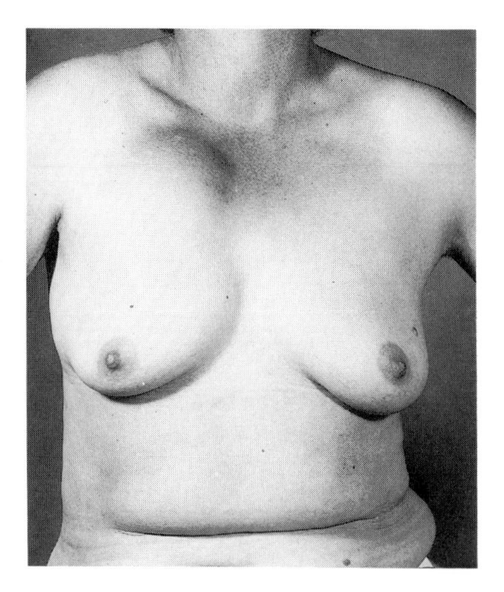

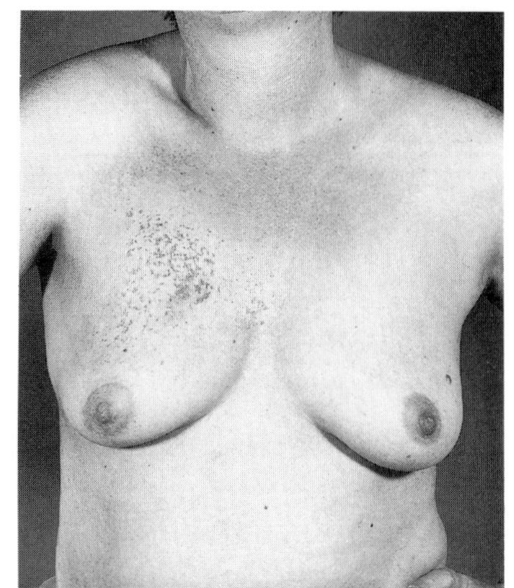

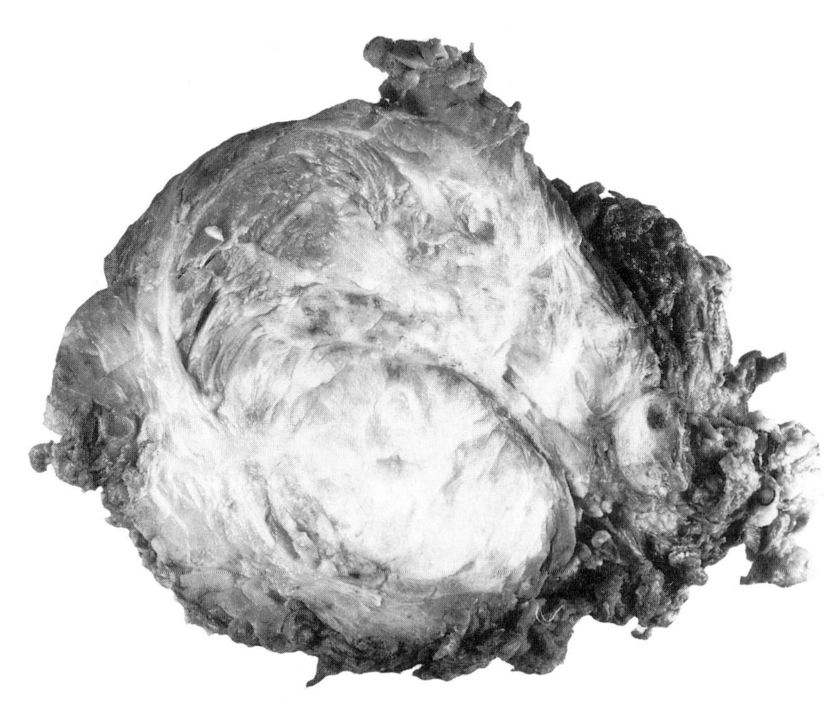

Figure 8.11 *Top left:* A 45-year-old female patient with a large swelling of 5 years' duration in the right chest wall. The right breast was normal. Biopsy showed a well differentiated fibrosarcoma. Preoperative radiotherapy with telecaesium was given for 43 days before the tumour was radically excised. *Top right:* The patient after excision of the fibrosarcoma, anterior segments of the 2nd, 3rd and 4th ribs and the intervening chest wall; the pleura was not opened. *Right:* The fibrosarcoma excised from the chest wall.

the radioactivity of uranium in 1896 and in 1900 Pierre and Marie Curie isolated radium from pitchblende.

The object of radiation is to destroy the tumour without affecting normal tissues, and modern high-voltage techniques have reached a considerable degree of perfection. Tumours vary in their radiosensitivity and therefore respond in different ways. We have acquired knowledge and experience which enable decisions to be made as to which tumours should be radiated. The search for radiosensitisers continues so that radioresistant tumours can be effectively treated by radiation techniques (see Chapter 15).

Chemotherapy and hormonal therapy

The medical treatment of malignant diseases with pharmaceutical preparations, including synthetic hormones, is of great present and potential future value. It has already cured patients with choriocarcinoma, leukaemias, lymphomas and seminoma. The search continues for new chemicals with specific tumour actions and no toxic side-effects.

Synthetic hormones are proving valuable, especially for tumours under hormone control systems, such as carcinoma of the breast and prostate. In some patients with hormone-related tumours their results are remarkable. Special mention is made of Nolvadex (tamoxifen), which is used in the treatment of breast carcinoma.

The concept that cancer might respond to medical treatment is not new, for many different medicaments, chiefly inorganic chemicals, which were applied locally or taken systemically, have been used for the treatment of tumours for many centuries. We now have an impressive list of organic chemicals which have an important place in cancer treatment when used alone or in combination with surgery and radiation.

The methods of administration of these pharmaceuticals have received much attention. In addition to the usual oral and intravenous routes, their delivery into the tumour-bearing area by surgical perfusion and infusion techniques has been developed. Clinical work continues concerning dosage schedules, toxicity and side-effects, their metabolism in the body and elimination.

The research effort to understand hormonal control mechanisms continues and already oestrogen, progesterone and other receptors have been discovered in the membranes of malignant cells, which indicate the responsiveness of the tumour to hormonal therapy (see Chapters 16 and 19).

TEAM-WORK IN ONCOLOGY

The magnitude of the multidisciplinary subject of oncology with its numerous subdivisions and scientific and clinical ramifications necessitates the joint efforts of many professionals in team-work of the highest quality. Team-work by clinicians, nurses and paramedical professionals for the total care of patients with oncological diseases is a fairly recent development. Communications with teams of research oncologists and scientists working in different disciplines should be established to provide a constant feedback between clinics and laboratories. Clinical oncologists can discuss important conditions and problems requiring solution in the laboratory with research oncologists, and they can apply new knowledge in patient care.

Team-work and the members of the oncology-rehabilitation-continuing care team are described further in Chapter 9.

It is clearly recognised that some other specialists have an important responsibility in the total care and management of certain cancer patients. Good examples are urological, chest and orthopaedic surgeons; many general surgeons and physicians also carry out much oncological work in addition to their other work.

Although clinical oncologists specialise in one particular discipline of surgery, medicine or radiation, they should be familiar with other treatment modalities, including their indications, side-effects, complications and end-results.

REFERENCES

Baldwin, R. W. (1977). Immunology of malignant disease. In Raven, R. W. (ed.) *Principles of Surgical Oncology*, pp 279–301. Plenum Medical Book Company, New York and London

Ellison, M. L. and Neville, A. M. (1973). Neoplasia and ectopic hormone production. In Raven, R. W. (ed.) *Modern Trends in Oncology*, Part 1: Research Progress, pp 163–81. Butterworth & Co., London

Goldenberg, D. M., Kim, E. E. and De Land, F. H. (1981). Human chorionic gonadotrophin radioantibodies in the radio-immune detection of cancer and for disclosure of occult metastases. *Proc. Natl. Acad. Sci. USA*, **78** (12), 7754–8

Raven, R. W. (1977). Oncology: attainment and anticipation (Bradshaw Lecture). *Ann. Roy. Coll. Surg. Engl.*, **59**, 210–21

CHAPTER NINE

Rehabilitation and Continuing Care

The concept of rehabilitation and continuing care for patients with oncological diseases is relatively new. The whole subject is being studied both nationally and internationally and developed practically in special units which are being established in the UK and other countries. The subject is discussed here in broad outline only; for details see, for example, Raven *(1986)*.

Rehabilitation begins with diagnosis and ends with the restoration of the patient to a life of good quality and duration. The programme therefore embraces the clinical examination, investigations and assessment of the patient for the definitive treatment of the disease by surgery, radiotherapy or chemotherapy, alone or in combination. After definitive treatment a further assessment of the "whole" patient is made: the patient's spiritual and physical needs are studied and measured, when this is possible, so that they can be adequately dealt with and deficits restored. Rehabilitation enables many patients to continue their usual life-style with their families at home, to resume their occupation and to enjoy their former recreations.

Patients can be divided into the different groups shown in Table 5, according to their various conditions for rehabilitation.

Table 5 Cancer patients for rehabilitation

State of cancer	*Objective for rehabilitation*
Patients with controlled cancer	
No disability is present.	Normal life-style
Disability is present from the treatment.	Life of good quality
Disability is present from the disease.	Life of good quality
Patients with uncontrolled cancer	
Disabilities are present from the disease and treatment.	Life of limited duration and quality

It is clearly apparent that effectual rehabilitation can be achieved for patients with cancer which has been controlled by definitive treatment, which is, in fact, the basis of the rehabilitation programme. Patients with a residual deformity, caused either by the treatment or by the disease, can be rehabilitated for a life of good quality and duration. However, life can never be the same again for those patients who require personal adjustments and alterations in their life-style. Nevertheless, substantial help and support are available for them which can be of real benefit. Even patients with uncontrolled disease and a short life expectancy can be made self-supporting and comfortable so that the length of the period of their eventual complete disability and dependency on others is considerably shortened. For these patients continuing care is highly essential, but of course all patients treated for cancer require continuing care of some sort, including follow-up supervision, for the rest of their lives.

The rehabilitation programme is shown in Table 6.

Table 6 The rehabilitation programme

Diagnosis of cancer
Assessment of the patient. General health. Local condition.

Definitive treatment
Surgery. Radiotherapy. Chemotherapy and hormonal therapy. Treatment triad (combination).

Rehabilitation
Restoration of the spirit and morale. Restoration of the nutritional state.
Restoration of haematological and biochemical deficits.
Restoration of mobility and functions.
Restoration of neurological deficits. Stoma care. Pain control.

Resettlement
Resumption of life-style at home. Resumption of occupation and recreations.

The diagnosis of the different oncological diseases, which must be accurate, has become a precise procedure with the available new methods of investigation (see Chapter 8).

DISABILITY CAUSED BY CANCER

The various, and in some cases serious, disabilities experienced by patients are caused either by the disease itself or by the treatment given, or by both. They are set out in Tables 7 and 8.

A survey of the numerous disabilities experienced by cancer patients

Table 7 Patients with disabilities caused by cancer

General effects
Cachexia. Malnutrition. Anaemia. Anxiety. Fear. Pain.
Social, vocational and economic problems.

Local effects
Destruction of soft tissue and bone.
Pathological fracture.
Dysfunction of bladder and rectum — incontinence.
Paralyses: Cranial nerves. Brachial and lumbo-sacral plexuses. Tetraplegia. Paraplegia. Hemiplegia. Cauda equina.

demonstrates their need for the advice and practical help of many professionals, who have to work together in a team.

Table 8 Patients with disabilities caused by treatment

Amputations
Major and minor. Upper and lower limbs. Breast. Genitalia.
Major excisions
Residual stoma. Tracheostomy. Colostomy. Ileal conduit. Ileostomy.
Facial with maxillary and mandibular defects.
Soft tissue defects. Plastic and reconstructive operations required.
Prostheses of various kinds provided. Speech therapy necessary.
Endocrine replacement therapy
Thyroidectomy. Adrenalectomy. Hypophysectomy.
Psychological effects
Restoration of spirit, morale, dignity.
Resettlement
Life-style. Family. Occupation. Recreations.

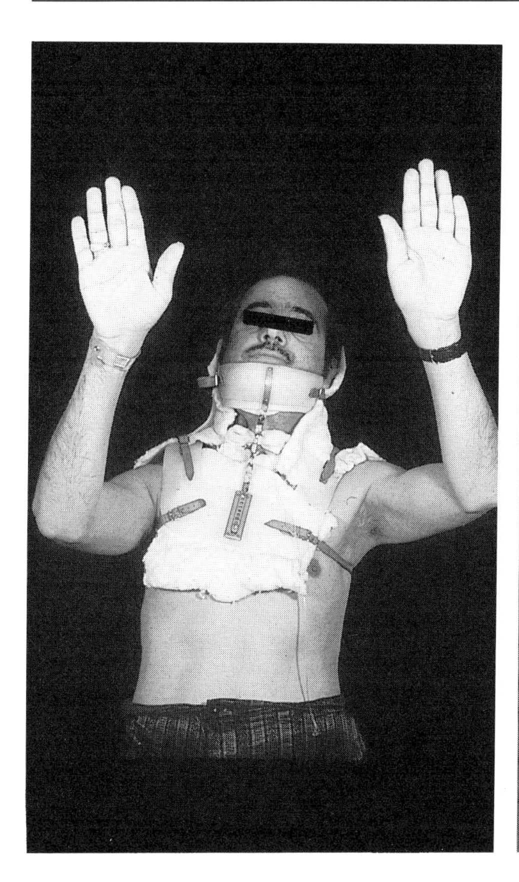

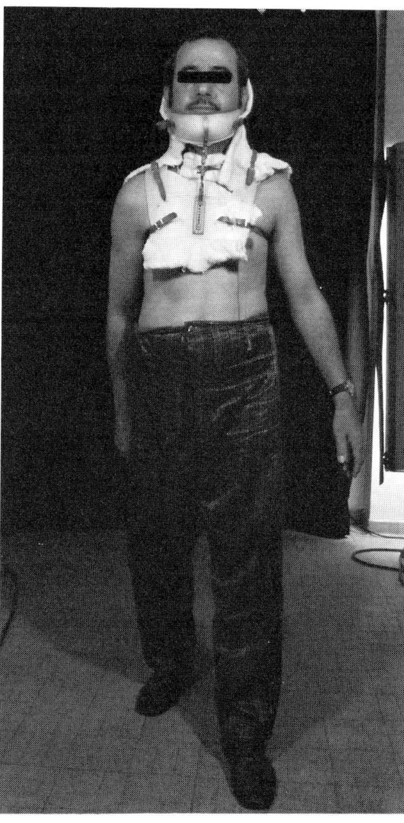

Figure 9.1 A male patient with tetraplegia from a chordoma of the nasopharynx. The chordoma was treated with radiotherapy, a cervical laminectomy was performed to decompress the spinal cord and a temporary tracheostomy was instituted. *Left:* The patient wearing a plaster collar after undergoing cervical laminectomy, being rehabilitated to recover the function of his upper extremities. *Right:* The patient recovered the use of his lower extremities and was able to walk again.

ONCOLOGY REHABILITATION TEAM

Efficient team-work is essential to achieve successful results in cancer rehabilitation and continuing care; the advice and skills of many professionals are necessary. The team includes the surgeon, physician, radiotherapist, anaesthetist, pathologist, radiologist, hospital and community nurses, family doctor, community physician, physiotherapist, occupational

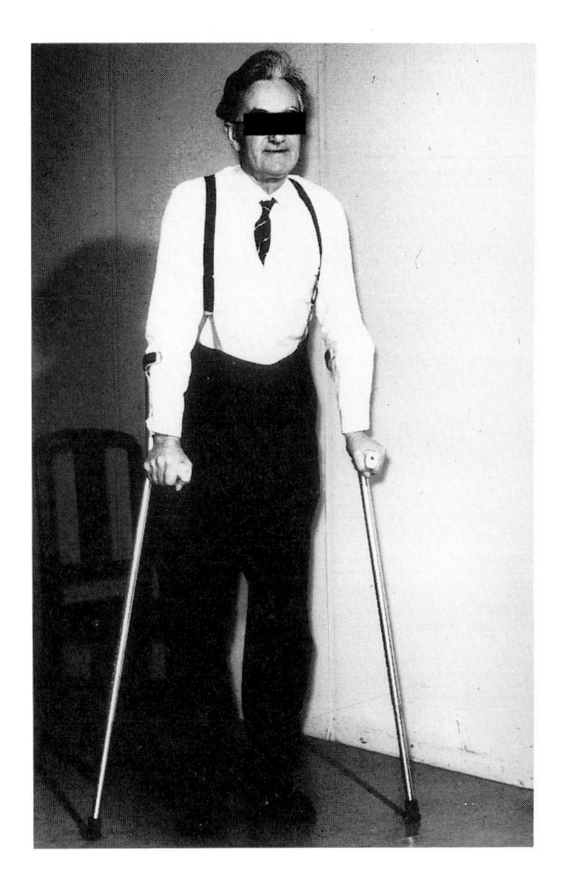

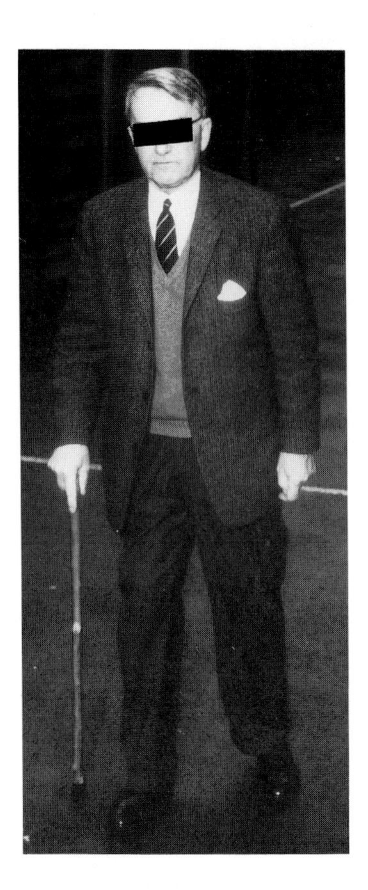

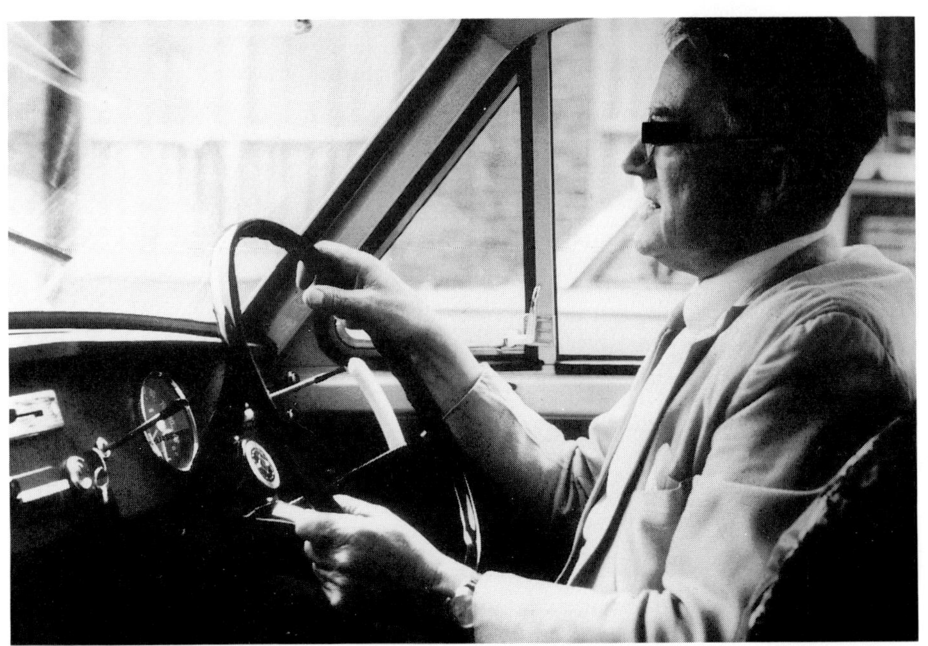

Figure 9.2 *Top left:* A patient undergoing rehabilitation consequent to paraplegia caused by a lymphoma compressing the 6th dorsal segment. The lymphoma has been successfully controlled by radiotherapy and the compression relieved. The patient is ambulant with the aid of elbow supports. *Top right:* The fully rehabilitated patient walking to work. *Right:* The patient, now resettled at work, driving his car with modifications for a disabled driver.

therapist, speech therapist, stoma therapist, nutritionist, medical social worker, prosthetist, resettlement officer, and the patient's own pastor.

It is most unlikely that all the members of the team will be needed at the same time, but each specialist must be available for consultation and to give treatment when necessary. Patients are often placed in groups according

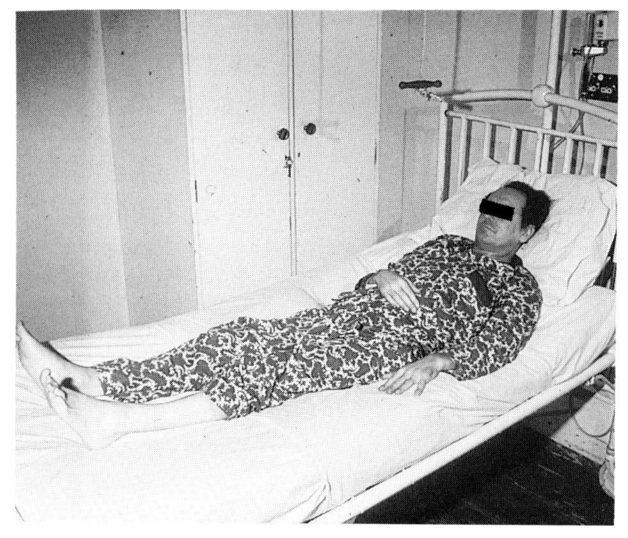
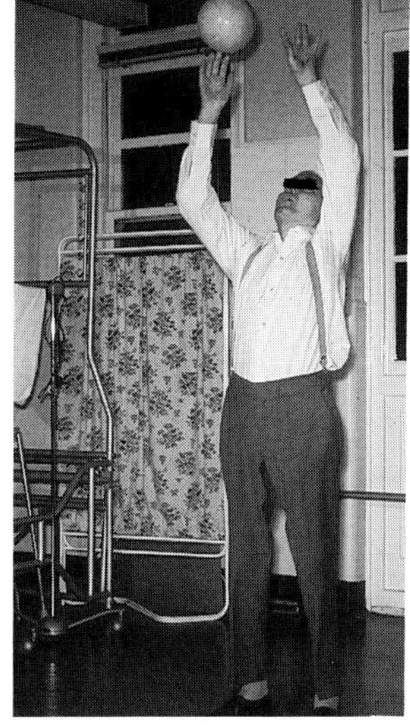

Figure 9.3 *Left:* A male patient with a right hemiplegia caused by a hypernephroma metastasis in the left parietal lobe of the brain. The metastasis was accurately localised and treated with radiotherapy. *Right:* The patient fully rehabilitated.

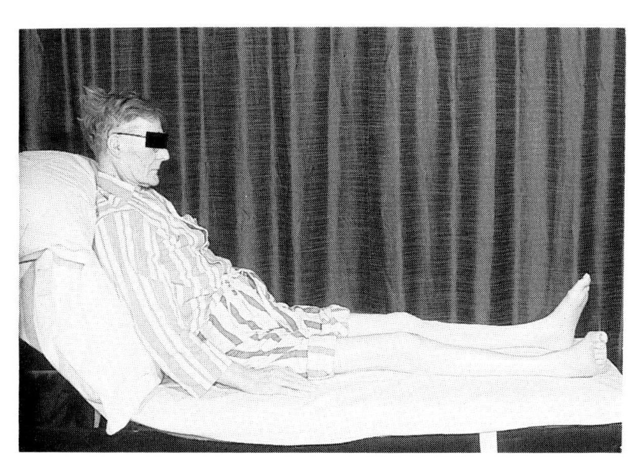
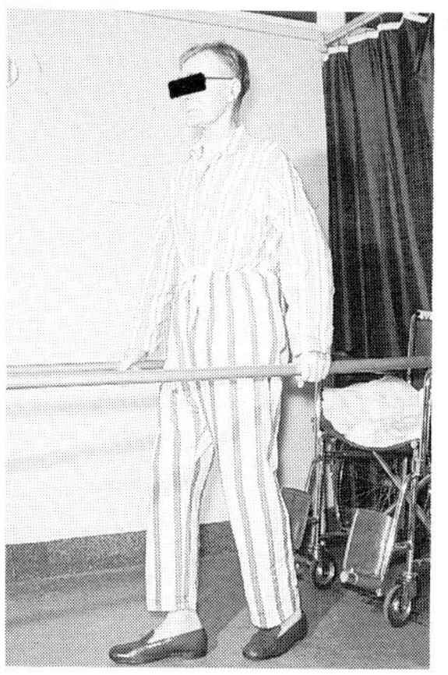

Figure 9.4 *Left:* A patient with a lesion of the cauda equina caused by a local recurrent carcinoma after abdominoperineal resection of the rectum for carcinoma. The recurrent tumour was treated by radiotherapy. *Right:* The patient during rehabilitation, walking between bars.

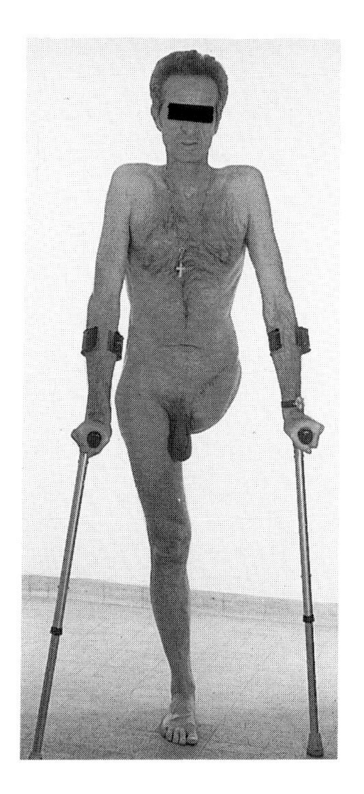
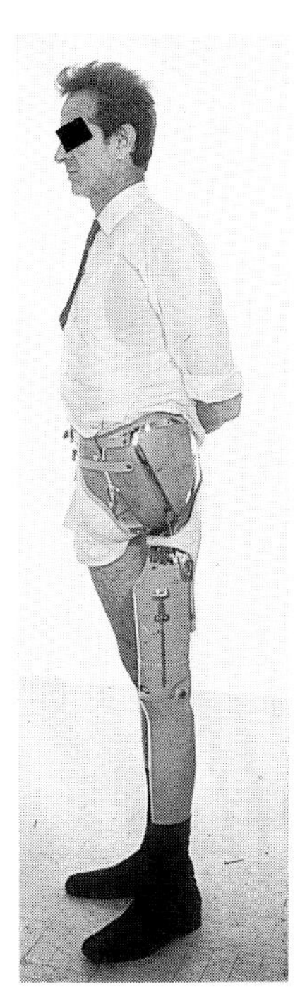
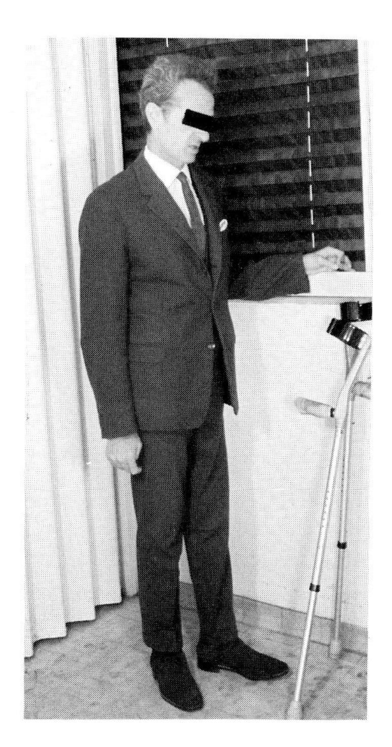

Figure 9.5 *Left:* A patient whose lower left extremity was amputated at the hip joint because of a sarcoma. The amputation stump healed well and rehabilitation has commenced. *Centre:* The patient fitted with a lower limb prosthesis. *Right:* The patient now fully rehabilitated, dressed normally, wearing his prosthesis and walking well.

to their requirements. The responsibility of being team leader is usually undertaken by the oncologist to whom the patient is first referred for diagnosis and definitive treatment — the surgeon, physician or radiotherapist.

Qualifications for team membership

The team members must have the necessary education, training and qualifications for their various specialities. They must have a knowledge of

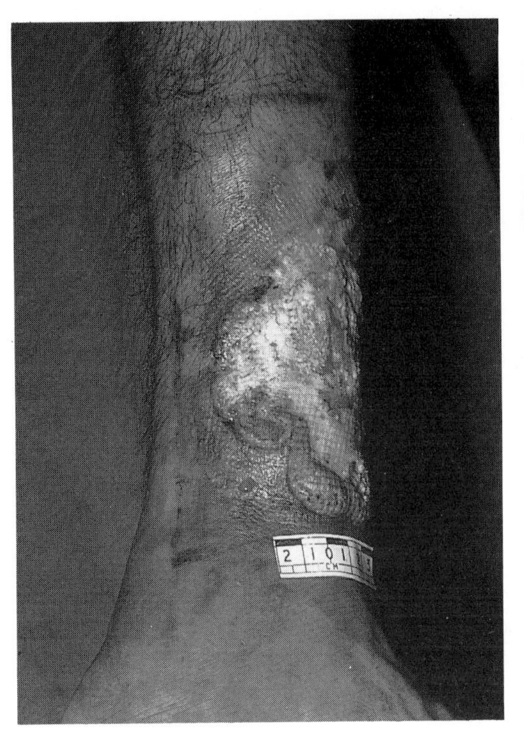

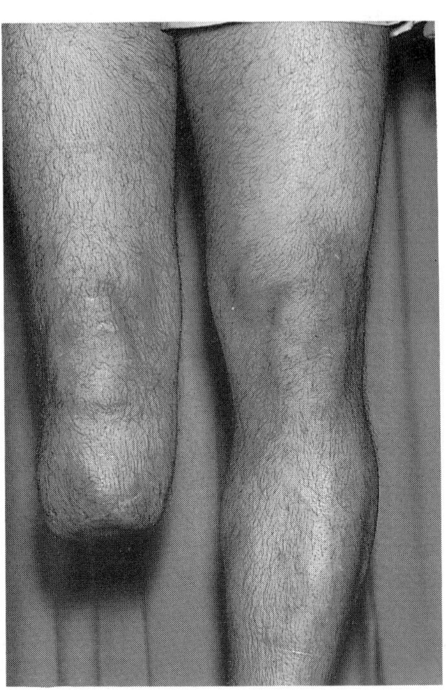

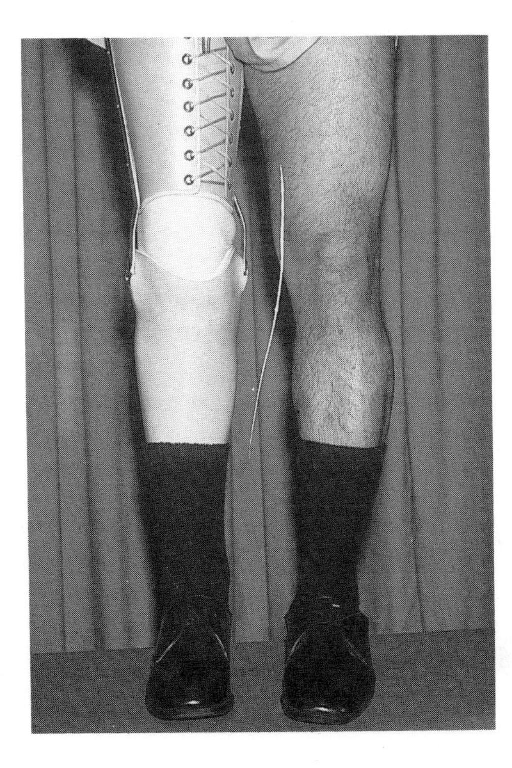

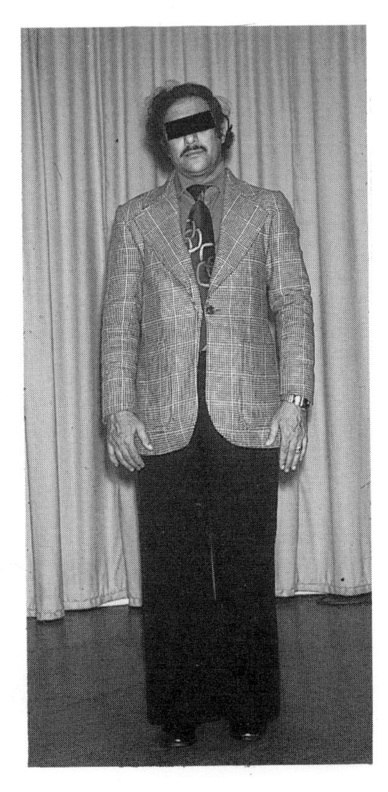

Figure 9.6 *Top left:* A male patient with an extensive squamous cell carcinoma of the right leg requiring a below-the-knee amputation. *Top right:* The amputation stump. *Bottom left:* The patient wearing his prosthesis. *Bottom right:* The patient fully rehabilitated and dressed. He returned to his usual work.

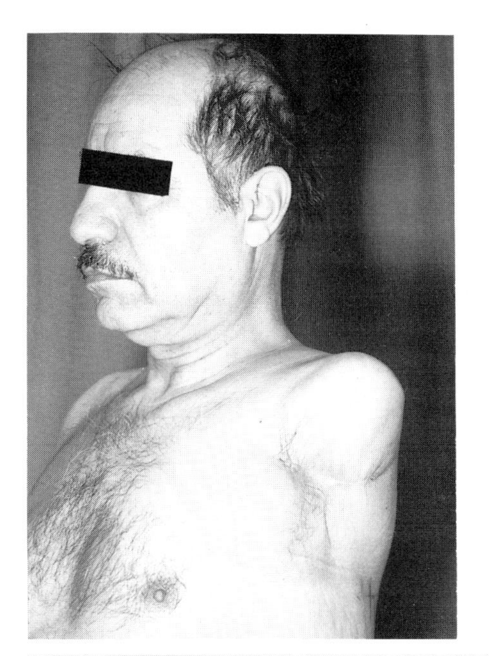
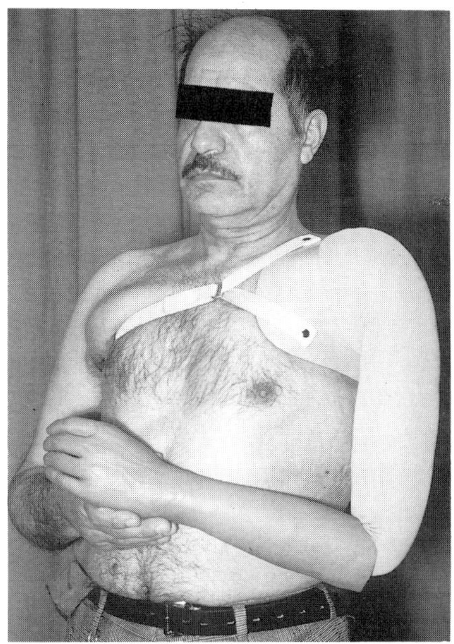
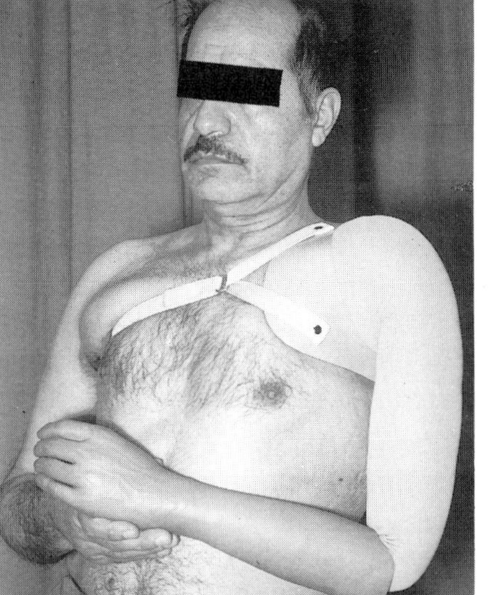
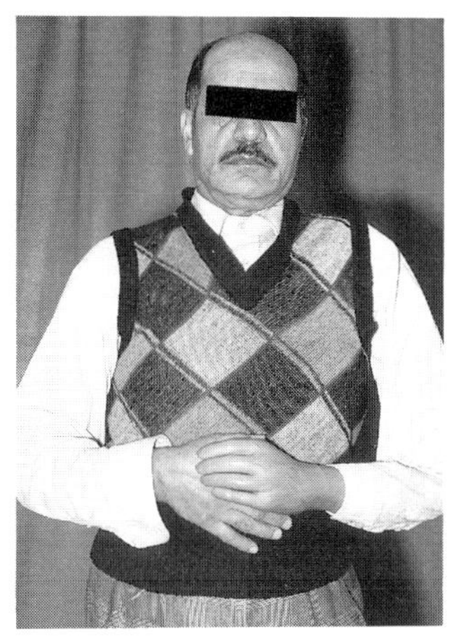

Figure 9.7 *Left:* A patient whose left upper extremity has been amputated by disarticulation at the shoulder joint because of a sarcoma of the arm. There is sound healing of the wound. *Centre:* The patient wearing an upper extremity prosthesis. *Right:* The patient fully rehabilitated, wearing his prosthesis and dressed normally.

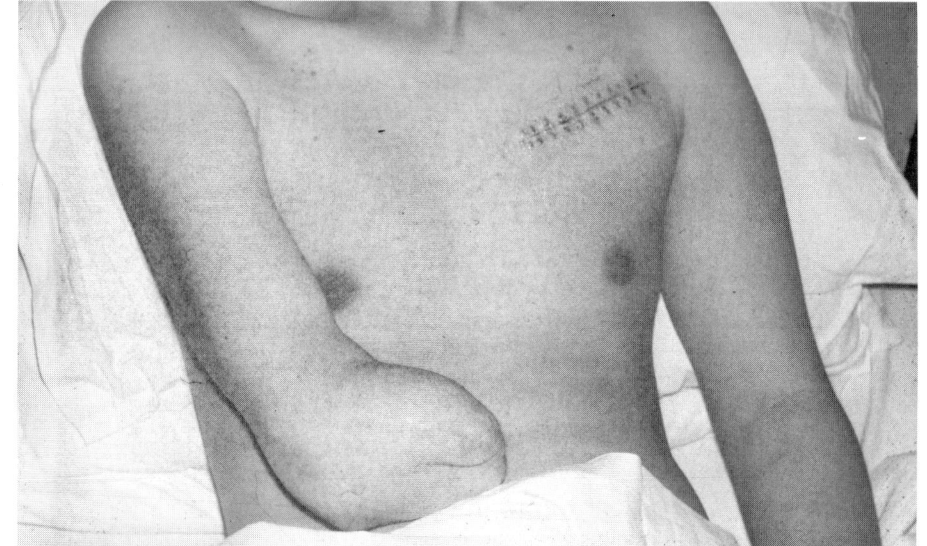
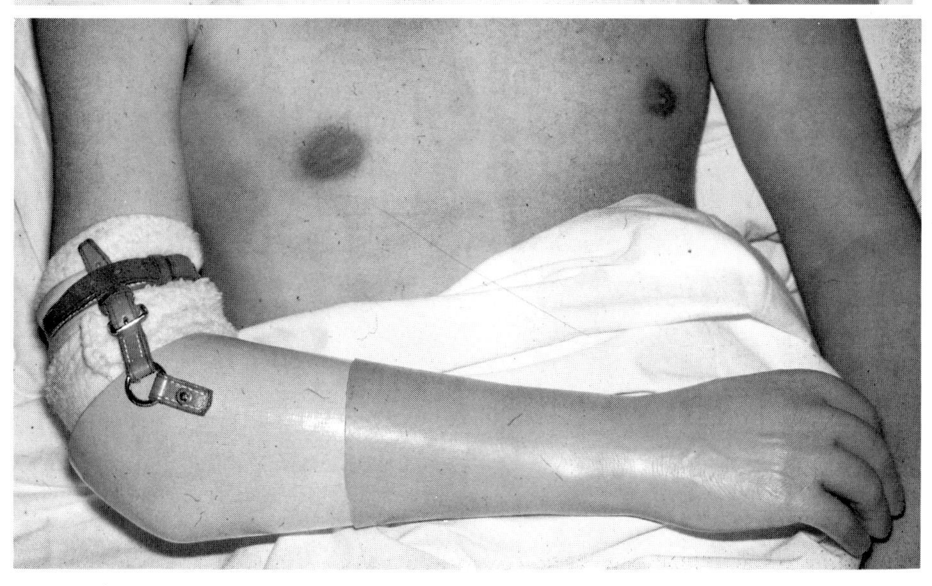

Figure 9.8 *Top:* A male patient after amputation of his right forearm. *Bottom:* The patient wearing his prosthesis.

oncology to enable them to make a maximum contribution to the work according to their special skills.

They must understand the meaning of team-work, for no oncologist can now work in isolation. This includes speaking the specialist language and therefore having an understanding of the technical terminology and methodology. The important art of communication with specialists, patients and families must be acquired by experience. There must be mutual respect between team members, so that each member is able to express an independent opinion in the joint consultation clinics and elsewhere. The team leader should welcome all contributions to discussions in order that a final consensus of opinion on the rehabilitation programme can be reached.

THE REHABILITATION AND CONTINUING CARE UNIT

This unit is an integral part of an oncology service and is sited in a hospital or in close proximity to a group of hospitals where a considerable amount of oncological work is done. It is also a necessary and valuable component of an oncology centre, special home for cancer patients or hospice where cancer patients are referred after their definitive treatment in hospital.

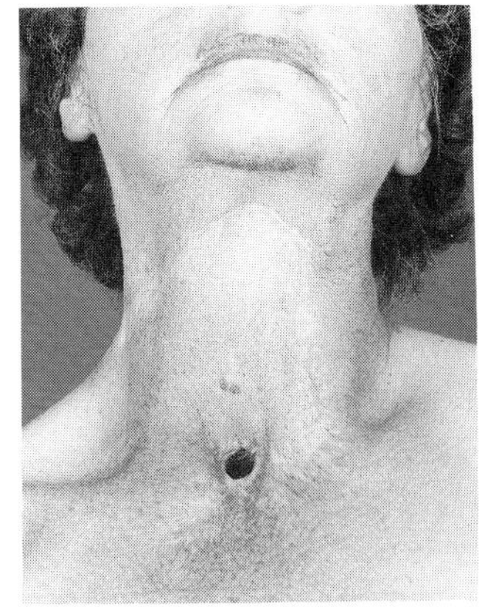

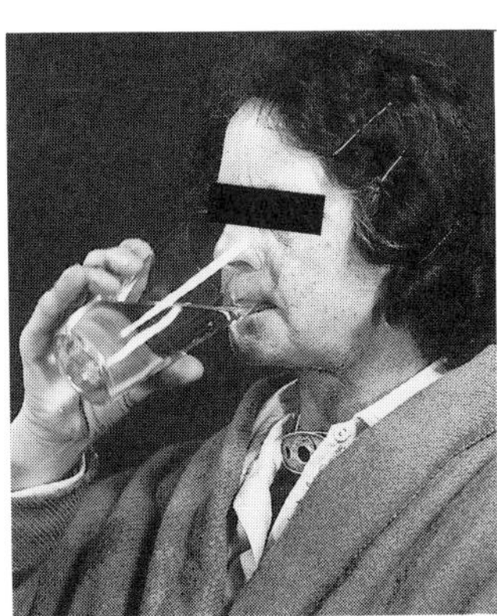

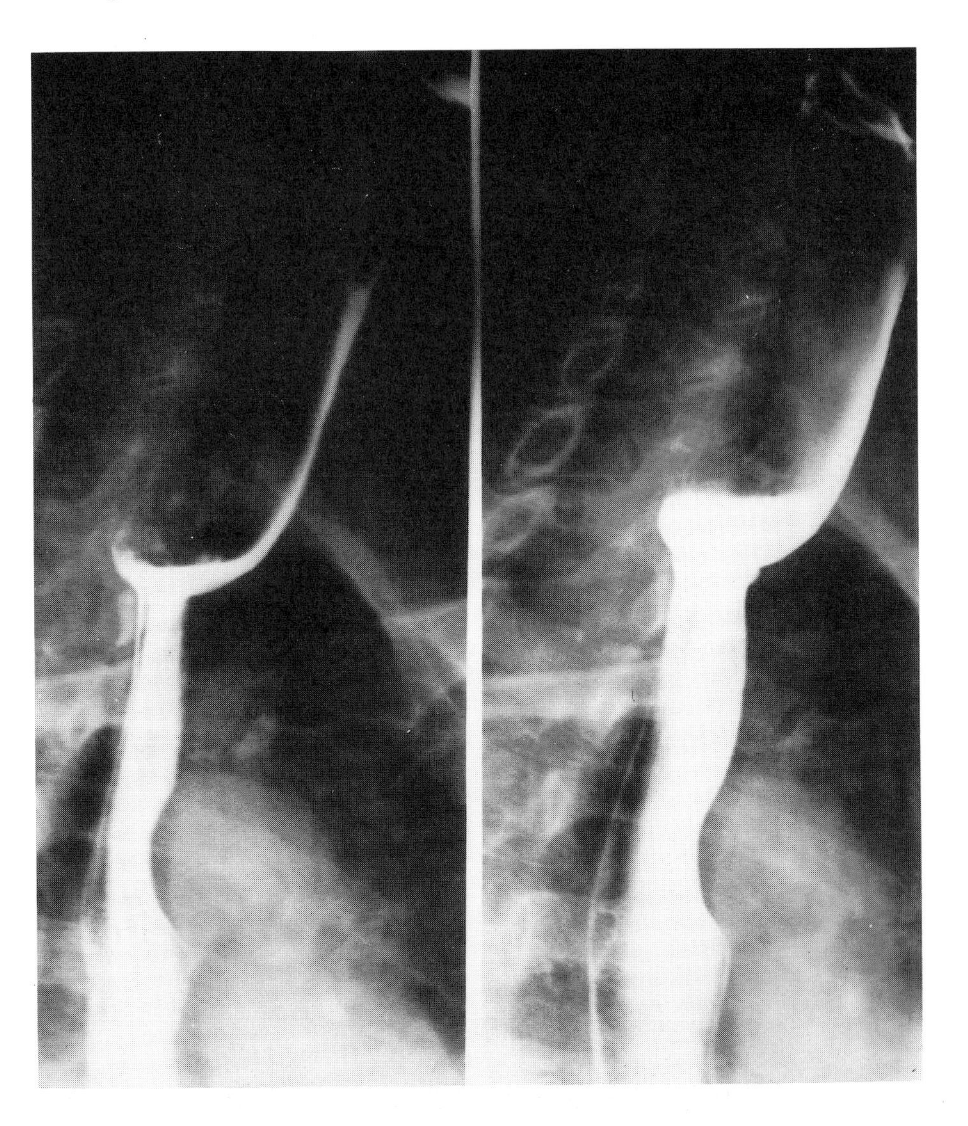

Figure 9.9 *Top:* The good cosmetic result and permanent tracheostomy in a female patient who has undergone a laryngo-oesophago-pharyngectomy in two stages for a carcinoma of the hypopharynx. *Above:* The patient fully rehabilitated, dressed normally and with deglutition fully restored. *Right:* Radiograph with a barium swallow showing the patient's new skin hypopharynx and its junction with the oesophagus.

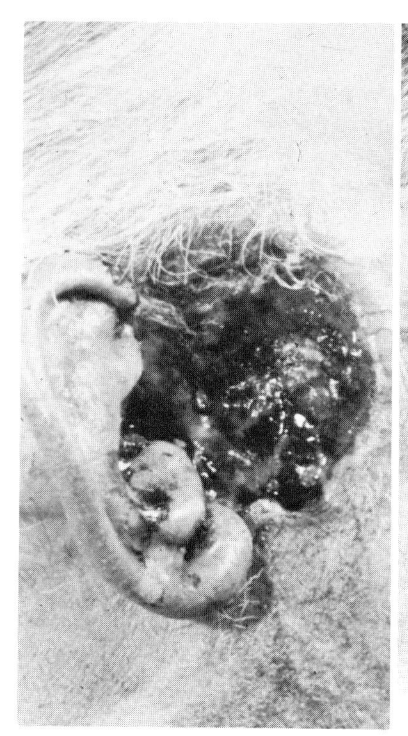

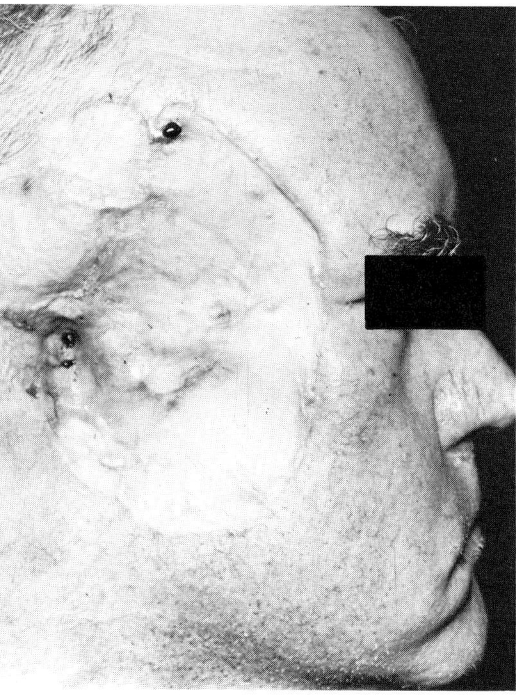

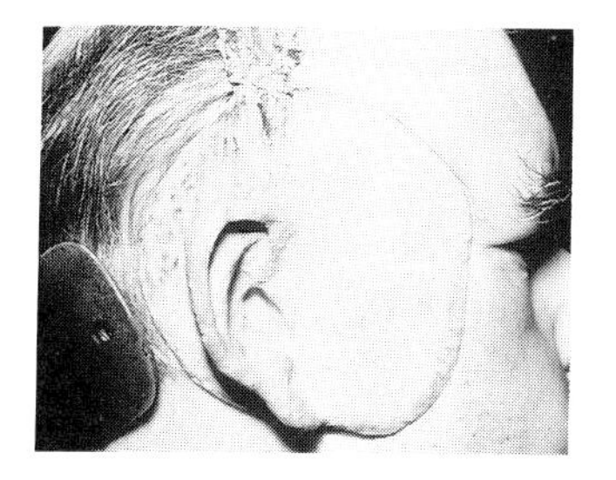

Figure 9.10 *Left:* A male patient with an extensive squamous cell carcinoma involving the skin of the face, pinna, middle and internal ear. This necessitated excision of the right temporal bone and a large area of skin. The defect was repaired with a split-thickness skin graft. *Right:* The patient after satisfactory healing of the excision wound. *Above:* The patient wearing the prosthesis which was specially designed and made for him.

The unit incorporates a day centre that cancer patients can attend from their homes several times a week, thus getting a change of surroundings, recreation, and an opportunity to be with other patients and giving their families a rest. Patients can also be assessed, advised and given appropriate treatment and care in these centres.

The unit provides adequate accommodation for all the different staff members, patients and their families, including beds for patients who need admission for special treatment, care, or other reasons.

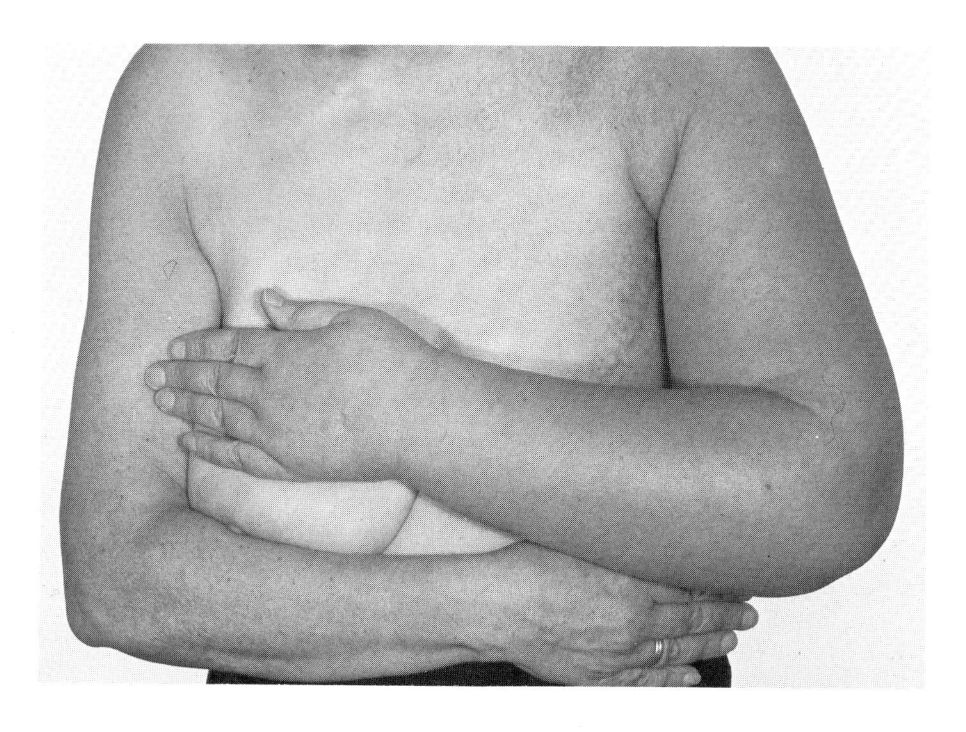

Figure 9.11 A female patient with lymphoedema of the left upper extremity, which is suitable for compression therapy.

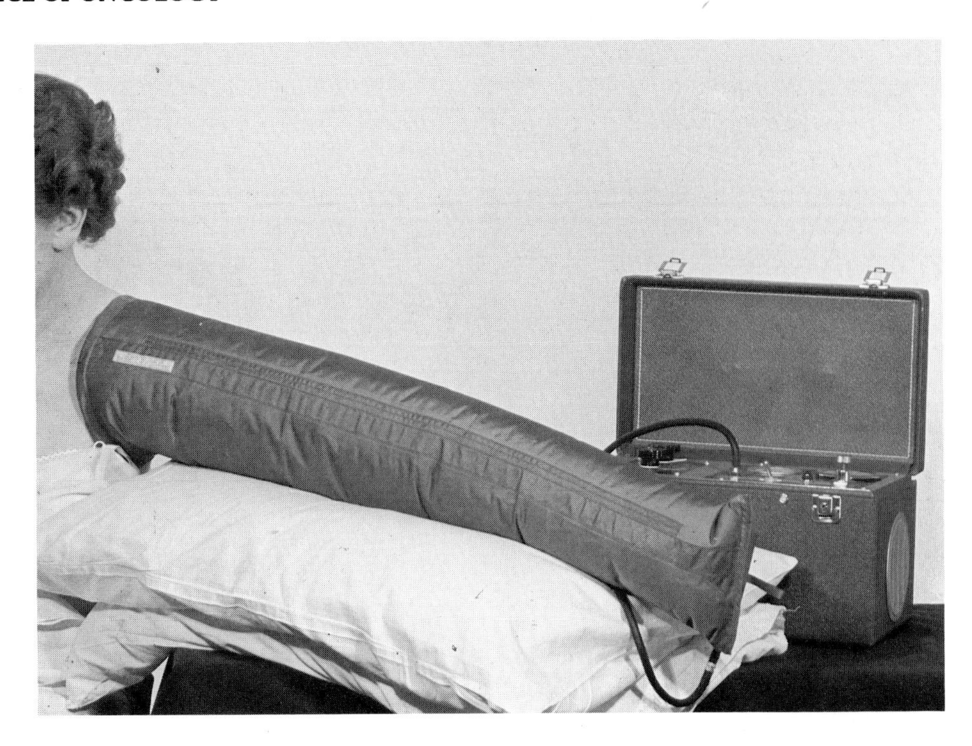

Figure 9.12 A Jobst Intermittent Compression Unit used for the treatment of lymphoedema of the upper extremity.

The reception area where patients register should have a clinical records system with computer facilities. Office accommodation is required for the medical, nursing, paramedical and administrative staff.

Rooms must be provided for consultation, examination and treatment, and have the appropriate equipment, apparatus and instruments for patient treatment and care. A small laboratory for haematology, biochemistry and other investigations is an advantage, especially when the unit is isolated from main laboratory facilities. A room which is suitably equipped for minor surgical procedures such as paracentesis and for wound dressings is a useful asset. Many patients require continuing chemotherapy with intravenous or intramuscular injections; these can be given in this sterile area.

The above general description is applicable when the unit is sited at a special cancer home or hospice. Modifications can be made, of course, when it is part of a hospital or hospital group. This applies also to the need for domestic arrangements, including feeding the staff and patients, and other facilities.

A Pain Control Clinic should be provided with the unit unless treatment of pain is readily available elsewhere. The control of cancer pain is an integral part of rehabilitation and continuing care. In recent years important progress has been made in our knowledge of the nature of cancer pain and in pain control methods.

Increasing numbers of voluntary workers are taking part in the work of continuing care units, especially in connection with patients attending day centres. The provision of transport for patients from their homes to the centres is a valuable service.

CONTINUING CARE

All cancer patients need continuing care. This forms an integrated process with rehabilitation, a process that is initiated at the time of diagnosis and which continues throughout the patient's life. The precise care which different patients need from different professionals varies considerably according to their state of health and local conditions. A system of continuing care for cancer patients must be clearly delineated, operational and available on a national scale. The demands for the appropriate facilities will increase in future years commensurate with the increasing incidence of various cancers throughout the world and the advances occurring in their treatment by surgery, radiotherapy, chemotherapy and combination treatment. The increasing use of cytotoxic medicines necessitates continuing care, especially of patients living at home who attend at regular intervals at hospitals or day centres for advice, treatment and assessment. The following groups of patients for continuing care are clearly identified.

Patients with controlled cancer

This group comprises many patients whose disease has been completely controlled and who are rehabilitated for a life of good quality and duration. These patients must not be lost sight of, but require follow-up supervision for the rest of their lives, though the interval between examinations can be gradually lengthened as they remain free of recurrent and metastatic cancer. Clinical records are compiled for each patient in the follow-up department so that statistical analyses can be made of survival rates for different cancers, correlated with the stage of the disease and the method of treatment.

Patients attending the department may have specific needs, such as replacement therapy for an endocrine imbalance and other imbalances caused by endocrine therapy. Adjustments and repair may be required for various prostheses, and amputation stumps can cause problems. Patients with stomas appreciate the routine surveillance and the opportunity to discuss their continued management.

Special follow-up clinics are arranged for patients with similar diseases. These include breast clinics; clinics for patients with head and neck cancers,

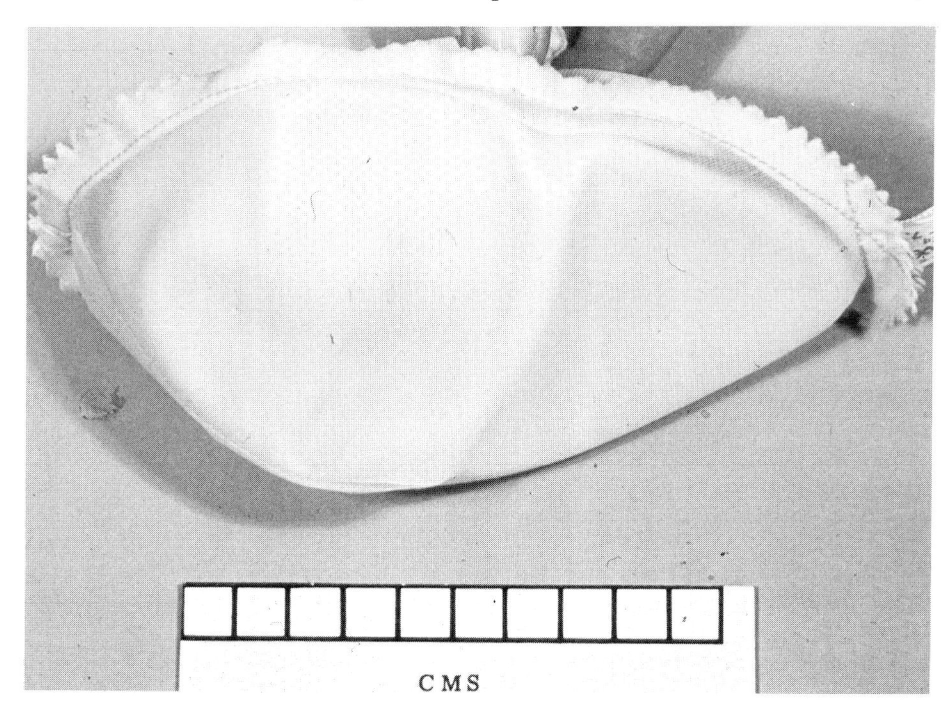

Figure 9.13 A breast prosthesis which is worn inside the patient's brassière. The patient is measured so that the correct size of prosthesis can be supplied.

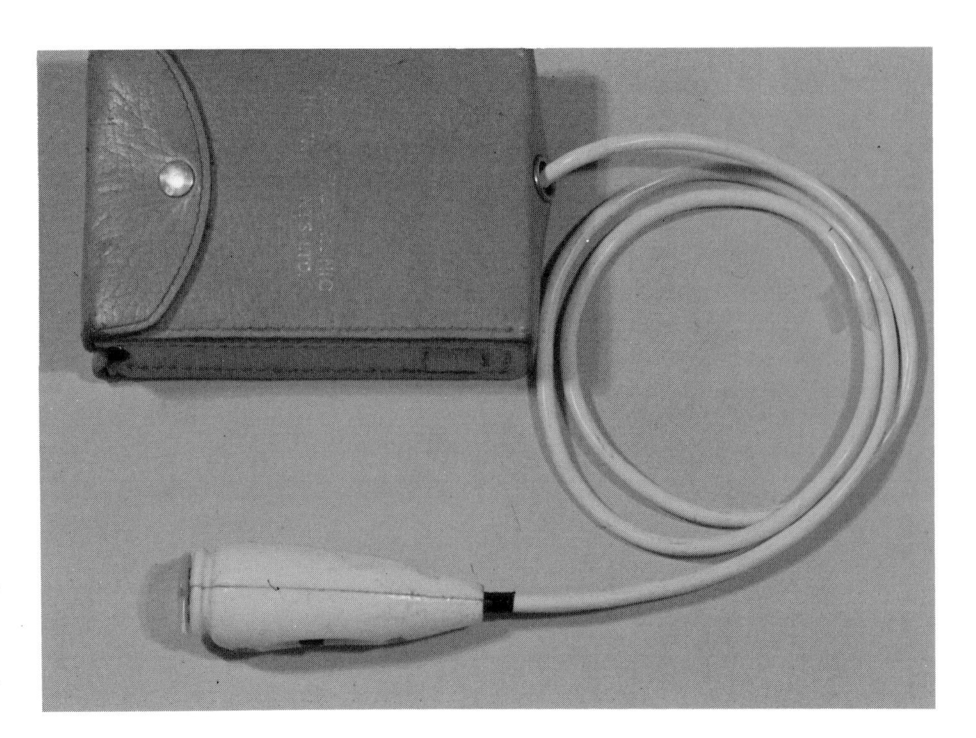

Figure 9.14 A pharyngeal vibrator used to aid voice production and speech after laryngectomy, laryngo-pharyngectomy and laryngo-oesophago-pharyngectomy operations.

especially those who have undergone laryngectomy or laryngopharyngectomy operations; paediatric clinics for the follow-up of children after their definitive treatment; and clinics for patients with gynaecological and dermatological cancers.

Patients with uncontrolled cancer

There are many patients with cancer which is uncontrolled by definitive treatment; some are rehabilitated to make them self-supporting for varying periods. It is a great benefit to them to be ambulant, able to feed themselves and undertake toileting. They all require constant supervision, treatment and care for different periods ranging from a few days to many months.

Many of these patients desire to remain at home with their family until they die. Continuing domiciliary care has therefore to be arranged for them in order that their wishes can be fulfilled. There is a special need for domiciliary nurses to care for these patients throughout the day and night. In the UK the Marie Curie Memorial Foundation provides a nation-wide domiciliary Day and Night Nursing Service, which has given enormous help and relief to many cancer patients and their families.

Family doctors also play a vital role in the domiciliary continuing care system.

Some patients require in-patient continuing care in hospitals, special homes or hospices. The Marie Curie Memorial Foundation has 11 homes for cancer patients, with a total complement of 400 beds, sited in strategic areas of the UK.

Symptom control is of crucial importance in the system of continuing care. Patients may suffer from a variety of different distressing symptoms of which pain might be an outstanding feature. Cancer pain is a global problem and details of its management and control should be made widely known, especially to members of the medical and nursing professions.

Important advances have been made in our knowledge of the causes and biochemistry of cancer pain, and effective methods of treatment, including physical and pharmaceutical means, are now available. Reference has already been made to the establishment of special Pain Control Clinics.

Patients may experience other symptoms and these need to be appropriately treated in order to make them comfortable. Various metabolic syndromes can develop, including hypercalcaemia, hypocalcaemia, the inappropriate antidiuretic syndrome, hypokalaemia, and hyperuricaemia, all of which require urgent treatment, or death could occur.

Finally, considerable attention has been given during recent years to the needs and the care of patients who are dying from cancer. Such patients may be at home with their families, where they receive the necessary special care. Others are admitted to special homes, hospices and hospitals. They all have spiritual as well as physical needs and they should all be given the tender, loving care which they require; here the patient's pastor can be of great help.

The ensuing family bereavement must be assuaged as much as possible by giving all necessary help and support.

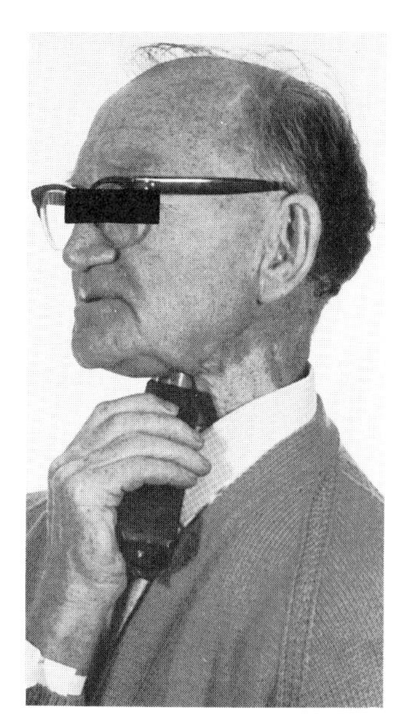

Figure 9.15 An elderly patient with a permanent tracheostomy after laryngectomy, using a pharyngeal vibrator in order to speak satisfactorily.

RESEARCH IN REHABILITATION AND CONTINUING CARE

There must be on-going research to find ways and means of improving the quality of life of patients with oncological diseases. This means there must be collaborative work betweeen cancer research institutes, biochemical engineering departments and rehabilitation and continuing care units.

Certain projects of the research effort are as follows.

Reactions of patients

Information is required about the reactions of patients to different conditions caused by cancer. Patients' reactions vary on hearing the diagnosis of cancer and can include shock, fear and even despondency. All the different reactions should be studied and measured to give guidance to members of the caring professions on how to deal with them. This includes the study of communication between doctors, nurses and patients.

Patients' reactions to proposed methods of treatment need more study. Information is required concerning the motivation of patients in accepting or refusing the treatment advised, for patient compliance is becoming increasingly important and necessary.

Patient dependency and social adaptation

A study should be made of methods of diminishing periods of hospitalisation and of ways to expedite the resettlement of patients in family life and appropriate work. More information is needed about the different work loads which cancer patients can undertake in various circumstances and about their adaptability to new employment.

Measurement of patient deficits

Certain deficits need to be measured and rectified in order that the patient can be restored to full mobility as soon as possible. For this work we need measurements of ambulation deficits, muscle power, and muscle wasting. The former are especially necessary in the case of patients who have undergone amputations of the lower limbs and have prostheses fitted.

The nutritional state of the patient should be measured by various parameters. These should include the degree of general and muscle wasting, loss of weight and functions of the alimentary system. Food values and caloric intake are measured to determine whether nutrition is adequate.

Estimates of renal and liver functions are made and the haematology and biochemical profiles are done. Endocrine deficits may be present, for example, after total thyroidectomy; these are measured and rectified.

Hormonal control mechanisms

These mechanisms play a vital role in the development and treatment of carcinoma of the breast and prostate and perhaps in other varieties of cancer too. We manipulate them by endocrine ablation procedures and by the administration of synthetic hormones, but we do not yet understand their working. Here much more scientific research work is required.

Pain control mechanisms

Considerable advances are being made to elucidate these mechanisms. We are learning more about pain mechanisms in the peripheral nervous system, with its pain receptors. The discovery of the brain receptor system of pain, with its opiate peptides, enkephalins and endorphins, is of immense importance. We are now seeking methods to stimulate this natural system so that the brain can provide its own opiates for pain relief. More accurate methods are needed for the measurement of pain, both by subjective and objective techniques. Similarly there is a need for the wider use of pain charts to record all observations and treatment.

Prostheses

Many different prostheses are required for cancer patients and they contribute considerably to the wearers' quality of life. There is on-going research to improve both their appearance and function.

Enormous advances have been made in limb prostheses since the original Chelsea Peg prosthesis was introduced. New materials are being used for their manufacture and the activation of prostheses is being studied so that "powered limbs" can be provided. Power systems are being sought for incorporation in upper limb prostheses to improve their functions and make their movements resemble the normal movements of the arm and hand. The latter is a difficult task but with the development of computer science and technology we can expect such improvements in coming years.

Incontinence

The presence of faecal or urinary incontinence adds very considerably to the suffering of cancer patients. Amelioration can be given by courses of electrical stimulation of the rectal and bladder muscle sphincters. The development of small electrical devices for placement in the appropriate sphincter mechanism is promising.

In all this important research close collaboration is necessary between researchers and clinicians, and essential help must be given by computer scientists, biomedical engineers and other professionals for progress to be made to help so many patients in their distress.

REFERENCE

Raven, R. W. (1986). *Rehabilitation and Continuing Care in Cancer*. Published on behalf of the International Union Against Cancer by Parthenon Publishing Group, Carnforth

CHAPTER TEN

Counselling Services

Counselling is a comparatively recent development and it is attracting an ever-growing amount of attention. Certainly both patients and their families have a great need for it. So many difficult problems, which have to be carefully considered and solved, are created by the oncological diseases and their treatment that patients and their families need considerable support and guidance during this time, which can be the most trying period of their lives. There are also many fears and much apprehension to be assuaged by helpful discussions with people who have the time to listen and who are able to give sound advice.

In addition to professionals who take part in counselling, some voluntary associations also participate in a most helpful way. The art of communication is involved in this work and in a general sense it should be acquired by professionals during their training in medicine, nursing and the paramedical professions. Counsellors need special qualities of heart and mind, so that they are capable of having an insight into the thoughts of other people and realising their problems, difficulties, hopes and fears. Following a correct appraisal of the situation, the counsellor should be able to suggest solutions and indicate the sources of help and means to attain them. He or she must create an atmosphere of sympathy and helpfulness which engenders trust. Different forms of counselling are discussed in the following paragraphs.

PROFESSIONAL COUNSELLING

Persons who undertake this work usually need special training and some knowledge of the oncological diseases to be able to function in a meaningful way. They should also be kind and sympathetic, able to understand and enter into the sufferings of others, and have a deep knowledge of human nature. The possession of a strong spiritual faith and belief in God is also a tremendous help.

Professional counselling is required during all the stages of cancer, for even when the diagnosis is first made problems arise for both patient and family. The clinician who makes the diagnosis of cancer will communicate the findings to the patient and near relatives in words that are carefully chosen so as not to alarm but to give hope for the future; he will assure them that everything possible will be done to get the patient back to good health. He will outline the programme of rehabilitation which should restore the patient to a life of good quality at home with his family and enable him to undertake work and enjoy recreations (see Chapter 9).

There has always been considerable discussion as to whether the patient should be told that he or she has cancer, because of possible unfavourable reactions to the diagnosis. The author believes that it is desirable for the majority of patients to know the truth, which should be expressed to them in the kindest terms in the presence of a spouse or near relative. He has found that in these circumstances complete trust is formed between the doctor and patient and they are then able to work together with the knowledge that the patient clearly understands the situation and will collaborate in carrying out the rehabilitation programme.

Patient compliance has assumed great importance in cancer work. If the patient is not told the diagnosis many difficulties can subsequently arise and confidence in the doctor may be weakened, especially if the patient's progress is poor.

It is realised that there are certain patients who cannot be told the truth for various reasons, including adverse psychological reactions; sometimes the patient's family makes a special request that the diagnosis be withheld. This may create a difficult situation when the patient has advanced cancer with a short prognosis and no marked improvement occurs with treatment but rather there is a constant deterioration of health. The result may be that the patient unfortunately loses confidence in the doctor and seeks advice and treatment elsewhere.

In counselling the patient and family about the diagnosis and rehabilitation, including the definitive treatment, it is very important that the doctor makes them clearly understand what will be done and the expected end-results. The majority of patients will accept all advice which is presented in this helpful way, but some patients and relatives may request a second opinion and this request should always be granted.

COUNSELLING BY PATIENTS

Patients can receive valuable help and support when they are visited by other patients who have undergone successful operations of the type that they themselves are contemplating. For example, it is very helpful for a patient with a carcinoma of the rectum which is to be treated by an abdominoperineal excision of the rectum and the institution of a permanent colostomy to be visited by a patient who has successfully undergone the same operation. The patient who has recovered is seen to be dressed normally, fully active and able to work without any interference from the colostomy. They can speak together in lay language about colostomy management and other subjects.

Similar counselling is very beneficial for patients who have to undergo an operation of laryngectomy, laryngo-pharyngectomy or laryngo-oesophago-pharyngectomy, which will mean that they have to be fitted with a permanent tracheostomy. They derive encouragement by seeing and talking to patients who have successfully undergone the same operation and who are able to dress normally and, in many cases, speak well. They can also discuss tracheostomy management from the patient's viewpoint.

Other patients who will benefit from this kind of counselling are those who have to undergo a major amputation; for example, of a limb or breast. When they see and talk to patients wearing a breast or limb prosthesis they are greatly helped and encouraged.

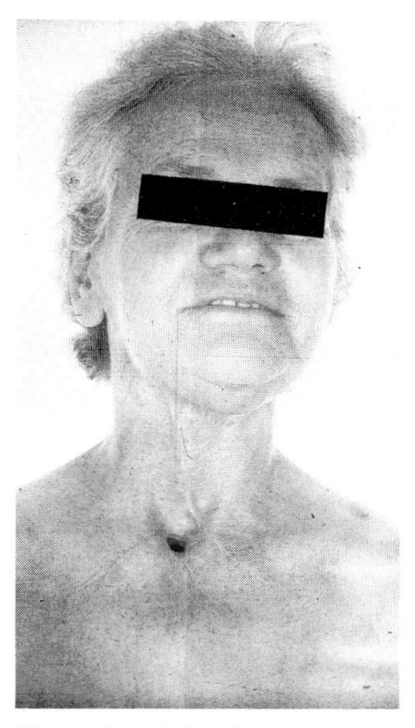

Figure 10.1 A female patient who has been rehabilitated and regained a good speaking voice after a laryngectomy operation. She took part in patient counselling of laryngectomy patients.

Special clubs for patients

A valuable extension of individual patient counselling is the formation of special clubs where group discussions can be held and patients can share their experiences with others. Patients who have undergone similar cancer operations can meet together regularly to help each other in various ways, including training. A good example is the laryngectomy club. This kind of work is incorporated into the functions of day centres.

FAMILY COUNSELLING

The family of a cancer patient have a number of problems to solve and they need help and support for different periods. They are concerned about the condition and progress of the patient during the short or long term and they may be experiencing economic difficulties because of the patient's inability to work. Advice might be required about the patient's likely physical and psychological state when he or she returns home after rehabilitation. The services of the medical social worker are valuable here. It is helpful to visit the family at home so that advice can be given and the appropriate arrangements made to receive the patient back into family life. If the patient has certain disabilities, alterations might be required in the house, and new accommodation might even be necessary if a patient cannot climb stairs. Means of locomotion and transport might need discussion and action, including altering a motor-car so that it can be driven by a disabled driver.

COUNSELLING OF THE BEREAVED

Bereavement can cause severe emotional reactions and illness. This is known as the grief process and is most distressing following the death of a loved relative or friend. It can also occur when there is loss of health and the diagnosis of cancer is made, when certain body functions are lost, or part of the body is amputated. Patients who are suffering bereavement and grief need careful medical observation, care and treatment.

Counselling of the bereaved is a delicate and special component of general counselling, whose objective is comforting bereaved individuals and families and assuaging their sorrow. It is a very important part of the work of doctors, nurses, pastors and other religious leaders, medical social workers and all members of the caring professions. Their sympathetic approach, sensitivity of mind and warmth of heart are basic requirements for such work and are enhanced by their own experience of sorrow, suffering and bereavement. The importance of their own spiritual faith is stressed when they seek to comfort others.

Suitable and adequate instruction and experience are required during the training period of these professionals, together with the strengthening of their personal faith in God. Special qualities can be developed in this way which are very valuable in caring for dying patients and bereaved families.

Bereaved persons and families greatly appreciate frequent visits by their doctor, who has become a trusted friend throughout the patient's illness. His visits should be special and unhurried and continued for a reasonable period of time, until there is amelioration of their grief and loneliness, which can be almost too great to bear.

Home visiting by their pastor or religious leader is also very important and much appreciated by families in their distress, for so many people feel the need for the spiritual help and support which these visits can give them.

While the effects of grief and bereavement can be serious and even devastating, it is well to remember that time is a good healer. The acute sense of loss is gradually ameliorated by the passage of time and the realisation that life must continue, even though it might never be the same again.

The subject of counselling has developed relatively recently and represents one particular advance which is being made in the total care of patients with cancer.

REFERENCES

Raven, R. W. (1975). *The Dying Patient.* Pitman Medical Publishing Co. Ltd, Tunbridge Wells

Raven, R. W. (1986). *Rehabilitation and Continuing Care in Cancer*, pp 33–9. Published on behalf of the International Union Against Cancer by Parthenon Publishing Group, Carnforth

CHAPTER ELEVEN

Education and Training in Oncology

EDUCATION

For the clinical oncologist, education is a continual learning process throughout professional life. It is distinguished from the training process, which involves acquiring skills in a treatment modality such as surgery, medicine or radiation techniques. During recent years increasing attention has been given to education and training, for many more graduates are enquiring about what is required to enable them to specialise in the different areas of clinical oncology and how to acquire the necessary knowledge and skills. Rapid advances are being made in understanding the biology of cancer and in the different treatments for the various diseases. It is now possible to delineate both the theory and the practice of oncology, subjects which are described in detail in Chapters 7 and 8.

Knowledge of the basic oncological sciences is essential for the clinical oncologist because of its value in illuminating the nature of the neoplastic diseases and its practical importance for their prevention, diagnosis, treatment, rehabilitation and continuing care. Graduate education commences during the period of training in the practice of oncology and continues through attendance at special courses in basis sciences and other subjects, lectures, symposia and seminars, and through keeping abreast of all the literature. Sufficient time should be allowed for trainees to attend such special courses and teaching sessions, which should be held in suitable centres to which they have easy access. All the above-mentioned types of teaching activity are being developed throughout the UK by universities, Royal Colleges, hospitals, postgraduate medical centres, and some charitable organisations.

Academic departments

It is noteworthy how many academic departments in clinical oncology are being established, and they are bound to increase in number. They are concerned with medical and radiation oncology and are headed by professors and their academic staff. They are responsible for patient care, education, training, and clinical research. It is hoped that clinical departments with professors and other staff will be established soon in surgical oncology. Already there are flourishing associations and societies, and some specialist clinical posts have been created.

Interdisciplinary education

There are many aspects of clinical oncology which require the attention of and need to be understood by all members of the caring professions who are responsible for the rehabilitation and continuing care of patients with cancer. In fact, the members of the oncology team are involved with the different professions they represent. The need for interdisciplinary education has been recognised by a number of organisations, which arrange special discussion programmes on subjects and problems of mutual interest and importance. Special courses, symposia, teach-ins and seminars are also arranged on a regular basis. There is a great demand for this kind of education in oncology, which will be used increasingly in the future.

Education of medical students

It is important for medical students to have a basic education in oncology, as many will become family doctors who have to care for patients with cancer in their own homes. In addition, they will have to play a vital role in the diagnosis of oncological diseases and should be able to advise people on the prevention of cancer. Oncology should be given a more prominent place in the medical curriculum, for in the past it has not been given the importance that it merits.

Community education

This subject, which is dealt with in Chapter 6, has developed in an impressive way in recent years. There was a time when there was considerable professional reluctance to speak publicly about cancer because it was felt that doing so would cause fear and despondency in people and even cancer phobia. Pioneering public education in cancer has been carried out by the Chelsea Cancer Education Committee *(Raven and Gough-Thomas, 1951)* and the subject has been clearly described by Wakefield *(1958)*, who did much important work with the Manchester Committee on Cancer.

TRAINING

The object of training for clinical oncologists is the development of clinical judgement and technical skills in the total management — including definitive treatment by the modalities of surgery, radiation and medicine — of patients with oncological diseases. Training is integrated with education and is an on-going process.

Considerable experience and skills are necessary in the general care and definitive treatment of patients, who often present difficult clinical problems. Combined surgical, radiation and medical treatment (the treatment triad) is used increasingly for many patients, so it is advisable for students to have periods of interdisciplinary training. There are well structured training programmes for medical oncologists and for radiation oncologists, but surgical oncology is still lagging behind, though it is hoped that relevant training programmes will be developed soon in the UK. For all trainees in oncology, general professional training in their particular discipline and the possession of high qualifications are essential. During their training they will gain experience in the investigation, diagnosis and management of cancer patients and become familiar with the indications for all methods of treatment which are used and the role, side-effects and complications of surgery, radiation and chemotherapy. The special skills and experience required by the three types of specialists are as follows.

Medical oncologists

Experience is acquired in all aspects of systemic therapy and supportive care of patients. This includes the study of the pharmacology of chemotherapeutic medicines, their modes of administration, dosage schedules and side-effects. Experience should be gained in the medical management of all forms of oncological diseases — leukaemias, lymphomas and solid tumours — including supportive care, the control and prevention of infections, cell component therapy, correction of nutritional and other deficits and the diagnosis and treatment of metabolic abnormalities and syndromes.

Paediatric oncology is a subspeciality of medical oncology which requires special training. It is justified by the importance of oncological diseases in children and the continuing progress which is being made in their diagnosis and treatment.

Radiation oncologists

Radiation oncologists need to have had a sound basic training and good experience in general medicine, followed by special training to obtain experience in the investigation and diagnosis of oncological diseases and the general management of patients. They should be familiar with the indications for the other methods of treatment. They frequently give chemotherapy when it is necessary. Experience and skill must be acquired in all the forms of radiation techniques which are used so often for cancer patients, both alone and in combination with surgery and chemotherapy.

Surgical oncologists

Both general and specialist surgeons will continue to be responsible for the investigation, diagnosis and surgical treatment of large numbers of patients with oncological diseases, which can affect many organs and tissues of the body. This responsibility will be additional to their other responsibilities, so special training in surgical oncology is very helpful for them. Some surgeons have a total or major interest in and commitment to surgical oncology and for these and more junior surgeons a training programme is essential. The surgical oncologist must be a well-trained technical surgeon who can competently perform many major, difficult surgical operations. Experience is acquired in the solution of clinical problems created by cancer and in the general management of cancer patients.

Some people training in general surgery today will later have to carry a heavy work load in surgical oncology and so would benefit from training programmes in surgical oncology. Such programmes should be arranged at hospitals where large numbers of cancer patients are investigated and treated by surgery, radiation and chemotherapy, for in addition to acquiring surgical expertise the trainee should have the opportunity to learn about the indications, side-effects and complications of radiation techniques and chemotherapy, alone or combined.

Trainees in all three disciplines must learn about the prevention of oncological diseases so that they can give the appropriate advice to people. Time should be allowed for them to attend clinico-pathological conferences, regular pathology review meetings and other multidisciplinary conferences.

Trainees should carry out a clinical or laboratory research project, especially if they plan to make a career in academic clinical oncology. They should also be given opportunities to develop their teaching abilities by lecturing, conducting clinical demonstrations and doing ward rounds. They should be encouraged and helped to write articles for publication in the medical literature.

REFERENCES

Raven, R. W. and Gough-Thomas, J. (1951). Cancer education of the public. *Lancet*, **2**, 495–6

Wakefield, J. (1958). Cancer education for the public in Great Britain. In Raven, R. W. (ed.) *Cancer*, Vol. 3, pp 407–16. Butterworth & Co., London

CHAPTER TWELVE

Cancer of the Breast: Historical Landmarks in Treatment

Carcinoma of the breast is the most freqently occurring malignant tumour in women in the Western world, though it is rarely found in men. The cause for this difference in incidence is unknown. Although other types of tumour, both benign and malignant, do occur in the female breast, carcinoma is the most common and is the main subject of this chapter in which the historical aspects of treatment are discussed.

Clinicians and researchers are rightly anxious to solve the problems connected with the aetiology and treatment of this disease which causes a high mortality and severe morbidity. The opinion is often expressed today that there has been no improvement in the results of treatment over many past decades, but a study of the end-results which have been published by many authorities in the literature does not substantiate this view. On the contrary, there is definite evidence that real progress has been made, as described in this chapter.

For many years there have been arguments as to what is the best treatment for breast carcinoma and the controversy still continues today. In fact, there is really no consensus regarding the advice that should be given to patients, and this can cause them concern. In order to clarify the situation and dispel the confusion, clinical trials continue to be carried out. The results are awaited with both concern and interest, for breast carcinoma is a dangerous and unpredictable disease.

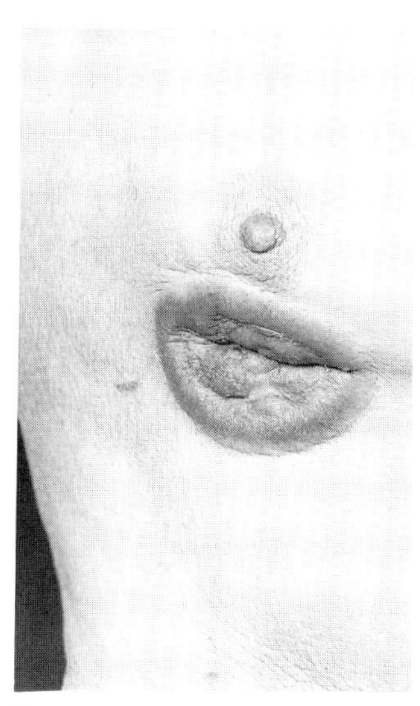

Figure 12.1 An unusual breast carcinoma – the keloid type.

SURGICAL TREATMENT

Different surgical operations have been advocated for breast carcinoma, which vary in their extent from local excision of the tumour to supraradical mastectomy. An examination of the end-results of these different procedures in their historical setting makes an interesting and salutary study, for important lessons can be learned which provide a valuable guide for our own treatment of carcinoma of the breast.

Operations for breast carcinoma in the 19th century

On 28 May 1867 Charles H. Moore, who was Surgeon to the Middlesex Hospital in London, addressed the Royal Medical and Chirurgical Society of London as its Vice-President. His talk was entitled "On the influence of inadequate operations on the theory of cancer", and was concerned mainly with cancer of the breast.

More than 100 years ago different operations were carried out for breast carcinoma — a comparable situation to that which exists today. Moore's description of these operations included the following words: "Sometimes the tumour only is removed, sometimes that segment of the breast in which the tumour lies is taken away with it; sometimes with the intention of extirpating the entire mamma, the failure happens that a portion of it is unwittingly left behind; sometimes the breast is carefully removed, but the propensity of cancer to extension in the skin is misapprehended, and, for symmetry's sake, a flap which even includes the nipple is preserved; and yet again, there being no definite plan in the mind of the operator but of cutting wide of the tumour, portions of the organ are left behind. The consequence of this last method of operating may be at once apparent, when, on examining the mass thus dug out of the centre of the breast, hard cancerous cords, continuous with the principal tumour are found to have been cut across. Their outer extremities, prolonged to the margin of the breast, remain behind, and it is fortunate if the discovery be made before the wound is closed and the patient replaced in bed." At that time there was no frozen section histopathology technique available to confirm the surgical clearance of the tumour.

Moore stressed the important rule that the whole tumour must be removed, since if the least remnant is left behind it is capable of growth and "may spring up into a new tumour with all the energy of the first". Referring to his own experience, he stated, "Five times within a couple of months I have found supposed extirpation of cancer to be demonstrably incomplete".

He illustrated his talk with case-records which showed the effects of "inadequate operations" for breast cancer. The patients concerned had developed recurrent cancer in the breast and axilla and also in breast remnants and scars. He concluded his address by stating, "... cancer of the breast requires the careful extirpation of the entire organ; that the situation in which this operation is most likely to be incomplete is at the edge of the mamma next the sternum; that, besides the breast, unsound adjoining textures, especially skin, should be removed in the same mass with the principal disease."

Results in breast cancer reported by Sir James Paget

Sir James Paget *(1856)* reported the end-results, including survival periods, of a series of 139 cases of scirrhous cancer of the breast. In the 75 cases in which no operation was carried out the average duration of life following the diagnosis was 48 months, while for the 64 patients who survived an operation the corresponding period was 52 months. The longest period of survival in the former group was 216 months and in the latter 146 months. The shortest periods were 7 and 7½ months, respectively.

These end-results in the treatment of breast cancer in London in the mid-19th century demonstrate the dangerous nature of this disease and show that the treatment which was given at that time was only a little more efficacious than leaving the patient untreated. The average survival period of untreated patients was only 4 months shorter than that of treated patients.

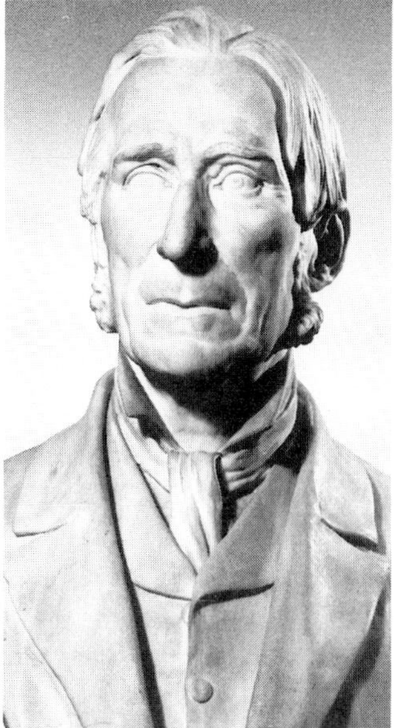

Figure 12.2 Sir James Paget (1814–1899), Sergeant-Surgeon to Queen Victoria and Surgeon to the Royal Hospital of St Bartholomew. He made important contributions to the understanding of several diseases, including osteitis deformans. He described certain chronic affections of the skin and areola of the breast which bear his name and are followed by the development of scirrhous carcinoma.

A new operation for breast cancer

Sweeting *(1869)* was impressed by the unsatisfactory results after "the ordinary operations" for cancer of the breast and noted that the disease generally returned after 6–8 months. He cited the observation of Sir James Paget that the disease usually recurred after 6 months, but that the patient might be considered safe in those very rare cases when the operation scar was soft and sound after 14 months. Sweeting commented, "This result is so rare that many experienced hospital surgeons have never seen it. If the disease returns so frequently, why not cut deeper?" It will be noticed that Sweeting was concerned only with the breast tumour and not with the regional lymph nodes in the axilla.

The operation he advocated consisted of the removal of a larger area of the skin covering the breast, and, instead of the breast being dissected off the underlying pectoralis fascia, the removal of the lower two-thirds of the pectoralis major muscle and all the tissues above it, except the skin. He described the results of three cases in which this new operation had "permanent success".

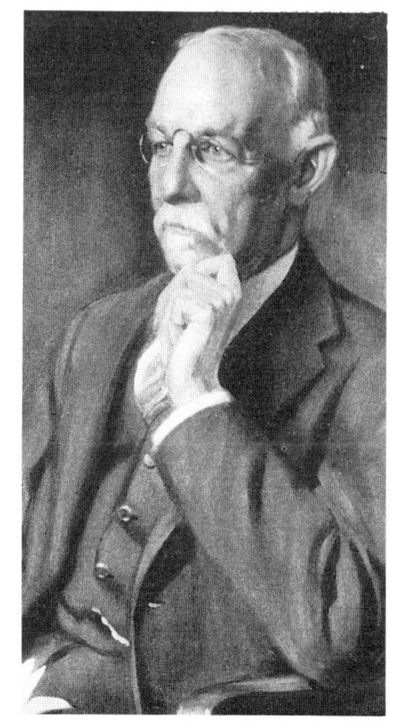

Figure 12.3 William S. Halsted (1852–1922).

Results in breast cancer treatment reviewed by William Halsted

The subject of carcinoma of the breast was of considerable interest to William Halsted, who was Surgeon to the Johns Hopkins Hospital in Baltimore, USA, and whose name is associated in perpetuity with the operation of radical mastectomy which he designed and practised.

Halsted *(1894)* reviewed the end-results obtained by different surgeons in the treatment of breast cancer and quoted the results 3 years after operations by the leading surgeons in Europe. The percentage 3-year survival rates were as follows:

Bergman, E., 30.2%; Billroth, V. W., 4.7%; Fischer, H., 9%; Güssenbauer, F., 16.7%; König, H., 22.5%; Küster, S., 21.5%; Lucke, D., 16.2%; and Volkmann, S., 14%.

Halsted stated that Volkmann and Güssenbauer were perhaps the first surgeons to suggest that it might be advisable to explore the axilla in every case, but that Küster was the first surgeon to advocate systematic axillary lymph node dissection (see Chapter 1).

The serious nature of cancer of the breast during that era is illustrated by Halsted's words: "Most of us have heard our teachers in surgery admit that they have never cured a case of cancer of the breast. The younger Gross did not save one of his first hundred cases." He also quoted the statement made by Haynes Agnew, in a lecture delivered a very short time before his death, that he operated on breast cancer solely for the morale effect on the patients, but believed the operation shortened, rather than prolonged, life.

Halsted referred to the end-results achieved by others too, including Nelaton, who had several patients who were permanently cured after an operation for breast cancer, and Velpeau, who knew of seven women—out of a series of 187 operated on for breast cancer—who lived for periods ranging from 5 to 20 years after the operation. He stated that Volkmann never performed a partial amputation of the breast, but made it his rule to remove the entire breast, even for the smallest tumour, together with a liberal piece of overlying skin and the fascia covering the pectoralis major muscle.

Halsted was impressed by the high rates of local recurrence in breast cancer after the operations which were performed, often without dissection of the axillary lymph nodes, by the following surgeons:

Billroth, 85% (180 cases); Czerny, 62% (102 cases); Fischer, 75% (147 cases); Küster, 60% (228 cases); Volkmann, 59% (131 cases); and Güssenbauer, 64% (154 cases).

Such high local recurrence rates of breast cancer are, of course, serious and quite unacceptable. The treatment of breast carcinoma should be designed, if at all possible, to at least prevent the growth of local recurrent disease. Halsted wrote: "Everyone knows how dreadful the end-results were before cleaning out the axilla became recognised as an essential part of the operation." In the same article he described the technical details of his radical mastectomy operation and stated that following this operation none of his patients developed local recurrent disease for a period of 3, or in some cases even more, years. His results were far superior to those quoted earlier in this chapter.

Breast cancer end-results at Johns Hopkins Hospital, Baltimore

The end-results achieved at this hospital after Halsted's important pioneer work there were reported in a review by Lewis and Rienhoff *(1932)*, which is of great value and interest. These authors described the results obtained

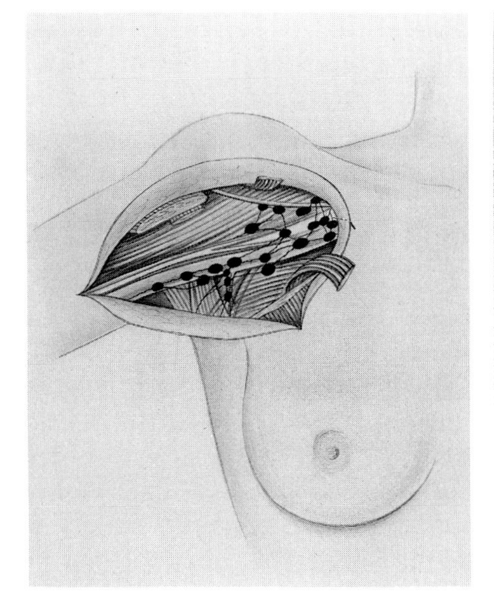

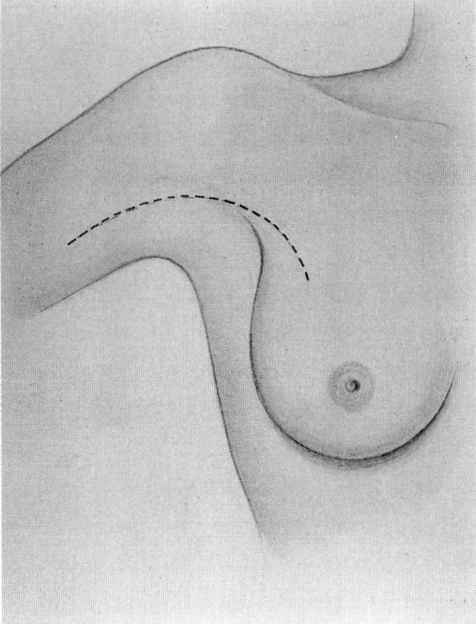

Figure 12.4 *Left:* The group of lymph nodes in the axilla after division of the pectoralis major and minor muscles. *Right:* The curved incision which might be necessary for the excision of the axillary lymph nodes when a malignant tumour in the upper extremity is treated, for example, a malignant melanoma of the skin.

in the treatment of breast cancer in the years 1889–1931. The hospital was opened in 1889 and their survey concerns 950 patients who were observed over a period of 42 years.

They explained that in the hospital's early years, before 1910, breast cancer was usually more extensive when the patients were admitted and the limits of operability were considerably wider than in 1932 when their report was published. In this series of 950 patients 72 (7.6%) were untreated because their disease was considered inoperable. In 21 cases (2.2%) an incomplete operation was performed to remove an ulcerated carcinoma or to prevent ulceration occurring. The ages of the patients ranged from 20 to 78 years. The authors state that breast carcinoma increases in frequency during the 2nd and 3rd decades of life and reaches its maximum incidence during the later years of the 7th decade.

There were nine cases of carcinoma of the male breast in this series. The marital status of the patients, compared with that in a series of non-cancer cases, was of no significance; 87.3% of patients were married, 12.4% were unmarried and the marital status of 0.1% was unknown.

The end-results reported in this series of 950 cases are as follows: known dead, 420 cases (44.2%); 209 cases (22%) were lost track of and presumed dead; 97 patients (10%) were alive and well and 65 (67%) of these had lived more than 5 years since their operation. Full details are found in the article by Lewis and Rienhoff.

The authors concluded from their studies that the large majority of patients with breast carcinoma died of it but quite a large number remained free of clinical cancer for a variable number of years after their operation. Undoubtedly, if operations were performed well the disease could be cured locally and this was the only result for which the surgeon should hold himself responsible. They pointed out that it was always possible that the disease could remain as a localised process which had not spread beyond the limits of operability, and this was especially true in the very early cases that were under observation at the time of their report. They advocated a thoroughly radical removal in all cases, whether the stage of cancer reached was early or late, because of the impossibility of foretelling the exact limits of the spread of the disease.

They also stated that it was a well-known and proved fact that patients who had had a primary tumour removed and who had lived without symptoms of clinical cancer for many years afterwards, then finally succumbed to some other malady, had been found to have regional metastases in which microscopical carcinoma could readily be demonstrated. It is interesting that the problem of micrometastases is well recognised today. In support of their statement concerning dormant tumour metastases Lewis and Rienhoff cited the case-record reported by Peugniez *(1924)*. In this case, the autopsy, which was performed 25 years later, showed carcinoma metastases in the liver and retroperitoneal lymph nodes, but the residual part of the stomach was normal following partial gastrectomy for cancer.

Lewis and Rienhoff point out that carcinoma appears to vary not only in its rate of growth, but also in its damaging clinical effects when the cells are removed from their primary site to a different type of tissue, such as a lymph node or other organ, when metastases develop. This idea is supported by the observation that the postoperative longevity of patients without local recurrent disease is greater than that of patients in whom a tumour recurs in the operation field. This is true despite the fact that in both groups there may be remote metastases.

Results of treatment of breast cancer at the Royal Hospital of St Bartholomew, London

The present author published a report on the end-results of the treatment of breast cancer at this hospital *(Raven, 1933)* in culmination of the work which had proceeded since 1922 when patients treated for breast cancer in the wards of the hospital began to be followed-up after their discharge.

The investigation included all the patients admitted to the wards during the years 1922–1932, who were followed-up to the end of 1932. The total number of 1009 patients included 894 with primary spheroidal carcinoma, 34 with primary columnar cell carcinoma, and 81 who were admitted for treatment after operations performed elsewhere. At that time three different operations for breast carcinoma were performed in this hospital, namely, radical mastectomy, mastectomy with excision of the axillary lymph nodes, and simple mastectomy. The survival rates at 3 and 5 years for the series of 394 patients who were treated by a radical mastectomy are given in Table 9. The numbers of patients who underwent treatment by the other operations were too small for comparison.

Table 9 Breast carcinoma treated by radical mastectomy

Stage of disease	*3-year survival rate*	*5-year survival rate*
Stage 1	65.4%	49.4%
Stage 2	34.5%	24.3%

It is interesting to compare the survival rates quoted in Table 9 with those that are published today, although it is now agreed that much longer periods must elapse after treatment for accurate assessments to be made. Thus survival rates of 10, 15 and 20 years are now studied.

The author pointed out as a result of these studies made more than 50 years ago that, however extensive the operation was, in many patients it was not extensive enough to eradicate the disease. He wrote that in many cases long intervals of time elapsed between the date of the operation and the appearance of metastases, so it must be assumed that the foci of disease were present when the operation was performed but were unrecognisable clinically. The modern concept of the presence of micrometastases was foreshadowed in this publication so many years ago. At that time synthetic hormonal therapy and chemotherapy were not available for the treatment of micrometastases.

CHANGES IN THE INCIDENCE AND MORTALITY RATES OF BREAST CANCER

This subject is under continual discussion at the present time and, as stated before, assertions are often made that the prognosis in breast carcinoma has showed no improvement over many decades. However, such assertions are very debatable, as a careful study of all the evidence does reveal a better prognosis for many patients, especially those with early disease, after adequate surgical excision, radiotherapy and hormonal therapy, as indicated for individual patients.

The incidence and mortality rates were studied and reported by Cutler, Christine and Barclay *(1971)*, who stated that mortality due to breast cancer had declined by a small amount since 1940 in spite of the evidence which indicated that there was a sizeable increase in the incidence of the disease, and that this contrasting trend had been observed in two areas with good cancer reporting systems. They suggested that the increased incidence might be due to better diagnosis or another cause, and reported that it occurred in each of the four decades from age 35 to 75; however, under the age of 35 the rate of incidence was decreasing. In one area they actually found an increase in women at and over the age of 75 years.

With regard to the decrease in mortality, they explained that it was due to an improvement in survival rates, and they quoted data from more than 100 hospitals which formed the "End-Results Group" *(1968)*. The 5-year survival rate increased from 54% in 1940–1949 to 61% in 1955–1959. The authors stated that the increase in survival rates was partly due to a shift in the distribution of cases according to the extent of the disease at diagnosis. For example, in the 1940s 38% of patients were classified as having localised disease, compared with 46% in the 1960–1964 period. There was also an increase in the survival rates of patients classified as having regional disease and more such patients were being treated by combined methods. For example, during the 1940–1949 period only 25% of patients were treated by combined surgery and radiotherapy and/or chemotherapy, whereas during the period 1960–1964 51% of patients were treated by combined modalities.

CHANGES IN THE TREATMENT OF BREAST CANCER

It is important for us to review at regular intervals the end-results of the treatment of breast cancer for this will lead to better treatment methods being evolved. It is probably true that the treatment of breast cancer has caused more discussion and argument than that of any other malignant disease. The debate continues at the present time and it is even suggested by some clinicians that alternative methods of treatment should be explained to the patient, so that she can decide which treatment to accept. Certainly each patient should be considered as a distinct individual and given clear explanations and advice about the appropriate treatment in her case. The subject of patient compliance is important nowadays.

With regard to the changes that have occurred in the treatment of breast cancer, Trimble and Trimble *(1962)* stated that in the 22 years after 1940 four challenges were made to the acceptance of radical mastectomy as the standard treatment for this disease. These included (1) that no surgical treatment should be carried out; (2) that such rigid criteria of operability were set up that an increasing number of patients were denied surgical treatment; (3) the substitution of simple mastectomy and radiotherapy for radical mastectomy; and (4) the revival and extended application of a more radical operation including the supraclavicular and internal mammary lymph nodes.

These authors expressed surprise that some people considered that the end-results in breast cancer were unaffected by the treatment and that

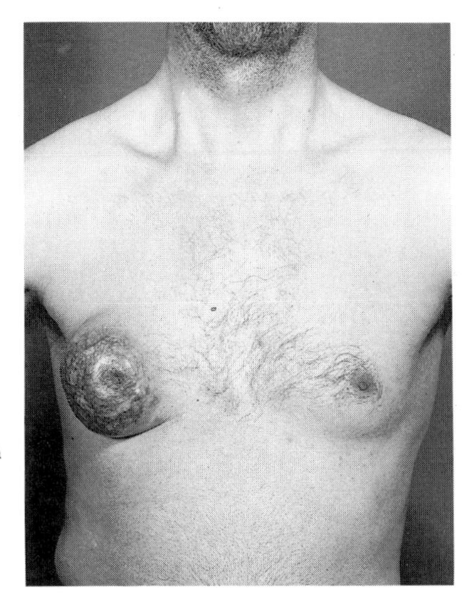

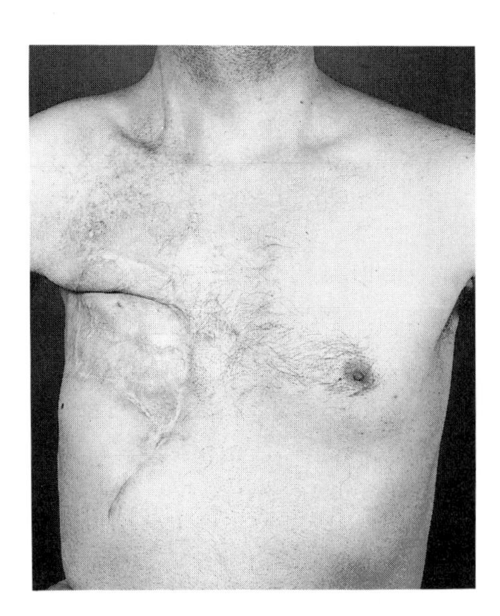

Figure 12.5 *Left:* A male patient with a carcinoma of the right breast. *Right:* The patient after a right mastectomy. A wide excision was performed, followed by an immediate skin graft to the wound.

no improvements in survival rates had occurred over many years. They stated: "It seems almost incredible in this day and age to read a statement seriously made that it is impossible to prove that the course of breast cancer is influenced by any form of treatment. This is based on a theory of 'biologic predeterminism' that the 'course of the disease depends chiefly on the biologic properties of the tumour and the resistance of the host'." They agreed that these factors are important, but stressed "we cannot refute the results of radical surgery demonstrated over and over again".

To support their views, Trimble and Trimble quoted evidence showing that the 5-year survival rate of all patients with primary operable breast cancer treated by radical mastectomy had doubled in the last 50 years. They pointed out that most American clinics currently reported a 5-year survival rate of about 55%, whereas Halsted's first results, published in 1907, gave a 5-year survival rate of 28.9%.

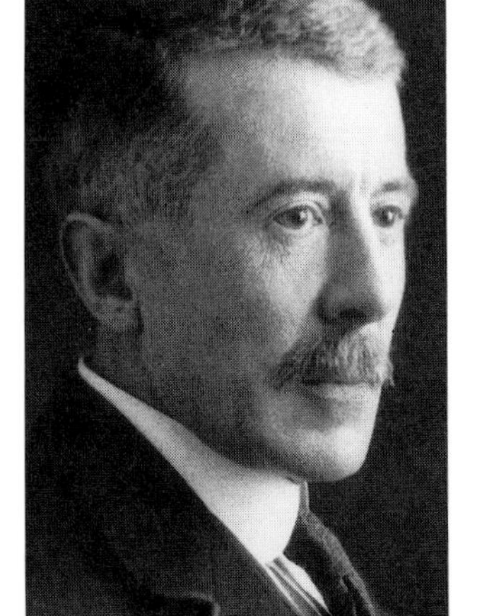

Figure 12.6 W. Sampson Handley (1872–1962), Surgeon to the Middlesex Hospital and author of *Cancer of the Breast and its Treatment*, which was published in 1906. He propounded the theory of "lymphatic permeation" in carcinoma of the breast whereby metastases are formed by extension of the disease through the lymphatic vessels to the nodes.

Extended radical mastectomy

A new procedure for the treatment of primary operable breast cancer, consisting of the removal of the internal mammary lymph nodes in continuity with a radical mastectomy, was described by Urban and Baker *(1952)*. They stated that the relatively poor results of radical mastectomy for primary operable breast cancer, especially in the inner half of the breast, were largely due to early involvement of the internal mammary lymph nodes. They felt that the new operation would remedy this particular defect in the classical radical mastectomy operation.

An initial report by Urban concerned 57 patients who had undergone the new operation; 28 patients had metastases in the internal mammary lymph nodes, while 33 had metastases in the axillary lymph nodes. In 24 patients both groups of lymph nodes were affected; in four only the internal mammary lymph nodes contained metastases, while in nine only the axillary lymph nodes had metastases. In 20 patients all the nodes were negative for metastases.

The extended radical mastectomy operation did not produce any better results than the classical radical mastectomy operation and it is no longer practised generally. Mention is made here of Urban's operation because of its historic interest. It is noteworthy that in many clinics today there is a movement away from Halsted's radical mastectomy. Finality has not yet been reached in the discussion concerning the best treatment for breast carcinoma; it is hoped that answers will be provided by the results of clinical trials which are now being carried out.

Radium treatment of breast carcinoma

Radiotherapy plays an important role in the treatment of breast carcinoma today, so it is of great historical interest to refer here to the use of interstitial radium needles more than 50 years ago. This treatment modality was well described by Sir Geoffrey Keynes *(1931)*, who had extensive experience using it with Professor G. E. Gask at St Bartholomew's Hospital, London. The present author was privileged to know both these surgeons and saw many of the patients with breast carcinoma who were treated by them.

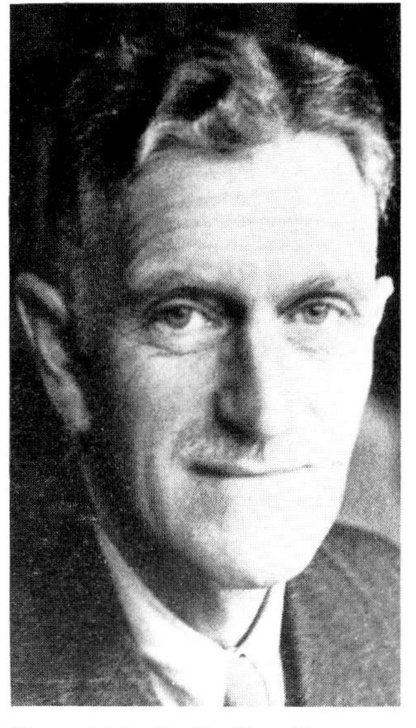

Figure 12.7 Sir Geoffrey Keynes.

In 1922 a small amount of radium was allocated for clinical use to the professorial surgical unit under the direction of Professor Gask, who, in consultation with Dr N. S. Finzi of the Radiology Department, decided to utilise it for the treatment of patients with breast carcinoma, by means of the interstitial radium needles technique.

Initially they selected patients with local recurrent breast carcinoma but when they had proof that the carcinoma nodules disappeared they decided to treat patients with primary inoperable carcinoma. In his report, which included clinical photographs, Keynes described the technique of interstitial radiation of breast carcinoma, the aftercare of the patients and the radiation effects in the tumours. An outstanding feature of the article is the large number of precise case-records presented. Keynes wrote: "The study of individual patients will throw more light than any figures." We must never forget the value of compiling accurate case-records and studying individual patients.

In his conclusions regarding radium treatment Keynes stated that no exaggerated claim was being made that it should supplant surgical treatment, but that in general the results compared favourably with those obtained by surgery. He pointed out that in the most successful cases of radium treatment patients remained virtually physically normal women and had a life expectancy at least as great as after a mutilating operation. He considered that the place of radium treatment varied according to the stage of the breast carcinoma. Thus he thought it the treatment of choice for very advanced or inoperable tumours, but that for the average intermediate operable carcinoma the psychology of the patient or other circumstances might call for orthodox treatment by radical mastectomy, followed perhaps by prophylactic radiation. He stated that for unprejudiced patients radical mastectomy was seldom necessary, as it was justifiable in most cases to use radium or radium in combination with a modified mastectomy. When radiation therapy was not entirely successful, conservative surgery could usually then be performed. Keynes pointed out that very adipose patients were probably unsuited for radium treatment and that the radical mastectomy operation was unnecessary for the earliest and smallest carcinomas. He stated that excellent results could be obtained by radium alone or combined with the most conservative operation.

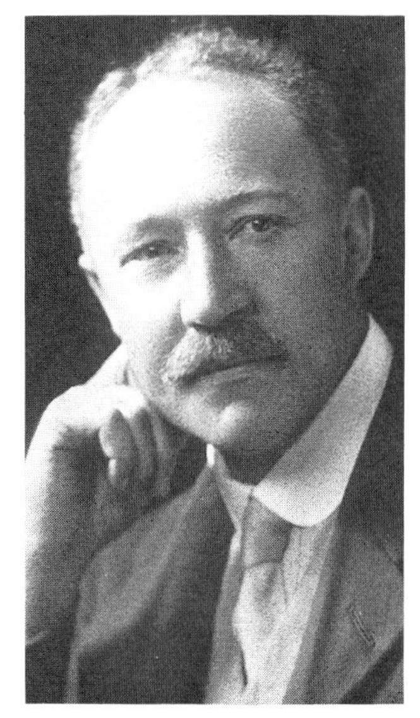

Figure 12.8 George E. Gask.

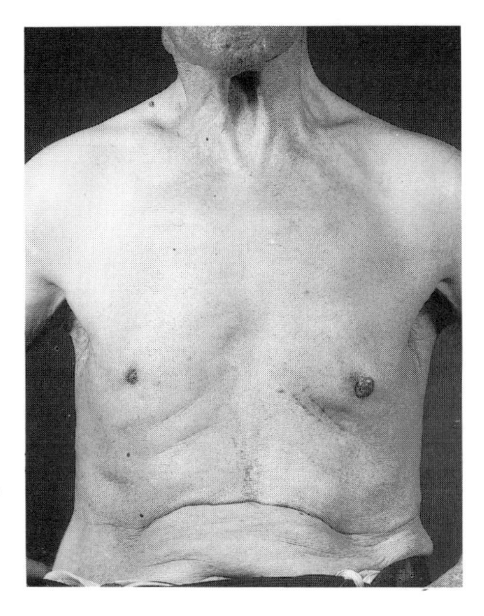
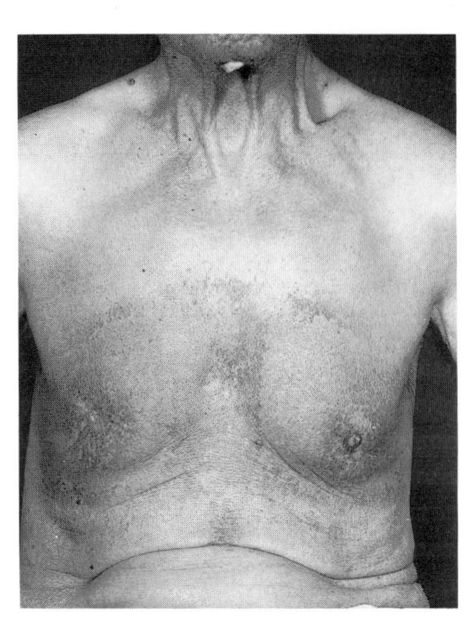

Figure 12.9 *Left:* A male patient with bilateral carcinoma of the breasts. Right: The patient 5 months after radiotherapy. Note the skin pigmentation over the treated area.

At the end of Keynes' article there is a detailed analysis of a series of 171 cases of breast cancer treated with radium. It includes a statistical analysis by Dr Janet E. Forbes, who points out that the most important group among these patients are those who survived 3 or more years after treatment. In this particular group there are only 46 cases, which is a small sample and does not contain sufficient data to show the differences in the results from radiation and combined treatments. However, with this reservation she gives the following statistics for the 3-year cases: Class 1 (operable, no lymph nodes), nine cases treated and seven cases (77.7%) alive at 3 years; Class 2 (operable, lymph nodes palpable), 11 cases treated and four cases (36.3%) alive at 3 years; Class 3 (inoperable), 26 cases treated and 12 cases (46.1%) alive at 3 years.

It is now accepted that 10-year survival rates or longer are necessary in order to be able to accurately assess the end-results of the treatment of breast cancer, and that the study must include an adequate number of patients for a significant statistical analysis to be made.

Keynes also called attention to the work carried out at the London Radium Institute and reported by Ward *(1929)*. During the period 1918–1927 633 patients with breast cancer were treated there by means of the external application of radium; 165 of these patients had primary inoperable tumours and the remainder had postoperative recurrent disease. The results were considered to be encouraging in that 26 patients out of a total of 128 survived for 3 years and 11 patients out of a total of 98 survived for 5 years.

Ward stated that there were reasons for supposing that many local carcinoma recurrences might be prevented if pre- and postoperative radiotherapy were used more often. He also pointed out that recurrent disease after prophylactic radiation is very refractory to further radiotherapy and furthermore that a second treatment of any neoplasm is less effective than the primary treatment. The first treatment which is given for cancer should always be as thorough and vigorous as possible and when a second treatment is required the dose of radiation should be relatively smaller.

This pioneer and important treatment of breast carcinoma with interstitial radium needles formed a landmark in the long history of the treatment of carcinoma of the breast. However, it did not receive wide approval and the method lapsed, especially after new techniques were developed with radiation apparatus that could deliver radiation from an external source such as X-ray tubes.

In this connection it is interesting to read the report by Baclesse *(1965)*, which included the 5-year results in a series of 431 patients with breast cancer who were treated solely with external radiation from the classical 200 kV apparatus. The following results were reported in groups of patients with breast cancer staged according to the Columbia-Clinical Classification. In Stage A 27 patients (54%) were alive and apparently cured after 5 years; in Stage B 58 patients (67%) were alive after 5 years, of whom 61% were clinically cured and 6% had persistent cancer; in Stage C there were 95 patients and a 41% 5-year survival rate; in Stage D, out of a total of 200 patients 27 (13%) survived 5 years, but six of these had persistent cancer.

PAGET'S DISEASE OF THE NIPPLE

Sir James Paget *(1874)* described certain chronic affections of the skin of the nipple and areola of the breast which are followed by the development of scirrhous carcinoma of the breast. He studied 15 patients, aged 40–60 or more, in whom the disease began as an eruption of the nipple and areola. In the majority of the patients this had the appearance of a "florid, intensely red, raw surface, very finely granular, as if nearly the whole thickness of the epidermis were removed; like the surface of a very acute diffuse eczema, or like that of an acute balanitis. From such a surface, on the whole, or greater part, of the nipple and areola, there was always copious, clear, yellowish, viscid exudation. The sensations were commonly tingling, itching, and burning, but the malady was never attended by disturbance of the general health. I have not seen this form of eruption extend beyond the areola, and only once have seen it pass into a deeper ulceration of the skin after the

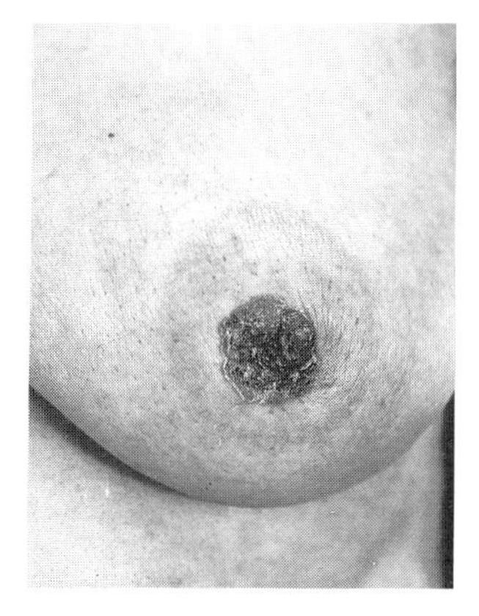

Figure 12.10 Paget's disease of the nipple.

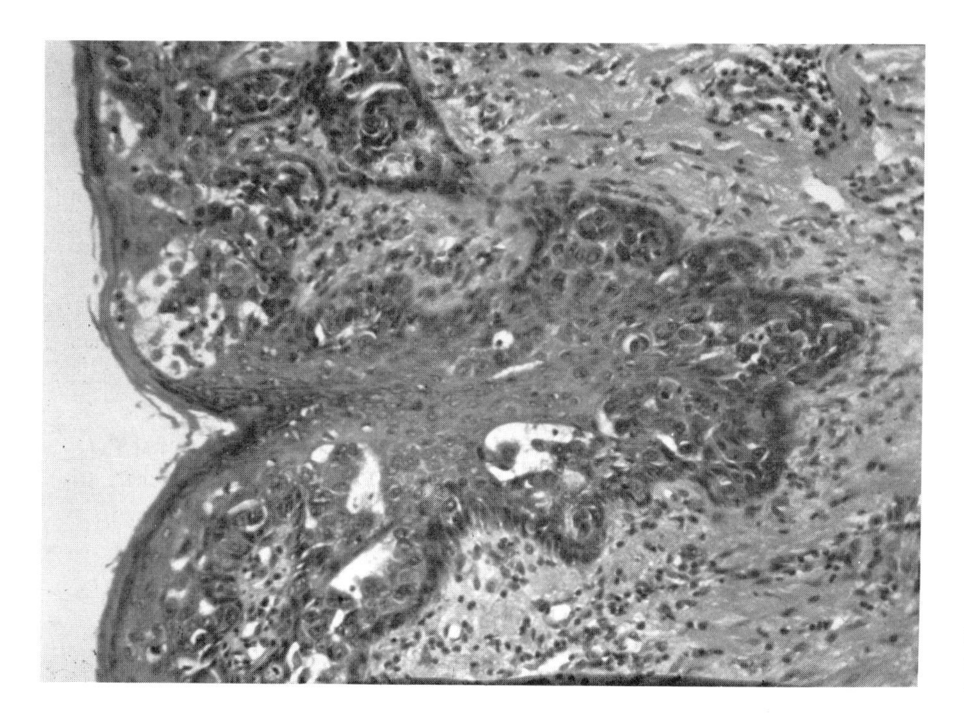

Figure 12.11 A histopathology specimen with Paget's disease of the nipple, showing the Paget's cells.

manner of a rodent ulcer." This is Paget's own clear description of this disease and he stated that in every patient he was able to observe breast cancer followed within at the most 2 years and usually within 1 year. The tumour always developed in the substance of the breast, beneath or not far from the diseased skin, and was always separated from that by apparently healthy tissue. The cancers themselves were in no way different from other forms of the disease.

In stressing the sequence of cancer developing so frequently after the chronic skin disease, Paget called attention to a nearly similar sequence in other parts of the body. He had seen a persistent "rawness" of the glans penis, which was followed after more than a year by cancer in the substance of the glans. A chronic soreness of the lower lip often precedes cancer in the substance of the lip and the superficial syphilitic diseases of the tongue are followed by cancers in the tongue. Paget posed the practical question as to whether a degenerate or diseased part where cancer is very likely to be induced should or should not be removed. On the whole, he was in favour of preventive treatment.

FURTHER DEVELOPMENTS IN TREATMENT

It is beyond the scope of this book to discuss in detail the present-day treatment of carcinoma of the breast, including hormonal therapy and chemotherapy. A study of the extensive experimental and clinical work which has been carried out over many decades is most indicative that breast carcinoma is chiefly an endocrine problem where we need to understand hormonal control mechanisms.

This subject was considered in the article by Trimble and Trimble *(1962)* which has already been referred to. These authors considered that the greatest advance in our understanding of breast cancer since the year 1940, that is, during a period of 22 years, resulted from the recognition of the hormonal influence of other glands on the breast. The application of the fact that breast epithelium possesses a total hormone dependence led to the supposition that hormonal imbalances must play a large part in the genesis of breast carcinoma, probably due to the unphysiological properties of the pituitary gland and ovarian hormones. They pointed out that the key hormone in the development of the breast seems to be prolactin, which is essential in all phases of breast growth, but this hormone cannot initiate breast mitosis without the ovarian hormones, oestrogen and progesterone. Full glandular differentiation requires the pituitary growth hormone, somatotrophin, and the adrenocortical hormone, in addition to prolactin. This action of the pituitary hormones is usually called mammotropic. Oestrogen is required for the ductal phase of breast development and progesterone for the development of the alveoli.

Trimble and Trimble recommended prophylactic oophorectomy for patients under the age of 30, irrespective of the condition of the axillary lymph nodes, and for patients with an inflammatory carcinoma. For patients over 30 years old and up to 5 years beyond the menopause they recommended oophorectomy when axillary lymph node metastases were present. Postoperative radiotherapy was advised for all patients with lymph node metastases.

Hormonal therapy for breast carcinoma is considered in greater detail in

Chapter 19 on endocrinology, where reference is made to oophorectomy, adrenalectomy and hypophysectomy, and to synthetic anti-oestrogens such as Nolvadex (tamoxifen).

At the present time there is considerable debate regarding the surgical treatment of breast carcinoma and the role of radiotherapy. It does appear, however, that the Halsted radical mastectomy is performed much less frequently nowadays, being replaced by the Patey modified radical mastectomy with conservation of the pectoralis muscles. The other operations which are done are simple mastectomy and local excision of the carcinoma (lumpectomy) with or without axillary node radiation according to the clinical findings. For a carcinoma in the upper, outer quadrant of the breast some surgeons perform excision of the outer part of the breast, with dissection of the axillary lymph nodes. A careful assessment of the end-results of all these different operations, with or without radiotherapy, hormonal therapy and chemotherapy, after periods of 5, 10 and 20 years will give future guidance. Finally, a new method of treatment, probably hormonal, is likely to be developed, and even preventive treatment is a possibility.

REFERENCES

Baclesse, F. (1965). Five-year results in 431 breast cancers treated solely by Roentgen's rays. *Ann. Surg.*, **161**, 103–4

Cutler, S. J., Christine, B. and Barclay, I. H. C. (1971). Increasing incidence and decreasing mortality rates for breast cancer. "End-Results Group" (1968) Cancer Report No. 3. *National Institutes of Health Publication No. 30*

Halsted, W. S. (1894). Operations for the cure of cancer of the breast. *Johns Hopkins Hospital Reports*, **4** (6), 1–54

Halsted, W. S. (1907). The results of radical operation for the cure of cancer of the breast. *Ann. Surg.*, **46**, 1–19

Keynes, Sir Geoffrey (1931). The radium treatment of carcinoma of the breast. *Br. J. Surg.*, **19**, 415–80

Lewis, D. and Rienhoff, W. F., Jr (1932). A study of the results of operations for the cure of cancer of the breast at The Johns Hopkins Hospital from 1889 to 1931. *Ann. Surg.*, **95**, 336–400

Moore, C. H. (1867). On the influence of inadequate operations on the theory of cancer. *Med.-Chir. Trans.*, **50**, 245–80

Paget, Sir James (1856). On the average duration of life in patients with schirrhous cancer of the breast. *Lancet*, **1**, 62–3

Paget, Sir James (1874). On diseases of the mammary areola preceding cancer of the mammary gland. *Saint Bartholomew's Hospital Reports*, Vol. 10, pp 87–9

Peugniez, P. (1924). Une gastrectomie pour cancer remontant à vingt-quatre ans. *Bull. Acad. Med.*, **92**, 831–3

Raven, R. W. (1933). Report from the Follow-up Department of St Bartholomew's Hospital. An investigation into the end-results in the treatment of cancer of the breast. *Saint Bartholomew's Hospital Reports*, Vol. 66, pp 45–64

Sweeting, R. (1869). A new operation for cancer of the breast. *Lancet*, **1**, 323

Trimble, I. R. and Trimble, F. H. (1962). Changes in the treatment of cancer of the breast. *Int. Abst. Surg.*, **114**, 103–29

Urban, J. A. and Baker, H. W. (1952). Radical mastectomy in continuity with en bloc resection of the internal mammary lymph-node chain. *Cancer*, **5**, 992–1008

Ward, R. (1929). Inoperable carcinoma of the breast treated with radium. *Br. Med. J.*, **1**, 242–4

CHAPTER THIRTEEN

Classical Oncological Operations

The design and development of the surgical operations for different forms of cancer have been impressive features in the history of surgery over the course of about a century. The design of the major operations is based on a precise knowledge of the local extensions of the tumour and of the presence of lymph node and other metastases. The basic medical sciences have made valuable contributions to this work, together with the new methods of screening used in preoperative patient assessment. The end-results of surgical treatment owe much to skilled operative techniques, modern anaesthesia and the use of antibacterial chemicals. Nurses play a fundamental role in the surgical team in postoperative and intensive care units and in hospital wards.

Rehabilitation and continuing care units are being developed, where patients are restored to a life of good quality after surgical and other forms of treatment.

Nine major operations for cancer in different sites, the names of the originators of the procedures and the dates when they were first performed are listed in Table 4 (Chapter 8).

The objective of a surgical operation for an oncological disease is to extirpate the local disease and its lymph node metastases in order to cure the patient, unless dissemination has occurred, producing metastases outside the field of operation. There are palliative surgical operations for the relief of different varieties of visceral obstructions — for example, intestinal occlusion — which are caused by malignant tumours which cannot be totally excised. Inoperable tumours are debulked to reduce their volume so that combination therapy with radiation and chemotherapy can be more effective.

The surgeons who initially designed and performed the radical surgical operations were concerned about the high local recurrence rates which had

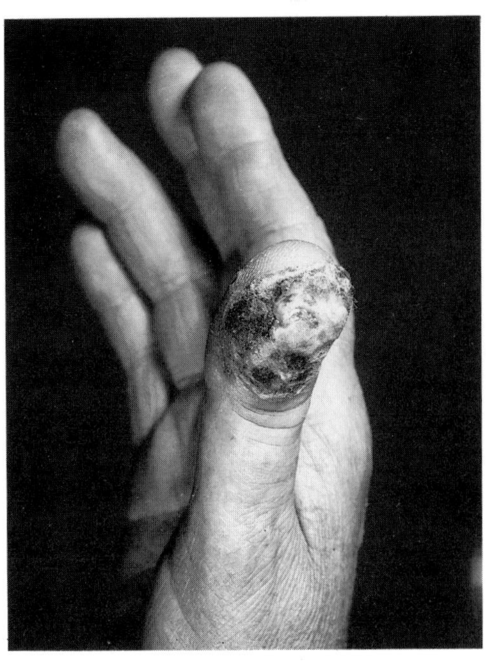

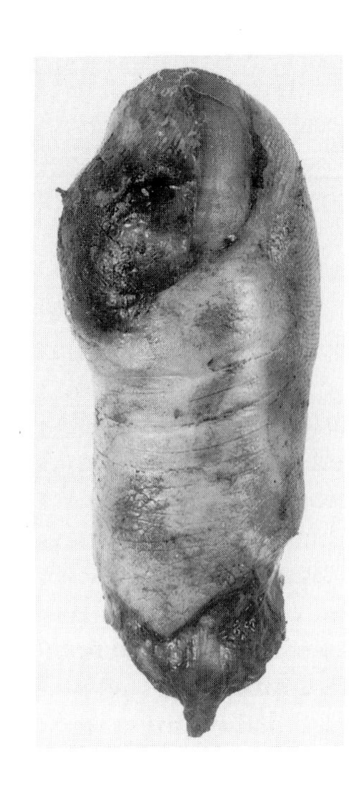

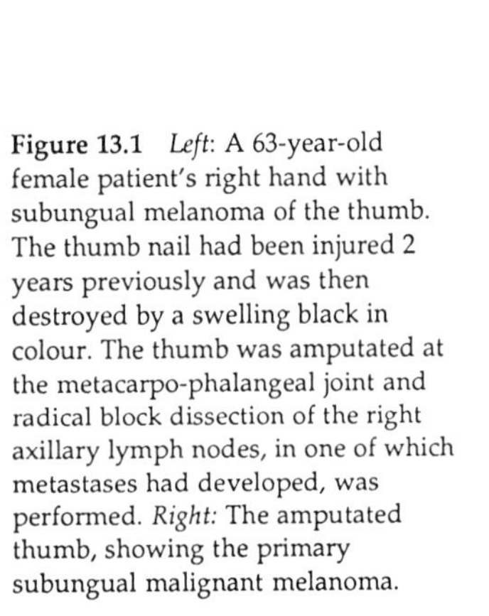

Figure 13.1 *Left:* A 63-year-old female patient's right hand with subungual melanoma of the thumb. The thumb nail had been injured 2 years previously and was then destroyed by a swelling black in colour. The thumb was amputated at the metacarpo-phalangeal joint and radical block dissection of the right axillary lymph nodes, in one of which metastases had developed, was performed. *Right:* The amputated thumb, showing the primary subungual malignant melanoma.

followed smaller operative procedures. Reference to their original descriptions shows the importance they gave to the pathology of solid malignant tumours in viscera and their mode of spreading into contiguous tissues and regional lymph nodes and forming more distant metastases. Their principles have stood the test of time and many of their radical operations or modifications remain as standard procedures today.

Surgeons who perform oncological operations must always be critical of their work and continue to study the end-results, including the survival rates and recurrence rates, in addition to measuring the quality of life of their patients. Controlled clinical trials can indicate that modifications are necessary and, indeed, certain changes have been made in these operations as experience regarding them has grown during recent years. Special reference is made later in this chapter to certain operations which are of historic interest.

DEVELOPMENTS IN SURGERY IN THE USA

Gross (1805–1884), Professor of Surgery in the Jefferson Medical College of Philadelphia, reviewed *(1876)* developments in surgery in the USA during the century 1776–1876. He wrote: "It is well that every profession once in a century should open its ledgers and examine its accounts to see how it stands with itself and with the world at large." He gives a fascinating account of outstanding American surgeons and their achievements during this epoch. He stated that the extirpation of tumours, even simple varieties, is often difficult, especially when the tumour is embedded in important structures, as in the cervical, axillary, inguinal, femoral and popliteal regions. He called attention to the celebrated clinical lecture delivered by Dr Stevens of New York at the New York Hospital on the operative surgery of tumours, in which two important rules were given. First, the surgeon should cut down fairly on the tumour before commencing the dissection, and, second, he should remove the diseased mass and nothing more. Gross added that since these suggestions were the result of extensive clinical experience, they were received with great respect and consideration by the medical profession at home and abroad. He stressed the importance of the curvilinear incision for removal of the mandible and various other tumours, instead of the straight incision which was advocated originally by Velpeau and Mott.

It is interesting to read his brief description of the treatment of carcinoma, sarcoma and other tumours of the tonsil. He states that when extirpation of these tumours is considered advisable, the operation is usually performed through the mouth, although there are difficulties with this approach. He called attention to an operation which was performed by Dr Cheever of Boston for "encephaloid of the tonsils", which Gross described as "working his way through the upper and lateral parts of the neck; necessitating the division of the stylohyoid and styloglossus muscles, together with the fibres of the superior constrictor of the pharynx, through the interspace of which the diseased mass was approached and removed. Twelve ligatures were applied. The wound was completely closed at the end of a month, unpreceded by any untoward occurrence."

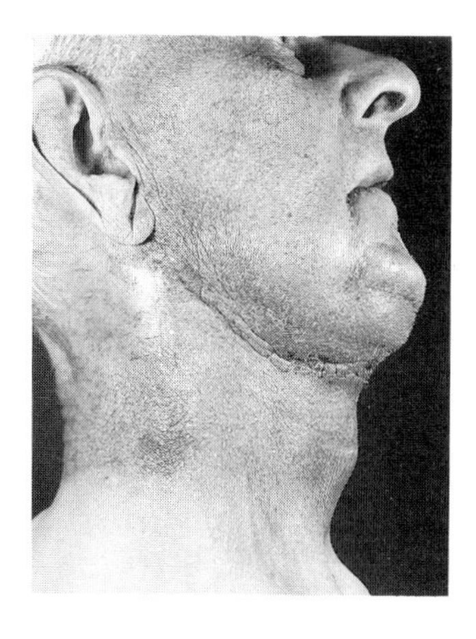

Figure 13.2 The healed submandibular curvilinear incision in a patient, made to remove his right mandible affected by carcinoma.

The subject of statistics was discussed briefly by Gross. He wrote: "Statistics, illustrative of the results of surgical operations, diseases and accidents, are, as is well known, often very troublesome and laborious undertakings, especially when attempted upon a large scale." The discipline of statistics has developed enormously during recent decades and is of vital importance in oncology work today.

Gross concluded his interesting review with the forecast: "The century closing with the year 1976 will open for medicine one of the brightest pages in the history of human progress." His forecast has been fully justified by the spectacular advances which have occurred.

The significant contributions from the USA to all branches of medicine are universally admired and acknowledged. However, no attempt is made here to deal in depth with this important and extensive subject.

CLASSICAL ONCOLOGICAL OPERATIONS

The classical oncological operations are listed in Table 4, and our attention is now focused on them because of their historic importance.

Abdominoperineal excision of the rectum

This major operation for carcinoma of the rectum was designed by William Ernest Miles *(1908)* and first performed by him in 1906. The present author enjoyed the friendship and teaching of Miles, and as his junior colleague on the surgical staff of the Gordon Hospital in London assisted him in performing this radical operation. Miles was also Surgeon at the Cancer Hospital in London (later the Royal Marsden Hospital). Visiting surgeons from all over the world came to both hospitals to watch Miles perform surgical operations and to discuss surgical problems with this master whose knowledge and surgical skill they greatly admired and appreciated. The present author recalls the advice he received from Miles regarding the surgical treatment of cancer: "Perform the biggest possible operation for

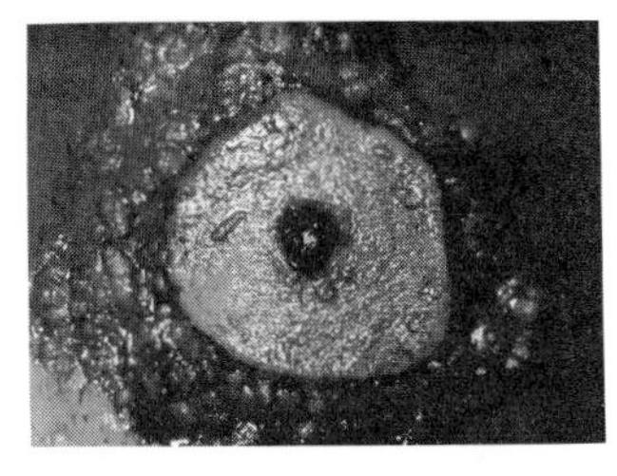

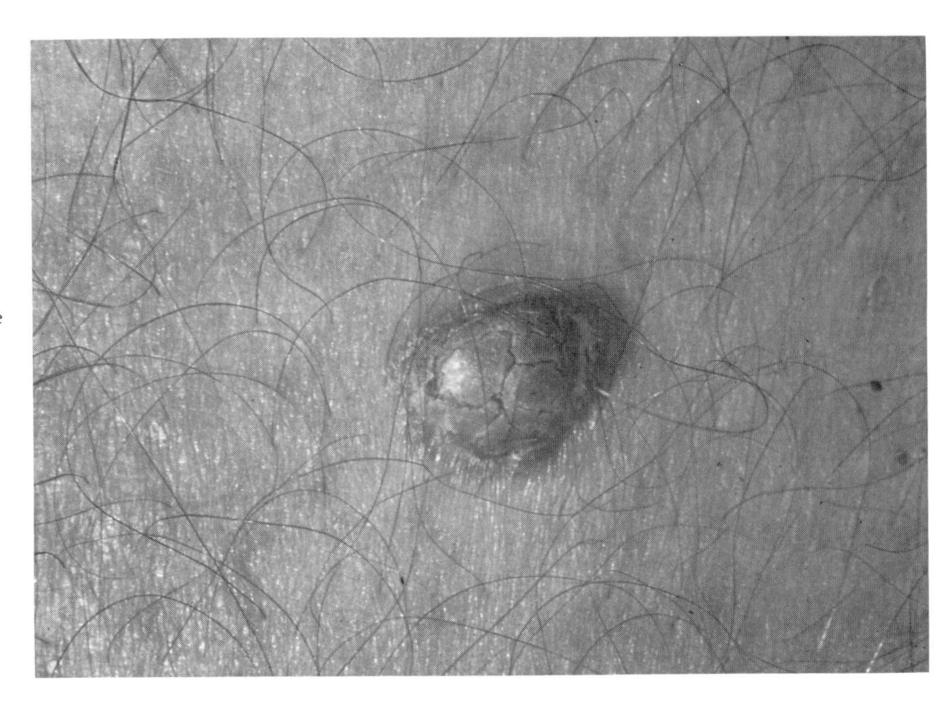

Figure 13.3 *Right:* A malignant melanoma of the skin treated by wide excision. *Above:* The specimen excised.

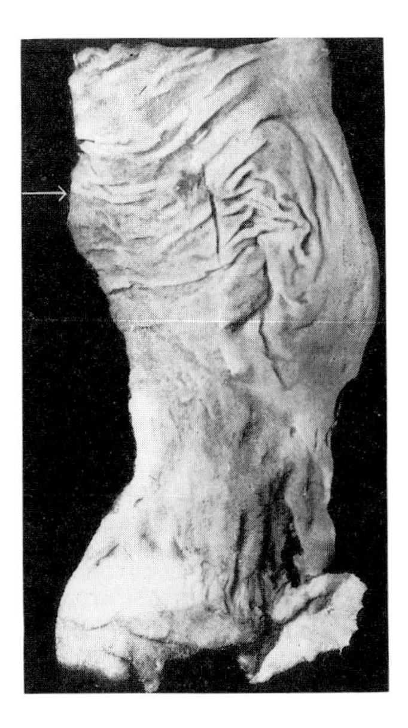

Figure 13.4 A rectum with an early carcinoma in the ampulla removed by the perineal operation.

the earliest possible case." He certainly carried out this dictum in practice.

A section of his book *Rectal Surgery (Miles, 1939)* describes earlier operations for cancer of the rectum. These were all restricted procedures and Miles was impressed by the frequency of local recurrent disease which followed perineal operations for the excision of rectal carcinoma. He studied the lymphatic drainage of the rectum in great detail in relation to lymph node metastases and also defined the sites of recurrent local carcinoma. Following this careful work he concluded that a satisfactory operation for the disease should include the removal of all the tissues which are known to be liable to be involved by the spread of carcinoma cells from the primary tumour. He stressed the importance of removing the tissues in the area at risk from the upward spread of the disease. It is interesting to compare his work with that relating to breast carcinoma.

Following the most extensive perineal excision operations there was considerable risk of local recurrent carcinoma after 6 months to 3 years. In order to include the tissues in the zone of upward spread of carcinoma Miles abandoned that operation and replaced it with his abdominoperineal operation, "thus bringing the operation of excision of the rectum into line with Wertheim's hysterectomy".

Wertheim's hysterectomy

The design and development of the radical operation for carcinoma of the uterus followed a similar pattern to those for the abdominoperineal excision of the rectum. The early hysterectomy operations were performed from the perineal region by the vaginal approach to the uterus. The surgery of the uterus in its historical context is described by Meade *(1968)*, to whom the present author is indebted for his information. According to Meade's account, it was Wrisberg who first suggested that vaginal hysterectomy should be performed for cancer of the uterus, in 1810, and in 1812 Paletta

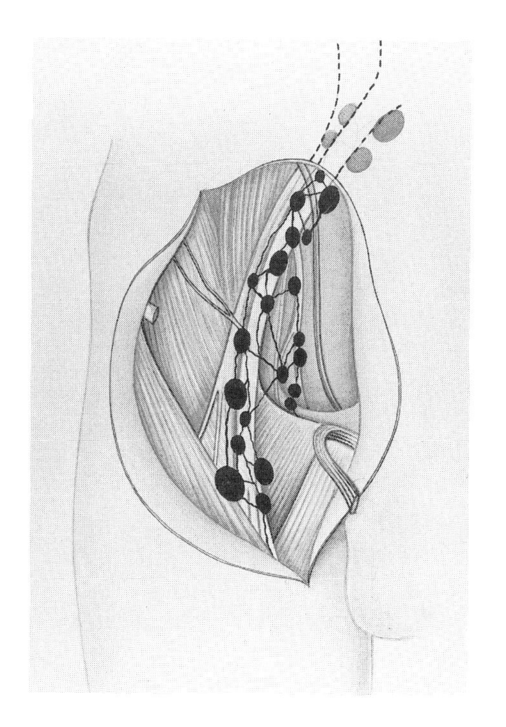

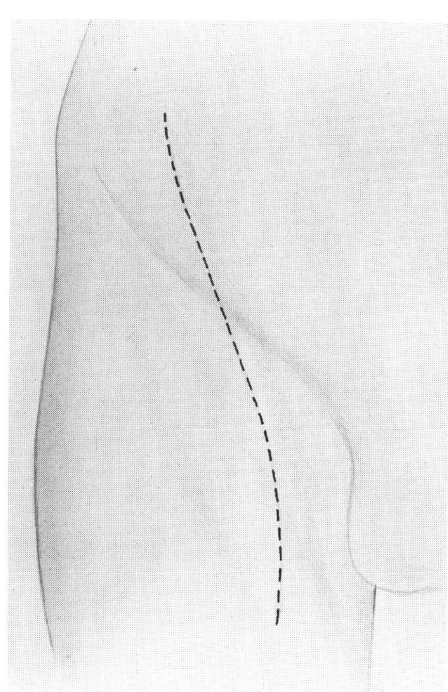

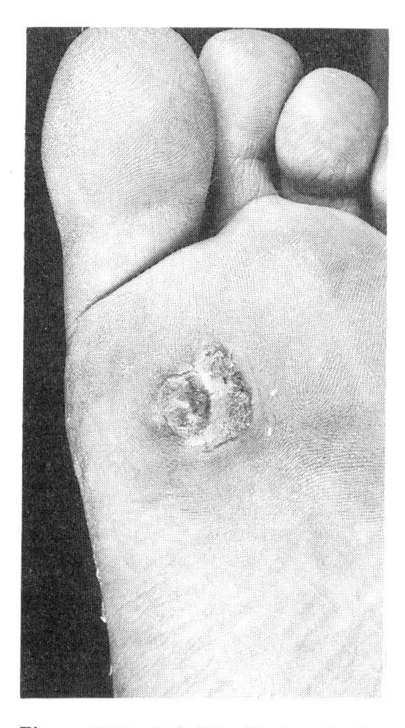

Figure 13.5 *Left:* The ilio-inguinal groups of lymph nodes where metastases occur from malignant tumours of the lower extremity. *Right:* The skin incision for radical ilio-inguinal lymph node excision. *Above:* A malignant melanoma in the skin of the sole of the left foot of a 27-year-old male which was treated with wide excision followed by a skin graft. The ilio-inguinal lymph nodes were excised but showed no metastases. The patient is still alive 8 years after his operation and has had no recurrent or metastatic disease.

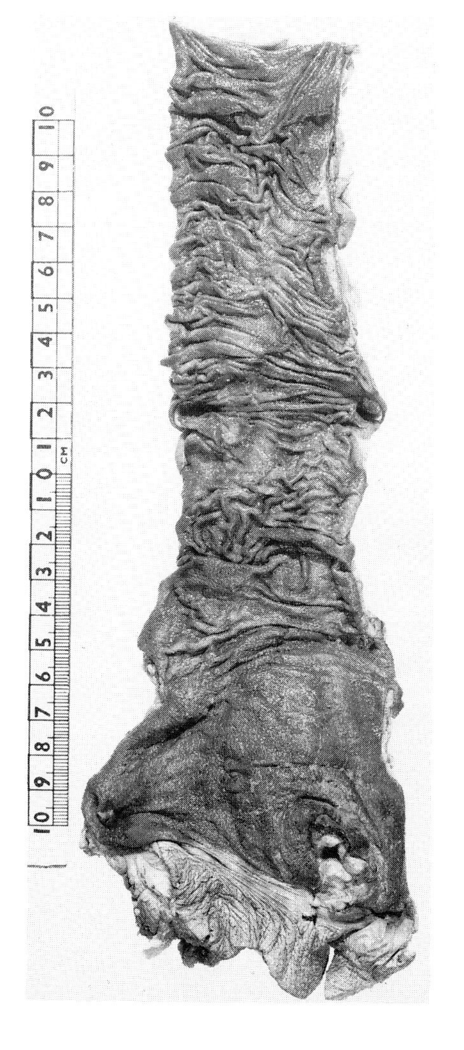

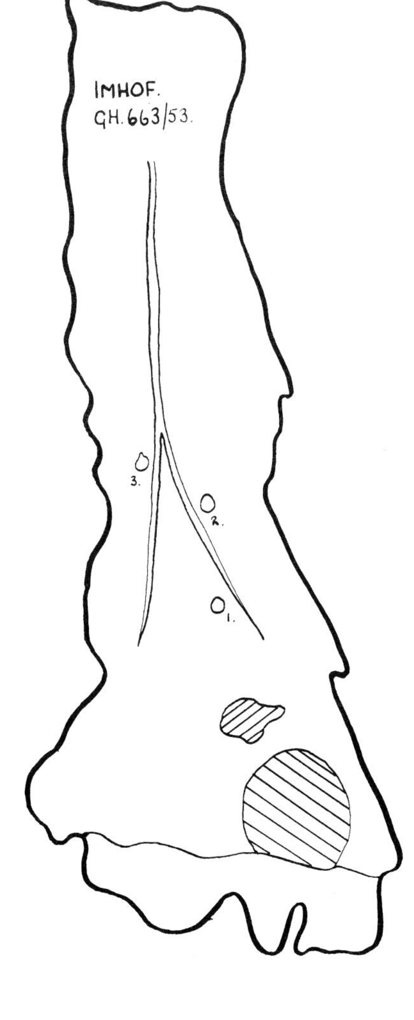

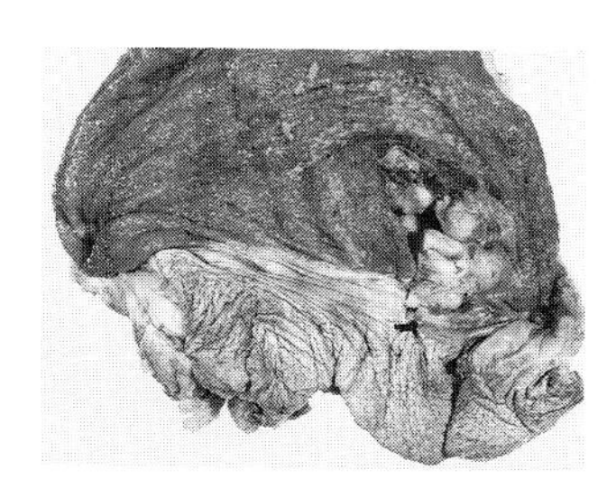

Figure 13.6 *Left:* A rectum with carcinoma, which has been removed by an abdominoperineal operation. *Right:* The method used in recording the primary carcinoma and the lymphatic nodes. *Above:* The carcinoma excised.

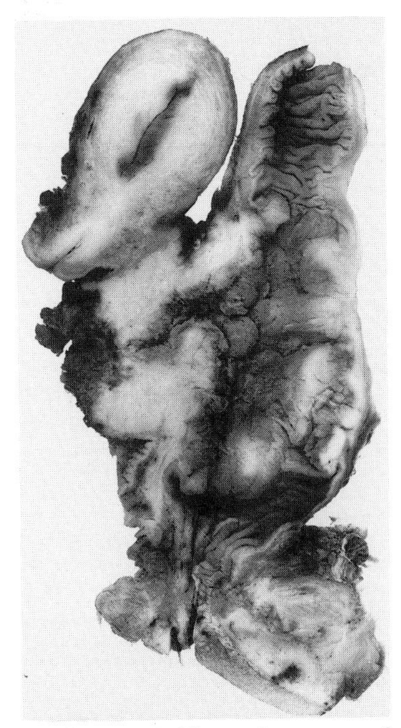

Figure 13.7 The specimen removed by combined abdominoperineal excision of the rectum and Wertheim's hysterectomy for an advanced carcinoma of the rectum invading the vagina and uterus.

carried out the operation. Meade stated that the first planned vaginal hysterectomy for cancer was performed by Von Langenback in 1813 and reported by him 4 years later. Again according to Meade, the first surgeon to carry out hysterectomy with any success in England was James Blundell, who worked at Guy's Hospital, London. He did his first vaginal hysterectomy for cancer in 1828.

Technical developments followed and the operation of abdominal hysterectomy began to be carried out for non-malignant conditions.

In 1898 Ernst Wertheim performed the first radical abdominal hysterectomy which now bears his name. In this procedure for carcinoma he removed the uterus and a large amount of parametrial tissues and the regional lymph nodes, especially in relation to the iliac arteries. Particular care has to be taken to avoid any injury to the ureters when performing this operation.

Since those early years when Wertheim's hysterectomy was first carried out, as with other radical operations for cancer, operative mortality has fallen considerably with the use of blood transfusion, modern anaesthesia, antibiotic therapy, and postoperative skilled nursing care in special units. The surgical treatment of carcinoma of the corpus and cervix uteri has undergone important modifications with the detection of premalignant lesions, early diagnosis of carcinoma and developments in radiation treatment.

Partial pharyngectomy

Important contributions to the surgical treatment of cancer of the mouth and pharynx were made by Wilfred Trotter *(1913)*, who was Surgeon to University College Hospital in London and highly respected for his great expertise. Trotter pointed out that an operation which is precisely

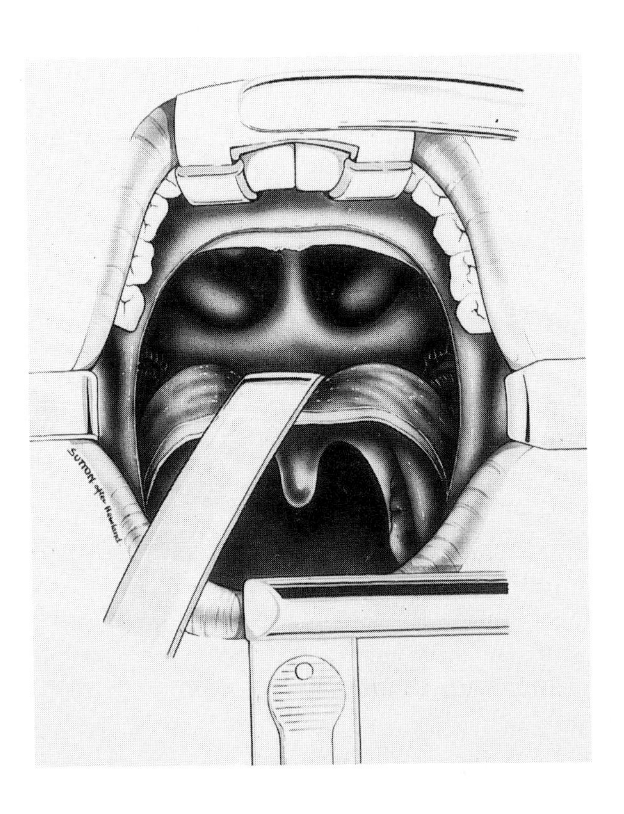

Figure 13.8 The surgical exposure of a tumour in the nasopharynx by detaching the soft palate from the hard palate and retracting the soft palate downwards. Described by C. P. Wilson.

designed anatomically is suitable for only a few patients with cancer. The operative requirements in order to cure the patient and limit the extent of mutilations due to the surgical operation are controlled by the pathology of malignant disease in the various parts of the body. He stressed the necessity of making a detailed clinical assessment of the extent of the malignant disease, to see whether a one- or two-stage operation was required. For the majority of patients he recommended a two-stage operation; at the first stage the primary tumour is excised and at the second stage a regional lymph node dissection is performed. He pointed out that every operation should commence with the complete exposure of the tumour so that an adequate margin of normal tissue can be excised with it. More recently this important principle was extended with the monoblock operation, designed to remove the primary tumour with its contiguous tissues and the regional lymph nodes en bloc. It was performed especially for malignant tumours situated in the head and neck.

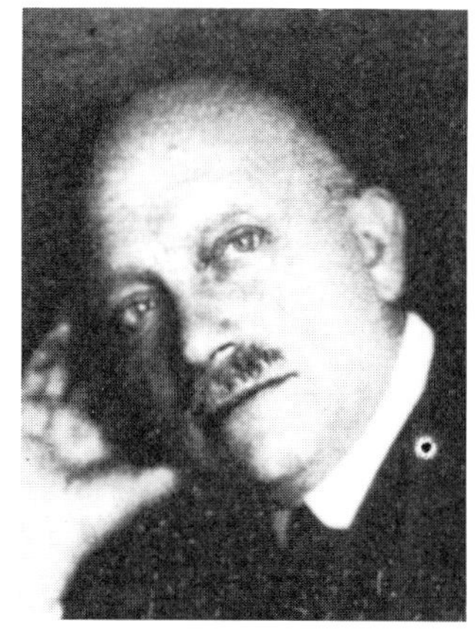

Figure 13.9 Ernst Wertheim (1864–1920).

The first pharyngotomy operation in England was performed by Edward Cock *(1856)* for the removal of a foreign body. The operation of transthyroid pharyngotomy for carcinoma of the hypopharynx was described by Trotter *(1913, 1926, 1929)*, who considered it to be the foundation upon which all the different surgical procedures, ranging from the simple to the elaborate, must be built, as it is primarily the method of gaining access to the tumour so that its precise extent in the pharynx can be determined by palpation and the decision made as to whether a radical operation can be done and, if so, what the attendant requirements are. Nowadays, in addition to actual palpation of the tumour to determine its local extent, multiple biopsies of contiguous tissues are performed for histopathology by the frozen-section technique.

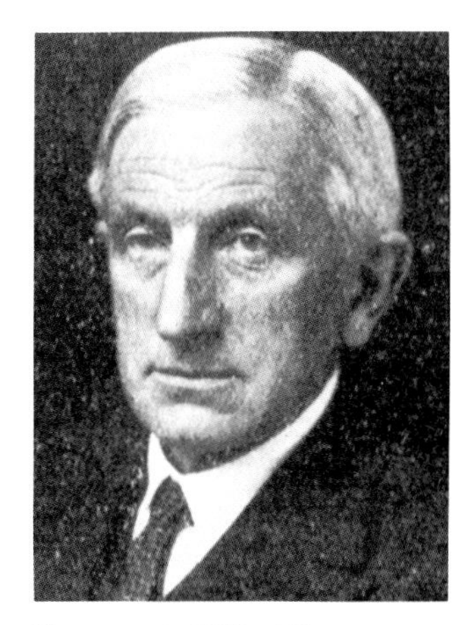

Figure 13.10 Wilfred Trotter (1872–1939).

In his 1929 publication Trotter described two operations for carcinoma of the hypopharynx, namely, median (anterior) translingual pharyngotomy for superior situated tumours and lateral transthyroid pharyngotomy for lateral tumours. He discussed the importance of controlling infections (antibiotics had not been discovered at that time); preservation and restoration of function; and the necessity for a temporary tracheostomy. These principles, he pointed out, were applicable in the surgical treatment of malignant tumours in the nasal cavity, mouth, pharynx and larynx.

Since this pioneer surgical work, the surgical operations for carcinoma of the pharynx and larynx have been considerably developed, to the great benefit of patients with these serious diseases. Many patients now survive for many years after radical surgical treatment, even for an extensive carcinoma with metastases in the cervical lymph nodes. A radical operation can be carried out on some patients when radiotherapy has failed to control the disease, but there are certain difficult technical problems to be solved in such cases. Some of the encouraging results in patients with carcinoma of the pharynx are recorded in Chapter 14.

Modern operations include partial pharyngectomy, with a radical neck dissection when metastases are present in the lymph nodes, for a carcinoma in the oropharynx. For a carcinoma in the hypopharynx and cervical oesophagus the operations of pharyngo-laryngectomy and laryngo-oeso-phago-pharyngectomy with a radical neck dissection are indicated. For a carcinoma of the larynx which is uncontrolled by radiotherapy a laryngectomy is performed, with a radical neck dissection when lymph node

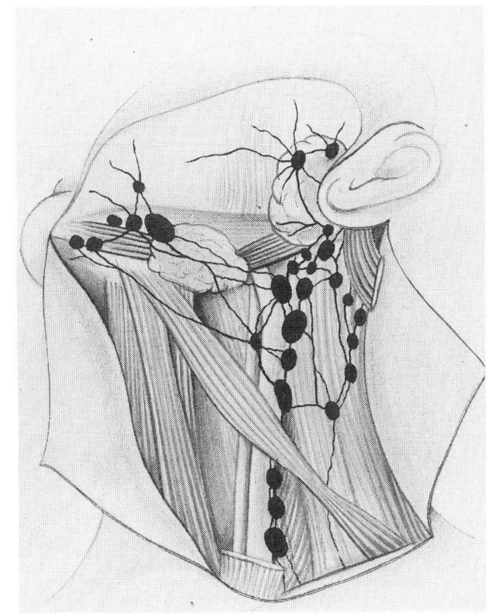

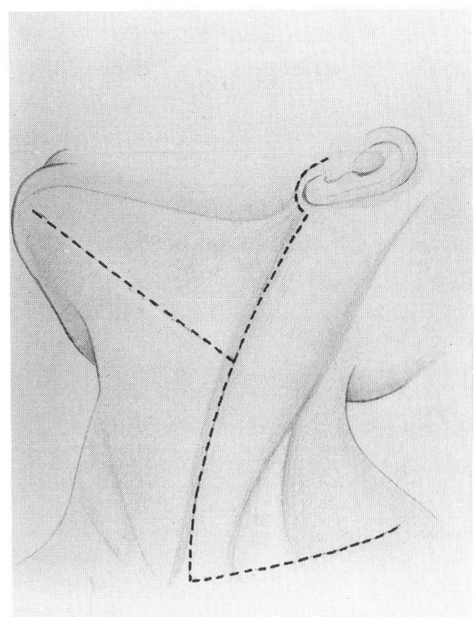

Figure 13.11 *Left:* The location of the pre-auricular, submandibular and deep cervical lymph nodes. *Right:* The incisions required for radical excision of these lymph nodes.

metastases are present *(Raven, 1958)*. Important contributions to the development of modern operations in these regions were made by Colledge *(1943)* and Wookey *(1948)*.

As a result of advances in plastic surgery various reconstruction methods are available to restore normal deglutition, but a permanent tracheostomy is necessary. The operations are performed with a great measure of safety; infection is no longer a problem as antibiotics are available and skilled nursing is provided in the postoperative period of care. A number of patients with serious carcinomas can be restored to lives of good quality and duration.

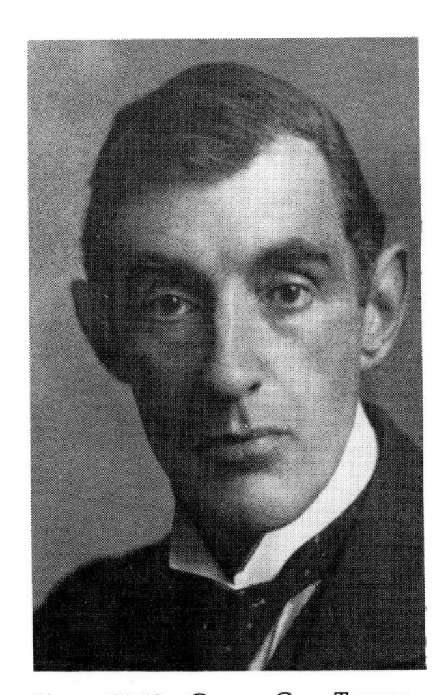

Figure 13.12 George Grey Turner, Surgeon to the Royal Infirmary at Newcastle upon Tyne and later Professor of Surgery in London. He also wrote *Hunterian Museum*, published in 1946, which described the museum's history from its foundation to its destruction during the aerial bombardments of May 1941.

Oesophagectomy

During the last 50 years important progress has been made in the surgery of cancer of the oesophagus. The first successful resection of the thoracic oesophagus for carcinoma was performed by Torek in 1913 *(Torek, 1913)*. There were many difficulties to be overcome by surgeons who performed oesophagectomy operations, including anaesthesia and the problem of infection. As long ago as 1877 Czerny *(1877)* carried out a successful operation for a cancer of the cervical oesophagus. The British surgeon Grey Turner was greatly interested in the surgical treatment of carcinoma of the oesophagus and made important contributions to the subject. He successfully removed the thoracic oesophagus by the collo-abdominal operation which he developed *(Turner, 1933)*. The present author recalls watching him perform the operation (the "pull through" method) at his clinic in Newcastle upon Tyne and his own abiding interest in the surgery of the oesophagus was greatly stimulated by this outstanding surgeon, who was later appointed Professor of Surgery at the Royal British Postgraduate Medical School in London.

At that time there were several problems to be solved, including an evaluation of the different methods of surgical exposure of the oesophagus. This particular work was carried out by O'Shaughnessy and Raven *(1934)*

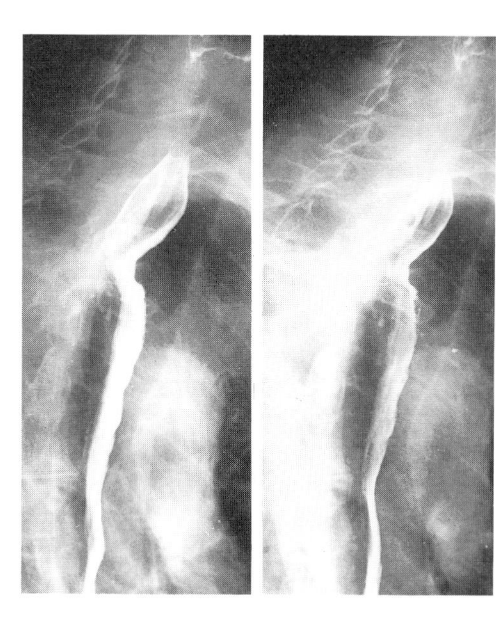

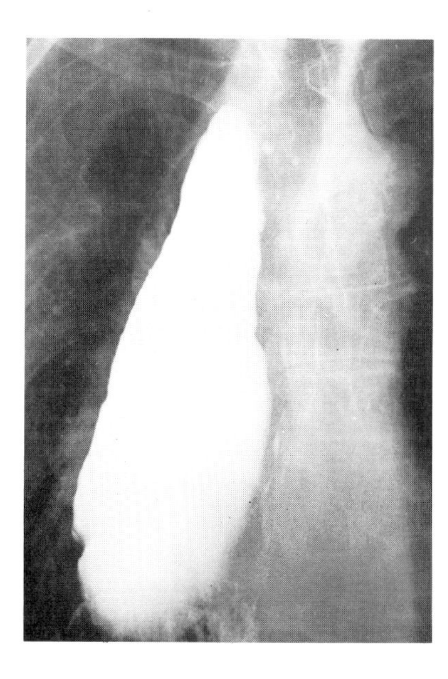

Figure 13.13 *Left:* A radiograph with a barium swallow showing a carcinoma in the middle third of the oesophagus. *Right:* A radiograph of the same patient following a subtotal oesophagectomy with the mobilisation of the stomach and its transposition into the right side of the chest with a high oesophago-gastric anastomosis.

by dissection on cadavers. They described the advantages over other methods which were gained by the right thoracotomy approach to the oesophagus, which gave an excellent exposure from the thoracic inlet to the diaphragmatic outlet following ligation of the vena azygos major.

An important surgical advance was made when Ivor Lewis *(1946)* described a new operation for tumours in the middle third of the oesophagus. There are two main steps in his operation. An exploratory laparotomy is done first, when the stomach is mobilised, the right gastric and right gastro-epiploic arteries being conserved, and a pyloroplasty is done to facilitate gastric emptying, when the stomach is placed in the chest. The second step of the operation is a right thoracotomy, as described by O'Shaughnessy and Raven, for excision of the thoracic oesophagus with the tumour and to establish an intrathoracic oesophagogastric anastomosis.

A number of other surgeons have made important contributions to oesophageal surgery, including the "three phase oesophagectomy" described by McKeown *(1976)*. A selected bibliography to earlier work has been compiled by the present author *(Raven, 1958)*, and a valuable book by Abel *(1929)* contains several chapters on cancer of the oesophagus.

Pneumonectomy

The incidence and treatment of malignant disease of the lung present a tremendous challenge to modern medicine and surgery, for this disease is both very frequent and dangerous. Since it is a "tobacco cancer", prevention holds the brightest hope for its control in the future. The surgical treatment of lung cancer by lobectomy and pneumonectomy can be curative, especially for relatively early disease, but the 3- and 5-year survival rates are still poor.

The first pneumonectomy for lung cancer was performed in 1933 by Graham and Singer, who in their published account *(1933)* called attention to several previous lobectomy operations for that disease. Their successful pneumonectomy was done for a squamous cell carcinoma which was situated almost at the bifurcation of the main bronchus into the bronchi

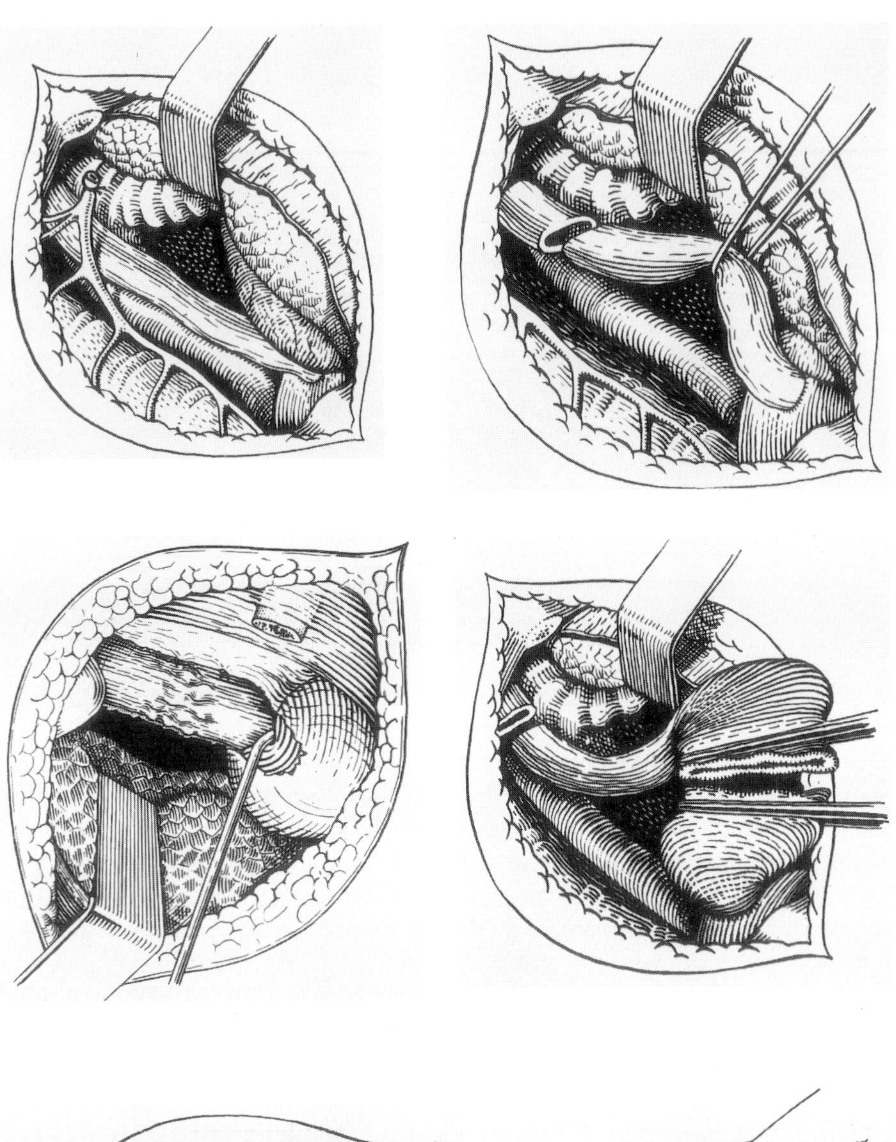

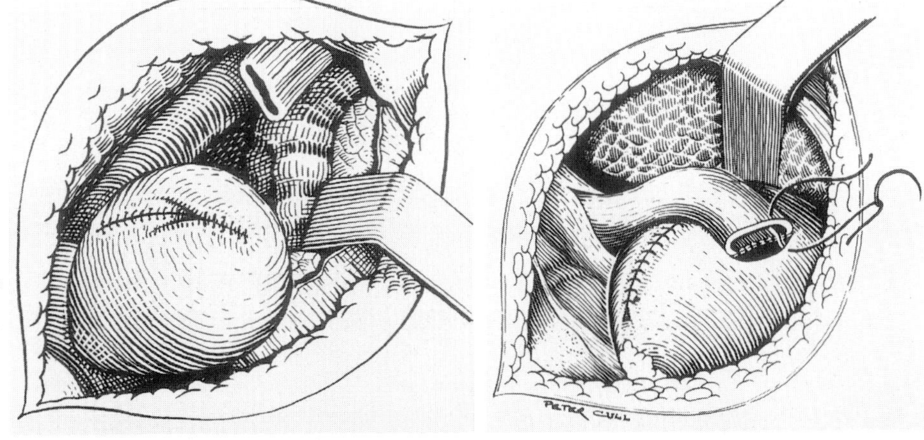

Figure 13.14 Partial oesophago-gastrectomy for carcinoma of the oesophagus. *Top left:* The exposure of the oesophagus by the right thoracotomy operation described by O'Shaughnessy and Raven. The entire oesophagus from the thoracic inlet to the outlet is exposed after the vena azygos major is ligated and exposed. *Top Right:* The mobilised oesophagus in a right thoractomy operation. *Middle left:* Dilatation of the oesophageal hiatus to allow transposition of the mobilised stomach into the right side of the chest. *Middle right:* The divided oesophagus above the carcinoma. The mobilised stomach has been transposed into the chest and the proximal part has been divided. *Bottom left:* Resection of the oesophagus with the carcinoma and the proximal stomach has been done and the distal stomach has been sutured. *Bottom right:* The oesophago-gastric anastomosis between the proximal oesophagus and the stomach in front of the closed resected portion to complete the operation (Ivor Lewis operation).

of the upper and lower lobes and which measured 1 cm in its longest diameter. There was no evidence of any local extension of the tumour and no metastases were present in the tracheobronchial lymph nodes.

Graham and Singer were of the opinion that pneumonectomy with excision of the tracheobronchial lymph nodes is entirely feasible in selected patients and that this operation is attended by less risk of recurrent disease than lobectomy or excision of a smaller segment of the lung. It must be conceded, however, that patient morbidity after pneumonectomy is considerable and there is a place for lobectomy in patients with an early carcinoma.

The great hope for the future is the prevention of cancer of the lung and other organs of the body by abolishing tobacco from human consumption.

Gastrectomy

During the last 100 years spectacular progress has been made in operations for diseases of the stomach, including cancer, which occurs frequently in this viscus. Nevertheless, mortality from gastric carcinoma unfortunately remains high in spite of treatment of the carcinoma by radical total gastrectomy.

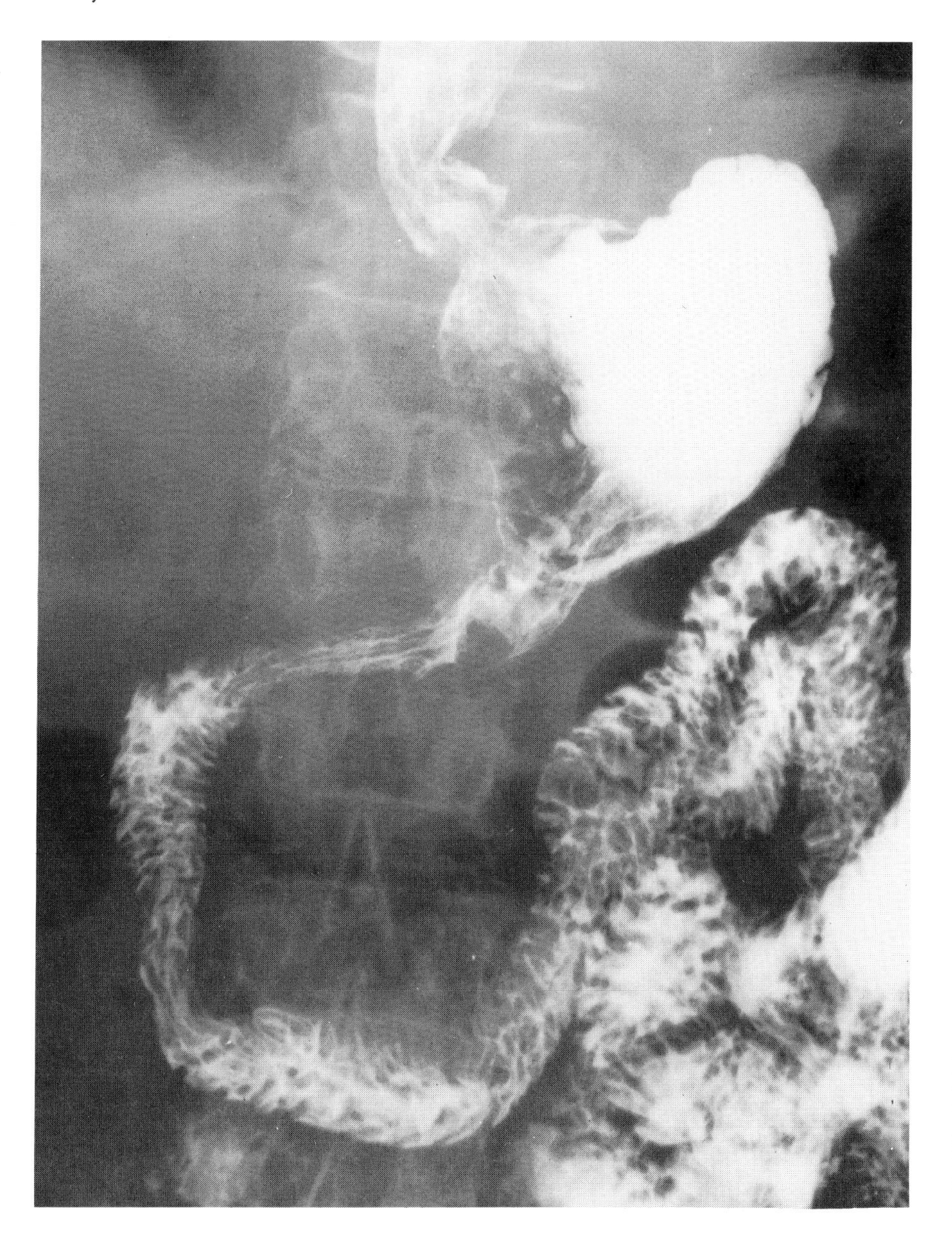

Figure 13.15 Radiograph of the upper gastrointestinal tract with a barium meal after a Billroth I partial gastrectomy. The proximal part of the stomach has been anastomosed to the duodenum after closure of a short segment of the stomach.

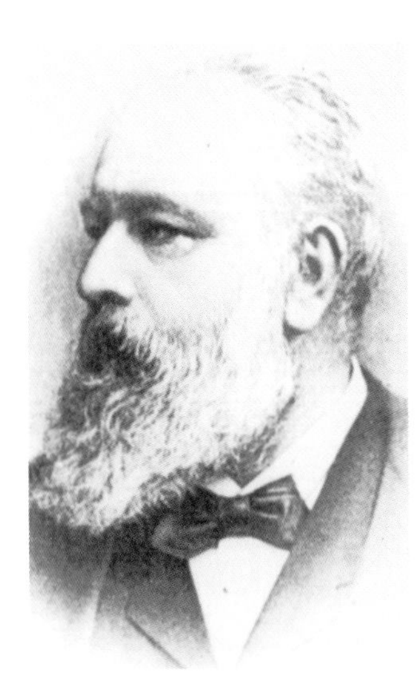

Figure 13.16 Christian Albert Theodor Billroth (1829–1894).

The first successful partial gastrectomy for cancer of the stomach was performed in 1881 by Billroth. In his account Meade *(1968)* states that the patient was a female with cancer of the pylorus and that following the resection Billroth made an anastomosis between the proximal part of the stomach and the duodenum after closure of a short segment of the stomach. The patient survived for 4 months. This operation is known as the Billroth I gastrectomy and has become a standard procedure.

Billroth later made an anastomosis between the stomach and the jejunum after the gastric resection. According to Meade, when this operation had been reported Von Hacker suggested an anastomosis between the divided stomach and the jejunum, and in 1888 Kronlein performed the operation with an antecolic gastrojejunal anastomosis. It is interesting to note that in later years the anastomosis was carried out by both the antecolic and retrocolic techniques. The operation of gastrectomy with a gastrojejunal anastomosis is known as the Billroth II operation.

The first total gastrectomy which was successful was performed by Schlatter in 1897, for gastric cancer. The whole stomach was removed and continuity re-established by anastomosis between the divided oesophagus and the jejunum. This operation, which has become a standard procedure for gastric carcinoma, includes resection of the great omentum and the regional lymph nodes. Continuity is re-established either by making an oesophagojejunal or an oesophagoduodenal anastomosis.

In modern times a more radical total gastrectomy is sometimes performed for an extensive carcinoma by including a splenectomy and partial pancreatectomy. A gastric resection which includes the lower end of the oesophagus is indicated when a carcinoma of the stomach extends to that

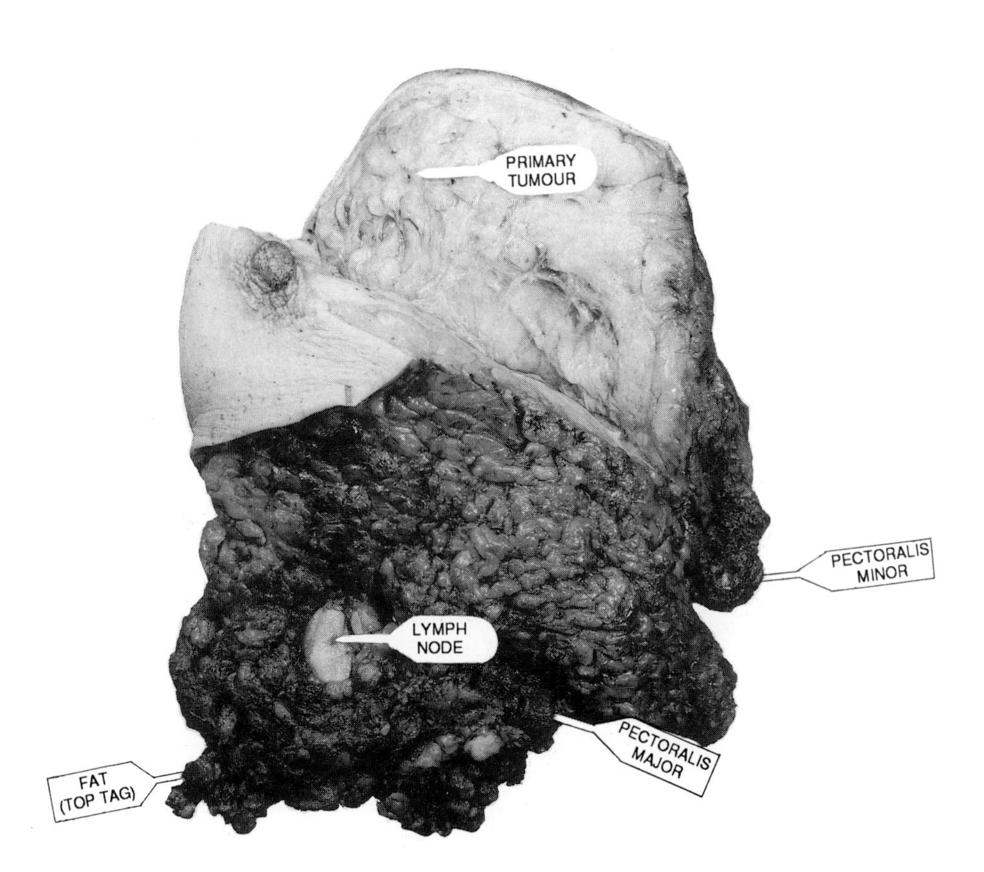

Figure 13.17 A specimen removed by a radical mastectomy with identification markers on tissues, including the apex of the axilla, for histopathology.

organ. The operation of oesophagogastrectomy was performed first by Von Mickulicz in 1898.

There are other standard operations for cancer whose design and performance are of considerable interest. The radical mastectomy operation for carcinoma of the breast was performed first by Halsted in 1890. This subject is discussed in Chapter 12.

All the major oncological operations are important features in the history of surgery.

REFERENCES

Abel, A. L. (1929). *Oesophageal Obstruction — Its Pathology, Diagnosis and Treatment.* Humphrey Milford. Oxford University Press, London

Cock, E. (1856). Case of pharyngotomy. *Lancet*, **1**, 125–6

Colledge, L. (1943). The pathology and surgery of cancer of the pharynx and larynx. *Trans. Med. Soc. London*, **63**, 306

Czerny, V. (1877). Nene Operationen (Resection des Oesophagus). *Zbl. Chir.*, **4**, 433

Graham, E. A. and Singer, J. J. (1933). Successful removal of entire lung for carcinoma of the bronchus. *J. Am. Med. Assoc.*, **101**, 1371–4

Gross, S. D. (1876). A century of American surgery. *Am. J. Med. Sci.*, **71**, 431–84

Lewis, I. (1946). The surgical treatment of carcinoma of the oesophagus with special reference to a new operation for growths in the middle third. *Br. J. Surg.*, **34**, 18–31

McKeown, K. C. (1976). Total three stage oesophagectomy for cancer of the oesophagus. *Br. J. Surg.*, **63**, 259–62

Meade, R. H. (1968). *An Introduction to the History of General Surgery*, pp 315–25. W. B. Saunders, Philadelphia and London

Miles, W. E. (1908). A method of performing abdomino-perineal excision for carcinoma of the rectum and of the terminal portion of the pelvic colon. *Lancet*, **2**, 812–13

Miles, W. E. (1939). *Rectal Surgery*, pp 244–51. Cassell and Company, London

O'Shaughnessy, L. and Raven, R. W. (1934). Surgical exposure of the oesophagus. *Br. J. Surg.*, **22**, 365–77

Raven, R. W. (1958). *Cancer of the Pharynx, Larynx and Oesophagus and Its Surgical Treatment.* Butterworth & Co., London

Torek, F. (1913). The first successful resection of the thoracic portion of the esophagus for carcinoma. *Surg. Gynecol. Obstet.*, **16**, 614–17

Trotter, W. (1913). Principles and technique of the operative treatment of malignant disease of the mouth and pharynx. *Lancet*, **1**, 1075 and 1147

Trotter, W. (1926). The surgery of malignant disease of the pharynx. *Br. Med. J.*, **1**, 269–72

Trotter, W. (1929). Operations for malignant disease of the pharynx. *Br. J. Surg.*, **16**, 485–95

Turner, G. G. (1933). Excision of the thoracic oesophagus for carcinoma with construction of an extra-thoracic gullet. *Lancet*, **2**, 1315–16

Wookey, H. (1948). The surgical treatment of carcinoma of the hypopharynx and oesophagus. *Br. J. Surg.*, **35**, 249–66

CHAPTER FOURTEEN

Long Survival after Cancer Surgery

Surgical treatment is the major treatment of patients with cancer today and it is most likely to remain so in the foreseeable future, either alone or in combination with radiotherapy and chemotherapy. The surgeon who is entrusted with the care of patients with any of the varieties of cancer, which can occur in all organs and sites of the body, carries heavy responsibilities and is confronted with many difficult problems. Due to the nature and behaviour of malignant diseases, the results of treatment can often be disappointing, but at the same time there is much encouragement when patients are seen to be restored to lives of good quality and duration. The great courage of patients suffering any of the various disablements due to cancer is a constant source of help to the surgeon who is responsible for their rehabilitation and continuing care.

It is unfortunate that many patients who present for treatment already have advanced local disease or metastases. Some other patients are referred to the surgeon when other treatment modalities have failed to control their disease. Special difficulties are caused when the malignant tumour is situated in an organ or tissue of the body where access for surgical extirpation and reconstructive procedures is difficult, and radiation effects in the skin and other tissues exacerbate operative difficulties.

In all these circumstances it is very helpful for the general and specialist surgeon and the surgical oncologist to have recourse to the experience of colleagues whose advice and support are valuable in the solution of difficult problems caused by cancer, in addition to learning from the wider field of experience which is available in oncology literature. The present author therefore decided to record some of his experience in the surgical treatment of some patients whose referral gave him many difficult problems to solve, including treatment decisions, surgical technique and the patients' rehabilitation. The study of individual patients, especially those with unusual forms of cancer, is very helpful. In the final assessment of our clinical work attention must be focused on the quality of life of the patient, including his freedom from suffering, life-style, ability to work, and period of survival after surgery. It is hoped that the case-records of patients treated by the present author, which embody helpful lessons concerning the management of malignant tumours in different parts of the body, will be interesting and valuable to colleagues, in addition to providing encouragement in cancer surgery. Many of the patients presented with advanced cancer, which, in some cases, radiotherapy had failed to control, nevertheless they all enjoyed long periods of survival after their treatment by surgery.

In recent years emphasis has been placed on the results, including survival rates, of clinical trials in cancer patients to compare the value of different treatment modalities. An outstanding example where the results of clinical trials are valuable is carcinoma of the female breast; these trials are still continuing, for the patients must be followed up for an adequate period of 5–10 years. There is much debate and concern today about the best treatment for this dangerous and unpredictable disease, so the results of the trials are awaited with interest.

In the last analysis of our work it is the well-being of the individual patient which concerns us and there is much to commend the individual experience of the clinician.

CARCINOMA OF THE FEMALE BREAST

Carcinoma of the breast is the most frequent variety of cancer in women in the UK and it continues to cause great concern today. Its treatment has been the subject of discussion and controversy for more than a century and the debate about it continues at the present time. Different surgical operations are being performed, ranging from local excision of the carcinoma to radical mastectomy. The role of radiotherapy is under consideration and our knowledge of hormonal control mechanisms and hormonal therapy is increasing. An important development in the treatment of breast carcinoma has been the introduction of new synthetic hormones, especially Nolvadex (tamoxifen). Consequently, operations for endocrine ablation, including bilateral oophorectomy, bilateral adrenalectomy and hypophysectomy, are now performed less frequently.

The present author has seen spectacular results in patients with advanced breast carcinoma whom he had treated by bilateral oophorectomy and bilateral adrenalectomy; there was complete regression of the disease and the patients survived for many years.

These impressive results achieved by manipulation of hormonal control mechanisms must never be forgotten, for they were important historic milestones in the development of our knowledge of the causation and treatment of breast carcinoma. It is visualised that eventually the hormonal control mechanisms will be clearly understood and it will be possible to manipulate them to prevent breast carcinoma or to reverse early carcinomatous changes in breast tissue back to normal and thus cure the disease. It has already been demonstrated that a reversal of advanced breast carcinoma can follow hormonal treatment; we need to know the reason why this occurs.

The subject of malignant disease of the breast is considered in greater detail in Chapter 12. Here below certain case-records are cited because of their individual interest and to give encouragement for the future.

Case-record 1

A female, aged 44, unmarried, was referred with a carcinoma measuring 3 cm in diameter situated in the upper inner quadrant of the left breast and a hard mobile lymph node in the left axilla. An aspiration biopsy of the breast tumour confirmed the presence of a carcinoma. The patient was treated by bilateral oophorectomy and radiotherapy to the left breast and regional lymph nodes.

Survival period. The patient is well 14 years later, with no evidence of local or metastatic breast carcinoma.

Case-record 2

An unmarried female, aged 46, was referred with a carcinoma measuring 2 cm in diameter situated above the nipple in the left breast. A left radical mastectomy was performed and postoperative radiotherapy was given. Histopathology showed an intraduct breast carcinoma with early infiltration of the perivascular lymphatics. The remaining breast tissue showed adenosis with occasional cyst formation. Metastases were present in the anterior lymph node in the left axilla, but the apical lymph nodes were free of disease. Breast carcinoma — stage 2.

The patient developed a carcinoma measuring 7 × 6 cm in the right breast 19 months later, for which a simple mastectomy with excision of the low axillary lymph nodes was performed after excision biopsy of the tumour had confirmed the carcinoma. Histopathology showed an intraduct breast carcinoma; no metastases were present in the right axillary lymph nodes. Breast carcinoma — stage 1.

This patient's family history is interesting. Her mother had a radical mastectomy for breast carcinoma at the age of 50 and died of cerebral thrombosis 18 years later having had no recurrent or metastatic breast carcinoma. Two paternal aunts also had a radical mastectomy for breast carcinoma.

Survival period. The patient is well 36 years after the first left radical mastectomy, with no recurrent or metastatic breast carcinoma.

Case-record 3

A married female, aged 39, was referred with a carcinoma measuring 4 cm in diameter in the upper outer quadrant of the left breast, and small lymph nodes in the left axilla. The carcinoma was confirmed by frozen-section histology and a left radical mastectomy was performed. Histopathology showed a breast carcinoma and metastases in the left axillary lymph nodes. Breast carcinoma — stage 2.

A bilateral oophorectomy was performed, the patient being premenopausal.

Subsequent history. The patient remained well with no recurrent or metastatic breast carcinoma until 20 years later, when she developed a tumour measuring 5 cm in diameter in the upper outer quadrant of the right breast. There were no palpable lymph nodes in the right axilla.

Excision biopsy of the tumour showed a breast carcinoma measuring 1.5 cm in diameter surrounded by fatty tissue. A modified right radical mastectomy was performed. Histopathology showed an invasive carcinoma and a microscopic focus of intraduct carcinoma; no metastases were present in the right axillary lymph nodes. Breast carcinoma — stage 1.

Survival period. The patient is well 23 years after the left radical mastectomy and bilateral oophorectomy and 3 years after the right modified radical mastectomy. It is noted here that bilateral oophorectomy did not prevent the development of a carcinoma in the opposite breast 20 years later.

Case-record 4

A female aged 36 was referred with a tumour measuring 5 cm in diameter in the upper, inner quadrant of the right breast. No palpable lymph nodes were present in the right axilla. In the left breast there was a tumour 1 cm in diameter medial to the areola. The tumour in the right breast was excised and histology showed an adenocarcinoma. The tumour in the left breast was excised and histology showed a fibroadenoma. The patient received postoperative radiotherapy for the carcinoma in the right breast.

It is noted that 9 years previously a mixed salivary gland tumour had been excised from the left parotid salivary gland, the excision being followed by a course of radiotherapy. Histology showed a mixed salivary gland tumour.

Subsequent history. The patient remained well with no recurrent or metastatic breast carcinoma or recurrent mixed salivary gland tumour until 26 years later, when she developed a hard tumour measuring 6 × 5 cm in diameter in the outer part of the right breast. (This breast was the site of the previous carcinoma.) Enlarged lymph nodes were palpable in the right axilla. Needle biopsy of the breast tumour showed a carcinoma — most likely a second primary carcinoma. A right modified radical mastectomy was performed.

Histopathology showed an infiltrating, moderately differentiated adenocarcinoma involving fat and lymphatic vessels. The main mass of the tumour was surrounded by mature collagenous tissue, evidently the result of radiotherapy. There were areas of intraduct carcinoma, suggesting a new primary lesion. Sections of the breast adjacent to the healed scar showed foci of calcification within mature fibrous tissue as well as normal breast ducts. Sections of the axillary lymph nodes showed that seven of the eight nodes were infiltrated by metastatic carcinoma. Tamoxifen therapy was instituted.

Survival period. The patient is well 31 years after excision of the first primary carcinoma in the right breast and postoperative radiotherapy and 4 years after the right modified radical mastectomy and tamoxifen therapy for the second primary carcinoma in the right breast. There is no recurrent or metastatic breast carcinoma. There is no recurrent mixed salivary gland tumour 40 years after excision.

Case-record 5

A female aged 64 years was referred following local excision, in another country, of a carcinoma measuring 3 cm in diameter in the upper, outer quadrant of the right breast. Histopathology showed a primary breast carcinoma composed of large polyhedral cells arranged as irregular groups in a fibroblastic stroma which displayed very heavy infiltration with lymphocytes and plasmacytes. Some of the lymphocytic aggregates had primitive reaction centres. This tumour was a medullary carcinoma with lymphoid stroma.

A right radical mastectomy was performed. Histopathology showed the changes of fat necrosis; metastatic polygonal carcinoma was present in two out of 18 right axillary lymph nodes. Postoperative radiotherapy was given to the scar and regional lymph node areas. Breast carcinoma — stage 2.

Subsequent history. The patient remained well for 18 years, then discovered a lump in the upper, outer quadrant of her left breast. A left modified radical mastectomy was performed in another country. Histopathology showed a scirrhous carcinoma of the left breast infiltrating the breast tissue; six nodes from the left axilla showed no metastases. Breast carcinoma — stage 1.

Survival period. The patient is well 19 years after the right radical mastectomy and postoperative radiotherapy for the stage 2 primary carcinoma and 1 year after the left modified radical mastectomy for the stage 1 primary carcinoma. There is no recurrent or metastatic breast carcinoma.

Case-record 6

A female aged 71 was referred with multiple carcinoma metastases in both lungs from a primary carcinoma measuring 2 cm in diameter situated in the lower, outer quadrant of the left breast. Another surgeon had performed an extended simple mastectomy 10⅔ years previously. Histopathology showed a mucoid carcinoma of the breast; three lymph nodes excised from the left axilla showed no metastases. A postoperative course of radiotherapy was given to the left axilla.

A radiological examination of the chest showed extensive metastases of breast carcinoma throughout both lungs. The patient was treated with tamoxifen 10 mg twice daily. A radiological examination of the chest 2¾ years later showed no evidence of lung metastases and the patient is well and has no cough, dyspnoea or pain. She continues with tamoxifen therapy.

Survival period. The patient is well with no evidence of recurrent or metastatic breast carcinoma 13 years and 5 months after the simple extended mastectomy and 2 years, 8 months, after the diagnosis of lung metastases and institution of tamoxifen therapy.

Combined cystosarcoma phyllodes and carcinoma of the breast

The occurrence of cystosarcoma phyllodes in one breast and a carcinoma in the other is extremely rare. One patient with these tumours has been under the care of the present author.

Case-record

A female, aged 23, was referred with a recurrent sarcoma phyllodes in the left breast. There had already been two recurrences and excision had been performed in another country. Histopathology showed the appearance of cystosarcoma phyllodes. There was a nodular tumour, 16 cm in diameter, occupying the whole of the left breast. This was carefully excised and a

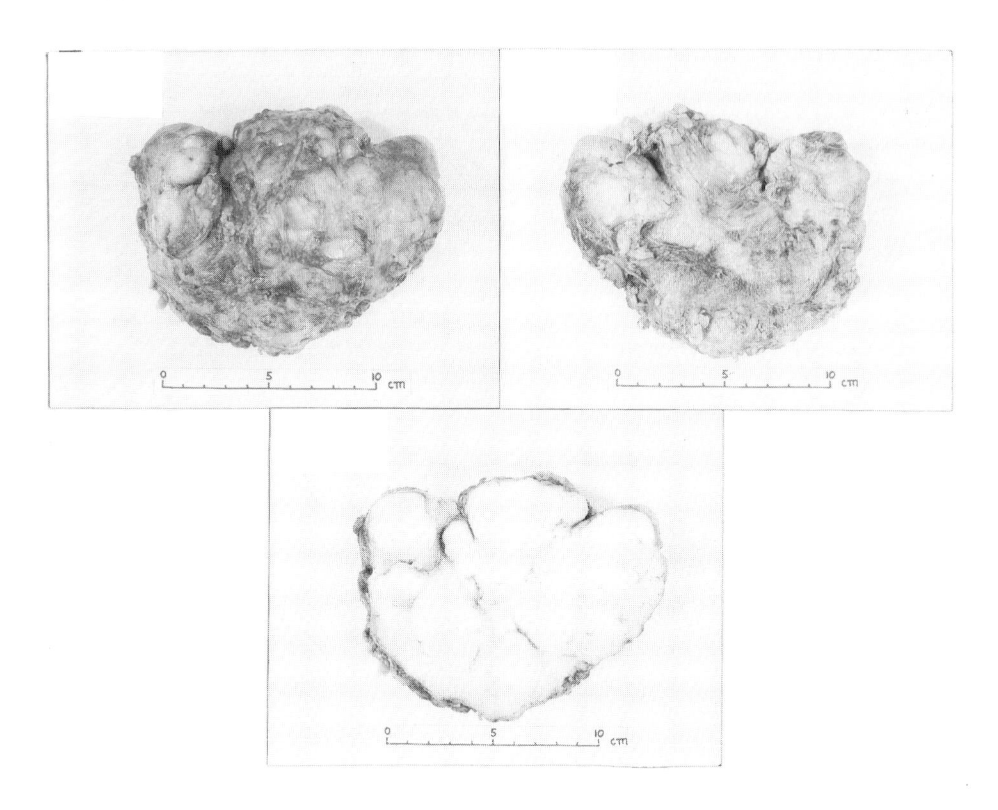

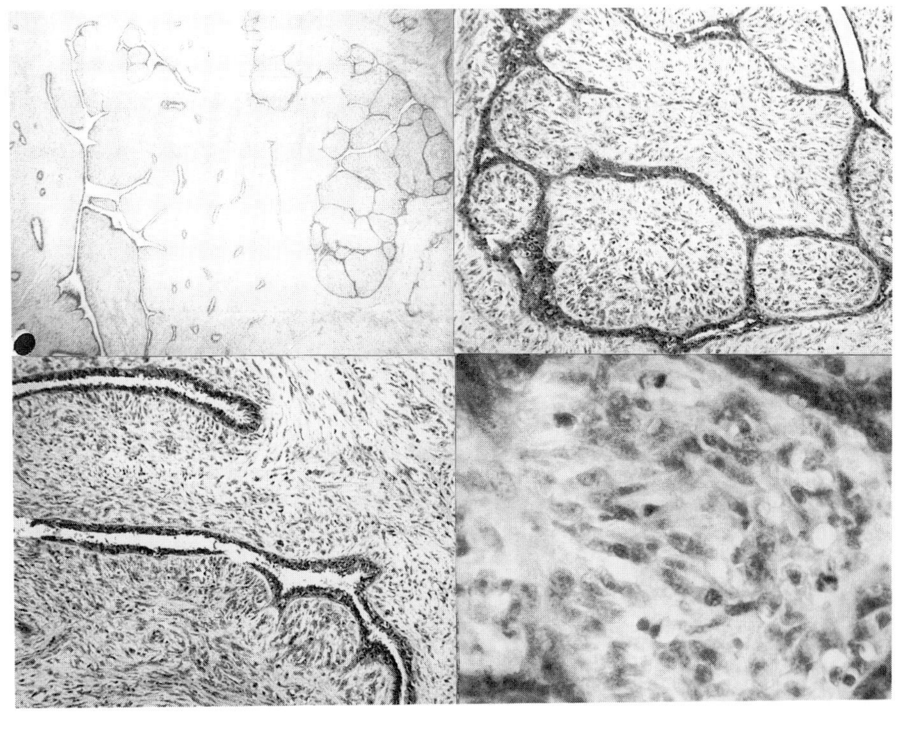

Figure 14.1 Cystosarcoma phyllodes (15.5 x 10.0 x 5.0 cm, weight 400 g) excised from the left breast of a female patient aged 23. Microscopy of multiple sections taken from various areas of the tumour show the features of a giant intracanalicular adenofibroma of the breast. In many areas there is a definite sarcomatous change with numerous giant cells, bizarre nuclei and atypical mitosis. The mitotic activity in those areas is of a high grade of malignancy. There is no suggestion of invasive tendency at the periphery of the mass, but within the tumour features of a rapid growth are evident.

silicone breast replacement was inserted. Histopathology showed a cystosarcoma phyllodes — grade 2.

One year later a recurrent cystosarcoma phyllodes appeared in the left breast and was excised, the silicone replacement being conserved. There was a swelling 5 cm in diameter in the upper, inner quadrant of the right breast. This tumour was also excised.

Histopathology showed there was a very large cell, highly malignant carcinoma in the right breast, with areas of necrosis and very poor stromal reaction. In the left breast there was a cystosarcoma phyllodes with an active stromal element but inactive duct element. It was encapsulated from the surrounding breast and did not appear likely to disseminate.

Postoperative radiotherapy was given to the right breast and regional lymph nodes and to the left breast — upper and inner aspect and the left internal mammary lymph nodes. Melphalan therapy was subsequently given.

Eight months later there was a recurrent cystosarcoma phyllodes in the left breast. This was excised and postoperative radiotherapy was given to the nipple and areola of the left breast. Six months later there were recurrent tumours in both the right and left breasts. After careful discussions with the patient and her family and joint professional consultations a right modified radical mastectomy was performed, the tumour in the left breast was excised and the prosthesis was removed.

Histopathology showed a cystosarcoma phyllodes of the right breast. There was no recurrence of carcinoma in the right breast, and no metastases in the right axillary lymph nodes, but there was a recurrent cystosarcoma phyllodes in the left breast. Postoperative radiotherapy was given to the right lateral chest wall and the left upper chest wall.

Eleven months later a recurrent cystosarcoma phyllodes was excised from the inner end of the right mastectomy scar and proved by histology. Postoperative radiotherapy was given to this area.

One year and 11 months later a recurrent cystosarcoma phyllodes was excised from the right chest wall and confirmed by histology. Local postoperative radiotherapy was given to the area.

Survival period. The patient is alive 4 years and 8 months after the last operation for recurrent cystosarcoma phyllodes of the right chest wall, but she has not been examined by the present author as she lives in another county.

Advanced carcinoma of the breast treated with endocrine surgery

The treatment of advanced carcinoma of the breast by oophorectomy and adrenalectomy has had spectacular results, including healing of the primary carcinoma and calcification, and control of osseous metastases. The following case-records are good illustrations.

Case-record 1

A female, aged 59, was referred with an advanced ulcerating carcinoma of the right breast. The tumour involved the whole breast. Histopathology showed a polygonal cell carcinoma — grade 3. The patient was treated at

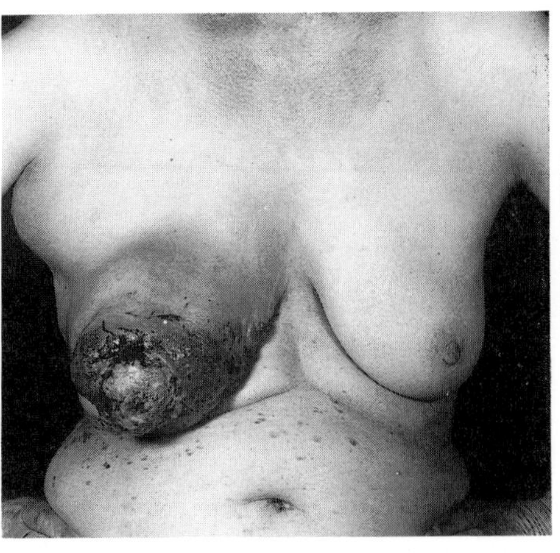
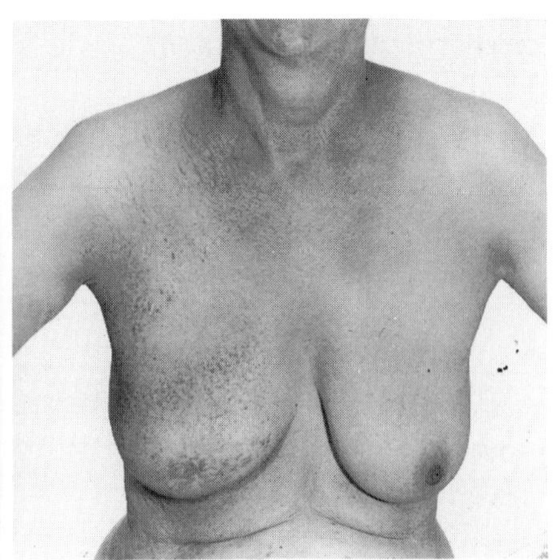

Figure 14.2 A female patient aged 59 (case-record 1) with an advanced ulcerating carcinoma of the breast. *Left:* Before treatment. *Right:* After radiotherapy, bilateral oophorectomy and adrenalectomy.

first by radiotherapy, with a tumour dose of 3100 rads. This was followed by bilateral oophorectomy and bilateral adrenalectomy. Postoperative radiotherapy was then given with a tumour dose of 4500 rads. In addition, fluoxymesterone and thyroxine were given.

A remarkable regression of the breast carcinoma occurred, with complete healing of the ulceration and disappearance of the massive carcinoma.

Survival period. The patient was well with no recurrent or metastatic breast carcinoma 11 years later. She died from a cerebral haemorrhage.

Case-record 2

A female, aged 44, was seen with a bone metastasis in the right acetabulum, which developed 6 years after a radical mastectomy for breast carcinoma. The patient was treated by bilateral oophorectomy and bilateral adrenalectomy. The bone metastasis was given local radiotherapy with a dosage of 2928 rads.

Survival period. The patient returned to an active life as a trainer of Arab horses. She died 3 years and 2 months later from carcinomatosis.

Synthetic hormonal therapy

Endocrine surgery has come to be performed less frequently with the development of synthetic hormonal therapy. Patients with advanced local breast carcinoma have been treated with synthetic oestrogens when they are in the older age groups. In some patients marked tumour regression has occurred.

Case-record

A female, aged 71, was referred because of an advanced carcinoma with massive skin involvement. Histopathology showed a carcinoma — grade 2. The patient was treated with local radiotherapy, with a tumour dosage of 5100 rads. In addition, she was given ethinyl oestradiol and thyroxine therapy.

Survival period. The breast carcinoma regressed completely and the skin healed. The patient was well 15 years and 8 months later and there was no recurrent or metastatic breast carcinoma.

Hormonal control systems

The close relationship of carcinoma of the breast with hormonal control systems is of great importance both in the prevention of the disease and in its treatment. At the present time we do not understand the mechanisms of these systems, although we see the clinical effects when they can be manipulated in various ways. The reversal of carcinomatous cells to normal cells that can be brought about in this way is of great significance. Hormone control systems are retained in about 40% of patients with breast carcinoma (hormone receptor sites can be demonstrated in the cell membrane and cytoplasm of the carcinoma cells), so appropriate biochemical reactions can be triggered off by the particular hormone. The presence of the receptors in a carcinoma is a good indication of the probable response of the tumour to endocrine ablation or the administration of synthetic hormones.

Hormonal control systems are being sought for tumours of the prostate gland, lung, kidney and other organs so that the appropriate endocrine therapy can be given.

CARCINOMA OF THE TONGUE

The prognosis for carcinoma of the tongue is usually poor, since many patients apply for treatment when they already have advanced local disease and metastases in the regional lymph nodes. Patients with earlier tongue carcinomas have been referred to the present author by dental surgeons, who have frequent opportunity to examine the buccal cavity of their patients.

Combined surgical excision and radiotherapy are frequently used for the treatment of tongue carcinoma and permanent cure can be achieved, even with extensive disease. The following case-records are good examples of what can be done for such patients.

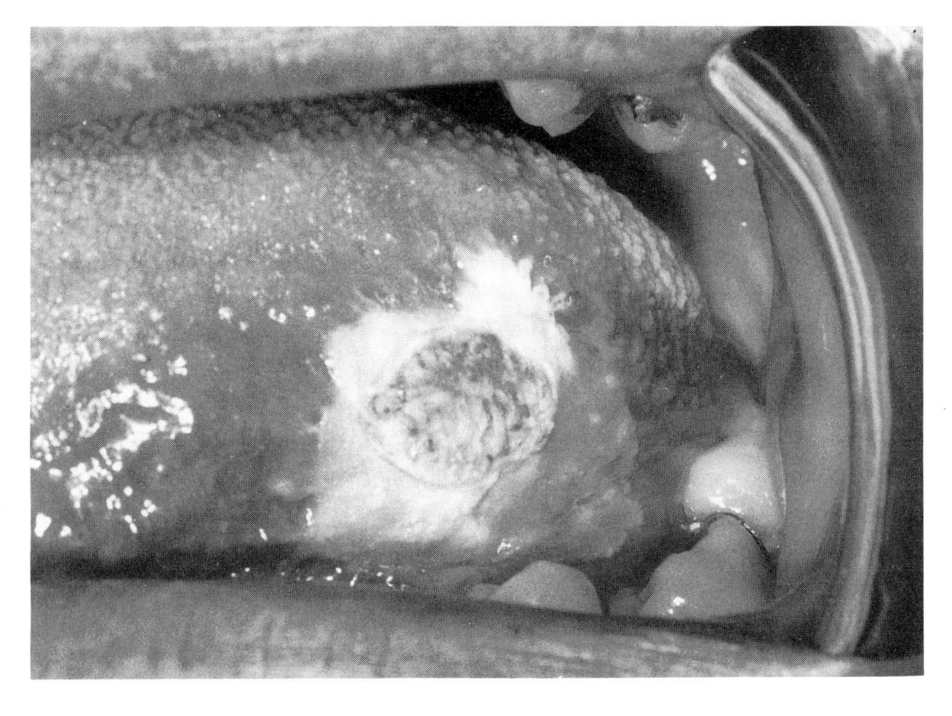

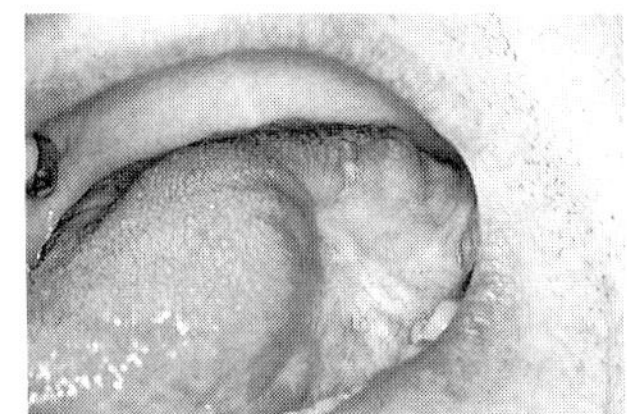

Figure 14.3 *Left:* A squamous cell carcinoma with an area of leukoplakia in the lateral border of the tongue of a 58-year-old male patient (case-record 1). *Above:* The healed tongue with no recurrent or metastatic carcinoma 10 years after excision of the primary carcinoma and postoperative radiotherapy.

Case-record 1

A male, aged 58, was referred with a superficial carcinoma of the tongue, situated in the left lateral border at the junction of the anterior two-thirds and the posterior third. There were no enlarged regional lymph nodes. The primary carcinoma was widely excised, then radiotherapy was given by means of an interstitial radium needle implant.

Histopathology showed a squamous cell carcinoma.

Survival period. The patient is well and there is no recurrent or metastatic carcinoma 22 years later.

Case-record 2

A male, aged 61, was referred with a carcinoma measuring 1 cm in diameter at the right side of the body of the tongue at the junction of the anterior two-thirds and the posterior third. The regional lymph nodes were not enlarged. There was an area of leukoplakia surrounding the primary carcinoma. The carcinoma was treated by a wide wedge resection of the tongue. Histopathology showed a superficial squamous cell carcinoma with no infiltration and chronic superficial glossitis.

Survival period. The patient is alive 17 years later and there is no recurrent or metastatic carcinoma.

A carcinoma of the tongue can be very extensive, in which case it requires a total glossectomy, especially if the carcinoma has recurred after a partial glossectomy or is uncontrolled by radiotherapy.

Case-record 3

A male with an extensive carcinoma of the tongue was treated by total glossectomy.

Survival period. The patient is well, with good speech and satisfactory deglutition, 10 years later. There is no recurrent or metastatic carcinoma.

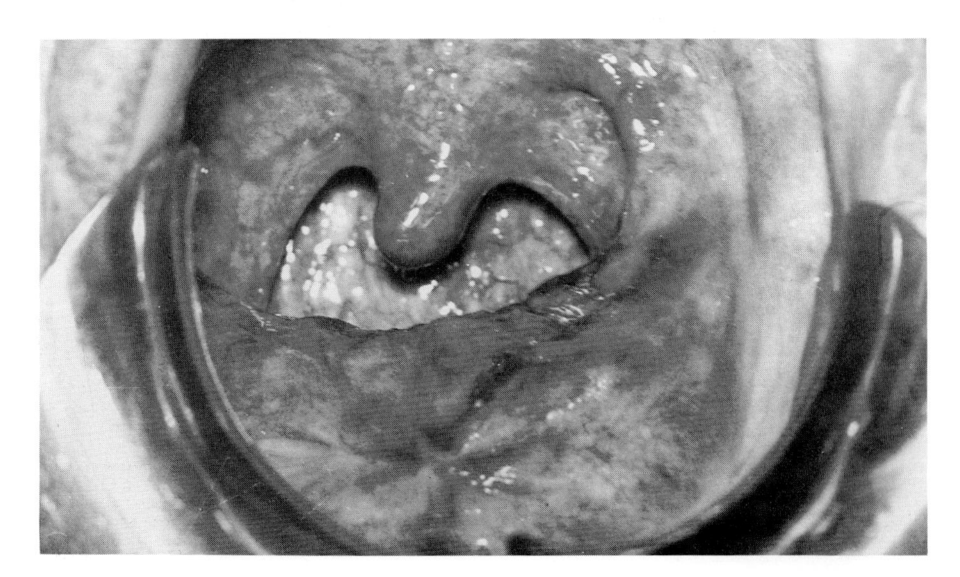

Figure 14.4 The mouth of a male patient (case-record 3) 10 years after a total glossectomy for an extensive carcinoma of the tongue. There is no recurrent or metastatic carcinoma.

A carcinoma of the tongue frequently invades contiguous tissues, such as the floor of the mouth, as shown in the following case-record.

Case-record 4

A male, aged 36, was referred with a carcinoma of the tongue and floor of the mouth. The carcinoma was advanced and affected the left lateral border of the tongue from the anterior faucial pillar to the second molar tooth, with medial spread to within 2 cm of the mid-line. There was a linear ulcer at the junction of the lateral border of the tongue with the floor of the mouth. The regional lymph nodes were not palpable. The carcinoma was treated with external radiation, with a tumour dose of 7361 rads. Oral methotrexate was given for 10 days. There was good regression of the primary carcinoma and the ulcer healed.

Six months later signs of residual carcinoma were seen, so the author performed a left hemiglossectomy and partial excision of the adjacent floor of the mouth; a reconstruction was made using a free split thickness skin graft.

Histopathology showed a poorly differentiated squamous cell carcinoma which had infiltrated the muscle for considerable distances.

Survival period. The patient was well with no recurrent or metastatic disease 20 years later. He then developed an inoperable carcinoma of the stomach, from which he died.

A carcinoma which affects the base of the tongue may extend into the larynx and hypopharynx, creating difficult treatment problems, and the prognosis is poor, especially when it fails to respond to radiotherapy. The following case-record is of much interest.

Case-record 5

A female, aged 49, was referred with an advanced carcinoma involving the base of the tongue and extending to affect the epiglottis. The primary

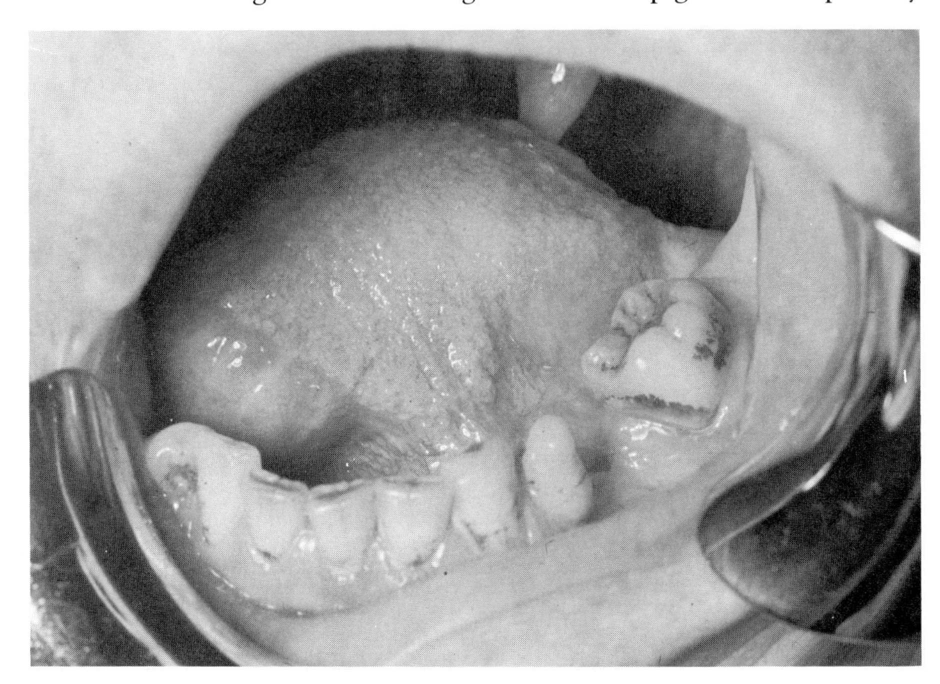

Figure 14.5 Poorly differentiated squamous cell carcinoma in the tongue of a male patient (case-record 4).

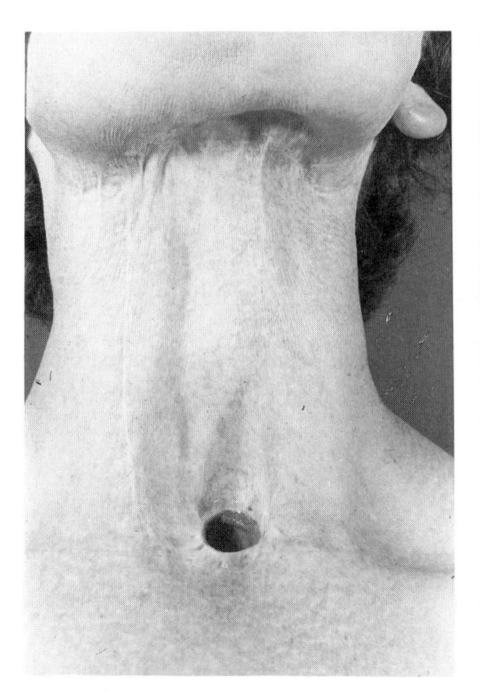

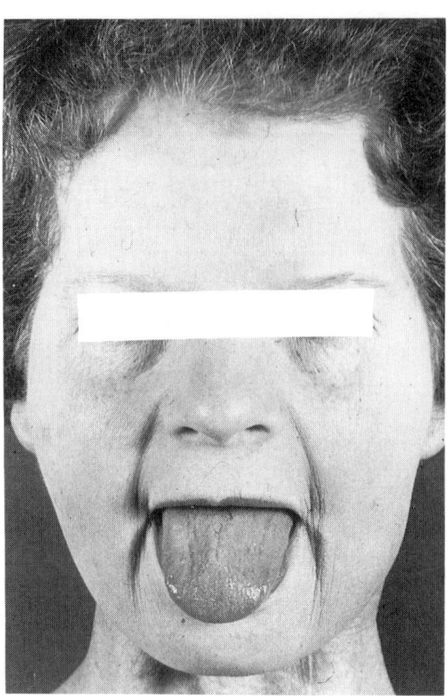

Figure 14.6 *Left:* The neck of a female patient (case-record 5) after laryngo-glosso-pharyngectomy and reconstruction of her hypopharynx. *Right:* The patient showing her functional tongue after the operation. *Below:* the advanced carcinoma removed extending from the base of the tongue to the epiglottis.

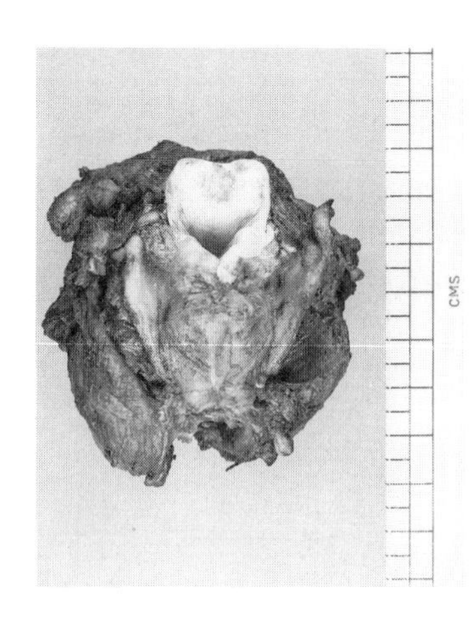

treatment was a course of radiotherapy with a full tumour dosage. This failed to control the carcinoma and the patient was referred for possible surgical treatment. The author carefully considered the problem and designed an operation to eradicate the disease and conserve a functioning tongue. He performed a laryngo-glosso-pharyngectomy as a 1-stage operation, conserving the anterior three-quarters of the tongue and the hypoglossal nerves, then immediately reconstructed the hypopharynx, with the provision of a permanent tracheostomy.

Histopathology showed a squamous cell carcinoma.

Survival period. The wounds healed perfectly and the tongue was fully functional. Deglutition was normal after excision of the posterior quarter of the tongue, the larynx and part of the hypopharynx. The patient is alive and well 17 years and 5 months later, and there is no recurrent or metastatic carcinoma.

CARCINOMA OF THE FLOOR OF THE MOUTH

Carcinoma in the floor of the mouth is a dangerous tumour and there are surgical difficulties to be overcome in its treatment. It spreads locally into the lower alveolus and the mandible, as well as into the tongue, and metastases are frequently present in the regional lymph nodes in the submandibular and cervical groups. Treatment is usually by radiotherapy in the first instance, but if the carcinoma is not controlled and there are lymph node metastases surgical treatment is necessary. The result achieved by combined radiation and surgical treatment is shown in the following case-record.

Case-record

A female, aged 40, was referred with an extensive carcinoma in the floor of the mouth, reaching from the left side over the mid-line for about 1 cm. It

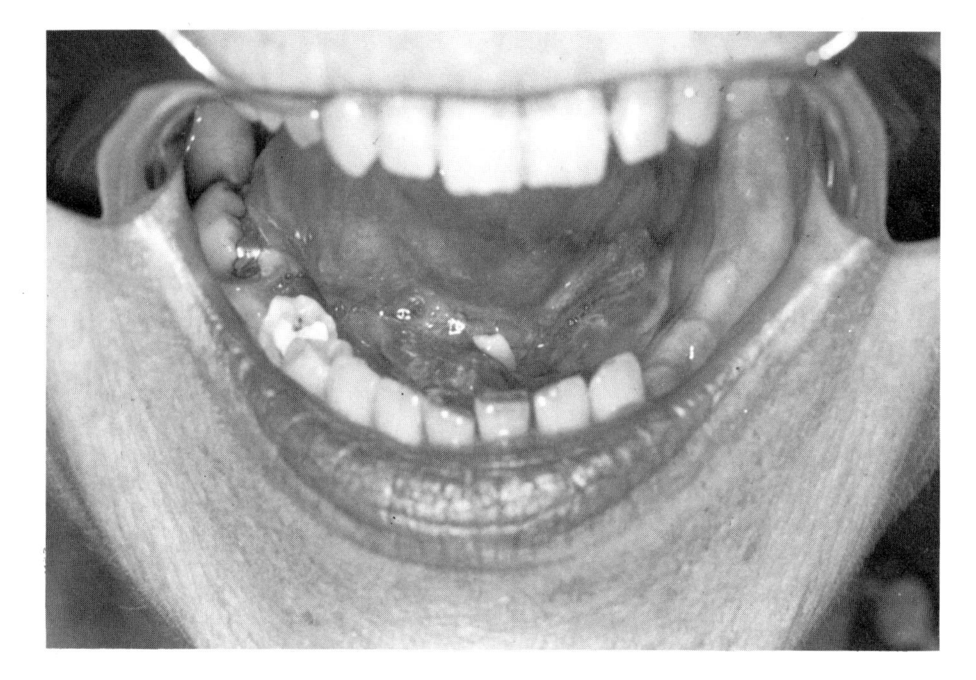

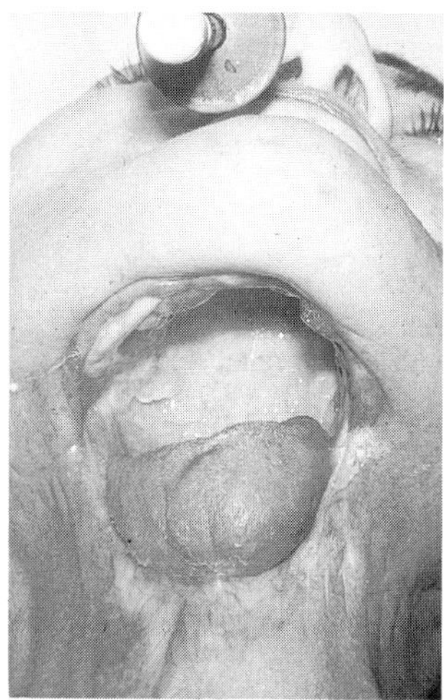

Figure 14.7 *Left:* The extensive carcinoma in the floor of the mouth of the case-record patient. *Above:* Before reconstruction of the floor of the mouth. *Below:* The healed reconstruction of the floor of the mouth 8 months later.

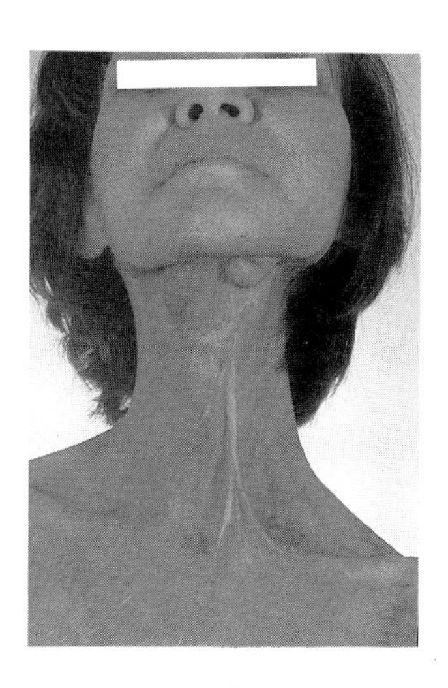

measured 5 × 2.5 cm anteroposteriorly and also involved the under aspect of the tongue and the mucous membrane on the inner side of the mandible. Movements of the tongue were limited and there was induration in the left submandibular region, extending into the right side. There was an enlarged hard lymph node measuring 1 cm in diameter in the left submandibular region and a smaller hard lymph node in the left upper deep cervical region. Radiological examination of the mandible showed no bone erosion.

The patient was treated with preoperative radiotherapy, a tumour dose of 6000 rads being given. There was some tumour regression but extensive induration remained.

The present author then performed a monoblock excision of the floor of the mouth and inferior aspect of the tongue, a modified upper right cervical lymph node dissection and a left radical suprahyoid lymph node dissection. Subsequently he reconstructed the floor of the mouth in stages, using the tongue for the inner aspect. Outer skin cover was obtained by acromio-pectoral tubed pedicle skin grafts. Perfect healing occurred.

The histopathology of the oral tissues showed a well-differentiated squamous cell carcinoma growing in an abundant, densely collagenised fibroblastic stroma, deep to the surface epithelium. The planes of surgical excision were clear by wide margins. There were no metastases in the lymph nodes.

Survival period. The patient is well and there is no recurrent or metastatic carcinoma 21 years later. She can eat satisfactorily, and speak quite well, even on the telephone.

CARCINOMA OF THE ALVEOLUS

Carcinoma of the alveolus is a serious tumour as it frequently invades the adjacent maxilla or mandible and affects contiguous soft tissues, in addition to forming metastases in the regional lymph nodes. When the underlying

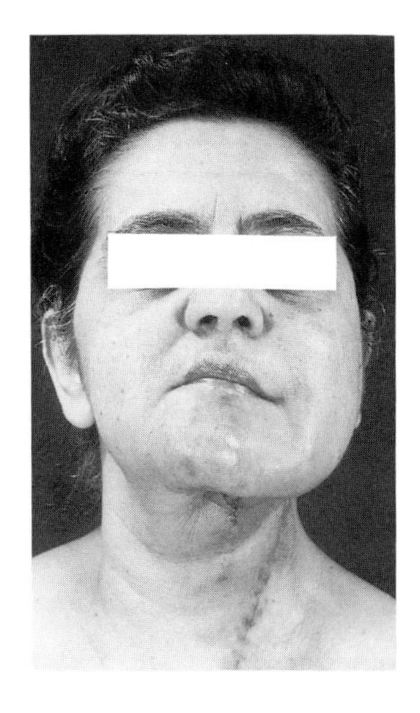

bone is involved surgical treatment is indicated, and if the mandible is affected a portion may have to be replaced by a prosthesis. The following case-record illustrates the solution of these treatment problems, followed by the long survival of the patient for 30 years.

Case-record

A female, 47 years old, was referred with a carcinoma arising in the left lower alveolus. A proliferative variety of carcinoma, measuring 5 × 2 cm, affected the left lower alveolus, being fixed to the mandible but not invading the floor of the mouth. The submental, submandibular and upper deep cervical lymph nodes were enlarged, hard and a little fixed. Radiological examination of the left mandible showed considerable absorption of the alveolar edge of the molar region and some rarefaction posterior to this near the base of the coronoid.

The present author performed a monoblock excision, including a left radical neck dissection and right submental lymph node, and resection of the left mandible from the angle to the symphysis menti, and the mucosa of the left side of the mouth floor. The left mandible was reconstructed with a polythene prosthesis but this was extruded 3 years later.

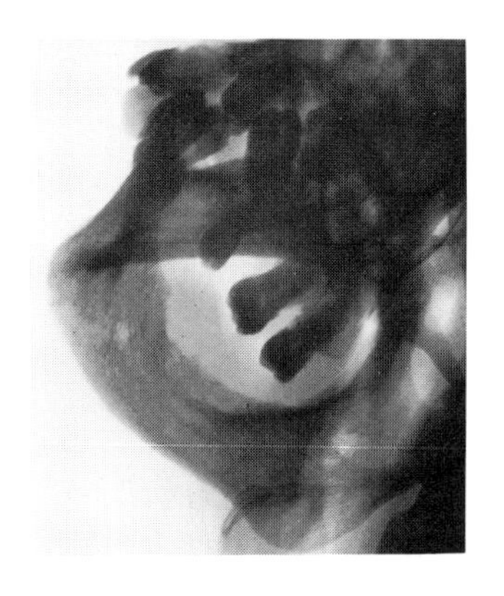

Histopathology showed an active, keratinising squamous cell carcinoma of the alveolus. Metastases were present in the submental and two upper cervical lymph nodes.

Survival period. The patient is well and there is no recurrent or metastatic carcinoma 30 years later.

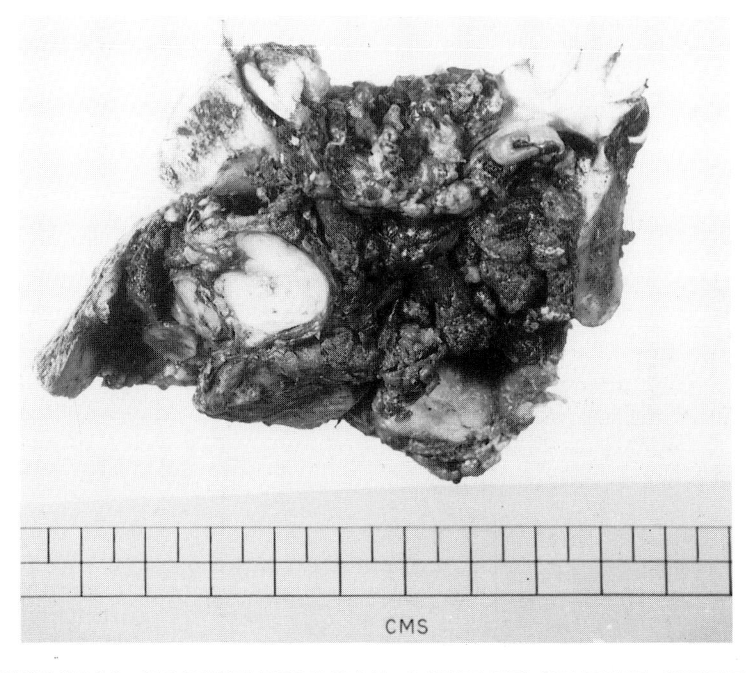

Figure 14.8 *Top:* A 47-year-old patient (see case-record) treated for a squamous cell carcinoma of the left alveolus, seen after left mandibulectomy, left radical neck dissection and the insertion of a polythene prosthesis to replace the left mandible. *Above:* A radiograph showing the polythene prosthesis. *Right:* The excised squamous cell carcinoma with metastases in the left submental and upper cervical lymph nodes.

CARCINOMA OF THE BUCCAL ASPECT OF THE CHEEK

The treatment of carcinoma of the buccal aspect of the cheek presents considerable problems, especially when the angle of the mouth is affected. If surgical excision is indicated, reconstruction of the cheek is necessary and some degree of deformity cannot be avoided. Radiotherapy is carefully considered and usually given as the primary treatment, but if it fails to control the carcinoma surgery is required. The problems created by this variety of carcinoma and their satisfactory solution are clearly exemplified by the following case-record.

Case-record

A female, aged 53, was referred with a carcinoma of the left cheek that radiation treatment had failed to control. For a period of 2 years the patient had injured the mucous membrane of her left cheek with her upper denture when eating. A small ulcer appeared, which gradually increased in size. A biopsy was done in another country and microscopy showed a highly differentiated squamous cell carcinoma, the cells being polygonal and growing densely. In some areas keratinised cells were present but there were only a few mitoses. A course of radiation treatment (Cobalt unit) was given, with a total tumour dose of 5000 rads. There was some initial regression but the carcinoma was not controlled.

Two months later clinical examination showed a carcinoma 6 × 5 cm in size, with a central necrotic slough, affecting the buccal aspect of the left cheek and extending to the alveolus. It was attached to the overlying skin, which was reddened. The left angle of the mouth was not involved. One firm submental lymph node was palpable.

Surgical treatment was carried out, with resection of the carcinoma and a portion of the overlying skin; a left suprahyoid block dissection was done, and the cheek reconstructed.

Histopathology showed a well-differentiated squamous carcinoma extending through the muscle of the cheek. Metastatic carcinoma was present in 1 upper deep cervical lymph node. A course of postoperative radiotherapy was given, with a dosage of 3000 rads.

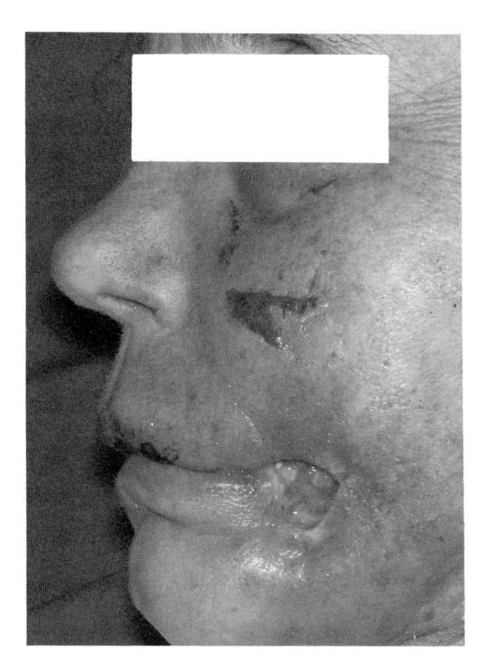

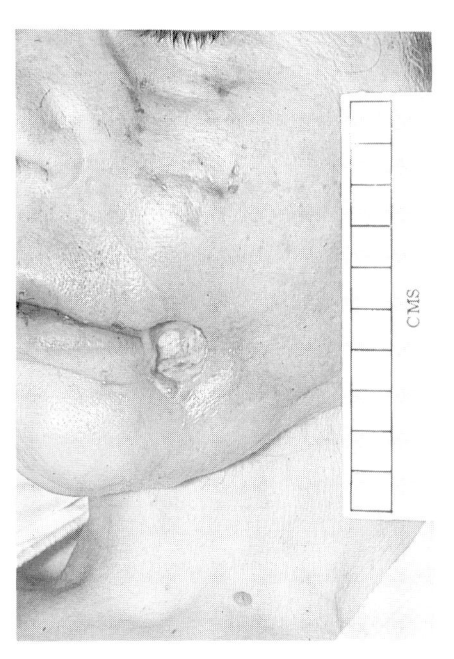

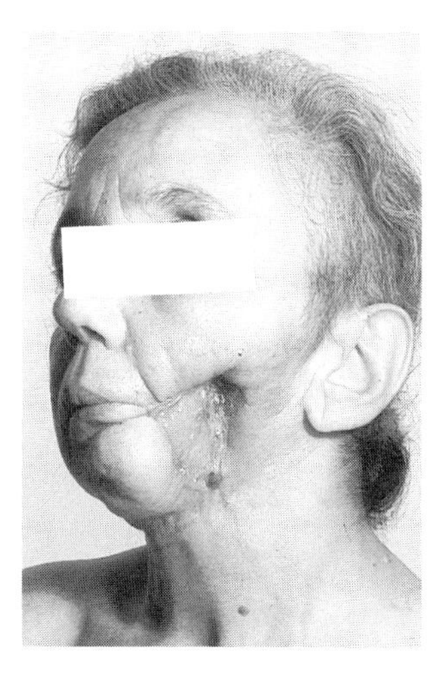

Figure 14.9 *Left:* A 53-year-old female patient (see case-record) with a squamous cell carcinoma of the buccal aspect of the left cheek, which was treated with radiotherapy, surgery and reconstruction of the cheek. *Right:* The patient with a recurrent carcinoma involving the whole thickness of the left cheek after regional perfusion chemotherapy. *Above:* After reconstruction of the left cheek 3 months after the regional perfusion chemotherapy.

After 5 months the patient was referred again with a large recurrent carcinoma of the left cheek, measuring 7.5 cm in diameter and involving the whole thickness of the cheek.

The treatment of this carcinoma, which appeared after two courses of radiation treatment and excisional surgery, presented a very difficult problem, which was solved as follows.

It was decided to administer a regional perfusion of methotrexate and nitrogen mustard. The present author inserted a cannula through the left superficial temporal artery into the external carotid artery. The correct site for the tumour infusion was determined by injecting dye to outline the soft tissues of the left side of the face. A continuous infusion was carried out for a period of 16 days, with a dosage of 350 mg methotrexate and 7.5 mg nitrogen mustard.

The treatment caused a remarkable regression of the carcinoma, which seemed to melt away completely, leaving a soft tissue defect at the left angle of the mouth. Reconstruction by surgery was carried out 3 months later.

Survival period. The patient is well and there is no recurrent or metastatic carcinoma 16 years later.

Comment. This is a remarkable case of a highly malignant carcinoma of the cheek, which was treated by radiation, surgical excision and reconstruction, and regional infusion with carcinostatic drugs.

MALIGNANT TUMOURS IN THE PHARYNX

The surgical treatment of malignant tumours in different parts of the pharynx presents many difficulties. Patients are usually seen when the disease is well established or advanced, with metastases in the regional lymph nodes. They are often referred for surgical operation after a full course of radiotherapy, which frequently causes degenerative changes in the skin of the neck and consequent surgical difficulties. In addition, such tumours are relatively inaccessible, so the surgeon has many technical problems to overcome. For many patients with pharyngeal malignant tumours the prognosis is grave and they have to endure much suffering.

The following section contains case-records of patients treated by the present author for malignant diseases of the pharynx which are of particular interest. The patients concerned enjoyed a life of good quality for many years after surgical treatment.

Malignant tumours of the oropharynx

These tumours are usually treated initially by radiotherapy, so case-records such as the following, where patients were treated surgically, are somewhat rare.

Case-record 1

A female, 44 years old, was referred with a malignant tumour which was situated in the retropharyngeal tissues and projected forward into the posterior wall of the left side of the oropharynx, with a superficial ulcer on the site of a previous biopsy. The tumour measured 3 × 2 cm and extended

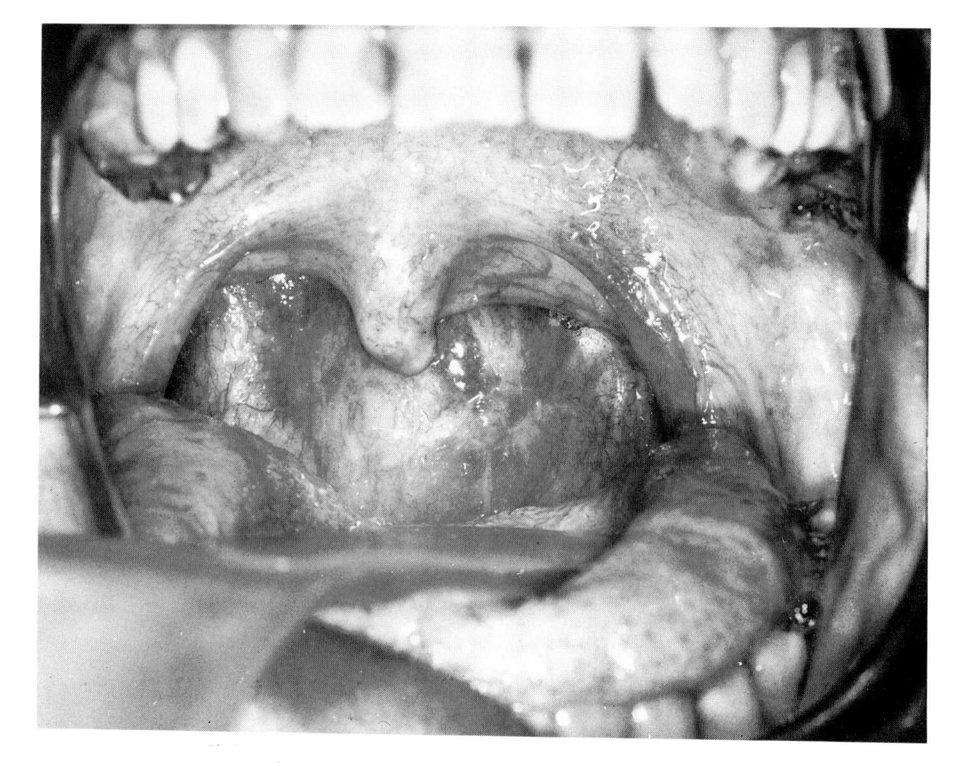

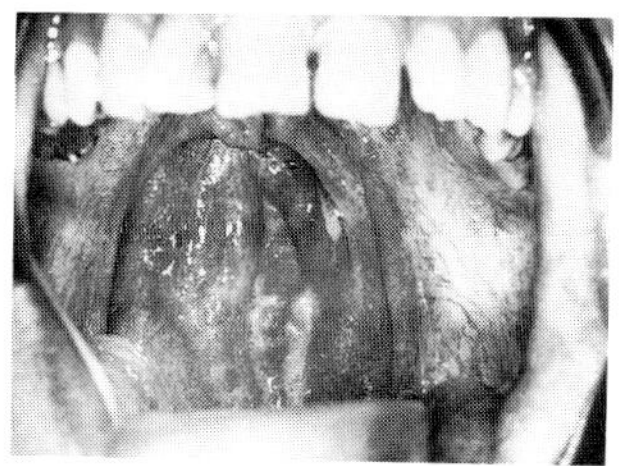

Figure 14.10 *Left:* Fibrosarcoma of the retropharyngeal tissues of the oropharynx of a 44-year-old female (case-record 1) . *Above:* The oropharynx after transbuccal excision of the fibrosarcoma. There is perfect healing of the posterior pharyngeal wall.

upwards into the nasopharynx. There were no enlarged cervical lymph nodes.

Careful consideration was given to the question of what would be the best surgical route of access to excise this tumour and it was decided to use the transbuccal approach. At operation the posterior wall of the oropharynx over the tumour was incised longitudinally and the flaps reflected to expose the tumour. This was then dissected off the anterior common ligament of the cervical vertebrae and removed. The posterior pharyngeal wall was sutured and a temporary tracheostomy was instituted. The patient made a good recovery from the operation and the tracheostomy closed spontaneously.

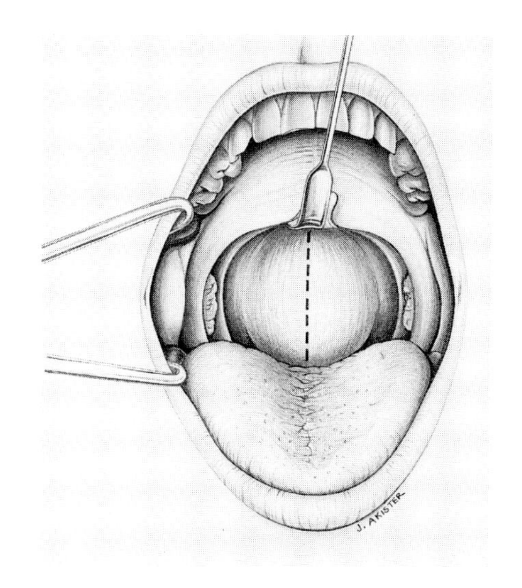

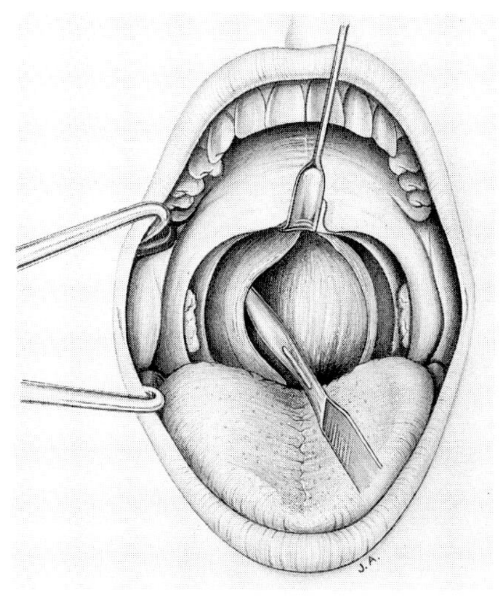

Figure 14.11 The transbuccal operation for excision of a fibrosarcoma. *Left:* The soft palate is retracted upwards and a longitudinal incision (dotted line) is made over the tumour. *Right:* The posterior wall of the oropharynx is reflected off the tumour.

(continued overleaf)

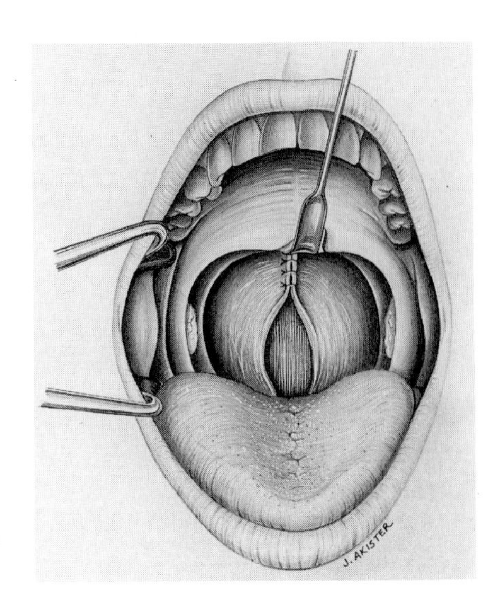

Figure 14.11 *(continued)*
Left: The fibrosarcoma is removed from its bed, which includes the anterior common ligament of the cervical vertebrae. *Right:* The incision in the posterior wall of the oropharynx is sutured with interrupted sutures of catgut and a temporary tracheostomy is formed.

A postoperative course of radiotherapy was given to the primary tumour site and the upper deep cervical lymph nodes.

Histopathology showed fibrosarcoma.

Survival period. The patient is well 26 years after the operation and there is no recurrent or metastatic disease.

Case-record 2

A male, 61 years old, was referred with an extensive malignant tumour involving the left tonsil, anterior and posterior faucial pillars, the adjacent soft palate and the base of the tongue. The left upper deep cervical lymph nodes were enlarged. The surgical operation performed to remove this tumour was a partial palato-glosso-pharyngectomy combined with a left radical dissection of the cervical lymph nodes. The defect in the oropharynx was repaired immediately with an inner mucous membrane lining and

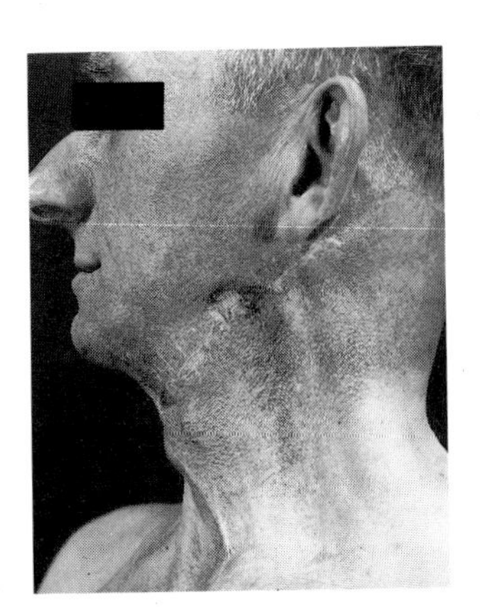

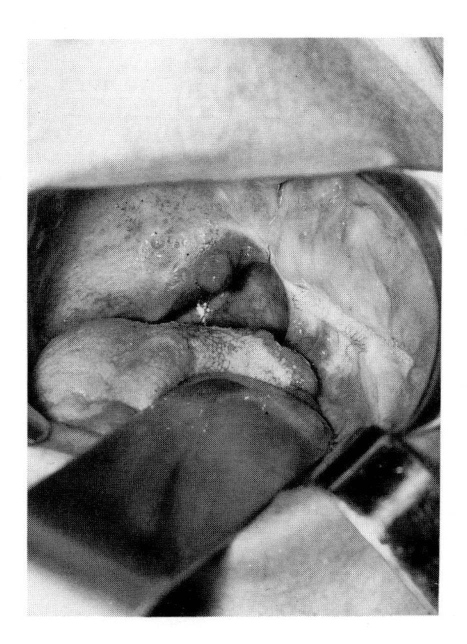

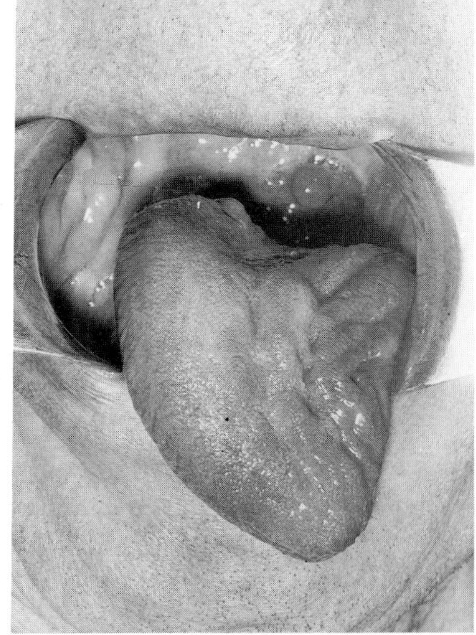

Figure 14.12 *Above:* A male patient (case-record 2) after a partial palato-glosso-pharyngectomy and left radical neck dissection for extensive carcinoma of the oropharynx. *Bottom left:* His healed left oropharynx. *Bottom right:* His functional tongue.

outer skin cover. A temporary tracheostomy was instituted. The patient made a good recovery and the tracheostomy closed spontaneously.

Histopathology revealed a squamous cell carcinoma of the oropharynx with metastases in the cervical lymph nodes.

Survival period. The patient survived for 10 years without recurrent or metastatic disease.

CARCINOMA OF THE HYPOPHARYNX AND CERVICAL OESOPHAGUS

The present author has had wide experience in the surgical treatment of carcinoma of the hypopharynx and cervical oesophagus, extending over many years. The end-results of surgical treatment and the long survival periods of the patients, who enjoyed a life of good quality, must be judged against this background.

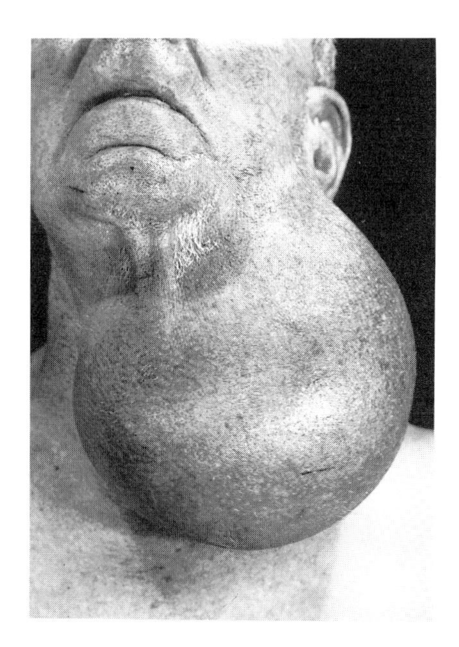

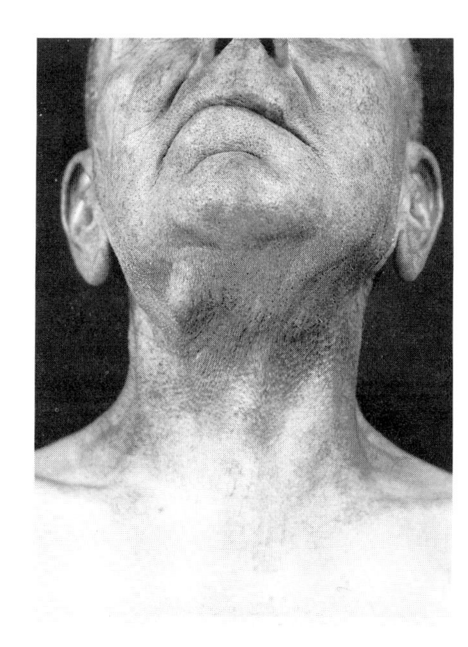

Figure 14.13 *Left:* A male patient with an enormous lipoma in the left side of his neck. *Right:* The patient after excision of the lipoma.

In a large series of cases, the majority of the patients had advanced carcinoma of the hypopharynx which had frequently infiltrated into the cervical oesophagus, larynx, trachea and thyroid gland. In 47% of the patients there were histologically proved carcinoma metastases in the cervical lymph nodes. The patients suffered severely from dysphagia, dyspnoea and stridor.

In some cases a palliative gastrostomy or tracheostomy had already been instituted in other clinics to provide relief. Some of the patients had been pronounced untreatable and were awaiting death with the aid of sedatives. Others had undergone a course of radiotherapy of the maximum tumour dosage, but this had failed to control the disease and the severe radiation effects in the skin and other tissues in the neck caused additional problems for surgical treatment.

In these difficult and serious situations the surgeon was greatly helped and encouraged by the splendid courage of the patients, with their strong will to fight for life and their desire, strongly expressed, that something be done to enable them to live.

Radical surgical treatment to extirpate an extensive carcinoma in this situation involved removal of the hypopharynx, larynx and cervical oesophagus, combined with a radical dissection of the cervical lymph nodes when metastases were present. Normal deglutition was restored by reconstruction of the hypopharynx and cervical oesophagus with a whole-thickness skin tube. A permanent tracheostomy was instituted, which gave complete relief from the respiratory difficulties.

The following case-records are cited to show the long survival periods of these patients, who enjoyed a life of good quality.

Case-record 1

An elderly female was referred with an extensive carcinoma of the hypopharynx and cervical oesophagus, which caused severe dysphagia. Another surgeon had already performed a gastrostomy. The present author carried out a two-stage operation, consisting of a laryngo-oesophago-pharyngectomy and reconstruction of the hypopharynx and cervical oesophagus with whole-thickness skin flaps. Normal deglutition was restored, and a permanent tracheostomy was instituted. The gastrostomy was allowed to close spontaneously.

Histopathology revealed a sqamous cell carcinoma, 7.5 cm wide, which extended from the cervical oesophagus to the arytenoid cartilages.

Survival period. The patient was alive 7 years and 7 months after the operation. Deglutition was normal and there was no recurrent or metastatic disease.

Case-record 2

An elderly female was referred with a carcinoma of the hypopharynx and cervical oesophagus which extended to the arytenoid cartilages. A laryngo-oesophago-pharyngectomy was performed as a two-stage operation, with reconstruction of the hypopharynx and cervical oesophagus with whole-thickness skin flaps. A permanent tracheostomy was instituted and normal deglutition was restored.

Histopathology showed the tumour to be a sqamous cell carcinoma.

Survival period. The patient was alive 7 years after the operation and there was no recurrent or metastatic disease.

Case-record 3

An elderly female was referred with an extensive carcinoma of the hypopharynx and cervical oesophagus, which caused considerable dysphagia. A laryngo-oesophago-pharyngectomy was performed as a 2-stage operation, with reconstruction of the hypopharynx and cervical oesophagus with whole-thickness skin flaps. A permanent tracheostomy was instituted and normal deglutition was restored.

Histopathology showed the tumour to be a squamous cell carcinoma.

Survival period. The patient was alive 22 years after the operation and there was no recurrent or metastatic disease.

Surgery following radiotherapy

The present author has successfully carried out surgical treatment for patients with an advanced carcinoma of the hypopharynx and cervical oesophagus after a complete course of radiotherapy of full tumour dosage had failed to control it. In addition, severe radiation changes had been caused in the skin and soft tissues of the neck and these made it considerably more difficult to carry out a radical operation, so several stages were necessary to reconstruct a new hypopharynx and cervical oesophagus with whole-thickness skin flaps in order to restore normal deglutition. Nevertheless, the following case-records show that, in spite of these difficult problems, surgical treatment can provide good results, giving patients complete relief from dyspnoea and dysphagia and enabling them to enjoy a life of good quality for many years.

Case-record 1

A male patient was referred with an extensive carcinoma of the hypopharynx which had been treated with a complete course of radiotherapy of full tumour dosage. This had failed to control the carcinoma and had caused severe radiation changes in the skin of the neck. A surgical operation was therefore specially designed for this condition. A pharyngo-laryngectomy was performed, leaving a temporary pharyngostome and a permanent tracheostomy. Later the pharyngostome was closed, using a tubed pedicle acromio-pectoral skin graft which provided both an inner skin lining and an outer skin cover, thereby restoring normal deglutition.

Histopathology showed the tumour to be a squamous cell carcinoma.

Survival period. The patient was alive 7½ years after the operation and there was no recurrent or metastatic disease.

Case-record 2

A male patient was referred with an extensive carcinoma of the hypopharynx which had been treated with a complete course of radiotherapy of full tumour dosage but had not been controlled. The patient had developed severe dyspnoea requiring an emergency tracheostomy. This had been carried out by another surgeon. There were very severe radiation changes in the skin of the neck, and extensive dermatitis was evident in the skin of the neck and the upper anterior chest wall. The patient's general condition was most serious, so careful study and care were required to build this up and to design the surgical technique of the operation necessary to restore him to health.

A multiple-stage operation was performed, which included a laryngo-oesophago-pharyngectomy and the reconstruction of a new hypopharynx and cervical oesophagus in stages, using two acromio-pectoral tubed pedicle skin grafts, which restored normal deglutition. A permanent tracheostomy was instituted.

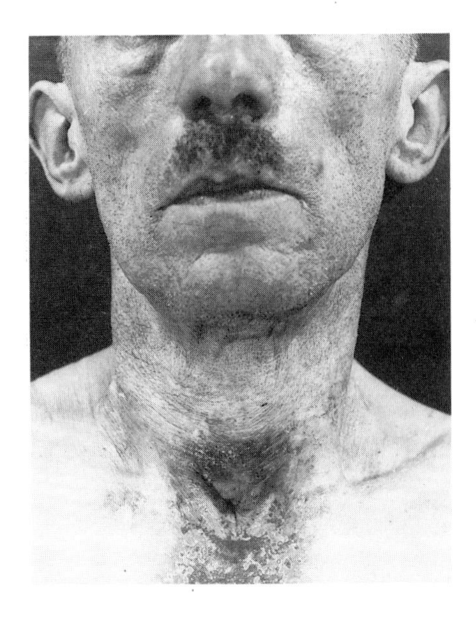

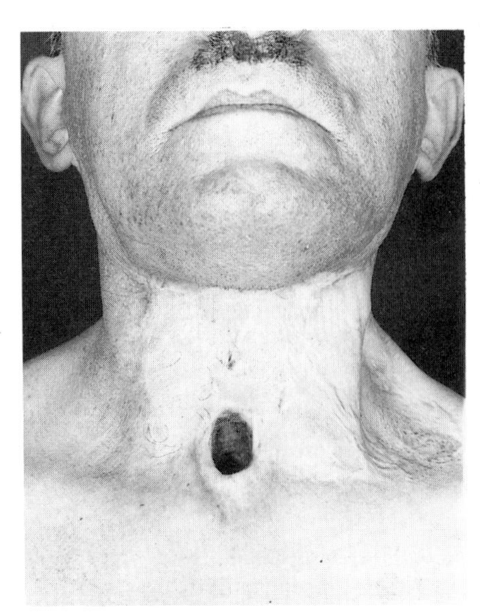

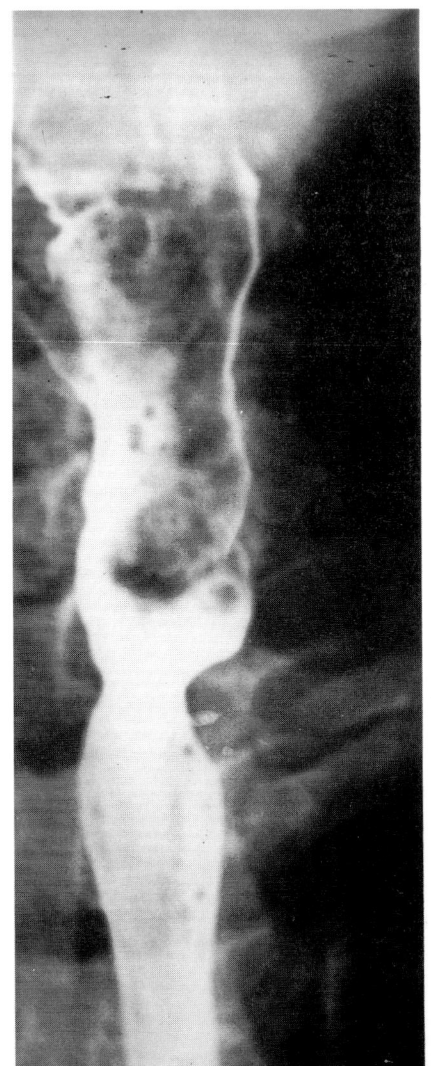

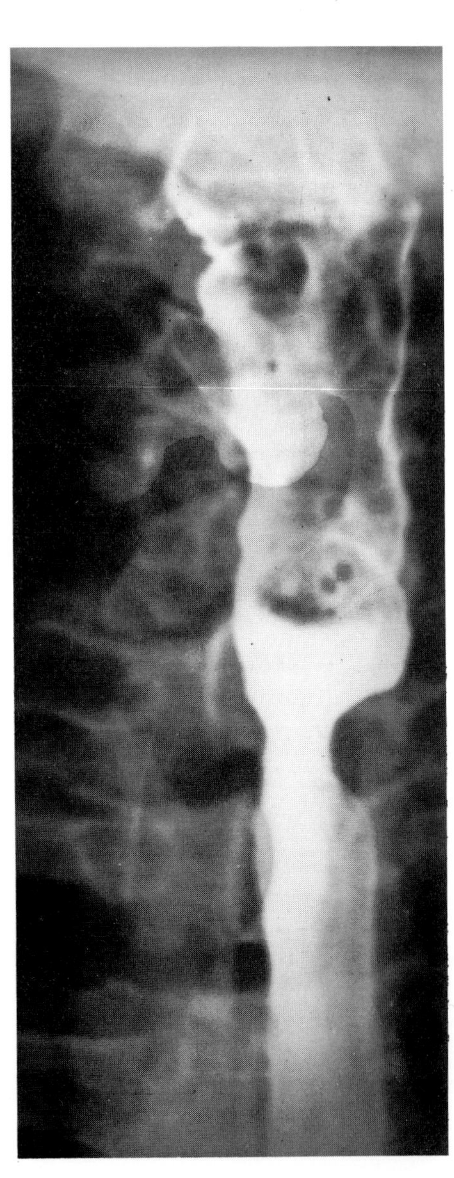

Figure 14.14 *Top Left:* A male patient (case-record 2) with an extensive carcinoma of the hypopharynx uncontrolled by a full tumour dose of radiotherapy which caused severe radiation changes in the skin of his neck. *Top right:* The patient after laryngo-oesophago-pharyngectomy, excision of regional cervical nodes and reconstruction of the hypopharynx and cervical oesophagus. *Bottom:* Radiograph with a barium swallow showing the skin hypopharynx and its junction with the oesophagus.

Histopathology showed the tumour to be an anaplastic ulcerating carcinoma occupying the right pyriform fossa. It extended into the larynx and involved the true and false vocal cords. Metastases were present in the regional cervical lymph nodes.

Survival period. The patient returned to his work as an architect and had no recurrent carcinoma in his neck. He died from a primary bronchogenic carcinoma 12½ years after the operation.

CARCINOMA OF THE OESOPHAGUS

Carcinoma of the oesophagus is a serious disease with a poor prognosis, especially when the tumour is situated in the upper and middle thirds of the thoracic oesophagus. Many patients apply for treatment when the tumour is well established and inoperable. In this case radiotherapy is instituted and can cause regression of the carcinoma for a period. The present author has found that when patients have dysphagia for 6 or more months and the X-ray filling defect shown by swallowing barium is longer than 7.5 cm the carcinoma is usually inoperable. A history lasting 3–6 months and a shorter filling defect indicate doubtful operability, but a thoracotomy should be done. A short history and a short filling defect usually mean that a tumour is operable.

The following case-records of patients with a squamous carcinoma situated in the middle third of the oesophagus who were treated surgically by the present author and who lived for many years after their operation are of interest and give encouragement in a difficult clinical situation.

The operation carried out consisted of a preliminary laparotomy to mobilise the stomach, the right gastric and right gastro-epiploic arteries being conserved, and a pyloroplasty. The abdomen was then closed. A right thoracotomy was next performed for a partial oesophago-gastrectomy and a high intrathoracic oesophago-gastric anastomosis was done.

Case-record 1

A male, aged 53, was referred with a squamous cell carcinoma, 7.5 cm long, in the middle third of the oesophagus. Its upper border was 30 cm from the incisor teeth. A partial oesophago-gastrectomy with an intrathoracic oesophago-gastric anastomosis was performed.

Histopathology showed that the tumour was a well-differentiated squamous cell carcinoma which was invading the oesophageal muscle. It was cleared above and below the resection. A para-oesophageal lymph node showed a metastatic carcinoma; the coeliac axis lymph node showed sinus catarrh only.

Survival period. The patient lived for 29 years after the operation and had normal deglutition. There was no recurrent or metastatic carcinoma.

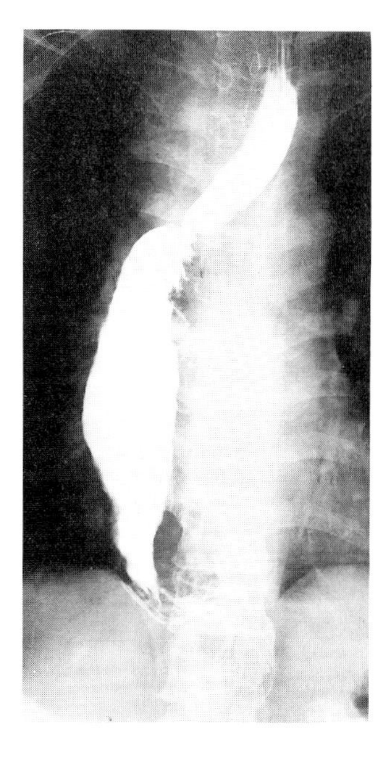

Figure 14.15 Radiograph of a male patient (case-record 1) showing the high oesophago-gastric anastomosis, with the stomach transposed into the right side of the chest.

Case-record 2

A male, aged 69, was referred with a squamous cell carcinoma situated at the junction of the middle and lower thirds of the oesophagus, with its

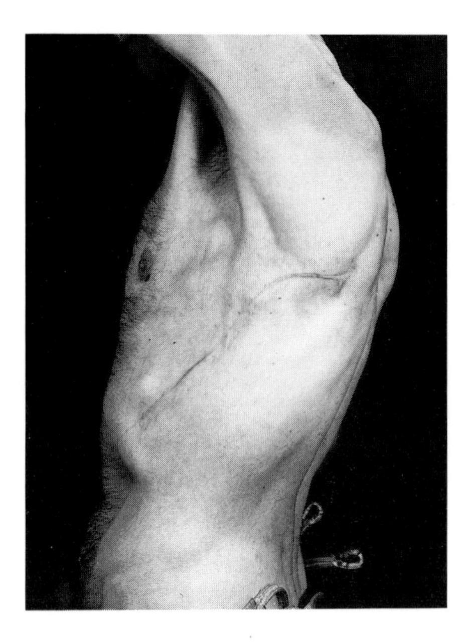

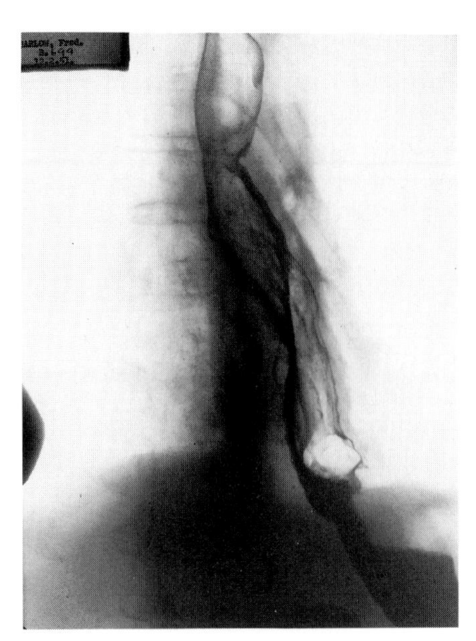

Figure 14.16 *Left:* A male patient (case-record 2) with a healed left thoracotomy incision made for a partial oesophago-gastrectomy with an intrathoracic oesophago-gastric anastomosis. *Right:* A radiograph with a barium swallow taken 3 years after the patient's operation. Gas is seen in the thoracic portion of the stomach on the left side.

upper border 33 cm from the incisor teeth. A partial oesophago-gastrectomy with an intrathoracic oesophago-gastric anastomosis was performed.

Histopathology showed that the tumour was a cornifying, but rapidly growing, squamous cell carcinoma which was invading all the coats of the oesophagus. It was 5 cm long and nearly encircled the lumen of the oesophagus. There was extension of infection into the peri-oesophageal tissues, with the formation of small abscesses accompanied by foreign-body giant cells and eosinophils.

Survival period. The patient lived for 10½ years, with normal deglutition. There was no recurrent or metastatic carcinoma.

Long survival after radical surgical treatment for carcinoma of the oesophagus, as shown in these case-records, is unusual. It is an unfortunate fact that many patients die within the first 2 years after their operation. Emphasis must be placed on the importance of early diagnosis before dysphagia occurs, when the patient notices the slightest abnormality in swallowing and an endoscopy is performed.

CARCINOMA OF THE THYROID GLAND

Carcinoma of the thyroid gland, accompanied by lymph node metastases, can occur in children, as shown in the following case-records where the patients survived many years after surgical treatment, with no recurrent or metastatic carcinoma.

Case-record 1

A female, 15 years old, was referred with an enlarged thyroid gland, the right lobe being much larger than the left, and marked enlargement of the isthmus. Enlarged hard lymph nodes were present on both sides of the neck but were larger on the right side. A chest X-ray showed evidence of large numbers of very small metastases throughout both lungs. At the age of 5 the patient had developed a swelling in the neck, which caused dysphagia and gradually increased in size. The present author performed a total thyroidectomy with a right radical neck dissection. The tumour was adherent to the larynx, trachea and both recurrent laryngeal nerves, from which it was dissected; however, a small portion of tumour was left attached to the right recurrent laryngeal nerve. A temporary tracheostomy was instituted because of the risk of laryngeal oedema. Postoperative radiotherapy and radioactive iodine and thyroxine replacement therapy were given. Four months later a left supraclavicular node was excised.

Histopathology showed a thyroid carcinoma of follicular type with colloid formation and involvement of the tracheal wall and right recurrent laryngeal nerve. The right cervical lymph nodes were invaded by a similar tumour. The left supraclavicular node which was removed later contained similar metastases.

Survival period. The patient is well and there is no sign of recurrent or metastatic carcinoma 13 years later. After her surgical treatment the patient gave birth to three healthy children, now aged 6, 5 and 1½ years, respectively.

Case-record 2

A female, aged 7, was referred with an enlarged thyroid gland and bilateral cervical enlarged lymph nodes which had been noticed 6 months earlier. Another surgeon saw the patient 2 months after their appearance and found enlarged tonsils, which he removed; 3¼ months later he performed a biopsy of a left cervical lymph node. Histopathology showed a metastatic papillary carcinoma of the thyroid gland. Clinical examination showed a hard swelling of the left lobe and isthmus of the thyroid gland and palpable bilateral cervical lymph nodes.

The present author performed a total thyroidectomy and a left radical neck dissection; no abnormality was found in the right side of the neck. The left recurrent laryngeal nerve was separated from the malignant tumour around it and marked for postoperative radiotherapy with a metal clip. A temporary tracheostomy was performed.

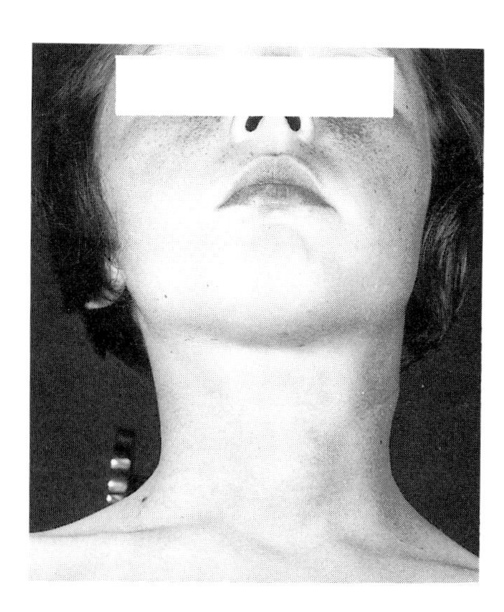

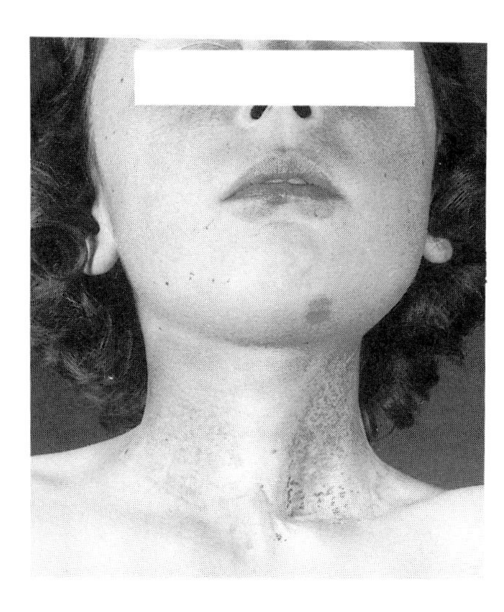

Figure 14.17 *Left:* A female patient (case-record 2) with an adenocarcinoma of the thyroid gland and metastases in the left cervical and prelaryngeal lymph nodes. *Right:* The patient after total thyroidectomy and left radical neck dissection.

Histopathology showed that the thyroid isthmus and left lobe had been replaced by a carcinoma; the bulk of the tumour consisted of a well-differentiated adenocarcinoma. There was progressive loss of differentiation in some areas to sheets of simple polygonal cells with no acinar arrangement or colloid secretion. Metastases were present in the middle deep cervical and prelaryngeal lymph nodes, but the highest and lowest were free of tumour.

Postoperative radiotherapy to a dosage of 4500 rads was given to the neck. The patient made an excellent recovery.

Survival period. The patient has developed normally and is well, with no recurrent or metastatic thyroid carcinoma 29 years after surgical treatment. She is married and has two normal children.

The case-records of individual patients reported in this chapter illustrate that surgical treatment even for the most dangerous malignant tumours can give long survival periods lasting many years, without recurrent or metastatic disease developing. This chapter could be entitled "Encouragement in cancer surgery".

CHAPTER FIFTEEN

Radiation and Cancer

The whole subject of radiation is of profound importance in oncology and the development of our knowledge is closely linked with the evolution of oncology. This is exemplified by the statement that radiation can both cause and cure cancer; hence its relevance to prevention and treatment.

This chapter is therefore divided into two main divisions, namely, radiation as a cause of cancer and radiation in the treatment of cancer.

RADIATION AS THE CAUSE OF CANCER

Radiation of the ionising and non-ionising varieties can cause different types of cancer in various organs and tissues of the body. Consequently the carcinogenic action of different radiations is the object of considerable study and research, which have already resulted in the institution of protection measures against radiation and in cancer prevention programmes for the population as a whole and for all workers who are exposed to radiation in their different employments.

Radiation carcinogenesis

The fact that non-ionising radiations can cause cancer is attracting considerable attention today because of the increasing incidence of various forms of cancer of the skin, including basal-cell carcinoma, and especially of malignant melanoma, which develops from overexposure to solar radiation. This serious tumour is often discovered in the skin of the head and neck and of the extremities, in addition to that of the trunk and other sites in the body.

There has been sustained interest in radiation carcinogenesis for about 100 years. According to Hueper *(1957)*, Unna, in 1894, was the first to associate chronic dermatitis with precancerous changes which occurred in workers in outdoor occupations who were exposed to solar radiation. In his very informative chapter on environmental factors in the production of human cancer, Hueper refers to the subsequent epidemiological studies which were carried out by many investigators in different countries of the world who confirmed the causal relationship between excessive exposure to sunlight and the development of cancer in the exposed skin. Cancer occurs in many workers who have outdoor occupations and also in people who indulge in sunbathing and overexpose their skin to the sun. People who live at high altitudes or in countries with a dry, sunny climate are also at risk. Hueper stated that individuals with a fair complexion are more susceptible to solar cancer than brunettes or members of the coloured races.

He also called attention to the potential risk of skin cancer developing as a result of the medicinal use of ultraviolet radiation for various non-cancerous conditions. He stated that the latent period for the development of ultraviolet radiation cancer is 15–40 years.

Developments in knowledge

The carcinogenic effects of radiation were discussed by Glucksmann, Lamerton and Mayneord *(1957)* in their most helpful contribution which includes a review of the literature on this subject.

These authors stated that the first case of cancer caused by X-radiation was described by Frieben in Hamburg in 1902. The victim was a male, aged 33, who had been employed in the manufacture of X-ray tubes and who had tested the apparatus with his hand. As a consequence of this exposure marked radiation dermatitis developed in the skin of the dorsum of his hand and small persistent ulcers occurred after 3 years. The edges of the ulcers became cancerous and eventually the skin on the dorsum of his hand was completely ulcerated. Metastases were present in the cubital and axillary lymph nodes. This extensive carcinoma necessitated amputation of the upper extremity through the shoulder joint.

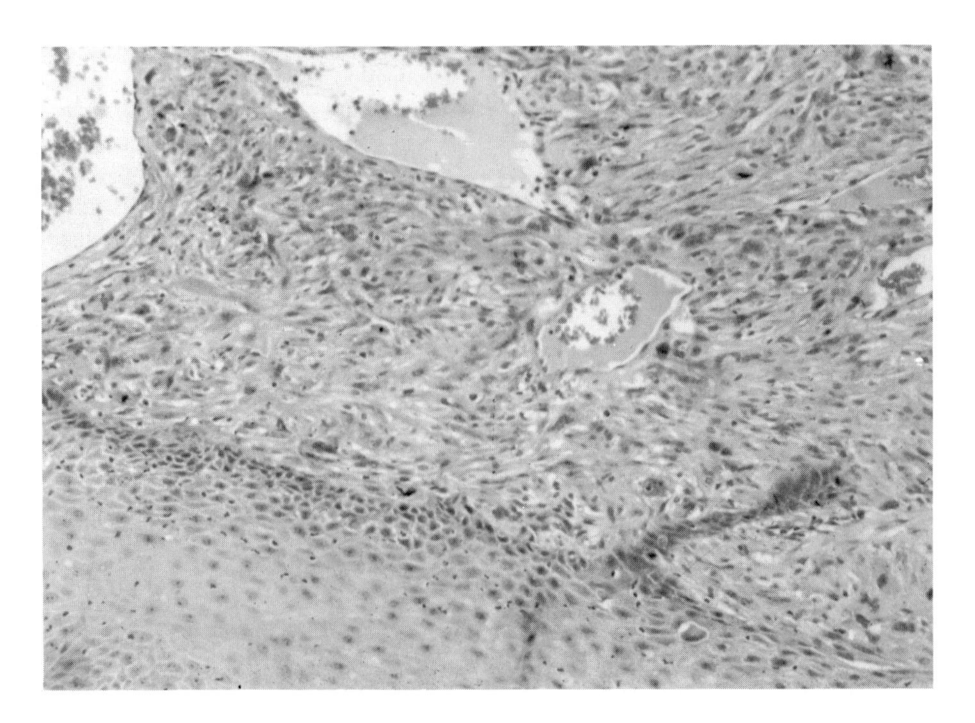

Figure 15.1 Radiation-induced carcinoma of the skin.

Glucksmann and his colleagues also quoted Hesse, who in 1911 reported 50 cases of cancer developing in previously normal skin in workers who were exposed to radiation in their employment and in four patients who had undergone radiation treatment.

The present author for several years treated a patient with squamous carcinomas of the skin of the hands. This patient had worked in radiodiagnosis during the early period of its development before radioprotection was introduced. The skin of the hands showed severe radiation changes and squamous cell carcinomas developed in several areas (Figure 15.2).

Other radiation cancers

Radiation-induced cancers have been described which affect different organs and tissues of the human body. A brief reference is made here to certain observations which are of historical interest and importance.

Lung cancer in uranium miners

From the 16th century onwards there have been reports of specific illness occurring in miners working in Schneeberg, now in East Germany, and in Joachimsthal, now in Czechoslovakia. It was recognised at the end of the 18th century in Schneeberg, and later in Joachimsthal, that many of these workers were dying from a malignant disease of the lungs. During their work the miners were exposed to a considerable amount of dust, which possibly contained traces of arsenic, cobalt and other metals, and it was thought that the inhaled dust caused lung cancer to develop. Later it was observed that a high level of radioactivity was present in the air in the mines and this was considered to be a possible cause of the lung cancer.

Glucksmann and his colleagues *(1957)* pointed out that radiation might not have been the whole cause of the cancer, for the miners inhaled dust

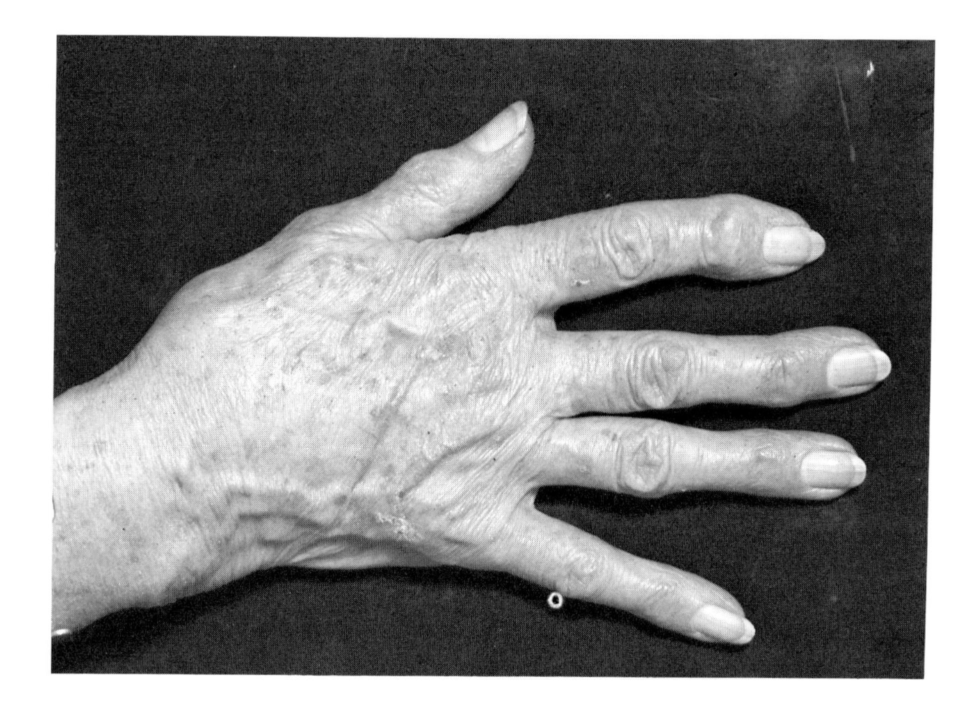

Figure 15.2 Radiation-induced squamous cell carcinomas in the hand of a patient who had worked in radiodiagnosis without any radioprotection.

containing traces of arsenic, cobalt and other metals which might have contained a carcinogenic or co-carcinogenic substance. Silicosis and tuberculosis of the lungs also occurred in the miners, and these diseases might have enhanced the carcinogenic action of radiation.

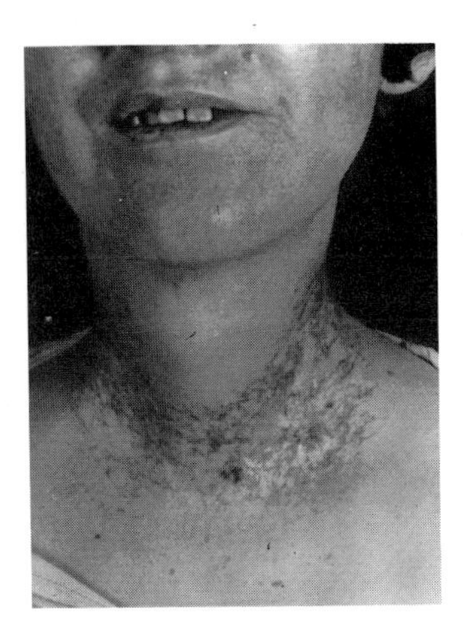

Figure 15.3 Radiation changes in the skin of the neck of a patient treated with large doses of radiotherapy 23 years previously. This patient developed carcinoma of the hypopharynx.

Radiation cancer of the hypopharynx

There are a number of reports in the literature about patients who have developed a carcinoma in the hypopharynx many years after having radiotherapy for a benign lesion in the neck *(Raven, 1958)*.

The subject was reviewed by Goolden *(1951)*, who cited nine patients who developed a carcinoma in the hypopharynx after having radiotherapy for thyrotoxicosis (five patients), goitre (one patient), and tuberculous cervical adenitis (three patients). The interval which elapsed between the radiation and the development of the carcinoma ranged from 18 to 30 years, the average being 25.2 years. No information is available about the dosage of radiation given, but as severe changes resulted in the skin of the neck it is assumed that large doses were used.

A case-record was reported by Raven and Levison *(1954)* of a female, aged 46, who had an inoperable extensive carcinoma of the hypopharynx. She had been treated with radiotherapy for thyrotoxicosis 23 years previously and these authors calculated that the dosage given must have been 8000 rads ± 10%, which means that 10 000 rads ± 10% would have been given to the hypopharynx. There were severe radiation changes in the skin of the neck which had been irradiated, and a wide band of telangiectasis in the skin covering the anterolateral area of the neck (Figure 15.3).

Holinger and Rabbett *(1953)* reported three patients who developed a malignant tumour in the hypopharynx after having radiotherapy for cervical tuberculous adenitis. In two patients it was a squamous cell carcinoma and in the third a fibrosarcoma. The tumours developed in irradiated areas at intervals of 32, 30 and 27 years after radiotherapy.

Ombrédanne, Poncet and Gandon *(1954)* reported the case-record of a 33-year-old male patient who developed an extensive carcinoma of the hypopharynx and larynx as a result of radiotherapy for a goitre 20 years earlier.

It is pointed out that these patients who developed radiation cancer in the hypopharynx were treated with radiotherapy for a benign condition many years ago when there were no accurate dosage measurements or any recognised unit of dosage. Benign lesions such as goitre, thyrotoxicosis and tuberculous adenitis are no longer treated with radiation techniques.

Radiation cancer of bone

Radiation treatment of benign osseous lesions can result in tumours in various bones. Thus bone tumours have been described in patients who have had radiotherapy for bone and joint tuberculosis, osteomyelitis, and chronic arthritis. In his review of the contribution of environmental factors to human cancer Hueper *(1957)* pointed out that osteogenic sarcomas might be caused by the action of hard X-rays penetrating the bone structures from the skin surface or they might result from the ingestion of radium or mesothorium, which is then stored in bones in a similar way to calcium.

The late effects of the early medical and industrial use of radioactive materials were studied in detail by Looney *(1955, 1956)*, who stated that he had concentrated primarily on individuals who had received radium for medical purposes and individuals who had been employed in the luminous-dial-painting industry. Radium salts had been given orally and intravenously for conditions such as hypertension, arthritis and anaemia from about 1915 to 1930. The painting of watch dials with luminous material containing radium, mesothorium and radioactive thorium had started in the USA in about 1915, but no adequate safety measures had been taken until about 1925–1927, when some of the workers died from bone tumours, crippling bone lesions and anaemia. Looney stated that bone tumours and skeletal changes have occurred 15–30 years after the administration or ingestion of radioactive materials. He pointed out that it is known that radium and plutonium are deposited primarily in bone, and that thorium is deposited in the liver, spleen and bone marrow. He discussed the clinical aspects of the problem in some detail and stated that any patient of middle- or old-age with significant skeletal changes, dental changes or skeletal tumours should be questioned about any previous radium administration or previous employment as a luminous-dial worker.

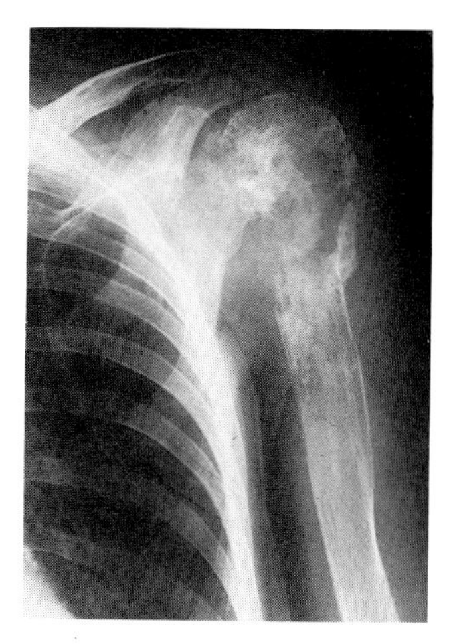

Figure 15.4 A radiation osteosarcoma in the upper end of a humerus.

Leukaemia

It was known many years ago that higher than expected rates of leukaemia occurred amongst radiation workers. The radiation dosages they received are not known, as records were not kept accurately at that time.

The distressing condition of ankylosing spondylitis was treated with radiotherapy several decades ago and it was found that a high incidence of leukaemia occurred in these patients.

A considerable amount of data concerning radiation-induced leukaemia has accumulated since the atomic bombing of Hiroshima and Nagasaki. The leukaemia induced in these areas was mainly of the myeloid variety and, as would be expected, the incidence of the disease was much greater amongst the survivors near the centre of the explosion than amongst those who were farther away.

Pochin *(1970)* stated that an excess incidence of leukaemia, and possibly of other malignant diseases, has been observed in children who have been exposed to only a few rads *in utero* in the course of diagnostic X-ray investigations of their mothers; this incidence seems likely to be attributable to the exposure received.

Protection from radiation

The lack of protection for individuals, nations and the whole of mankind from the effects of radiation, and today especially from the lethal effects of the explosion of atomic bombs and major and minor leakages of radioactive materials from nuclear plants, is a matter of great concern and anxiety on an international scale.

Reference is made here to the early work on radiation protection and the safeguards which were then introduced. This subject was considered in detail by Osborn *(1959)*. Soon after the discovery of X-rays and radium it was found that they had harmful biological effects and unfortunately many of the early pioneers in this work died from radiation injuries. Osborn quoted Spear, who stated that a monument commemorating 170 such workers was unveiled in Hamburg on 4 August 1936 and that in 1938 27 more names were added. In 1956 steps were taken to bring the list up to date.

In tracing the development of radiation protection, Osborn stated that the British X-ray and Radium Protection Committee was formed shortly after World War I and that their first report was published in July 1921. Other countries formed similar committees soon afterwards. The International Committee on Radiological Protection presented its first report to the International Congress of Radiology in Stockholm in 1928. New knowledge was quickly acquired, necessitating frequent revisions of their recommendations.

It is interesting that the protection of whole populations against the hazards of exposure to ionising radiation was being carefully studied 30 years ago. Osborn stated that at the request of the government the Medical Research Council in 1956 published a report entitled "The hazards to man of nuclear and allied radiations". Similar reports were published in the USA and in India.

Hospital radiation protection services have been efficiently organised and detailed instructions have been issued regarding the protection of people working with all forms of radiation. The protection of patients undergoing radiotherapy, and the therapeutic dosages to be given, have been carefully considered and controlled. The general and local radiation reactions and effects and their treatment are now clearly understood.

There must be no complacency concerning the enormous lethal effects which can follow nuclear radiation pollution, including that of the atmosphere, the sea, the earth and our food. We cannot accept that there is any "completely safe" level of radiation contamination.

Diagnostic radiation

The possibility that even the small dosage of radiation given to the body by X-ray diagnostic procedures might cause cancer has attracted considerable attention. It is inadvisable for a pregnant woman to undergo an X-ray examination because of the risk of radiation injury to the developing foetus. Mayneord *(1967)* cited reports published in *U.N. Report 1964* which confirmed a higher incidence of malignant disease, including leukaemias, in children who received radiation in this way. He suggested that under certain conditions low doses of only a few rads of radiation can induce malignancy in the foetus. He also stated that irradiation should be avoided in small children, where it cannot be expected to substantially help in the medical care of the patient.

The role of ionising radiation in the causation of specific varieties of malignant disease is now well recognised and special interest — heightened since the introduction of mammography as a diagnostic procedure — has been focused on cancer of the breast. This subject was dealt with by Samuel *(1973)*, who called attention to the reported increase in breast cancer in the survivors of the atomic explosions in Japan some 20 years after the explosions had taken place, showing that the long-term effect of radiation should always be considered. He thought that, with our present state of knowledge, it would probably be advisable to confine repetitive mammography to females over the age of 50.

A very interesting contribution to the subject of breast cancer following radiation was made by Mackenzie *(1965)*, who gave details of 40 patients with this disease who for varying periods had received either unilateral or bilateral artificial pneumothorax therapy for pulmonary tuberculosis. The treatment was accompanied by fluoroscopy, which was usually carried out before and after each chest refill, the number of treatments varying with the length of time the treatment was given. Mackenzie stated that if irradiation played a part in the appearance of tumours, these would be more likely to occur in the inner half and central areas of the breast, since the X-ray beams would tend to be focused more over the medial aspect of the chest wall on the side of the pneumothorax. This supposition was borne out by the figures; over two-thirds of the tumours were in the inner half and central areas of the breast, in contradistinction to the usual distribution of cancer in the outer half of the breast. The time-interval between the institution of the pneumothorax and the onset of breast cancer in these cases varied from under 10 to over 20 years.

Mackenzie also quoted Smith *(1962)*, who called attention to the possible role of irradiation in patients with carcinoma of the rectum who had been treated with irradiation for carcinoma of the cervix uteri.

In conclusion, after these considerations of the risks of cancer developing as a consequence of exposure to ionisation radiation, it is reasonable to advise that caution be had in subjecting patients to diagnostic procedures where radiation is used. Thus pregnant women should be excluded from such investigations; so should young children, unless an X-ray examination is essential in their management. Radiological diagnostic examinations are necessary for adults, but their frequency should be carefully controlled.

RADIOTHERAPY IN CANCER

The radiation treatment of cancer is a major modality today; it is curative for many patients, and palliative for others with advanced disease. The history of its development is very interesting. The background was clearly described by Russ *(1959)*, who stated that the first reported successful radiation treatment of cancer was carried out in the USA in 1899 for a malignant tumour of the nose; the patient was still apparently disease-free in 1920. Russ then described subsequent developments, including the use of radiotherapy in Germany before 1914 and the Erlinger method used after World War I. In this method a large single dose of radiation was given, consequently many patients with breast carcinoma suffered severe damage to the skin and other healthy tissues. Russ also described the Paris technique based upon the research of Regaud, Nozier and Lacassagne *(1912)*, who developed the principles of preserving the patient's tissues in the radium treatment of uterine cancer by extending low dosage treatment over several days. About the same time Coutard treated a variety of malignant tumours with subdivided doses of X-rays spread over several weeks.

Russ then described the methods of radiotherapy used nearly 30 years ago. These included the use of a moderately high voltage of 200–250 kV, with filtered doses given at intervals over several days or weeks. Other

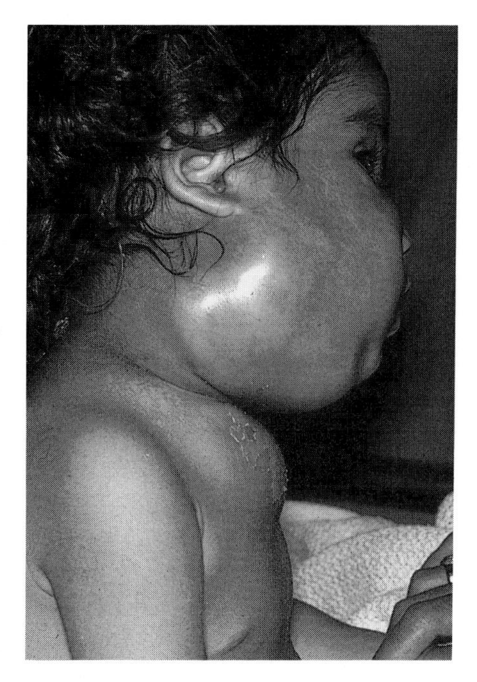
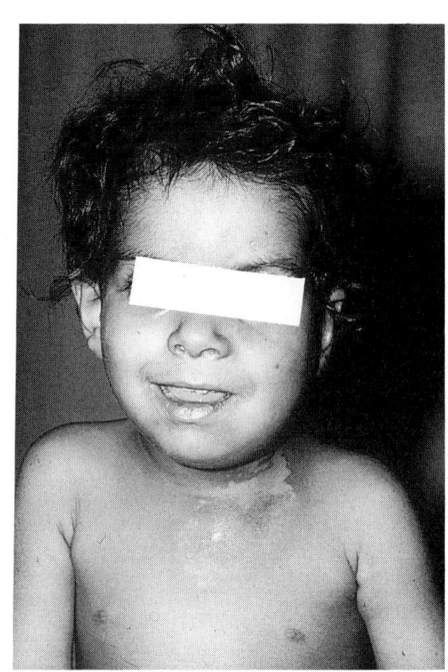

Figure 15.5 *Left:* A child with a massive lymphoma of the right cervico-facial region which was treated with radiotherapy. *Right:* The patient seen after radiotherapy had induced complete regression of the lymphoma.

methods included the use of a million or more voltages with X-rays, massive units of radium, cobalt or caesium, giving a greater percentage depth dose to deep-seated tumours; the use of a rotating tube or rotating table for the irradiation of deep-seated tumours, with minimal exposure of the superimposed tissues; and the Jolles method, where a sieve or grid was placed between the X-ray source and the body surface to lessen the reaction in normal tissues during and after treatment. Russ also called attention to the enhancement of the radiation action on the tumour that was achieved by giving the patient Synkavit, the treatment developed by Mitchell, and oxygen therapy to increase the oxygen tension in the tumour.

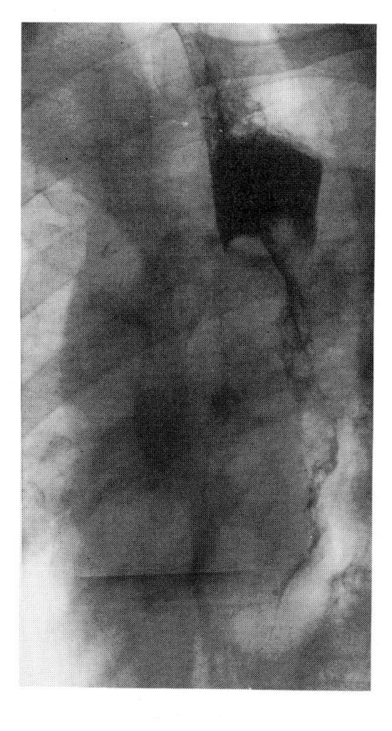
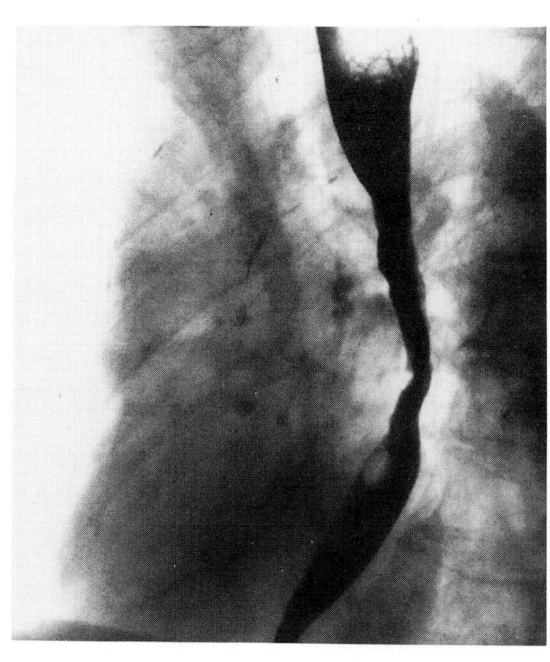

Figure 15.6 *Left:* Radiograph with a barium swallow of a male patient's oesophagus, showing an advanced carcinoma which caused him severe dysphagia. *Right:* 6 weeks after the completion of radiotherapy there was marked regression of the carcinoma and relief of the dysphagia.

The discovery of radium

A brief reference is made here to the historic discovery of radium by Pierre and Marie Curie, who on 22 April 1898 announced that pitchblende ores probably contained a hitherto unknown element with powerful radioactivity. This was the first stage of their important discovery (see the biography of Madame Curie by Eve Curie). The Curies had been greatly impressed by Henri Becquerel's discovery that, without exposure to light, uranium salts spontaneously emitted some rays of unknown nature. The nature of the radiation and its origin remained unknown until through their extensive research on radioactivity and radioactive substances they isolated two radioactive substances from pitchblende. The first they named polonium. On 26 December 1898 they announced the second radioactive substance, which they called radium.

Marie Curie was awarded the Nobel Prize in Physics and the Nobel Prize in Chemistry for her memorable scientific work and outstanding discoveries. She died at Sancellemoz on 4 July 1934. Her devoted husband, Pierre Curie, the scientific genius, had died on 19 April 1906 as the result of a tragic accident in Paris.

The introduction into the UK of the treatment of cancer by radium techniques is described later in this chapter.

Modern radiotherapy

Radiotherapy is a major method of treatment of cancer today, both alone and in combination with surgical and medical treatments. Impressive technical developments have occurred since the discovery of X-rays, and there are now a number of sophisticated methods from which to select the most suitable for cancer in specific organs and tissues.

Surgical and medical oncologists need some knowledge of radiation oncology in the practical management of cancer patients in order to establish meaningful collaboration with radiation oncologists.

The subject of radiotherapy was described in a very helpful way by Deeley *(1977)*, who dealt with the important aspects of the indications for radiotherapy; tumour types showing radiosensitivity or radioresistance; the tissue reactions to radiation and methods whereby they can be modified.

The radiotherapy equipment used for cancer treatment depends on the variety of the lesion. Thus very superficial malignant skin lesions can be treated with low-energy electrons from linear accelerators or radioactive strontium. More penetrating rays are produced by cobalt machines, which Deeley states are the mainstay of most radiotherapy departments. For deep-seated tumours linear accelerators in the range of 4–10 MV are used; and betatrons with energies of up to 35 MV are used to give high-power beams of electrons.

Fast-neutron therapy, which was made possible by the introduction of the cyclotron, has attracted considerable interest during recent decades. This subject was dealt with in some detail by Morgan *(1973)*, who stated that fast neutrons are arbitrarily defined as having energies greater than 10 KeV and that the principal problem in the production of these beams for radiotherapy is the generation of beams of sufficient intensity and energy to effectively penetrate tissues. Morgan concluded his review by stating there is good reason to believe that neutron therapy will be able to

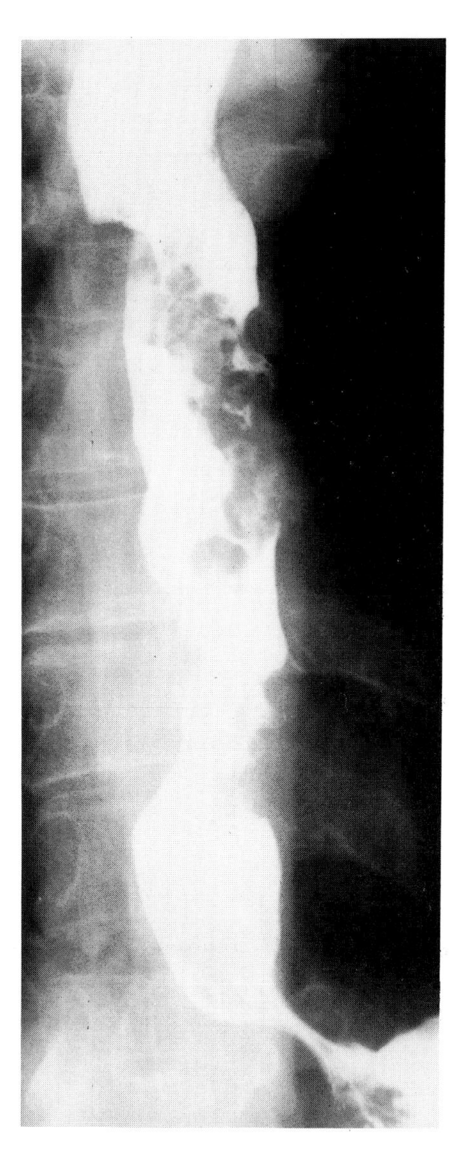

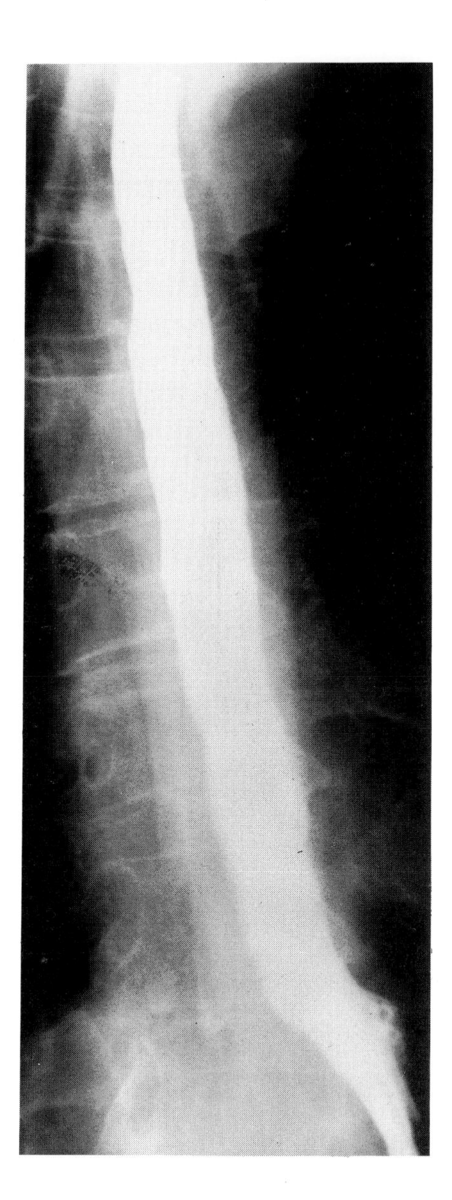

Figure 15.7 *Left:* Radiograph with a barium swallow of the oesophagus of a 54-year-old male patient, showing an extensive undifferentiated carcinoma extending from the level of the carina to the cardia.
Right: Radiograph of the same patient 56 days after completion of radiotherapy with a maximum tumour dose of 6392 rads, administered by a linear accelerator, and chemotherapy with intramuscular bleomycin. There is marked regression of the carcinoma.

achieve better tumour control, at least in certain sites, and that further clinical trials should be encouraged.

Tumour oxygenation

The subject of radiosensitivity and ways to increase it has attracted considerable attention and the classification of tumours as radiosensitive or radioresistant is of obvious great practical importance. It is recognised that from the histology viewpoint anaplastic tumours are usually more radiosensitive than well-differentiated tumours. The degree of oxygenation of the tissues is also important, for it is known that anoxic cells are relatively radioresistant; on the other hand, well-oxygenated cells are more responsive.

This subject was dealt with by Henk *(1973)*, who described methods to overcome the adverse effect of hypoxic tissues on radiotherapy results. He stated that fractionation of the radiotherapy treatment over a period offers the simplest and probably the most effective method of overcoming the oxygen effect. The most obvious method to counteract the radioresistance of hypoxic cells is to increase the oxygen inhaled by the patient. Henk called attention to the use of normobaric oxygen and hyperbaric oxygen techniques. The former method is simple; the patient breathes pure oxygen from a mask for about 15 minutes before each treatment and whilst the radiotherapy is given. The use of hyperbaric oxygen is time-consuming and the technique is more complex. Henk stated that controlled clinical trials were necessary and outlined many difficulties in their execution and in the assessment of the results obtained from various techniques of treatment.

Research, present and future

The development and growth of the treatment of cancer by radiation have been most impressive. This modality is a major form of therapy today and is likely to remain so in the future. Research in the science of radiobiology will continue to be carried out, especially by radiation oncologists, but also by other clinical oncologists. This subject is concerned with cell kinetics and the characterisation of normal and neoplastic cells, the cell cycle and cell division, cell loss and multiplication, and the method of cell repair.

Radiation physics is another important science of which radiation oncologists must have an in-depth knowledge, for it is concerned with the safe and effective radiotherapy of patients with cancer. This includes knowing the physics of ionising radiations and their interactions with cells, tissues and various other materials.

Computers have contributed greatly to all aspects of oncology, both research and clinical. In radiotherapy the complexity of the calculation of dosages of treatment has been simplified by using computer techniques, and the isodose distribution in various places can now be investigated.

The availability of artificial radioisotopes for the diagnosis and treatment

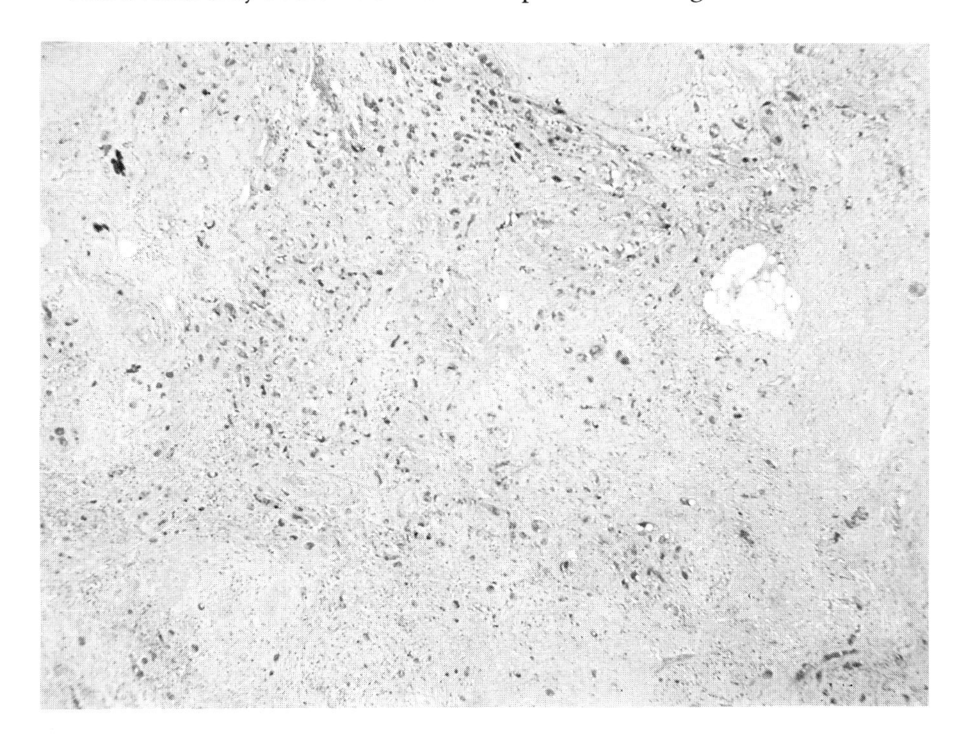

Figure 15.8 An irradiated carcinoma showing isolated tumour cells.

of several malignant tumours and for radiation research purposes suggested hopeful possibilities in radiation therapy, including the systemic treatment of tumours by their selective take-up capacity for certain isotopes. The clinical use of radioiodine in thyroid carcinoma is an important example. The subject of artificial radioisotopes in cancer was clearly described by Ellis *(1959)*, who gave a long list of references to the earlier literature.

THE TREATMENT OF CANCER BY RADIUM IN THE UK

The introduction into the UK in 1929 of the treatment of cancer by radium and its organisation were landmarks in oncology that were of outstanding importance and historic interest, so they are described here in some detail. The author has abstracted the relevant information from the *First Annual Report of the National Radium Trust and Radium Commission 1929–1930.* He can also claim a special knowledge of the subject, as he was Registrar of Statistics to the National Radium Commission during the years 1931–1934.

The National Radium Trust and the National Radium Commission were established by Royal Charter issued under Letters Patent of 25 July 1929. "The main functions of the Trust are to take charge of the funds which were raised by public subscription and voted by Parliament for the provision of radium, and to arrange for the purchase of radium therewith. The Committee have the duty of making arrangements for the proper custody, equitable distribution and full use of the radium purchased by the Trust." The Trust appointed the Right Hon. Viscount Lee of Fareham as Chairman of the Commission. The members of the Commission included G. E. Gask (Professor of Surgery at St Bartholomew's Hospital, London), who was well known to the present author and responsible for his appointment as Registrar of Statistics to the Commission. Another member was the well-known surgeon W. E. Miles.

Soon after their appointment the Trust considered what steps should be taken to begin the purchase of radium at the earliest practicable date with the funds at their disposal, which included £100 000 (at least) from *The Times* newspaper appeal (part of the thank-offering fund for the King's recovery from illness) and £100 000 voted by Parliament. In addition to problems regarding the price of the radium, its quality and the early delivery of the large quantity required, a particular problem concerned the filling of the radium in containers, because of the limited facilities for such work in the UK. An agreement was made with the Union Minière du Haut Katanga for the purchase of 10 g of radium at 50 USA dollars per mg, approximately £10¼ per mg.

The Union Minière also loaned to the Trust, free of charge, for a period of 3 months a "bomb" of approximately 4 g of radium, giving them the option to purchase it at the end of that period at the same cost. The option was subsequently exercised and the only other purchase made by the Trust at that time was that of the small quantity of 186.5 mg of Cornish radium from the British and General Radium Corporation Limited for £1920 and 19 shillings. The Radium Commission had recommended that a supply of radium be acquired for the preparation of radon emanation, so the Trust communicated with the Union Minière regarding the purchase of 3 g of radium for this purpose.

The *Report of the Radium Commission (31 August 1930)* detailed the duties of the Commission, which included making arrangements for the proper custody, equitable distribution and full use of the radium to promote the treatment of the sick throughout Great Britain and advance the knowledge of the best methods of treatment. The Scientific Secretary of the Commission was Sidney Russ (Professor of Physics at the Middlesex Hospital, London), with whom the present author subsequently worked in close collaboration. It was decided that a special programme of radium therapy suggested by the Commission should be carried out at the Westminster Hospital, London, using the 4 g radium "bomb".

National radium policy

The Commission decided to adopt a policy of concentrating the radium in centres possessing a university with a medical school and complete clinical courses and that only one hospital nominated by the medical faculty of the local university and approved by the Commission should be recognised as the national radium centre for the area concerned. In this way the Commission would retain control over the distribution and use of the radium committed to its charge.

National centres

The following national centres were selected for the geographical distribution of the radium: England (seven centres) — Birmingham, Bristol, Leeds, Liverpool, Manchester, Newcastle upon Tyne and Sheffield; Scotland (four centres) — Aberdeen, Dundee, Edinburgh and Glasgow; Wales (one centre) — Cardiff. London, which was to be a separate and special case, was to have a treatment centre with a national school of radiotherapy to serve the whole country.

In organising the national radium service the Commission established effective relationships with other important bodies who were interested in the medical uses of radium, namely, the Medical Research Council, King Edward's Hospital Fund for London and the British Empire Cancer Campaign. It also agreed to cooperate with the Cancer Commission of the League of Nations by recommending to all national centres that they should complete the international gynaecological record for all cases of cancer of the uterus. The 4 g radium "bomb" at the Westminster Hospital was under the control of a distinguished and highly experienced team who were to investigate the method of "distance radium therapy" or "mass irradiation" practised in other countries with undetermined results. It was considered that, if successful, this method might make surgical interference unnecessary in many patients.

The National Physical Laboratory undertook the important work of measuring the radium purchased from abroad, testing it for purity and providing custody until the centres were ready to receive it.

Technique of radium therapy

During the early years of the use of radium therapy for cancer much work was being done in many countries to develop methods of treatment. The National Radium Commission was therefore concerned with evaluating

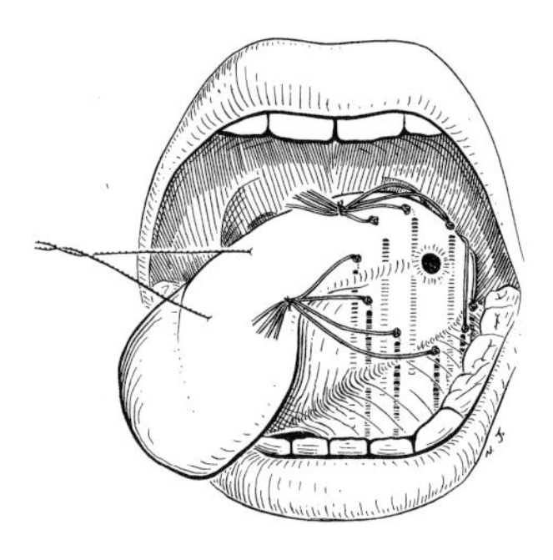

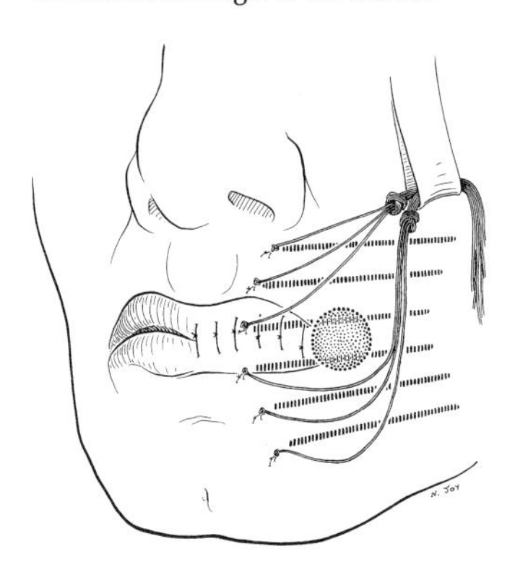

Figure 15.9 *Above:* The insertion of radium needles to treat a squamous cell carcinoma of the tongue. *Below:* The upper and lower lips are sutured together to form a solid block of tissue for interstitial radiation with radium needles to treat a squamous cell carcinoma of the buccal aspect of the cheek and angle of the mouth.

these techniques. At that time there were four main ones available.

(1) The use of radium in containers (needles, tubes, etc) which are inserted surgically into the tumour tissues or placed in natural body cavities.

(2) Surface therapy, where the radium containers are placed in external contact with the body or very close to it.

(3) Distance radium therapy (mass irradiation) by means of a "bomb" containing a large quantity of radium, placed at a distance of some inches from the body.

(4) Radon therapy, which is similar to (1) except that "radon" (the gas emanating from radium) is collected and sealed in small tubes or "seeds" which are inserted into the tumour tissues, instead of radium.

The National Commission arranged that all national centres should be equipped to practise methods (1) and (2), that some centres should also be equipped for the production of radon, and that the Westminster Hospital should try out method (3).

The Commission emphasised the importance of protection against radiation by stating that so far as possible the radium should be concentrated in one place, or in one hospital, and the patients should be brought to the radium centre, instead of the radium being sent to the patient. The care and custody of the radium should be entrusted to a physicist or radiologist. Furthermore, workers and patients should be safeguarded against dangers arising from the misuse of, or unnecessary exposure to radium.

Clinical records

The National Commission clearly understood the necessity of compiling accurate and detailed clinical records for all cancer patients who were treated with radium. The national radium centres were instructed to keep their records on standard forms which had been jointly agreed upon by the Commission, the Medical Research Council, the British Empire Cancer Campaign and King Edward's Hospital Fund. The Commission hoped that in this way truly national statistics, on a uniform basis, would become available.

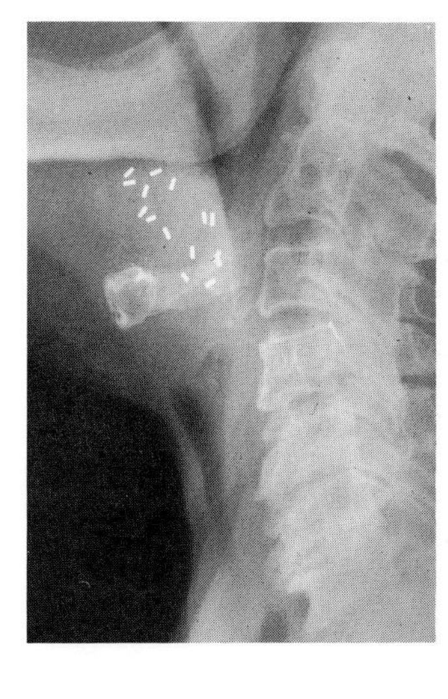

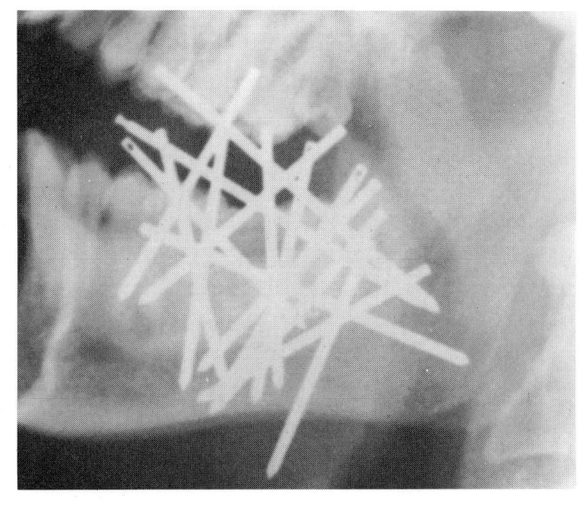

Figure 15.10 *Left:* A radiograph of the lateral aspect of the upper part of a neck, showing interstitial radon seeds inserted to treat a carcinoma in the base of the tongue. *Right:* A radiograph of the lateral aspect of the upper part of the neck, showing interstitial radium needles inserted to treat a carcinoma in the base of the tongue.

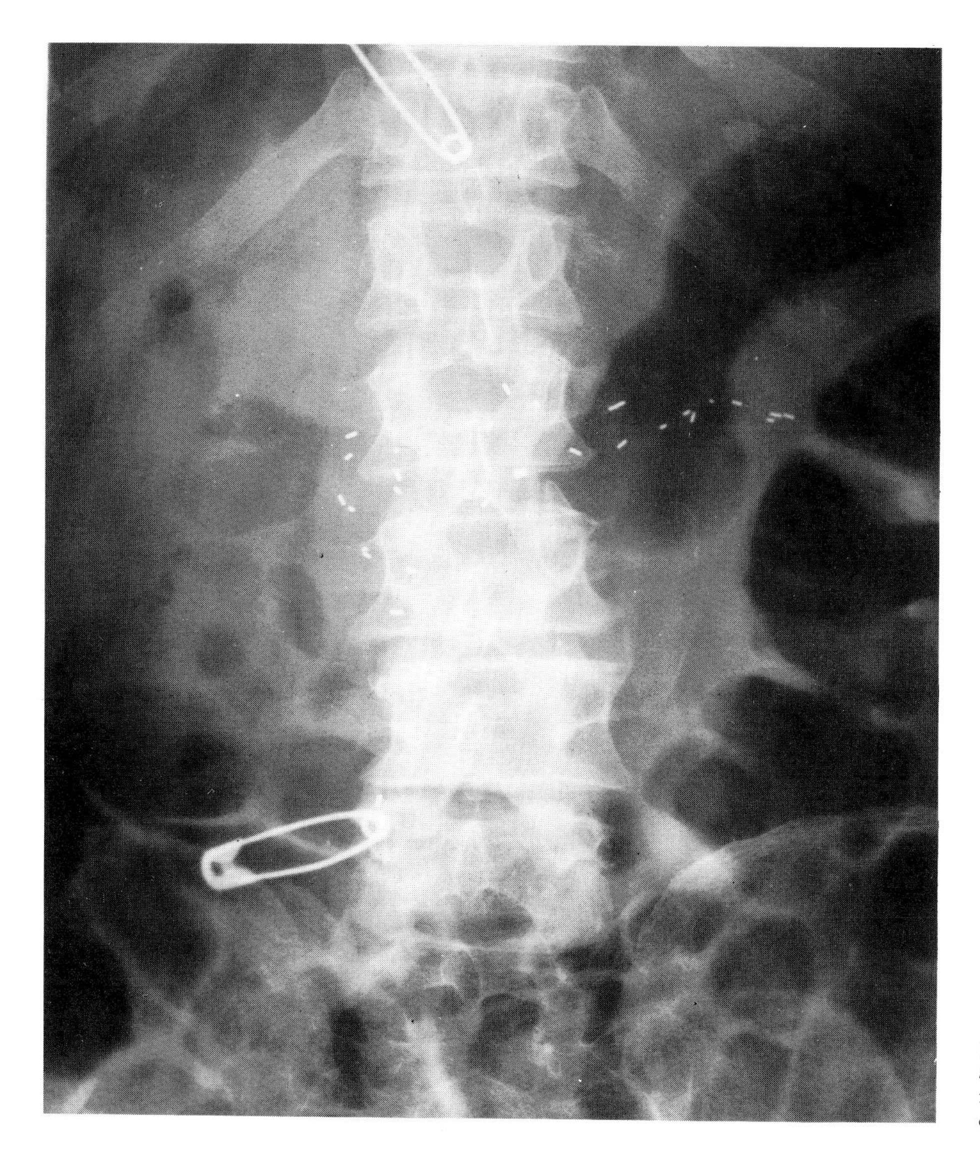

Figure 15.11 A plain radiograph of an abdomen showing interstitial radon seeds implanted to treat a carcinoma of the pancreas.

The *First Annual Report* contained details about the record forms. The analysis of the data was entrusted to the present author on his appointment as Registrar of Statistics to the National Radium Commission in 1931. This work is described in detail later on in this chapter.

Conclusion to the *First Annual Report*

The *First Annual Report* contains certain conclusions that are both interesting and important, especially when considered against the background of more than 50 years ago. It was emphasised that great caution was necessary in estimating the value of radium treatment for cancer and that false hopes should be avoided. Much time and experience would be needed to solve many problems, using a sufficient supply of statistical and scientific data, to reach positive conclusions and publish them to the world. The Commission had made their first duty the organisation of a concentrated and controlled national radium service with a programme to be carried out at selected centres supervised by recognised experts, the progress and results of which would be recorded on a uniform basis. It warned that radium was not yet established as a "cure" for cancer, but gave good promise of beneficial results and certainly of alleviation of suffering. However, it was a very dangerous weapon which must be used with the greatest skill and care, for it could easily produce more harm than good. It was visualised that at least 5 years of further experience and coordinated research would be required before any final verdict could be reached.

"PRELIMINARY REPORT ON RADIUM TREATMENT OF CANCER OF CERTAIN SITES"

The policy of the National Radium Commission has been described earlier in this chapter, including the establishment and work of the national radium centres. Detailed case-records were compiled for patients with different varieties of cancer treated by radium techniques. The clinical data included the history of the disease, clinical examination, method of radium treatment and the results of treatment as observed on clinical examination in the Follow-up Department at regular intervals.

It is emphasised that the evaluation of the treatment of cancer by radium techniques on a national scale was a new task of tremendous importance and great potential value for the future, all of which implications were fully realised by the National Radium Commission. The statistical basis of the vital project and the results of the statistical analysis are therefore worthy of record and consideration here.

The national survey

The present author, who was Registrar of Statistics to the National Radium Commission from 1931 to 1934, and A. E. C. Hare, Statistical Assistant, had the responsible task of furnishing to the Commission a report on radium treatment of cancer in certain sites of the body.

It was arranged that at each national radium centre all the relevant clinical data for analysis should be transferred from the patients' case-records to a special system of cards designed for the purpose. The total number of cases for analysis was augmented by the collaboration of King Edward's Hospital Fund for London, which requested the hospitals to which it had loaned radium to furnish their clinical data in the same way for the purpose of this statistical research.

It is pointed out that modern sophisticated methodology, including the use of computers, was not available at that time, neither had the Hollerith Punch Card system been introduced for statistical analysis. The task of the Registrar of Statistics and the Statistical Assistant was to carry out a detailed examination of all the cards and to make an analysis of the extensive data that were provided. This involved sorting all the cards by hand and extracting all the data for each patient.

The research was concluded when the preliminary report was published in 1934 *(Raven and Hare, 1934)*. This Report dealt only with patients with cancer in certain sites of the body who were treated with radium techniques in 1930, as their 3-year survival rates could be determined. The National Radium Commission quite rightly felt that 5-year survival rates were the minimum required to accurately assess the results of treatment, but the 3-year survival rates gave a useful guide to the progress of patients after their treatment. Nowadays, with increasing experience in this work, it is accepted that periods of 3 and even 5 years following treatment are too short and that it is necessary to have survival rates at 10, 15 and 20 years to evaluate the results of cancer therapy with different treatment modalities.

Definitions and results of treatment in the report

Net survival rate

The definition in the report is stated as "the proportion of patients who are alive, irrespective of the presence of disease, to the total number of patients treated, including those who have died of operation, but deducting from the sample the number of patients dead from causes other than cancer and patients lost sight of".

Stage of disease

A detailed definition of each stage of disease is given in the section concerning each site. It is pointed out that the clinical stage, unconfirmed by the histopathology of the regional lymph nodes, might cause a degree of error. Thus a patient might have clinically enlarged axillary lymph nodes which are negative on microscopical examination, and metastatic axillary lymph nodes are not always palpable.

Clinical staging is relied on for patients who are undergoing radiation treatment, in the absence of biopsy material for histopathology. It is stated that the stage of disease markedly influences the prognosis and that, in general, invasion or otherwise of the regional lymph nodes is the touchstone by which the prognosis is judged.

Results of treatment

The Report gives the results of radium treatment for cancer in various sites of the body, as assessed at the end of the 3rd year after treatment. These 50-year old results are of historic interest today, so they are dealt with here in some detail.

Carcinoma of the breast

The Report gives the results of the various radium treatment methods that were used for 557 patients with breast carcinoma. The 3-year survival rates obtained for each stage of disease are listed in Table 10. As stated already, 3-year survival periods are too short to adequately assess the results of treatment, nevertheless they do reveal a trend. The rates shown in Table 10 are inferior to those which are achieved with our modern methods of treatment for breast carcinoma.

Table 10 Carcinoma of the breast. 3-year net survival rates with all methods of treatment where radium was used

Stage of disease	*Number of patients treated*	*3-year net survival rate*
Stage 1	116 (20.0%)	64.0%
Stage 2	171 (30.7%)	39.9%
Stage 3	270 (48.5%)	24.9%

Carcinoma of the cervix uteri

The results are shown for a total number of 590 patients with primary carcinoma of the cervix uteri who were treated with various methods of radium treatment.

The disease was staged according to the method defined by the Radiological Sub-Commission of the League of Nations Health Organization. This classification is as follows:

Stage 1. The carcinoma is strictly limited to the cervix uteri.

Stage 2. The carcinoma is spreading into one or more fornices.

Stage 3. There is nodular infiltration by carcinoma of the parametrium on one or both sides.

Stage 4. There is massive carcinomatous infiltration of both parametria.

It is important to note the proportion of patients applying for treatment in each stage and to compare this with the position today, more than 50 years later, when many more patients are diagnosed with precancerous disease and in the early stages of carcinoma as the result of cytology and other screening techniques. Such tests were not carried out in 1930.

The proportion of patients in each stage of carcinoma of the cervix uteri and the 3-year net survival rates with all methods of treatment where radium was used are given in Table 11.

Table 11 Carcinoma of the cervix uteri. 3-year net survival rates with all methods of treatment where radium was used

Stage of disease	*Number of patients treated*	*3-year net survival rate*
Stage 1	123 (20.9%)	60.8%
Stage 2	148 (25.1%)	48.1%
Stage 3	241 (40.8%)	32.6%
Stage 4	78 (13.2%)	11.8%
All stages	590 (100%)	39.4%

A comparison was made in the Report between the 3-year survival rates of treated and untreated patients. For all patients who were treated (590 patients) the 3-year survival rate was 39.4%, whereas according to Greenwood *(1926)* only 10.5% of untreated patients were alive at the end of 3 years, the average survival rate being 20.9 months. A plea was made in the Report for earlier diagnosis to be made, for only 46% of the patients reviewed were at stages 1 or 2 of the disease when they applied for treatment.

The age incidence of 605 patients with carcinoma of the cervix uteri showed that in 1930 this disease was infrequent in patients under 30 years of age and that about 6% of all patients were in the age-group 30–39 years. The incidence rose sharply after the age of 40 years and reached a maximum of 18.2% in patients aged from 45 to 49 years. The situation has changed markedly today, for an increasing number of patients are now seen in the younger age groups (i.e., under 30 years), due to early sexual experience and promiscuity.

Carcinoma of the mouth

It is of much interest to take a retrospective look at the results achieved over 50 years ago by radium treatment alone or by radium combined with excisional surgery, in patients with carcinoma of the lip, tongue and floor of the mouth.

Carcinoma of the lip

The report gives the 3-year net survival rates for 94 patients, 44 of whom were treated with interstitial radium for primary lip carcinoma. This form of radiation has now been replaced by external radiation. The disease was assessed as stages 1 and 2 according to the clinical enlargement of the regional lymph nodes. The enlarged nodes were treated with interstitial or surface radium or by excision. The 3-year net survival rates for the 94 patients are listed in Table 12.

Table 12 Carcinoma of the lip. 3-year net survival rates with all methods of treatment where radium was used

Stage of disease	*Number of patients treated*	*3-year net survival rate*
Stage 1	50	75.0%
Stage 2	44	40.0%
Total	94	60.0%

Carcinoma of the tongue and floor of the mouth

The treatment of patients with carcinoma of the tongue and floor of the mouth has changed considerably since 50 years ago. The Report states that in 1930 there were 406 patients with these diseases who were treated with radium alone or radium combined with X-radiation or excisional surgery. The regional cervical lymph nodes were affected in 52.8% of the patients with carcinoma of the tongue and in 64.3% of the patients with carcinoma of the floor of the mouth.

Carcinoma of the tongue. The disease was assessed in stages as follows: stage 1 — carcinoma is limited to the tongue; stage 2 — carcinoma involves the tongue and floor of the mouth; stage 3 — the regional lymph nodes are enlarged clinically; stage 4 — carcinoma involves the tongue, floor of the mouth and the mandible.

The 3-year net survival rates for 322 patients are set out in Table 13.

The prognosis was serious for all this series of patients with carcinoma of the tongue. The spread of the carcinoma to the regional lymph nodes made a profound difference to the survival rates.

Table 13 Carcinoma of the tongue. 3-year net survival rates with all methods of treatment where radium was used

Stage of disease	*Number of patients treated*	*3-year net survival rate*
Stage 1	84 (26.1%)	40.0%
Stage 2	31 (9.6%)	23.4%
Stage 3	170 (52.8%)	12.9%
Stage 4	37 (11.5%)	2.9%
All stages	322 (100%)	19.6%

Carcinoma of the floor of the mouth. The Report dealt with 84 patients who had a primary carcinoma of the floor of the mouth. The disease was assessed as stage 1 or stage 2 according to the absence or presence of clinically enlarged regional lymph nodes. The 3-year net survival rates are given in Table 14.

The serious effect which the involvement of the regional lymph nodes had on the survival rate is clearly shown. The 3-year survival rate is better for patients with this disease than for those with carcinoma of the tongue.

Table 14 Carcinoma of the floor of the mouth. 3-year net survival rates with all methods of treatment where radium was used

Stage of disease	*Number of patients treated*	*3-year net survival rate*
Stage 1	30 (35.7%)	60.7%
Stage 2	54 (64.3%)	25.0%

Conclusion of the Report

It was stressed in the Report that the results given concerned patients who were distributed throughout England, Scotland and Wales, and that they therefore provided a representative picture of the results of radium treatment for cancer in these special sites in the year 1930. The authors stated that the results of radium treatment were encouraging and they felt it would be interesting to see if they improved during subsequent years.

FIFTH ANNUAL REPORT OF THE NATIONAL RADIUM TRUST AND RADIUM COMMISSION 1933–1934

Reference is made to the statistical work of the Commission, which included the compilation of adequate clinical records of patients treated in the various clinics and ensured easy transcription of the essential data from these records to appropriate forms for analysis. It was concluded that no less than 5 years would have to elapse before a reply could be given to the question: "Of how much value is radium in the treatment of cancer?" The Commission felt that an interim report, as described here, in 1934 would be valuable in differentiating on a broad basis, without attention to variations in technique, between the results of the several methods of cancer radiation in various sites in the body. It was pointed out that in this evaluation of radium treatment it would be necessary to use comparable data from surgical treatment.

One-gramme unit therapy

It is important to note the reference in the Report to this form of radium treatment and its development. One-gramme radium units were placed at the disposal of the Cancer Hospital (now the Royal Marsden Hospital), the Middlesex Hospital and University College Hospital for their use to be investigated. The Commission learnt that they were likely to be valuable in treatment and they visualised that, as more experience was acquired, larger units would be used, with greater probability of success.

The National Radium Trust was interested in this new method, known as "beam therapy", whereby a highly penetrating beam of rays was directed on the malignant tumour, from a large quantity of radium (a "bomb") not in contact with the body. The Trust recognised that the results of this external radiotherapy would largely influence the quantities of radium required on a national scale.

REFERENCES

Curie, E. *Madame Curie. A Biography* (translated by Sheean, V.). International Collectors Library, New York

Deeley, T. J. (1977). Radiotherapy. In Raven, R. W. (ed.) *Principles of Surgical Oncology*, pp 379–404. Plenum Medical Book Company, New York and London

Ellis, F. (1959). Artificial radioisotopes in cancer. In Raven, R. W. (ed.) *Cancer*, Vol. 5, pp 93–116. Butterworth & Co., London

First Annual Report of the National Radium Trust and Radium Commission 1929 to 1930. Presented to Parliament by the Financial Secretary to the Treasury by command of His Majesty, October 1930. HMSO, London

Glucksmann, A., Lamerton, L. F. and Mayneord, W. V. (1957). Carcinogen effects of radiation. In Raven, R. W. (ed.) *Cancer*, Vol. 1, pp 497–539. Butterworth & Co., London

Goolden, A. W. G. (1951). Radiation cancer of pharynx. *Br. Med. J.*, **2**, 1110–12

Greenwood, Major (1926). A report on the natural duration of cancer. *Report on Public Health and Medical Subjects No. 33.* Ministry of Health

Henk, J. M. (1973). Tumour oxygenation and radiotherapy. In Raven, R. W. (ed.)*Modern Trends in Oncology*, Part 2: Clinical Progress, pp 217–36. Butterworth & Co., London

Holinger, P. H. and Rabbett, W. F. (1953). Late development of laryngeal and pharyngeal carcinoma in previously irradiated areas. *Laryngoscope*, **63**, 105–12

Hueper, W. C. (1957). Environmental factors in the production of human cancer. In Raven, R. W. (ed.) *Cancer*, Vol. 1, pp 404–96

Looney, W. B. (1955). Late effects (twenty-five to forty years) of the early medical and industrial use of radio-active materials. *J. Bone Joint Surg.*, **37A** (6), 1169–87

Looney, W. B. (1956). Late effects (twenty-five to forty years) of the early medical and industrial use of radio-active materials. *J. Bone Joint Surg.*, **38A** (2), 392–405

Mackenzie, I. (1965). Breast cancer following multiple fluoroscopies. *Br. J. Cancer*, **XIX** (1), 1–8

Mayneord, W. V. (1967). Cancer hazards in diagnostic and therapeutic irradiation. In Raven, R. W. and Roe, F. J. C. (eds) *The Prevention of Cancer*, pp 53–9. Butterworth & Co., London

Morgan, R. L. (1973). Fast neutron therapy. In Raven, R. W. (ed.) *Modern Trends in Oncology*, Part 2: Clinical Progress, pp 237–70. Butterworth & Co., London

Ombrédanne, M. M., Poncet, E. and Gandon, J. (1954). Cancer pharyngo-laryngé et sténose oesophagienne chez un homme irradié pour goitre 20 ans auparavant. *Ann. Oto-Laryngol.*, **71**, 94–6

Osborn, S. B. (1959). Radiation protection. In Raven, R. W. (ed.) *Cancer*, Vol. 5, pp 117–33. Butterworth & Co., London

Pochin, E. E. (1970). The hazard of cancer induction by radiation. In Raven, R. W. (ed.) *Symposium on the Prevention of Cancer*, pp 29–37. Heinemann Medical Books Ltd, London

Raven, R. W. (1958). *Cancer of the Pharynx, Larynx and Oesophagus and Its Surgical Treatment*, pp 32–4. Butterworth & Co., London

Raven, R. W. and Hare, A. E. C. (1934). Preliminary Report on radium treatment of cancer of certain sites. Appendix to the *Fifth Annual Report of the National Radium Commission*. HMSO, London

Raven, R. W. and Levison, V. B. (1954). Radiation cancer of the pharynx. *Lancet*, **2**, 683–4

Regaud, C., Nozier, T. and Lacassagne, H. (1912). Sur les effets redoutables des irradiations étendues de l'abdomen et sur les lésions du tube digestif determinées par les rayons de Röentgen. *Arch. d'Elec. Méd.*, **21**, 321–34

Russ, S. (1959). Historical background of radiation in cancer. In Raven, R. W. (ed.) *Cancer*, Vol. 5, pp 1–13. Butterworth & Co., London

Samuel, E. (1973). Mammography. In Raven, R. W. (ed.) *Modern Trends in Oncology*, Part 2: Clinical Progress, pp 69–77. Butterworth & Co., London

Smith, J. C. (1962). Carcinoma of the rectum following irradiation of carcinoma of the cervix. *Proc. Roy. Soc. Med.*, **55**, 701–2

CHAPTER SIXTEEN

Cancer Chemotherapy

It is generally agreed that Ehrlich (1854–1915) is the father of chemotherapy when this term is used in a general sense. In a lecture to the Berliner Medizinis Gesellschaft on 13 February 1907 he stated, "What we want is a chemotherapie specifica, that is, we are looking for chemical agents which, on the one hand, are taken up by certain parasites and are able to kill them, and, on the other hand, in the quantities necessary for this lethal action, are tolerated by the organism without too much damage."

This was a historical pronouncement by a man of vision and its fulfilment has saved countless lives. The most fruitful application of Ehrlich's work up to the present time has been in the treatment and cure of microbial diseases, and the term "chemotherapy" became almost synonymous with the treatment of infections which was based upon the sound foundations of theory and practice.

The history of the medical conquest of diseases makes an impressive and fascinating study. The outstanding achievements of the past include the successful chemotherapy of malaria, syphilis and trypanosomiasis. These developments in controlling spirochaetal and protozoal diseases were followed by the spectacular introduction of the sulphonamides by Domagk *(1935)*, which brought bacterial diseases into the realm of chemotherapy.

The next important milestone on this historic road of medical achievement was the discovery of penicillin by Alexander Fleming in 1929. This was followed by the outstandingly important work of Florey, Chain and their colleagues in the development of its therapeutic application *(Florey, 1946)*. The present author recalls the enormous value of the use of penicillin in the surgical treatment of soldiers wounded in the battles of World War II.

Since that time an ever-increasing range of powerful antibiotics has been used throughout the world, saving countless lives, and this has completely revolutionised the medical treatment of bacterial diseases.

CANCER CHEMOTHERAPY

The concept that cancer might respond to medical treatment is not new, for throughout many centuries attempts have been made to treat cancer with various kinds of medicaments. These have been either applied locally to the tumour or administered orally with the objective of producing systemic effects in the body. Many different chemical substances have been used, which have contained arsenic, mercury and antimony. It seems that arsenical preparations were the most popular medicaments, since arsenic had the most efficacious effect on tumours.

The popularity of arsenic in cancer therapy was greatly increased by Lissauer, who in 1865 described the marked symptomatic improvement brought about in leukaemia by the administration of potassium arsenite (Fowler's solution). A few years later Billroth, quoted by Haddow *(1947)*, published the case-record of a patient with lymphoblastoma who showed repeated and dramatic responses after the administration of Fowlers's solution. The tumours and enlarged lymph nodes entirely disappeared.

In the context of cancer chemotherapy it is pertinent to refer to the opinion of Percivall Pott, which was quoted by Haddow: "We are not yet so happy as to be possessed of any medicine which will cure a cancerous habit. When the constitution is thoroughly infected, neither our knives or caustics will avail; they can only remove the local mischief but can have no effect on the general one in the constitution."

This statement succinctly expresses our modern dilemma, for we now recognise that cancer is not a single disease entity but is the name which is given to a large number of different, dangerous diseases which require diverse methods of treatment. Furthermore, these diseases are often generalised when patients first apply for diagnosis and treatment. Studies of their life-histories showing their metastatic potential have stimulated a constant search to find specific medicines which will exert a systemic effect in the body without causing deleterious general reactions and side-effects.

During the last 50 years impressive progress has been made in finding pharmaceutical agents for the treatment of different varieties of cancer. There has been an enormous research and clinical effort, so that today chemotherapy can be said to cure patients with certain cancers. These include some patients with leukaemia, lymphomas and solid tumours such as choriocarcinoma and seminoma of the testicle. Many other patients enjoy relief, with regression of their tumours.

The meaning of cancer chemotherapy

The term "cancer chemotherapy" has aroused considerable discussion in the past, which has included the question whether such a treatment modality really exists in the light of our ignorance concerning the nature and aetiology of the cancerous diseases and the availability of non-specific chemical substances for clinical use. It is arguable whether hormonal therapy should be included under the title of chemotherapy. In hormonal therapy the rationale and clinical approach are different. Some tumours, such as carcinoma of the breast and prostate and probably others, are under hormonal control and their treatment involves the manipulation of hormonal control mechanisms by endocrine surgery such as oophorectomy and adrenalectomy, or the administration of synthetic hormones. By these means a change in the general hormonal environment of the tumour and its metastases is effected which influences the ability of the carcinoma cells to survive or reverses them back to normal cells. In contradistinction, chemotherapy involves the administration of chemical substances which will directly attack and kill malignant cells.

Reference has been made to the important pioneer work of Ehrlich, who was seeking chemical agents which could be absorbed by parasites and kill them, but who also clearly realised that the lethal parasite dosage should not be too damaging to the host's normal tissues. Chemicals were therefore sought which had a specific action on abnormal tissues without damaging normal tissues. This is the original conception of chemotherapy for microbial infections.

According to Lourie *(1946)* the term "chemotherapy" should be restricted in its meaning, as Ehrlich intended, to "the treatment of infections by chemical compounds", but Lourie added the very significant phrase "and perhaps cancer". He quoted the important statement by Schulemann *(1939)*, "The investigator in chemotherapy strives after the somewhat different aims (from those of the pharmacologist). He is not concerned with restoring diseased cells to their normal function, or with bringing about a reversible alteration of the cell functions. He aims at reaching the parasite cells and at throwing their function so irreversibly out of order that the parasite dies, but the host remains as unharmed as possible."

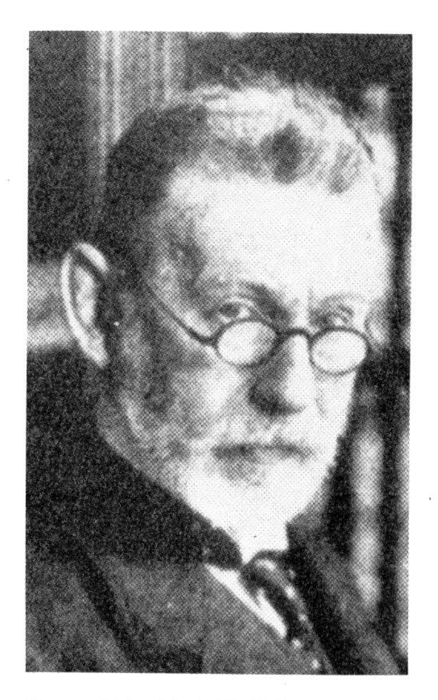

Figure 16.1 Paul Ehrlich (1854–1915), the recognised father of chemotherapy.

Relevance of chemotherapy in virus diseases

Although our knowledge about oncogenic viruses and their role in the aetiology of the cancerous diseases is still limited, can we learn any lessons from the chemotherapy of virus diseases? This subject was considered in detail by Andrewes and King *(1946)*, who stated that if the viruses consist largely of a lipid–nucleoprotein complex they should be vulnerable to chemotherapy. Such a complex can be disintegrated by denaturants and detergents, but this approach to their control is excluded because viruses are intracellular, or even intranuclear, so their metabolism is closely linked with that of the cell. Andrewes and King introduced the interesting hypothesis that a virus might at times multiply within a limited number of cells and destroy them, thus becoming liberated to invade more cells and then destroy them too. This would mean that the virus could be attacked with a viricidal drug in its extracellular environment. Andrewes and King considered that for an attack on the intracellular virus to have the best chance of success it must interfere with the sequence of processes in its multiplication. They suggested that it should be possible to specifically inhibit the essential metabolites by presenting to the cell foreign substances which bear a resemblance to the essential metabolites. Another possibility they put forward is to present to the cell substances which are foreign to it, in the hope that they will be incorporated into the structure of the virus and result in a non-self-reproducing unit.

Andrewes and King also described a different approach depending upon the discovery of chemicals to combine with those substances which are essential for viral reproduction, or with the enzymes which control the synthetic processes by selectively blocking their activity.

They also suggested a visionary approach to the whole problem by stating that it might be possible to take advantage of the "interference phenomenon". They pointed out that there are many examples in which infection of a host with one virus can suppress the activity of a second virus added with, or even before, the "interfering" virus, and that it had been found that a bacterial virus (bacteriophage) inactivated by ultraviolet radiation could thus block the activity of a living virus. They postulated that if the interfering principle in the killed virus particles could be isolated, chemically identified and initiated, important new therapeutic possibilities would result.

These opinions of Andrewes and King are of great historic interest, for now, 40 years later, we are using interferons especially in virus diseases, and their possible role in treating cancerous diseases is being actively explored.

The early conceptions of chemotherapy of parasite diseases which have been referred to here have an important relevance to the development of modern cancer chemotherapy, to which they have contributed ideas and principles.

EARLY DEVELOPMENTS IN CANCER CHEMOTHERAPY

The treatment of cancer with lead preparations

The present author remembers the enormous interest and enthusiasm that were engendered by the new treatment of cancer with lead preparations when he was a student at St Bartholomew's Hospital, London, where some of the clinical work was carried out and evaluated.

This treatment was introduced and developed by Professor Blair Bell and his colleagues working in Liverpool and was an important landmark in cancer chemotherapy, as it was an effort to treat malignant tumours by the systemic administration of a chemical compound.

In an article published in *Lancet (1922)* Blair Bell stated that much time and labour had been expended on this subject for more than 3 years, but it was still in the experimental stage. He summarised the relevant work in the following terms. Lead combines, probably chemically, with lecithin and therefore affects those normal tissues of the body in which lecithin, or similar lipids, are present in greatest quantity. Malignant tumours contain lecithin in direct proportion to their rate of growth. The intravenous injection of colloidal preparations of lead, whilst not without danger, can with experience be so regulated that little or no disturbance is caused. After an intravenous injection of the colloid preparation, lead can be recovered from the tumour in a quantity proportionately greater than that contained in the rest of the body. Lead in suitable doses appears in nearly all cases to arrest the growth of malignant tumours. In some cases lead treatment can result in the disappearance of the tumours, possibly by the action of normal tissues on arrested cell development, and this possibility appears to depend on the vascularity of the parts. At the same time the patient's general condition improves. It is desirable, when possible, that the bulk of the tumour be removed, then injections made immediately, while the blood supply is increased to the part concerned.

Previous injections of a colloidal lead preparation seem to increase the beneficial effects of X-ray therapy, owing to the promotion of secondary radiation. Finally, in this 1922 article, Blair Bell indicated the possibility that prophylactic lead treatment following complete excision of a tumour might be of considerable value in preventing recurrent disease.

Another important communication by Blair Bell and his colleagues, published in 1926, presented the conclusions they had reached after further experience with lead therapy for malignant tumours. They stated that there was additional evidence to support their views regarding the nature of malignant neoplasia but that more work was required to discover a more therapeutically active lead preparation that was less toxic generally. They thought that all varieties of malignant tumours are probably amenable to the beneficial influence of lead, provided this metal can reach the malignant cells in sufficient quantity. Adjuvant surgical and radiation treatments can be used with considerable advantage in suitable cases. When the tumour has been partly or apparently entirely removed, lead should be given intravenously within a few days of the operation, if this is possible. They concluded that lead treatment is difficult and to some extent dangerous, and it can be used safely only by those who are highly experienced in this work and have the necessary laboratory facilities.

Further experience

The treatment of cancer with preparations of lead created a lot of interest and it was investigated by a number of different centres. It was used with the greatest care because there was much concern regarding its dangers for patients. Reference is made to the investigations carried out by Wyard and King *(Wyard, 1928)* at the Cancer Hospital (now the Royal Marsden Hospital), where the staff considered that a clinical evaluation should be made. The method adopted at Liverpool was used for the treatment of 56 patients, but only one patient showed definitive improvement. This patient had undergone a mastectomy operation for breast carcinoma a year earlier but had later developed an enlarged supraclavicular lymph node which was visible and the size of an almond. The swelling was presumably due to a metastasis, but there was no tissue diagnosis. After lead therapy it diminished in size until it was only just palpable. Wyard stated: "From these observations there was no support for the statement that colloidal lead exerts a beneficial effect on the progress of a malignant growth. Moreover, it is a difficult and dangerous therapeutic method."

Whilst the clinical use and value of lead therapy for cancer was widely criticised, Canti *(1926)* wrote in the *British Medical Journal* that for the "first time in history ... a generalised treatment has been found to cause local disappearance of a cancerous growth". He advocated further investigations and stated: "Blair Bell and co-workers never claimed that lead is an infallible cure for malignant disease, but they have approached the matter from a scientific standpoint." Following the critical clinical evaluations, lead treatment for cancer was discarded.

It is there we shall have to leave this detailed account of the investigations concerning the systemic treatment of cancer with lead which were carried out by Blair Bell and his colleagues carefully and scientifically, with the expenditure of a considerable amount of time and effort. Although lead therapy caused much disappointment over 50 years ago, it remains a historic landmark in the development of cancer chemotherapy.

The treatment of cancer with bacterial toxins

This treatment was used by William B. Coley and based on observations that many varieties of neoplasms regressed when acute bacterial infections, principally erysipelas, were present in the patients. In many patients the inhibitory action was sufficiently strong to cause complete disappearance of the tumour without any recurrence. This novel method of treatment attracted the interest of Coley, who subsequently had extensive experience of its use, but he never recorded his work in a monograph. We are therefore indebted to Helen Coley Nants, Walker E. Swift and Bradley L. Coley *(1946)* for their valuable review article about the subject.

The author acknowledges his particular indebtedness to these writers for he has taken much of his information from their article, which gives a thorough record of reports about this treatment in the literature and an analysis of Coley's and other investigators' case-records of their patients. In addition, it contains a review of the experimental work on the subject. Following the introduction of this treatment modality in 1892 at least 15 different preparations of Coley's toxins were used, three being more potent than the rest, and the methods of treatment varied considerably with regard to dosage, frequency and duration.

According to the article by Nants and colleagues, Coley's interest in this form of treatment was aroused by the experience of a patient with an inoperable lymphosarcoma of the neck, which had recurred three times, who had recovered after an attack of erysipelas. Searching the literature he found case-records of 38 patients with inoperable malignant tumours who suffered an attack of erysipelas as a result of an accident or inoculation. Amongst these patients there were 17 with carcinomas, three of whom had permanent regressions; another 17 patients had sarcomas and seven of these had permanent regressions.

Nants and colleagues stated that the factors which hindered the acceptance and development of toxin therapy were as follows. It could be argued that the disappearance of tumours was due to spontaneous regression, the toxin therapy being incidental. Such criticism, however, seemed not to take into account that the majority of so-called spontaneous tumour regressions recorded in the literature had occurred during, or following, an acute bacterial infection, such as erysipelas, pneumonia, pyaemia, typhoid fever and others. Furthermore, the criticism was weakened by the fact that the neoplasms did not recur after the administration of Coley's toxins. Coley had a microscopical examination made of the tumours he treated, which excluded the possibility that they were benign.

Later it was argued that if toxin therapy was as valuable as Coley claimed it would have been adopted universally. To this particular criticism Coley answered, "I will call attention to one fact apparent to anyone familiar with the history of medical discoveries, that the relative value of such discoveries bears not the slightest relation to the rapidity of acceptance by the medical profession." It was noted also that the discovery of X-rays and radium very soon after toxin therapy was introduced might have influenced its acceptance, as the methods of treatment by radiation attracted considerable attention.

Another factor to consider, as these authors pointed out, is the possible effect which other treatments, given before or during toxin therapy, have on the latter treatment. It was found that any agent which alters or destroys the vascular or lymphatic channels through which the toxins must reach the tumour, or whereby the regeneration of normal tissues is sought, such as heavy radiation, or repeated incomplete surgical procedures, appears to limit the effectiveness of subsequent toxin therapy. These factors are important in modern chemotherapy and have influenced its combined use and effectiveness with preradiation and presurgical treatments. Nants and colleagues stated that cytological studies indicated that the neoplastic cell is most responsive to toxin therapy during its division, so that any inhibition of the rate of cell mitosis during toxin therapy may retard or minimise the destruction of tumour tissue by this treatment.

They advised that toxin therapy should be completed before radiotherapy was given, and since any process that decreases tissue permeability can have a deleterious effect on toxin therapy, they recommended further study, with a view to using invasive strains of bacteria, including a "spreading factor", such as hyaluronidase, as a means of possibly enhancing the effects of bacterial products. They concluded by stating that their study had provided sufficient clinical and experimental evidence that toxin treatment had clinical value and that more extensive research was warranted to provide better preparations of toxins and further refinements in the techniques of administration.

It is important that we should consider the lessons to be learnt from toxin therapy, especially with the help of modern scientific knowledge and methodology. It seems likely that it has general effects in the body which are probably mediated through the immunological system, in addition to any local effects it may have on the tumour.

PROGRESS IN CANCER CHEMOTHERAPY

Cancer chemotherapy was discussed in detail by Haddow *(1947)*, who with his colleagues at the Chester Beatty Research Institute played a leading role in the establishment of this new treatment modality for cancer. He stressed the almost insuperable difficulties which had to be overcome. It was always doubtful, he said, whether a therapeutic agent could be found which could impair the growth of malignant cells without at the same time equally damaging the normal cells of the body, especially those which are undergoing active division, such as cells in the intestinal mucosa, bone marrow and the generative organs.

Another serious obstacle is the fact that the malignant variant of the normal cell is permanent and irreversible. Haddow pointed out that even if its growth is impeded by any agent except the most specific, so far unknown, it is likely to recover and recur. (The present author notes that the malignant cell might be reversible.)

Haddow felt that the best prospect for successful cancer chemotherapy was to understand the mechanism of carcinogenesis and its deliberate reversal which could be effected by substances sufficiently powerful to inhibit cell division occurring in tumours directly or indirectly, without unduly affecting normal cells.

To illustrate his views he gave as examples of the progress made in cancer chemotherapy the treatment of carcinoma of the prostate with oestrogens, the action of chloroethylamines in treating certain patients with Hodgkin's disease, and the effects of urethane on the immature cells in leukaemia.

None of these particular drugs, however, are curative and their effects are usually only temporary.

Nevertheless, this early work pointed in the right direction for ultimate success, and continuing research during succeeding decades has resulted in considerable progress, so that today we can speak about curing certain cancerous diseases with chemotherapy. Successful treatment results occur in patients with Hodgkin's disease and other lymphomas, leukaemias, and other diseases too. For example, the addition of chemotherapy to surgery and radiotherapy for patients with Wilms' tumour has added considerably to the cure rate.

Nitrogen mustards and related compounds

The way by which these chemical substances were introduced into cancer chemotherapy is of much historical interest and illustrates the fact that good can sometimes come for the human race even from the horrors of warfare.

During World War I it was learnt that the nitrogen mustard chemicals used in chemical warfare caused a vesicant lesion on the skin and mucous membranes of the body, in addition to having a toxic action on other tissues, especially those of the haemopoietic system.

Subsequently Pappenheimer and Vance *(1920)* carried out experimental investigations on the effects which followed the intravenous injection of dichloroethylsulphide into rabbits and they found that the lethal dose was 0.0005–0.01 g per kilo weight. The rabbits which died within 24 hours showed extensive haemorrhage and oedema of the lungs and severe lesions of the intestinal tract occurred in two-thirds of them.

It was found that this chemical is specifically poisonous for the haemopoietic system, for it causes severe damage to the bone marrow and a marked diminution of the blood leucocytes. In the surviving animals regeneration occurred, but the granular cells of the bone marrow seemed to be more sensitive to dichloroethylsulphide than the lymphoid cells and erythrocytes.

Later work

Interest in the nitrogen mustard group of chemicals deepened in subsequent years and was heightened during World War II. An increased amount of research was carried out on experimental animals, the results of which showed that there had been a rapid destruction of lymphocytes in the lymph nodes, spleen and thymus, a reduction in granulocytes, and cytotoxic effects in the epithelial cells of the intestinal mucosa. It seemed to be a reasonable deduction that this group of chemical substances which caused such cytology changes should be used for the treatment of patients with selected cancerous diseases.

Clinical use

Clinical work was carried out by Goodman and colleagues, who in a preliminary communication *(1946)*, reported the results obtained with the clinical use of halogenated alkylamines in the treatment of patients with lymphosarcoma, Hodgkin's disease, and leukaemia, and a limited number of patients with allied or miscellaneous disorders.

They described the encouraging results, particularly in patients with Hodgkin's disease, lymphosarcoma, and chronic leukaemia. There was a dramatic improvement in a few patients, but others failed to derive any benefit from the treatment, for no apparent reason. Various responses were observed in patients with acute and chronic leukaemias. The investigators concluded that diseases other than those of the blood-forming organs did not appear to be indicated for treatment with the nitrogen mustard group of chemicals.

Much encouragement was gained from this work, however, for in an impressive proportion of patients who were considered to be in the terminal phase of their illness with so-called resistant disease, especially Hodgkin's disease and lymphosarcoma, the nitrogen mustard treatment caused remissions which lasted for weeks and in some cases even months. There was also evidence that nitrogen mustard therapy could occasionally restore the responsiveness of the disease to radiotherapy.

Goodman and colleagues wisely gave the warning that since the margin of safety in the use of nitrogen mustard chemicals is so narrow, caution is necessary in their clinical use and haematology monitoring must be done at frequent intervals during treatment.

Serious toxic side-effects which affect the blood-forming organs can occur after treatment, but it is possible to avoid them by using safe dosage schedules.

Whilst these chemicals do not cure malignant diseases, Goodman and colleagues recommended that further clinical trials should be carried out. They also pointed out that chemicals which are discovered to be therapeutically active in malignant diseases deserve to be studied carefully by clinicians, experimental pathologists, enzymologists and others who are interested in cancer and cellular biology.

Histological effects

It was a logical and necessary development of these important clinical observations that the histological changes that occur in human tissues and tumours after the administration of nitrogen mustard compounds should be studied. This was done by Sophie Spitz *(1948)*, who published the results of an intensive autopsy study of 57 cases of leukaemia, lymphoma and other malignant tumours treated with nitrogen mustard compounds.

Cytological changes were particularly marked in Hodgkin's disease and reticulum-cell sarcoma and were considered to be a direct effect of the nitrogen mustard rather than spontaneous changes which can occur in lymphomas. All cells were not equally affected and some cells appeared to completely escape any injury. After their recovery from the effects of the nitrogen mustards, many of the tumours seemed to be more pleomorphic than before the treatment. No cytological effects were found in a variety of malignant epithelial tumours. An additional effect attributed to the nitrogen mustard therapy was a constant apparently cumulative hypoplasia of the bone marrow, associated with the disappearance of granulocytes and the persistence of small numbers of erythroblasts and megakaryocytes.

Effects of the nitrogen mustard compounds on human tumours

These effects differ from those in experimental animals, the main difference being an absence of demonstrable changes in the gastric and intestinal mucous membrane. Atrophy of the testes seems to be more frequent after nitrogen mustard therapy than after other forms of therapy in control cases.

The chloroethylamines are toxic to those cells which are undergoing active proliferation. With a low dosage of chemicals cell mitosis is arrested in the resting stage, but with higher dosages gross abnormalities occur in cell division. The chemicals cause a characteristic fragmentation of the chromosomes, similar to the effects of radiation, hence the name given to these effects is "radiomimetic" *(Dustin, 1947)*.

Elson *(1963)* discussed in detail the actions of radiation and radiomimetic chemicals and compared their physiological effects. He called attention to the initial chemical changes which are induced in cells and tissues by radiation and which result in metabolic derangements that can cause cellular damage and lead to the death of the cells and the organism. Such radiation damage is associated with changes in nuclear material, including chromosome breaks in dividing cells, fragmentation and bridge formation at the anaphase stage.

Elson pointed out that very similar cellular changes are induced by certain chemicals including the nitrogen mustards. These chemicals can therefore be used clinically as an adjunct to, or as an alternative to, radiotherapy. He stated that, with regard to their biological action, alkylation was the most important reactivity. The term "alkylation" is applied to chemical reactions which involve the replacement of a hydrogen atom by an alkyl group; we now know that alkylating agents prevent replication of nucleic acid by cross-linking base parts.

The early work on the use of the nitrogen mustard compounds in the treatment of cancer has been discussed here in some detail as it shows the careful way in which cancer chemotherapy has developed. Other important members of the nitrogen mustard series have been produced and used

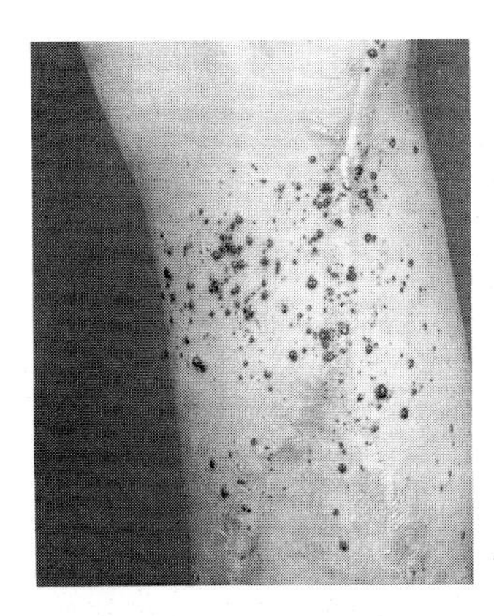

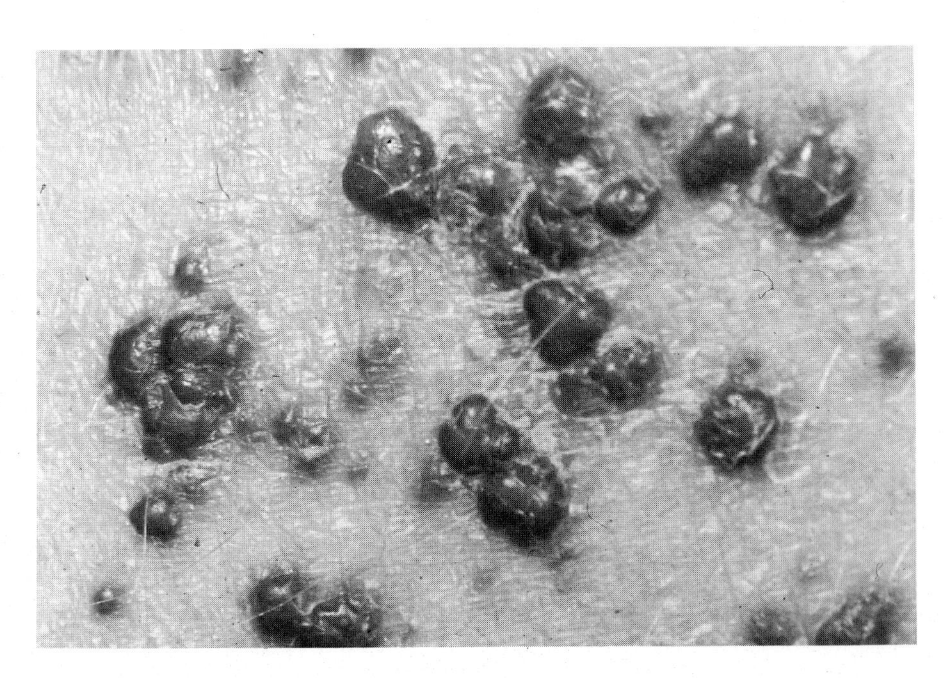

Figure 16.2 *Above:* Multiple metastases of malignant melanoma in the skin of a leg of a female patient after the excision of a primary malignant melanoma. *Right:* Good regression of the tumours after treatment of the affected limb with regional perfusion of phenylalanine mustard.

clinically with some success. These include chlorambucil and melphalan. The former has proved useful in the treatment of lymphocytic leukaemia, Hodgkin's disease and lymphosarcoma.

A valuable contribution to many early aspects of the chemotherapy of cancer is found in *Cancer*, which was edited by the present author *(Raven, 1959)* and contains chapters on various aspects of the subject by recognised authorities.

The antimetabolites

The development of this group of chemical compounds and their clinical use in cancer represented another major advance in cancer chemotherapy. Their action depends upon successful competition with normal metabolites for particular enzymes. The metabolite is the substrate which is loosely bound to the corresponding enzyme and normally enables it to function in the required utilisation of the substrate. Since the antimetabolite displaces the substrate, the enzyme cannot function normally.

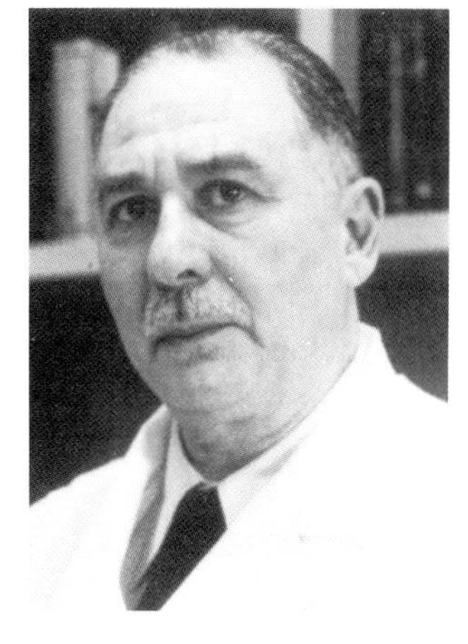

Figure 16.3 Sydney Farber.

The antimetabolite approach to cancer chemotherapy has been described in a most instructive book by Timmis and Williams *(1967)*, both of whom were colleagues and friends of the present author. In his Foreword to their book Sydney Farber stated that in the mid-1940s the first remissions in childhood leukaemia by therapeutic means were achieved by antagonists to folic acid using the antimetabolites aminopterin and methotrexate. A few years later similar temporary successes both in children and adults with acute leukaemia were obtained with a purine antagonist, 6-mercaptopurine. Farber called attention to the gift of Timmis to clinical oncology of Myleran (busulphan), which has been of great value in the control of chronic leukaemia.

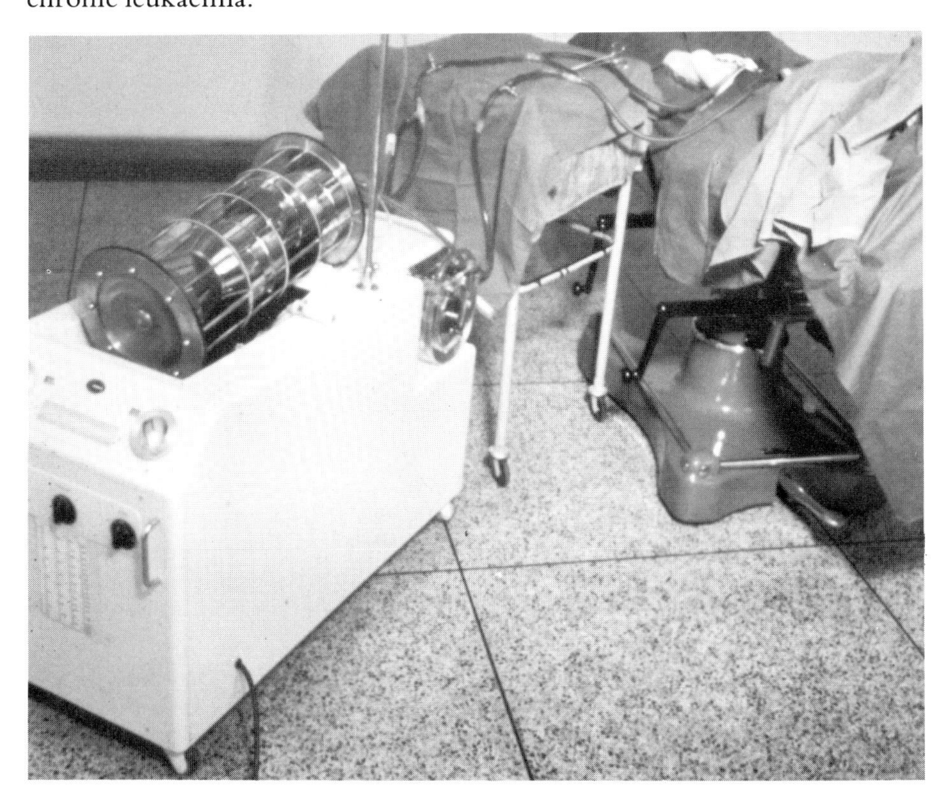

Figure 16.4 The regional perfusion apparatus used at the Royal Marsden Hospital.

A study of the book written by Timmis and Williams demonstrates the enormous research and clinical work on which the antimetabolite approach to the treatment of cancer is based. The foundation which was securely laid in those early years of development now bears a superstructure of great importance. The authors discuss antagonists to purine metabolism and state that 6-mercaptopurine was the first antipurine to be used clinically with very encouraging results in the treatment of acute leukaemia. Patients who had developed resistance to methotrexate often responded to 6-mercaptopurine.

It is interesting to see that in the chapter devoted to antagonists of pyrimidine metabolism the authors state that 5-fluorouracil is the most useful and widely investigated drug of the pyrimidine series. The appreciation of the value of this drug in the treatment of certain cancers has been enhanced by subsequent experience up to the present day. It is chiefly used for solid tumours, including carcinoma of the colon, rectum and pancreas.

The chapter on antagonists to folic acid is full of interest and is important, as it describes their mechanism of action and their clinical uses. The authors state that folic acid antagonists were first used by Farber and his colleagues in the treatment of acute leukaemia where children are highly responsive to amethopterin (methotrexate) and aminopterin.

The great value of methotrexate is in the treatment of choriocarcinoma of the uterus, especially with higher doses of the drug. Remissions of the disease have occurred over many years and in some women they have been recorded as complete.

The authors call attention to the promising use of folic acid antagonists by regional infusion. The tumour-bearing part of the body is infused with the drug and the non-malignant tissues are protected from its toxic effects with folinic acid. Subsequent experience with regional infusion has proved the value of this method of administration. For example, the present author had a patient with a squamous cell carcinoma of the cheek which regressed to such an extent that excision of the tumour and reconstruction of the cheek became possible and the patient has now remained without recurrent disease for 16 years. Regional perfusion of tumours of the lower limb has proved valuable.

SUBSEQUENT DEVELOPMENTS IN CANCER CHEMOTHERAPY

During the last two decades important progress has been made in cancer chemotherapy, so that it is now an established treatment modality, used either alone or combined with surgery and radiation, in the management of many varieties of cancer.

New chemicals with stronger cytotoxic action on tumours are being produced; for example, vincristine, vinblastine, bleomycin, mustine, adriamycin, thiotepa and cisplatin, to mention but a few. Combination chemotherapy, where several drugs are administered simultaneously, is very often given.

Much work is being done regarding dosage schedules, including the effects of the administration of high doses in certain cases.

Considerable experience has been acquired concerning adverse reactions to the carcinostatic agents and the avoidance and treatment of side-effects.

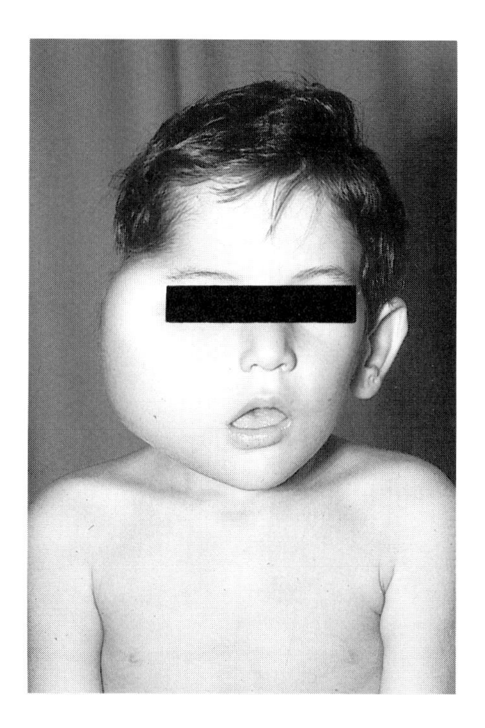
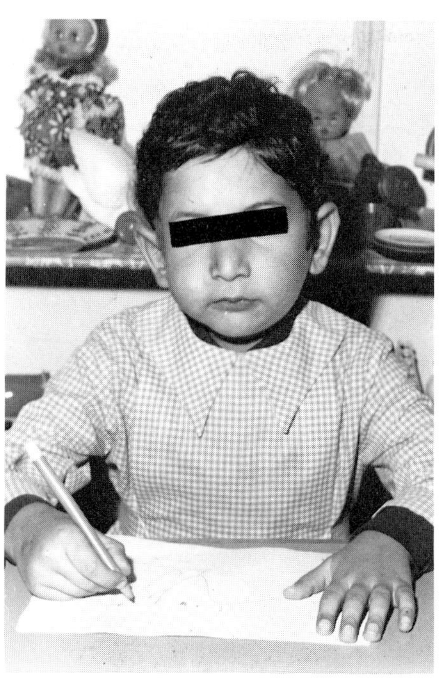

Figure 16.5 *Left:* A male patient aged 3½ years with a large embryonal sarcoma projecting from the right side of his face. Tomography showed that the whole of the ascending ramus of the mandible, the lateral wall of the right antrum and the posterior part of the alveolar portion of the right maxilla had been destroyed. There was also evidence of destruction of the anterior part of the lateral wall of the right orbit and of the inferior wall of the orbit and malar bone. The patient had a maximum tumour dose of 4732 rads radiotherapy by linear accelerator and chemotherapy with vincristine, adriamycin, methotrexate and bleomycin. Thiotepa was injected into the tumour and treatment with methotrexate was continued. After further quadruple chemotherapy and treatment with cyclophosphamide there was remarkable regression of the tumour. *Right:* The results achieved 1½ years after the combined radiotherapy and chemotherapy. Chemotherapy was continued, using actinomycin D, vincristine and cyclophosphamide. At age 5½ there was no evidence of the primary tumour or metastases and the patient was well at age 16.

Many of the drugs are very toxic and must be used with great skill and care. Doctors and nurses who handle them and administer them in various ways have to be protected from possible effects on themselves.

The subject of tumour resistance to various drugs is important, including the reasons why certain tumours are completely or partially resistant. We need to understand the reason why combined chemotherapy and radiotherapy can in some cases increase tumour susceptibility to treatment.

Another important question which is being asked today is whether children who are successfully treated with carcinostatic chemicals will be more susceptible to another cancer developing in later life.

Finally, new carcinostatic chemicals are required which have a specific antitumour action but do not affect normal tissues. In addition, simple methods of administration would be more advantageous than intravenous injections.

The emergence of the chemotherapy of cancer as an established treatment modality was a major event in the history of medicine. We anticipate with confidence that the careful, combined work of scientists and clinicians in many disciplines will result in further important advances being made.

REFERENCES

Andrewes, C. H. and King, H. (1946). Chemotherapy of Rickettsial and virus diseases. *Br. Med. Bull.*, **4** (4), 272–5

Blair Bell, W. (1922). The influence of saturine compounds on cell-growth. *Lancet*, **2**, 1005–9

Blair Bell, W. and colleagues (1926). An address on the treatment of malignant disease with lead. *Lancet*, **1**, 537–44

Canti, R. G. (1926). Lead treatment of cancer. *Br. Med. J.*, **2**, 1135–6

Domagk, G. (1935). Ein Beitrag zur Chemotherapie der bakteriellen Infektionen. *Dtsch. Med. Wochenschr.*, **61**, 250–3

Dustin, P. (1947). The cytologic action of ethyl carbamate (urethane) and other carbamic esters in normal and leukaemic mice and in rabbits. *Br. J. Cancer*, **1**, 48

Elson, L. A. (1963). *Radiation and Radiomimetic Chemicals* (Raven, R. W., consultant ed.). Butterworth & Co., London

Florey, Sir Howard, (1946). Steps leading to the therapeutic application of microbial antagonisms. *Br. Med. Bull.*, **4** (4), 248–58

Goodman, L. S., Wintrobe, M. M., Dameshek, W., Goodman, M. J., Gilman, A. and McLennan, M. T. (1946). Nitrogen mustard therapy. *J. Am. Med. Assoc.*, **132**, 126–32

Haddow, A. (1947). Note on the chemotherapy of cancer. *Br. Med. Bull.*, **5** (6), 417–26

Lourie, E. M. (1946). A sketch of the history of chemotherapy. *Br. Med. Bull.*, **4** (4), 243–8

Nants, H. C., Swift, W. E., and Coley, B. L. (1946). The treatment of malignant tumours by bacterial toxins as developed by the late William B. Coley, M.D., reviewed in the light of modern research. *Cancer Res.*, **6**, 205–16

Pappenheimer, A. M. and Vance, M. (1920). The effects of intravenous injections of dichloroethylsulfide in rabbits with special reference to its leucotoxic action. *J. Exp. Med.*, **31**, 71–92

Raven, R. W. (ed.) (1959). *Cancer*, Vol. 6. Butterworth & Co., London

Schulemann, W. (1939). Problems and progress in chemotherapy. *Ann. Trop. Med. Parasit.*, **33**, 171–95

Spitz, S. (1948). The histological effects of nitrogen mustards on human tumours and tissues. *Cancer*, **1c**, 383–98

Timmis, G. M. and Williams, D. C. (1967). *Chemotherapy of Cancer. The Antimetabolite Approach* (Raven, R. W., consultant ed.). Butterworth & Co., London

Wyard, S. (1928). Report on the treatment of malignant disease by colloidal lead. *Br. Med. J.*, **1**, 838–40

CHAPTER SEVENTEEN

Carcinogens and Carcinogenesis

For more than a century active research has been carried out to discover the aetiology of cancer. During recent decades the volume of work has increased enormously with the opening up of new avenues of clinical and laboratory investigations. The increase and maintenance of cancer research require the expenditure of considerable amounts of money, much of which is given by individuals and voluntary organisations. In spite of all the international effort a lot more on-going work must be done to solve the relevant, difficult biological problems and unveil the secrets of Nature.

We are still unable to understand the mechanism of carcinogenesis, although we have succeeded in identifying a considerable range of carcinogens. If this mechanism were understood, the whole problem of cancer would be illuminated, with profound implications for both prevention and treatment.

The term "carcinogen" is given to an agent, either chemical, physical or viral, which is capable of inducing neoplastic changes in a normal cell. Carcinogens are either exogenous or endogenous, the former being more common. There are many different carcinogens in the human environment which affect people because of their life-style and occupation. In contradistinction, there are endogenous, naturally occurring carcinogens in the human body.

Carcinogenesis is the mechanism whereby a normal cell is converted into a malignant cell following the application of a carcinogen to the cell. It is uncertain whether a malignant tumour is derived from a single cell or a clone of cells that have undergone malignant transformation. It remains unknown which component of the cell is the actual target for the carcinogen and whether total intracellular malignant change occurs.

This chapter describes the early work which led to the beginnings of our knowledge of this subject and outlines the developments which then

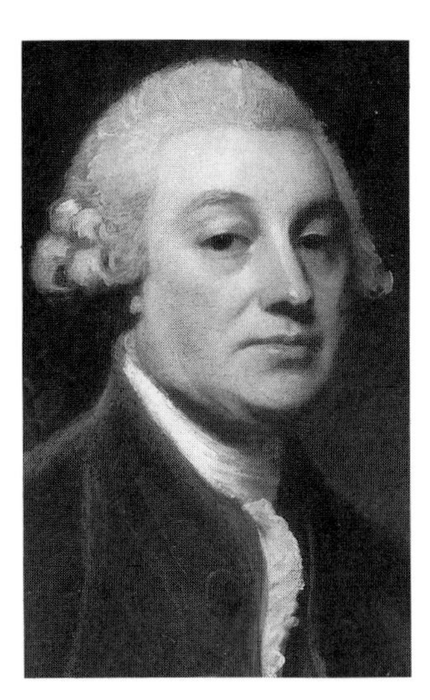

Figure 17.1 Percivall Pott (1714–1788).

occurred over many decades, enabling the subject to reach its present, central position in oncology.

EARLY OBSERVATIONS BY PERCIVALL POTT (1714–1788)

Percivall Pott was a distinguished surgeon on the staff of the Royal Hospital of St Bartholomew in the City of London. He possessed notable powers of observation, allied with keen clinical acumen, which enabled him to describe several conditions which were given his name, by which he will always be remembered by posterity. He described the fracture-dislocation of the ankle (Pott's fracture), which he himself sustained when he fell off his horse in the Old Kent Road in London on his way to see his patients in St Bartholomew's Hospital. He also described the paraplegia which is caused by pressure on the spinal cord from tuberculosis of the spine (Pott's paraplegia).

CANCER OF THE SCROTUM

Special attention is given here to the recognition by Pott of an occupational cancer called "the chimney-sweepers' cancer". In his book on the subject *(Pott, 1775)* he recorded that "everybody is acquainted with the disorders to which painters, plummers, glaziers and other workers are liable". At that time, however, according to Pott, no-one had noticed the disease which is peculiar to a certain occupation, that is, chimney-sweepers' cancer. He described this as a disease which always first affects the inferior part of the scrotum, where a "superficial, painful, ragged, ill-looking sore with hard and rising edges is produced. The trade call it the soot-wart and I never saw it under the age of puberty."

He pointed out that this disease was supposed to be venereal in origin and was treated with mercurial medicaments. He described the spread of the disease through the scrotal skin to "involve the testicle and later invades the spermatic cord, inguinal glands, and finally the abdominal viscera and very soon becomes painfully destructive."

Regarding the treatment of the disease, Pott advised early excision of the affected part of the scrotum; if the testicle was affected, castration would not be curative, because recurrent disease was common.

It is of historical importance to record that Pott held the opinion that this cancer was caused by the lodgement of soot in the rugae of the scrotal skin because of the occupation of the patients. He felt that the development of the disease was a "singularly hard fate for these chimney-sweepers who are young and poorly nourished (and who are) thrust up narrow and sometimes hot chimneys where they are bruised, burned, and almost suffocated, and when they get to puberty, become liable to a most noisome, painful and fatal disease."

Pott's observations naturally attracted considerable professional interest and we can see today, in retrospect, that his work was the first step in the scientific study of chemical carcinogenesis.

Additional observations

Further studies of chimney-sweepers' cancer were carried out by Butlin *(1892)*, who was also a distinguished surgeon on the staff of St Bartholomew's Hospital in London. He delivered three lectures on the subject at the Royal College of Surgeons of England, in which he stated that an extensive international literature about the subject had built up, and he examined in detail the following three important aspects of the disease:

(1) The disease was seldom seen in any part of the civilised world except Great Britain. At first the evidence seemed to show that the immunity of chimney-sweeps in other countries was due to the innocuous qualities of the soot there, but after making considerable investigations Butlin concluded that it was due to the care which foreign sweeps took to protect their bodies from contact with soot by daily washing from head to foot and by wearing protective clothing carefully designed for the purpose.

(2) The disease was generally considered to be a comparatively mild malignant disease. Butlin believed that the prognosis was very good after excision of the uncomplicated scrotal carcinoma, but he had no doubt that the disease was cancer and he described its clinical features as follows: "A wart, or warts, may exist for many years, in fact the whole scrotum may be covered with warts and no malignant change occurs. In other patients, after a period, one wart, due to scrotal irritation, grows larger and is fixed deeply. The centre ulcerates, the disease spreads steadily along the skin, penetrates deeply into the tunica vaginalis and then into the testicle, which is gradually destroyed. In more serious cases everything is destroyed between the anus and pubes. The inguinal glands are enlarged at first from infection, but later are affected by metastases, causing ulceration which spreads to the femoral and iliac glands. The patient's general condition deteriorates gradually due to pain and the profuse discharge from the ulceration of the scrotum and groins, but death may be long delayed until the patient is worn out by the disease." Butlin stated that whilst metastases in other organs and tissues were uncommon, they did occur, and he cited the case of a patient of Travers who developed cancerous nodules in the peritoneum.

(3) It was being said that the incidence of the disease was diminishing in Great Britain, but Butlin produced strong evidence that this statement was not true.

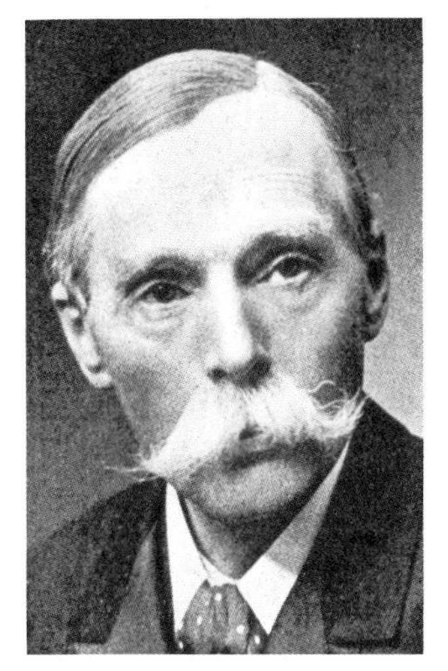

Figure 17.2 Sir Henry T. Butlin.

He also made the following important observation: "Now here we have a curious kind of experiment which has been conducted before the eyes of surgeons for at least one hundred years and which continues to be conducted year by year upon the human body, namely, the repeated application of a chemical substance, or of a mixture of chemical substances, to a particular part of the integument which is not at all predisposed to cancer, with the effect of rendering it pre-eminently disposed to the occurrence of cancer in a certain number of persons experimented on."

The observation is relevant today that Nature continues to carry out these large-scale experiments on the human race throughout the world and especially on those nations who live in an environment which is polluted by an increasing number of chemical substances, of which many are known to be carcinogenic. Such experiments merit our earnest consideration and scientific study for thereby important clues about the aetiology of cancer will be discovered. The method of clinical observation which was used with excellent results by Pott and Butlin has great merit in our own work.

In addition to this fruitful approach, we now have modern scientific methodology to assist us in our difficult task of wresting the obscure secrets about cancer from Nature.

These original, fundamental observations by surgeons who associated certain cancers with the occupations of patients have been extended and synthesised into the important modern discipline of occupational and industrial cancer, which forms part of epidemiology, one of the basic oncology sciences. The range of carcinogens to which workers in industry are exposed continues to expand with industrial growth, and from their identification and measures for protection the prevention of cancer has become an important practical modality with great present and potential value.

Further studies on cancer of the scrotum

A significant and valuable contribution to our knowledge of scrotal cancer was made by S. A. Henry *(1946)*, who held the post of H.M. Medical Inspector of Factories in England. His monograph was based on the results of the analysis of a series of more than 700 patients with this disease. He described the different varieties of scrotal cancer which occurred in men in different occupations, where exposure to certain specific agents was the main causative factor. In those case-records where the exact position of the epithelioma in the scrotal skin was given, he found that the tumour occurred in the left side of the scrotum in about 60% of patients when the worker was in contact with tar or mineral oil. He suggested that the reason for this might be that the usual way of dressing on the right side caused intimate contact between the scrotum and the left thigh, which resulted in the retention of moisture and extraneous matter.

The monograph contains some important statistical data. Since the year 1920, when skin epithelioma was added to the list of notifiable diseases under the Factories Act, 3333 cases of skin cancer, of which 1355 (40.6%) were of scrotal cancer, were notified up to the end of the year 1943. It is noteworthy that 1892 cases (56.7% of all the cases) were attributed to exposure to pitch and tar, probably because these were regarded as the causal agents for the longest period, but the scrotum was not the main site for the epithelioma.

Henry investigated a series of 1631 patients who died of scrotal cancer; the average age at death was 61.6 years, the youngest patient being 25 and the oldest 91. The induction time (incubation period) for scrotal cancer in mule-spinners was 49–50 years after they had commenced work in the majority of cases; the minimum period was 16 years.

Henry described the preventive measures needed to protect workers from developing this disease. These included education about the warning symptoms and signs, the wearing of protective clothing and undergoing periodic medical examinations to ensure early diagnosis and treatment of the disease.

The monograph also contains a bibliography of the medical literature about this subject.

TUMOURS OF THE URINARY BLADDER

The German surgeon Rehn *(1895)* observed that an unduly high incidence of tumours of the urinary bladder occurred in men working in the manufacture of fuchsine (magenta). He concluded that aniline was the most suspicious element amongst the chemical substances they were using in their work. As a result of his observations the term "aniline tumour of the bladder" was incorporated in the medical literature, which has now become voluminous through additions from many manufacturing countries.

After these initial clinical observations by Rehn several decades elapsed before the responsible chemical carcinogens were identified by experimental research. Many chemical substances used in the dye industry were suspected, but only a few proved to be carcinogenic. In 1947 Goldblatt stated that tumours in workers in the dyestuffs industry were caused by β-naphthylamine and benzidine; other possible and perhaps probable causes were aniline and α-naphthylamine. He also referred to the nature of the industrial processes associated with the problem of bladder tumours and the ways by which the amino-bases are absorbed. He stated that it was not improbable that in the latter part of the 19th century and the first two decades of the 20th century absorption through the skin and mouth would occur daily.

Absorption of the dust and fumes of these chemical substances was also considerable through the respiratory system. This proved to be the most difficult route of absorption to control, even in later years.

The latent period (incubation period) between the first exposure to the chemical substances and the onset of symptoms and signs of bladder disease was stated by Goldblatt to vary from about 4 years to 48 years in his series of cases. He described the method of medical control in the factories and stressed that the workers should be kept under medical supervision throughout their working lives in order to detect any evidence of bladder disease.

Valuable contributions to our knowledge of this subject are based on the research of Case and his colleagues *(1954)*, carried out at the Chester Beatty Research Institute in London. They found that the chemical substance β-naphthylamine was the most potent cause of occupational bladder tumours between the years 1915 and 1951. The tumours appeared after an average incubation period of 16 years for β-naphthylamine and benzidine and 22 years for α-naphthylamine. There were also some exceptional incubation periods of less than 2 years and more than 45 years after the first exposure to the chemical carcinogen. According to Case and colleagues, the average incubation period is not influenced appreciably by the severity or duration of the exposure, but is apparently a characteristic feature of the causal chemical agent. Older men seem to be more susceptible to the action of these carcinogens and the length of the exposure affects their chances of developing a tumour, but exposures of less than 1 year to β-naphthylamine or benzidine, or mixed exposures, do carry a definite risk of bladder tumours.

Experimental cancer of the bladder

During recent decades considerable research work has been carried out on experimental bladder cancer, using different chemical substances, including β-naphthylamine, 2-acetylaminofluorene and azo compounds. This work has been helpfully summarised by Bonser *(1947)*, who pointed out the difficulties which were encountered in the research, including the complicated factors of species, strains and diets in the experiments. She considered trials of different species and strains to be essential, in spite of the considerable expenditure of labour entailed, and stated that, in addition to its value concerning the relation of bladder cancer to the dye industry, the research seemed likely to provide an important link in the investigations of cancer in general.

It has been possible to reproduce cancer of the bladder in a number of experimental species by using aromatic amines. Clayson *(1970)* stated that all chemicals of the aromatic amine type which induce tumours in animals are likely to induce tumours in humans also, so that workers in industries where these chemicals are used must be adequately protected against their dangerous potential action. He pointed out that there is no guarantee that an animal carcinogen will necessarily be effective in humans and that direct inspection of its chemical structure is of little or no value. Some aromatic amines require metabolic activation to make them effective carcinogens. He illustrated his observation by the fact that tumours induced by aromatic amines do not arise on the route of entry into the experimental animal, that is, in the mouth, larynx, oesophagus and stomach, but along the routes of excretion, in the urinary tract, including the bladder, the liver and the intestines. He stated that when a pellet containing an aromatic amine suspended in paraffin wax or cholesterol is implanted surgically in the lumen of the bladder of the mouse, relatively few tumours are produced, but if certain metabolites are similarly implanted many tumours develop. In addition, on systemic administration to animals, certain of the activated metabolites have been shown to be more potent carcinogens than the amines.

THE BROAD SPECTRUM OF OCCUPATIONAL CANCER

The early clinical observations and research concerning cancer of the skin and urinary bladder are considered here in some detail because of their historical interest and importance, for they describe the development of occupational cancer as a distinct subject. Kennaway *(1957)* stressed the immense practical and academic value of the research, calling attention to the data concerning the incubation period of cancer, which he defined as "the time of exposure to the carcinogen and of any interval after it before neoplasia begins".

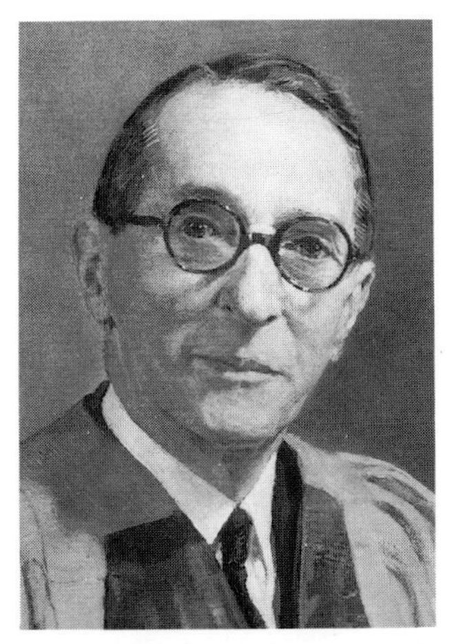

Figure 17.3 John T. Ingram (1899–1972), Professor of Dermatology, University of Newcastle upon Tyne.

The subject of occupational skin cancer was discussed in detail by Ingram and Comaish *(1967)*, who stated that every consideration of industrial carcinogens must include the environmental influences from social, domestic, therapeutic and industrial sources, because of their additive and summation effects. They called attention to the large number of cases of skin cancers recorded in England, which were caused chiefly by contact with coal-soot, tar pitch, creosote, anthracene oils, wax and arsenicals.

Mule-spinners' cancer of the scrotum and vulva in the cotton industry, caused by mineral oils, paraffin, or their residues, became a notifiable disease in 1926. Ingram and Comaish pointed out that the largest incidence of occupational cancer occurred in workers in industries concerned with coal-tar and its derivatives: pitch, tar oils and creosote.

The effects of arsenic are seen in metal workers and smelters, handlers of insecticides and sheep dip and in vineyard workers. Ingram and Comaish stated that the danger arises more from inhalation and ingestion than from skin contact. They called attention to the fact that Jonathan Hutchinson was the first to describe the carcinogenic effects of the treatment of psoriasis with arsenic in the year 1887.

Ionising radiation is also a risk in medical practice and in industries, but monitoring the dosage and good protection arrangements against exposure have practically eliminated it.

Hueper *(1957)* wrote a valuable and comprehensive account of industrial and occupational cancer and included many references to the literature on the subject. He described in detail the significance and scope of the environmental cancer problem, including the nature of the exposure and the organs affected. In addition to the organic chemical carcinogens, there are several inorganic chemical carcinogens, including asbestos, chromates and nickel, as well as arsenic.

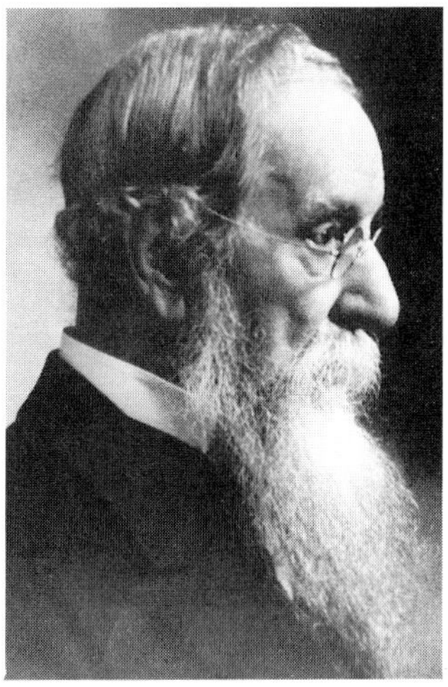

Figure 17.4 Sir Jonathan Hutchinson (1828–1913).

The cancer risk from exposure to asbestos is well recognised today and every effort is taken to protect people from its serious effects. Newhouse *(1970)* stated that the association between lung cancer and asbestos was already known in 1935 and she quoted the work of Doll and his colleagues, who in 1955 published the results of the analysis of deaths at a large textile asbestos factory, which showed that the risk of developing lung cancer was about 10 times higher in the factory workers than in the general population. Asbestos Industry Regulations were brought into effect in 1931. Newhouse studied factory workers first employed between the years 1933 and 1948 (after regulations were introduced) and found that the risk of dying of lung cancer amongst those in dusty work was still very high, not only in those who had long exposure but also in those who worked at the factory for only short periods.

Mesothelioma is another dangerous malignant tumour associated with exposure to asbestos. It can affect both the pleura and the peritoneum and is mainly occupational in origin. This subject was considered by Harington *(1967)*, who pointed out that the measures taken to prevent lung cancer

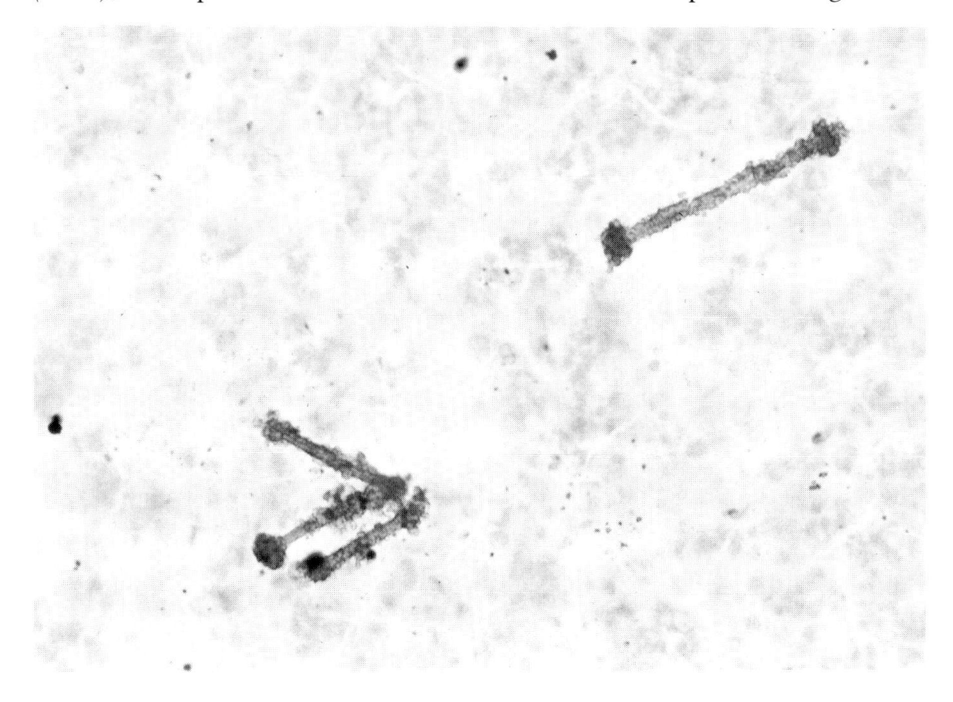

Figure 17.5 Asbestos bodies associated with the development of cancer of the lung.

arising from exposure to asbestos should be used, with stricter application, to prevent mesothelioma. Such measures consist in the suppression of asbestos dust and air pollution from it, wherever asbestos is used, even in limited quantities and on limited occasions.

CANCER CAUSED BY MEDICAMENTS

It has been known for more than 100 years that certain substances which are used as medicines can cause cancer at various sites, and during recent decades this risk has attracted more attention. The screening of new pharmaceutical products and the observation of their effects are necessary today, when an ever-increasing number are prescribed. There is a wide range of products, which includes hormones, antimicrobial medicines, cancer chemotherapy agents and several metals. This subject was reviewed by Roe *(1967)*.

The earliest observations which concern us here were related to arsenical cancer and emphasised the importance of recognising cancers which are caused by medicaments. Special reference is made to Neubauer's review of arsenical cancer, published for the Medical Research Council in 1947, which also contains a valuable list of references on the subject.

Neubauer *(1947)* stated that Sir Jonathan Hutchinson first directed attention to the role of arsenical drugs in the origination of skin cancer (already alluded to earlier in this chapter), when in 1887–1888 he described five cases which indicated that large doses of arsenic administered internally over long periods might cause cancer with certain peculiarities. In three patients local keratosis preceded the development of cancer. In one patient the cancerous ulcer had developed in rough skin situated at the side of the trunk; in another patient on a corn in the skin of the scrotum; and in others in keratotic areas in the skin of the hands or feet.

Neubauer noted that before Hutchinson made his observations Pozzi (1874), Tillaux (1877), Cartaz (1878), White (1885) and Hebra (1887) had reported cases of skin cancer occurring in psoriasis, but they had not associated the development of cancer with the previous administration of arsenicals for the treatment of psoriasis.

Neubauer's review contains a table which lists 143 patients with arsenical cancer, 125 of whom had a known disease that had been treated with arsenic. Eighty-nine patients (71.2%) had skin diseases and 67 of these (53.6%) had psoriasis. Thirty-six patients (28.8%) had other diseases which had been treated with arsenic, including epilepsy and "fits" (11 cases); asthma and bronchitis (six cases); complexion complaints for which arsenic had been given as a "tonic" (four cases); and others.

Arsenical cancer can occur in organs other than the skin, for Neubauer reported the association of skin cancers with cancers of the stomach, tongue, buccal mucosa, uterus, bronchus, urethra and oesophagus. He also mentioned the occurrence of papilloma of the ureter and bladder. In some cases, after the administration of arsenic cancers occurred in different organs, such as the breast and pancreas, without the development of skin cancer, but these patients had skin keratosis.

Neubauer discussed the incubation period, that is, the time interval between starting arsenical medication and the beginning of cancer. This period showed a wide variation, from 3 years to 40 years, the average being

18.1 years. There was no marked difference in the incubation period for the different forms of cancer.

Other forms of arsenical cancer were also described by Neubauer and he quoted Eggers, who stated that Lambe in 1809 believed that arsenic in potable water might cause malignant disease. He considered that cancer caused by the arsenical content of drinking water is apparently identical with medicinal arsenical cancer.

Neubauer states that there is no satisfactory theory concerning the pathogenesis of arsenical cancer in spite of all the clinical observations and experimental work devoted to the subject. To explain the predilection of arsenical cancer for the skin, he stated that arsenic has a special affinity for structures of epidermal origin, and that after its ingestion it accumulates in the epidermis, sweat and sebaceous glands and ducts, hair follicles and hairs. It may affect these tissues as an irritant, causing keratosis and malignancy. He postulated, however, that arsenic is not the only causative factor; others include a variability in the sensitivity of the individual to arsenic; variations in the excretion of arsenic, with longer retention in the epidermis; predisposition of the skin, such as local sensitivity; and hereditary factors.

Finally he quoted Eggers *(1932)*, who summarised the facts and concluded: "Arsenic is an agent that seems to cause a decided increase in the predisposition to cancer, so that an added element of irritation, which under ordinary conditions would be inadequate, comes into operation."

The early observations which are described here were largely concerned with cancers of the skin and urinary bladder. They form a valuable and firm foundation upon which the subject of carcinogens and carcinogenesis has been gradually built. Later observations regarded the relationship of environmental carcinogens with cancers of the respiratory system and other organs. The great importance of life-style, habits and customs in the risk of cancer is clearly understood today. History also shows how cancer hazards have become more serious due to the expansion of industries, with the use of an ever-increasing number of different chemical substances and radioactive materials. The recognition of environmental cancer hazards has presented us with the valuable and practical concept of cancer prevention.

EARLY EXPERIMENTAL RESEARCH IN CANCER

Experiments with coal-tar

A fundamental contribution to our knowledge of exogenous carcinogens was made through research carried out by the Japanese scientists Yamagiwa and Ichikawa. They commenced their work in 1914 and published their first account of it both in Japanese and in English in 1918. They made their experiments in accordance with the viewpoint of Yamagiwa that "the repetition or continuation of chronic irritation may cause a precancerous alteration in epithelium previously normal. If the action of the irritant continues, carcinoma may be the outcome, even though no particular agent has been interpolated" *(Yamagiwa, 1905)*.

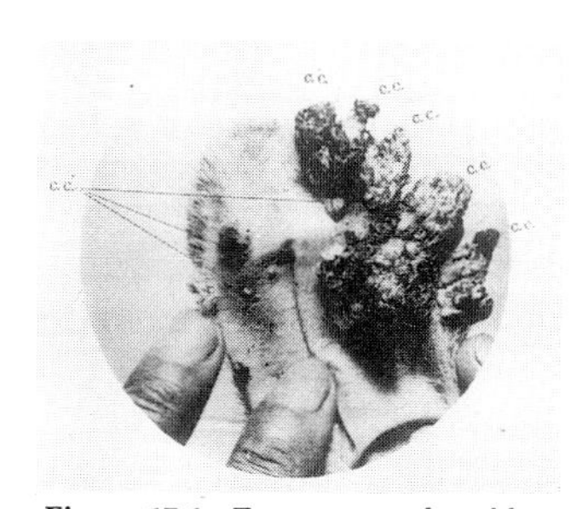
Figure 17.6 Tumours produced by Yamagiwa and Ichikawa in the skin of the ear of a rabbit by painting it with coal-tar (1918).

For their experiments they selected the ear of the domestic rabbit, where no spontaneous neoplasm has ever been reported, and they painted coal-tar on its inner surface. This is a simple technique and a method of causing mechanical or chemical irritation which they found to be most efficacious in producing carcinoma. They were already familiar with the occurrence of carcinoma in workers with coal-tar and they cited the investigations of Vollkmann, Liebe, Tillmanns and Schuchardt, pointing out that coal-tar carcinoma had not yet been produced by the experimental method.

Their expectations from these experiments were rewarded when it was proved that folliculoepitheliomas developed in nearly all the ears of the animals, after a period of over 100 days had elapsed from the time of the first application of coal-tar. In the ear of one animal 20 neoplasms developed. They recorded that the size of the tumours varied from that of a grain of rice to that of a sparrow's egg. Later, when some of the tumours showed a more malignant character, they proved both macroscopically and microscopically that they had produced eight cases of carcinoma in its earliest stage, 16 cases of carcinoma in its early stage, and seven cases of carcinoma which was more fully developed. In addition to the local malignant disease, they also demonstrated metastases in the lymph nodes at the root of the ear and in the submaxillary region in two of the last seven animals with carcinoma.

The same researchers studied the histology of these lesions in the ear and described in detail four periods of development. In the first period there was an atypical growth of epithelium with hyperplasia, which was especially marked at the periphery of the hair follicles. The duration of this period varied from 30 to 350 days, the average being 100 days. The second period was characterised by the appearance of folliculoepithelioma with a marked degree of hyperplasia and hyperkeratosis and from the affected areas neoplasms arose which they divided into pedunculated and sessile folliculo-epithelioma. In the third period carcinoma was produced. The fourth period was the stage of metastases which developed in the regional lymph nodes of two animals.

The description given by Yamagiwa and Ichikawa of the earliest stage of carcinoma is so interesting that it is quoted in detail here. "All or a part of the epithelium of these new growths assumes a fainter stain with hematoxylin than does normal epithelium, or that of benign folliculoepithelioma; the sprout-like processes developed by atypical proliferation of the basal epithelium of the hair follicle become more angular at their basal layer and the processes grow very irregular in thickness; the interstitial connective tissue becomes looser, or shows a slight mucous degeneration; lateral and downward penetration of the cancerous epithelium can be demonstrated."

These researchers also produced seven carcinomas on the inner surface of the ears of seven rabbits after further applications of coal-tar; histologically these tumours closely resembled the spontaneous carcinomas that occur in humans.

In the summary of their article, they stated that Yamagiwa's hypothesis, which is quoted earlier in this chapter, had been confirmed.

The identification and synthesis of 3:4 benzpyrene

After the successful and fundamental research work in rabbits carried out by Yamagiwa and Ichikawa, several decades elapsed before the next big advance was made by Kennaway and his colleagues at the Cancer Hospital and Chester Beatty Research Institute (now the Royal Marsden Hospital and Institute of Cancer Research, London). These scientists isolated and synthesised the carcinogenic chemical in coal-tar. Their brilliant research is an outstanding landmark in the history of experimental cancer research and it is an abiding witness of the results that can be achieved by the coordinated efforts of a team of scientists with able and imaginative leadership.

The leader of this particular team, Sir Ernest Kennaway, wrote an authentic account of their research work towards the close of his career *(Kennaway, 1955)*.

The present author enjoyed the friendship of Kennaway and the members of his scientific staff at the Chester Beatty Research Institute, when he was working as Surgical Registrar at the associated Cancer Hospital. He vividly recalls those exciting years of discoveries in cancer research and shared the staff's enthusiasm engendered by the outstanding research carried out during the decade 1930–1939.

Kennaway compiled his narration of the research in consultation with his collaborators, for he fully recognised the important contributions made by each member of his team and he desired that the honours for the work should be shared by all concerned.

The present author has drawn freely from the writings of Kennaway and his colleagues and acknowledges his great indebtedness to them in this chapter. He recognises the importance of accuracy in recording historical events and data which are of outstanding interest to posterity. This is indeed a fascinating record of scientific achievement which will interest readers in the years to come.

Earlier research

In 1922 Kennaway joined Archibald Leitch on the staff of the Research Institute of the Cancer Hospital (Free), as this combined institution was originally called. It later became known as the Royal Marsden Hospital and Institute of Cancer Research, and in the interim as the Chester Beatty Research Institute.

Kennaway then began his research to identify the cancer-producing chemical compound in coal-tar. He had learnt about its properties which had been discovered by Bruno Bloch, a dermatologist in Zurich *(Bloch and Dreifuss, 1921)*. These were: a high boiling point; neutral reaction; nitrogen and sulphur free and the substance was able to form a picrate. With his customary thoroughness Kennaway collected from the literature all the known data about those substances in coal-tar which possessed these particular properties and he also obtained specimens of those constituents.

During the next 2 years he carried out experiments with animals by applying anthracene, phenanthrene, retine, fluorene, acenaphthene, chuprene, truxene and picine to the skin of mice. The results were negative, but in a subsequent experiment chrysene produced one carcinoma on the 853rd day after its first application. These preliminary studies suggested that exposure to temperatures above a certain level was a factor in conferring carcinogenic activity on the chemical substances in question.

The temperature factor was investigated next by Kennaway and Frank Goulden, whose technical skill he commemorated in his article. They found that when pitch from gasworks was heated to 500 °F it produced a strongly carcinogenic distillate and they also obtained carcinogenic products by heating various substances to temperatures of 700–900 °F in an atmosphere of hydrogen. These substances included a non-carcinogenic sample of petroleum, isoprene ($CH_2:C(CH_3)CH:CH_2$) and acetylene. In addition, there were various biological products, including cholesterol, yeast, human skin, hair and muscle.

The details of the experimental work are clearly described in an article by Kennaway *(1925)*, where he also stresses the earlier classical experiments of Berthelot, carried out in 1866, and their relevance to his own work. He quoted Berthelot's original and concise account of his research *(Berthelot, 1866)*: "L'acetylène chaliffé dans une cloche combe à une température voisine de la fusion du verre, se transforme peu à peu en polymères ... après une suite fastidieuse de manipulations méthodique ... j'ai isolé ... benzene, styrolène, carbures fluorescents, rétène ..."

At that time Kennaway related his experimental work on tar carcinogenesis not only to industrial cancers in humans, but also with the possible explanation of more important cancers which are caused by internal factors. He postulated that those chemical reactions which require high temperatures *in vitro* must, if they occur within the body, be brought about by other means.

The Schroeter reaction

Kennaway states that in 1923 he had read an article by Schroeter, written in 1920, which described the production from tetralin (tetrahydronaphthalene), at a temperature of 30–40 °F, by the action of 1.5% aluminium chloride, of a number of more complex compounds, amongst which benzene, octahydroanthracene, octahydrophenanthrene, a-phenyl-g-2-tetralyl-butane, 2:6-ditetralyl, and dodecahydrotriphenylene were identified. The low-temperature products were tested for their carcinogenicity and within 2 years, using preparations made by Schroeter's method and its modifications, Kennaway and his colleagues obtained 110 cancers in 496 mice. He considered that although the carcinogen in the mixture had not been identified, in all probability it was 3:4 benzpyrene.

In 1924 Kennaway was joined in his research work by Izrael Hieger, who studied the Schroeter reactions with him. They made variations in the technique for obtaining Schroeter preparations, in addition to carrying out other research projects. They were encouraged in their work by the fact that a carcinogen could be prepared without recourse to pyrolysis, or even by the use of temperatures above body temperature.

The importance of a single scientific observation is illustrated by subsequent events, for Kennaway states that their work would have ceased at this stage had they not noted that the one vital feature of the Schroeter products was that they are vividly fluorescent in both ultraviolet light and in daylight. They made numerous entries in their notebooks concerning the frequency with which they were impressed by the beautiful blue-violet fluorescence of the distilled Schroeter fractions.

Fluorescence spectroscopy

It was most fortunate for Kennaway and his team at this crucial period of their research work that W. V. Mayneord (later Professor of Physics as applied to Medicine at the Institute of Cancer Research) joined the Depart-

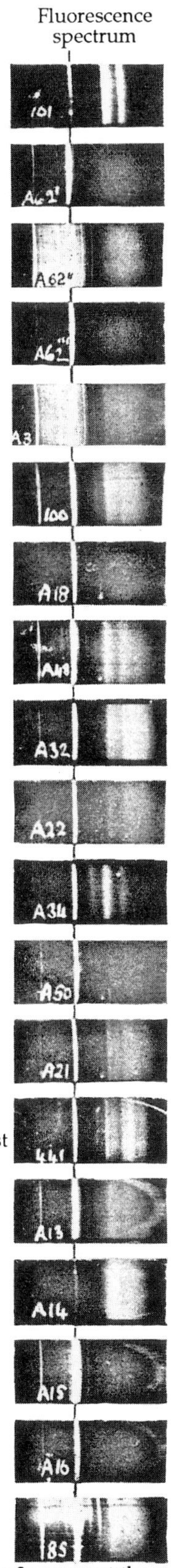

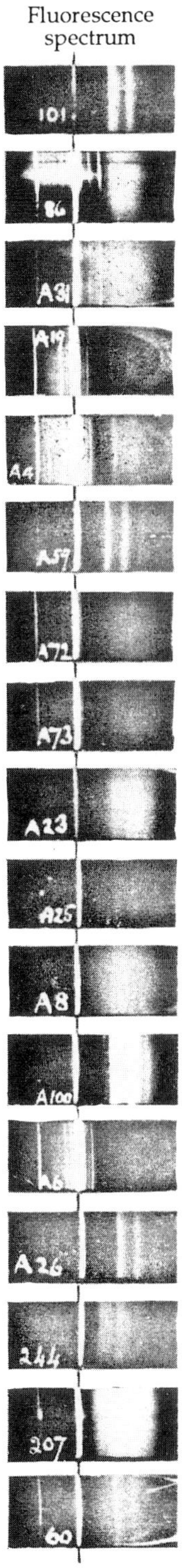

	Substance	Carcinogenic activity	Fluorescence spectrum
101	$AlCl_3$-treated tetralin	Active	
A62	Durham Holmside gasworks tar 450°	Active	
A62"	Durham Holmside gasworks tar 600°	Active	
A62'''	Durham Holmside gasworks tar 1250°	Active	
A3	Ether extract of gasworks tar	Active	
100	1% gasworks tar	Active	
A18	Blast furnace tar	Inactive	
A48	Creosote oil	Active	
A32	Anthracene oil	Active	
A22	Green oil	Active	
A34	Anthracene 85%	?	
A50	Pitch (medium soft)	Active	
A21	Pitch distillate	Active	
441	Pitch distillate 300–345°/ 4mm.	Under test	
A13	Shale oil (Pumpherston S)	Inactive	
A14	Shale oil (blue oil)	Active	
A15	Shale oil (Pumpherston R)	Inactive	
A16	Refined lubricating oil	Inactive	
85	Low temperature tar 350°	Active	
101	$AlCl_3$-treated tetralin	Active	
86	Spindle oil	Active	
A31	Unheated Californian petroleum	Inactive	
A19	Heated Californian petroleum 880°	Active	
A4	Acetylene tar	Active	
A50	Chlorinated acetylene tar	Active	
A72	Yeast tar	Active	
A73	Muscle tar	Active	
A23	Hair tar 800°	2/94	
A25	Cholesterol tar	Active	
A8	$AlCl_3$-treated naphthalens	1/50	
A100	Undistilled $AlCl_3$-treated tetralin	Inactive	
A6	Commercial tetralin	1/30	
A26	Tetroyl-propionic acid mother liq.	Inactive	
244	Residue from preparation of phenylnaphthalene	Active	
207	Oleic acid ("redistilled")	Inactive	
60	Benzyl oleate	Inactive	

The fractions in column 3 represent the ratio of tumour-bearing mice to total mice tested

Figure 17.7 The spectra of cancer-producing tars and oils and of related substances. *(From Hieger, I.)*

ment of Radiology at the Cancer Hospital in 1926 as part-time physicist, and became a full-time member of the staff in 1927.

Kennaway and his colleagues had in their laboratory a number of various higher-boiling fractions of coal-tar, including green oil, anthracene oil and the different Schroeter preparations. Mayneord was impressed by their conspicuous fluorescence and examined it by spectroscopy. He then observed that the same characteristic bands were to be found in the spectra of tars and other carcinogenic substances such as the Schroeter mixture. It is perhaps needless to record here that this contribution by Mayneord was acclaimed by his colleagues as the major fundamental observation.

Further developments

Early in 1927 Mayneord found that on spectroscopy the Schroeter products showed two very distinct bands in the blue and violet regions of the spectrum. He photographed more than 100 fluorescence spectra of various non-carcinogenic hydrocarbons and those of the carcinogenic preparations and found that the same bands were seen in the spectra of the majority of the latter group.

He was then joined by Hieger and they examined the spectra of all the tars made in the laboratory from acetylene, human tissues, shale oil, pitch distillate and various fractions and extracts of coal-tar. None of these substances showed these bands as distinctly as the Schroeter preparations. They next examined the fluorescence spectra of as many types of the hydrocarbons present in tar as were available, to find some hint of the source of the specific "cancer bands", but unfortunately without any success.

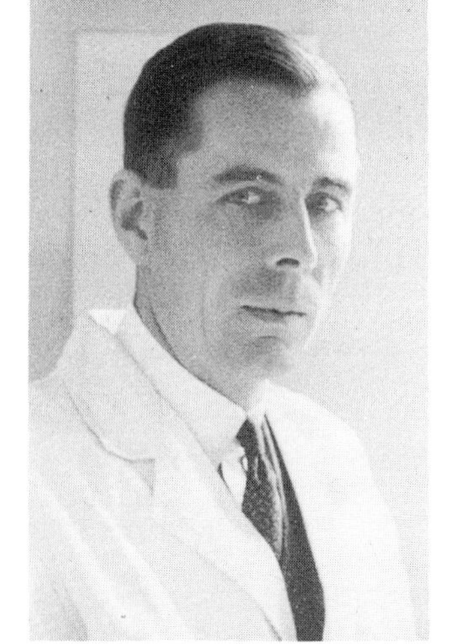

Figure 17.8 Sir James Cook.

In 1928 Hieger consulted E. de Barry Barnett about the problem. The latter was the author of a standard work on anthracene and anthraquinone and Head of the Department of Organic Chemistry at the Sir John Cass College. This proved to be a most valuable connection, as J. W. Cook (later Sir James Cook), who was Barnett's assistant at that time, sent Hieger some samples of polycyclic hydrocarbons for fluorescence spectroscopy. One of these was 1:2 benzanthracene, the fluorescence of which was so similar to that of the Schroeter mixture that there was no doubt that they were closely allied compounds. The two spectra are practically identical, but that of the hydrocarbon lies in the region of the longer wavelength.

Kennaway states that the next move at this exciting stage of their researches was to seek some derivative of 1:2-benzanthracene which by an intramolecular addition would show the vibration of fluorescence and cause a shift to a longer wavelength.

THE FIRST SYNTHETIC CARCINOGENS

In 1929 Kennaway read an article in *British Chemical Abstracts* about the work of E. Clar *(1929)* of Dresden, who synthesised 1:2:5:6-dibenzanthracene. Kennaway's assistant Goulden then prepared this compound and its 3′-methyl derivative by using the method of Fieser and Dietz *(1929)*. It was found that both compounds were carcinogenic when applied to the skin of mice. The fluorescence spectrum consisted of the Schroeter bands in a position intermediate between those of Schroeter and 1:2-benzanthracene.

These were the first carcinogens to be synthesised and they were prepared later by Cook in a highly purified form.

Additional papers were published by Clar and his colleagues *(1929)* on the synthesis of polycyclic hydrocarbons, and their methods were used by Goulden during the same year to prepare a number of chemical compounds for preliminary tests for carcinogenicity in mice. Three of them were found to be carcinogenic, namely, 1:2:5:6-dibenzanthracene and its 3′-methyl derivative, and 1:2:3:4-dibenzanthracene. The compound 1:2:5:6-dibenzanthracene was found to possess undiminished carcinogenicity in very high purification, it was active in nine different media and produced skin cancer in a concentration of 0.003% in benzene *(Kennaway and colleagues, 1932)*.

Fractionation of pitch

No less than 2 tons of pitch were fractionated by the Gas Light and Coke Company at their Becton works through W. Gordon Adam. The resulting soft, reddish-black, heavy extract was sent to Kennaway's laboratory, where it was fractionally distilled at low pressure, differentially extracted, picrated, and crystallised. This was a task of considerable magnitude and was guided by the fluorescent spectrum and the assay of carcinogenicity by application to the skin of mice. The various fractions showed a correspondence between the intensity of the Schroeter bands and the carcinogenic potency. Kennaway stressed the value of the fluorescence spectrum and this directed attention to the benzanthracene type of molecular structure.

Identification and synthesis of 3:4 benzpyrene

In 1931, during the final stage of their series of experiments, the Kennaway

1.2-Benzanthracene

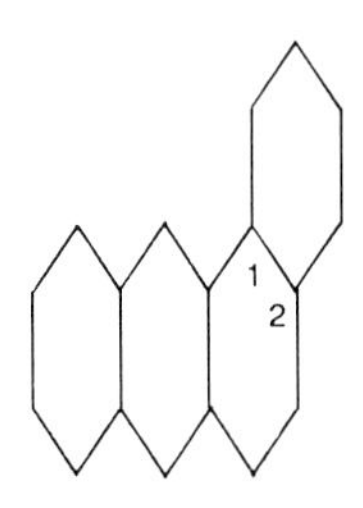

Dibenzanthracenes

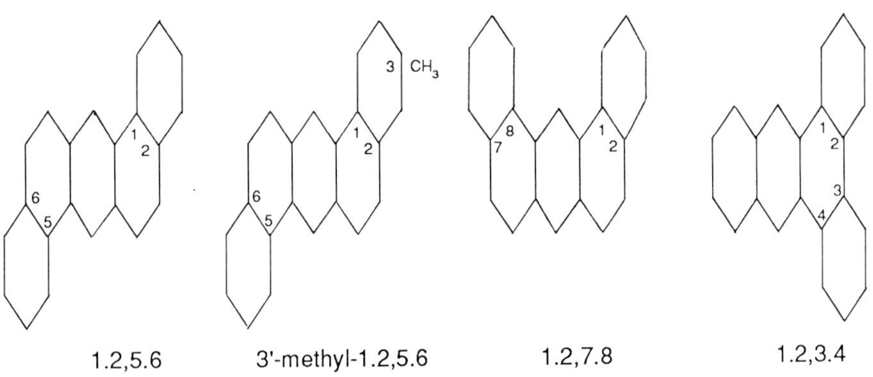

Figure 17.9 The chemical formulae of 1:2 benzanthracene and the dibenzanthracenes. *(From Kennaway, E. L., and Hieger, I.)*

group of scientists was joined by C. L. Hewett, and a batch of crystalline material was fractionated further under the direction of Cook. Several other compounds (2:3-benzcarbazole, chrysene and perylene) were separated from the final fractions of crystals, which melted at 160 °F. The crystalline material with this melting point was of dubious homogeneity. Cook *(1932)* isolated from it two pure crystalline products with melting points of 176 °F and 187 °F, respectively. These were found to be uncommonly rich in carbon and both appeared to be isomeric with the highly condensed pentacyclic aromatic hydrocarbon, perylene. The major component, the one with the melting point of 176 °F, showed the characteristic spectrum discussed already, in high dilution.

Cook and Hewett concluded that they might find it easier to identify the two hydrocarbons if they prepared for comparison synthetic specimens of the then unknown pentacyclic hydrocarbons isomeric with perylene, 3:4 benzpyrene and 1:2 benzpyrene. They did this by methods which established unequivocally the structure of the synthetic products. It was shown that 3:4 benzpyrene was identical with the strongly fluorescing major component of the crystals prepared from pitch distillate. The synthetic preparation (3:4 benzpyrene), with a melting point of 177 °F, was also highly carcinogenic. The synthetic 1:2 benzpyrene was identical with the minor component (the melting point 187 °F) of the original crystallate.

For their remarkable achievements the five members of the research team were awarded the first Anna Fuller Memorial Prize in 1939 "in recognition of their notable accomplishments in the fields of Cancer Research, specifically for the isolation and synthesis of cancer-producing hydrocarbons from coal-tar, the identification by fluorescence spectroscopy, and for the study of the biological effects of these substances".

The present author has quoted freely above from Kennaway's own description of the research work *(1955)*. Other references consulted were Kennaway *(1925)*, Kennaway and Hieger *(1930)*, Hieger *(1930)*, Cook and colleagues *(1932)* and Cook and colleagues *(1933)*.

THE MECHANISM OF CARCINOGENESIS

For many decades research scientists have sought the solution to this perplexing and intricate problem. Our knowledge on the subject 30 years ago was summarised in a helpful review by Peacock *(1957)*. It has increased considerably since then, especially during recent years noteworthy with studies concerning cell cycle genes and oncogenes. Peacock suggested that the induction of a malignant tumour depends on more factors than the actual contact between the carcinogen and the living cell. He considered that most tumours arise from a number of cells in an organ or tissue as a result of a locally-acting carcinogenic factor to which many more cells are exposed without undergoing any neoplastic change. He stated that various changes might follow contact between the carcinogen and the living cell: the cells might die; other cells might successfully metabolise the carcinogen into a harmless derivative; cells might be permanently changed but never be able to reproduce themselves; or they might start to reproduce but be controlled before a tumour is recognised. A recognisable tumour proves that cellular carcinogenesis has occurred.

Haddow *(1958)* (later Sir Alexander Haddow), who succeeded Sir Ernest Kennaway as Director of the Chester Beatty Research Institute, called attention to the importance of considering genetics in any study of the mechanism of carcinogenesis. He explained that there can be little doubt about the importance of the combination of the carcinogens with genetic material, or its precursors, especially those which function as carcinogens through biological alkylation. He stated that the primary step might be the inhibition of certain fundamental processes of genetical or enzyme synthesis, followed by the generation of new self-duplicating fibre or template chemically modified and hence genetically modified also.

The subject of carcinogenesis was reviewed by Warwick *(1973)*, who included an extensive list of references in the literature. He stated that cancer must not be regarded as an inevitable result of the aging process and he pointed out that carcinogenesis is grossly modified by different variables, including age, diet, hormones, immunological status and the presence of conditioning factors such as pre-existing diseases and chemical additives. He reported that many workers think that the interaction of carcinogens with DNA is responsible for at least the first stage of carcinogenesis, but others consider that cancer is caused by a fault in cellular differentiation and therefore that the interaction of carcinogens with one of the various forms of RNA might be most important. He called attention to the importance of cell proliferation in carcinogenesis and its possible involvement in the process of tumour initiation and he pointed out that human tumours often occur in areas of higher than normal proliferative activity, such as hyperplastic nodules, cirrhotic nodules, leucoplakia and tropical ulcers.

The influence of diet on carcinogenesis

For many years much consideration has been given to this important aspect of carcinogenesis. Warwick deals with it in some detail, stating that there is little doubt that protein levels and vitamin concentrations can influence carcinogenesis at least at the level of enzymatic activation of carcinogens. Attention has been focused on vitamin A deficiency, for it can give rise to squamous metaplasia of epithelial tissues and it is necessary to maintain the integrity of certain varieties of epithelium. It is known that vitamin A has an inhibitory effect on the development of cancers induced by chemicals at various sites.

Viral carcinogenesis

Warwick *(1973)* also discussed aspects of viral carcinogenesis and stressed its importance. He stated that Huebner and Todaro in 1969 propounded the oncogene hypothesis in an attempt to explain various aspects of carcinogenesis, including the fact that cancer is caused by virus in some animals. He explained, as the basis for the hypothesis, that mammalian cells contain genes (oncogenes) which when expressed release the particular cells from the constraints regulating their normal growth pattern, so that they become malignant. Further reference is made to this subject in Chapter 22.

Carcinogenesis is a multidisciplinary subject, for valuable information can be obtained from several basic sciences, including virology, immunology and epidemiology, and this re-emphasises the fact that the oncologist should have a broad spectrum of knowledge embracing many different sciences.

REFERENCES

Berthelot, M. (1866). Les polymères de l'acetylène. I: Synthèse de la benzine. *Compt. Rend. Acad. Sci. (Paris)*, **63**, 479–84

Bloch, B. T. and Dreifuss, W. (1921). Experimental tar cancer. *Schweiz Med. Wochenschr.*, **51**, 1033–7

Bonser, G. M. (1947). Experimental cancer of the bladder. *Br. Med. Bull.*, **4**, 379–85

Butlin, H. T. (1892). Cancer of the scrotum in chimney-sweeps and others. *Br. Med. J.*, **1**, 1341–6

Case, R. A. M., Hosker, M. E., McDonald, D. B. and Pearson, J. T. (1954). Tumours of the urinary bladder in workmen employed in the manufacture and use of certain dyestuff intermediates in the British chemical industry. *Br. J. Indust. Med.*, **11**, 75–104

Clar, E. (1929). Polynuclear aromatic hydrocarbons and their derivatives. I. Dibenzanthracene and its quinones. IV. Naphthaphenanthrones and their quinones. *Br. Chem. Abstracts*, Vol. A, pp 435 and 922

Clar, E. (1929). Zur Kenntnis mehrkerniger aromatischer Kohlen-Wasserstoffe und ihrer Abkömmlinge. I. Dibenzanthracene und ihre Chinone. *Ber. Dtsch. Chem. Gesselsch.*, **62**, 350–9

Clar, E. (1929). Zur Kenntnis mehrkerniger aromatischer Kohlen-Wasserstoffe und ihre Abkömmlinge. IV. Naphthophen-anthrene und ihre Chinone. *Ber. Dtsch. Chem. Gesellsch.*, **62**, 1574–82

Clayson, D. B. (1970). Industrial bladder cancer induced by aromatic amines. In Raven, R. W. (ed.) *Symposium on the Prevention of Cancer*, pp 46–57. Heinemann Medical Books, London

Cook, J. W. (1932). The production of cancer by pure hydrocarbons. Part II. *Proc. Roy. Soc.*, **BIII**, 485–96

Cook, J. W., Hewett, C. L. and Hieger, I. (1933). The isolation of a cancer-producing hydrocarbon from coal-tar. Parts 1, 2 and 3. *J. Chem. Soc.*, April, 395–405

Cook, J. W., Hieger, I., Kennaway, E. L. and Mayneord, W. V. (1932). The production of cancer by pure hydrocarbons. *Proc. Roy. Soc.*, **BIII**, 455–84

Eggers, H. E. (1932). The etiology of cancer. *Arch. Path.*, **13**, 296–320

Fieser, L. F. and Dietz, E. M. (1929). Beitrag zur Kenntnis der Synthese von mehrkernigen Anthracenen (Bemerkungen zu einer Arbeit von E. Clar). *Ber. Dtsch. Chem. Gesellsch.*, **62**, 1827–33

Goldblatt, M. V. (1947). Occupational cancer of the bladder. *Br. Med. Bull.*, **4**, 405–17

Haddow, A. (1958). Chemical carcinogens and their modes of action. *Br. Med. Bull.*, **14**, 79–92

Harington, J. S. (1967). Mesothelioma. In Raven, R. W. and Roe, F. J. C. (eds) *The Prevention of Cancer*, pp 207–11. Butterworth & Co., London

Henry, S. A. (1946). *Cancer of the Scrotum in Relation to Occupation.* Oxford University Press, London

Hieger, I. (1930). The spectra of cancer-producing tars and oils and of related substances. *Biochem. J.*, **24** (2), 505–11

Huebner, R. J. and Todaro, G. J. (1969). Oncogenes of RNA tumor viruses as determinants of cancer. *Proc. Natl. Acad. Sci., USA*, **64**, 1087–94

Hueper, W. C. (1957). Environmental factors in the production of human cancer. In Raven, R. W. (ed.) *Cancer*, Vol. 1, pp 404–96. Butterworth & Co., London

Ingram, J. T. and Comaish, S. (1967). Occupational cancer of the skin. In Raven, R. W. and Roe, F. J. C. (eds) *The Prevention of Cancer*, pp 216–25. Butterworth & Co., London

Kennaway, E. L. (1925). Experiments on cancer-producing substances. *Br. Med. J.*, **2**, 1–4

Kennaway, E. L. (1955). Identification of carcinogenic compound in coal-tar. *Br. Med. J.*, **2**, 749–52

Kennaway, E. L. (1957). The incubation period of cancer in man. In Raven, R. W. (ed.) *Cancer*, Vol. 1, pp 6–23. Butterworth & Co., London

Kennaway, E. L. and Hieger, I. (1930). Carcinogenic substances and their fluorescence spectra. *Br. Med. J.*, **1**, 1044–6

Kennaway, E. L. (1932). See under Cook, J. W. *et al.* (1932)

Neubauer, O. (1947). Arsenical cancer; review. *Br. J. Cancer*, **1**, 192–251

Newhouse, M. L. (1970). Industrial hazards of cancer including skin. In Raven, R. W. (ed.) *Symposium on the Prevention of Cancer*, pp 38–45. Heinemann Medical Books, London

Peacock, P. R. (1957). Carcinogenesis. In Raven, R. W. (ed.) *Cancer*, Vol. 1, pp 32–75. Butterworth & Co., London

Pott, P. (1775). *Chirurgical Observations Relative to the Cataract, the Polypus of the Nose, the Cancer of the Scrotum etc.* Hawes, Clarke and Collins, London

Rehn, L. (1895). Uerber Blasentumoren bei Fuchsinarbeitern. *Arch. klin. Chir.*, **50**, 588–600

Roe, F. J. C. (1967). Pharmaceutical products. In Raven, R. W. and Roe, F. J. C. (eds) *The Prevention of Cancer*, pp 34–42. Butterworth & Co., London

Warwick, G. P. (1973). Newer aspects of carcinogenesis. In Raven, R. W. (ed.) *Modern Trends in Oncology*, Part 1: Research Progress, pp 61–97. Butterworth & Co., London

Yamagiwa, K. and Ichikawa, K. (1914). *Verhandl d. japanischen path. Gesellsch.* Tokyo

Yamagiwa, K. and Ichikawa, K. (1918). Experimental study of the pathogenesis of carcinoma. *J. Cancer Res.*, **3**, 1–21

Yamagiwa, K. (1905). Zur Histo- und Pathogenese des Magencarcinoms. *Nisshin-Igaku*, Vol. 3, No. 4. Tokyo

CHAPTER EIGHTEEN

Epidemiology

This scientific discipline has grown rapidly and considerably during recent decades and it has contributed substantially to oncology. It has provided many important clues regarding the aetiology of the oncological diseases and will doubtless continue to do so in the future. We recall again the original observations made by Percivall Pott in 1775 concerning the occurrence of scrotal skin cancer in chimney-sweeps, which eventually led to the identification and synthesis of chemical carcinogens.

Epidemiology is a very important scientific discipline today, which is divided into the following three main sections:

(1) Descriptive epidemiology studies and evaluates cancer risks occurring in large population groups, and the geographical incidence of different forms of cancer.
(2) Analytical epidemiology studies and investigates the causes of different cancers in specific individuals and the reasons for cancer aggregations in different people.
(3) Metabolic epidemiology is concerned with the study of physical and chemical environmental factors which cause cancer.

A detailed review of the subject was given by Steiner *(1958)*, who summarised the position of this basic science 30 years ago. He stated that it is concerned with the aetiology and nature of cancer and also with the size and composition of the detection and therapeutic problem for cancer control. He discussed important aspects of the subject, including geographical, ethnic, occupational, social and economic, age, sex and intrinsic factors, which clearly illustrate how it had begun to illuminate the cancer problem. He stated that a valuable result expected from geographical studies was the separation of environmental from intrinsic factors and their identification. (During succeeding decades our knowledge of these different factors has developed well.) He called attention to the discovery by Maxwell in 1879 of the Kangri skin carcinoma in Kashmir, one of the many important early contributions on the subject of causative factors.

Regarding social and economic factors, he made the interesting comment that this was a relatively new field in cancer epidemiology. As new knowledge has been gained since that time, considerable emphasis is now placed upon these factors, for life-style is extremely important in cancer causation and prevention.

Steiner included in his review the subject of "cancer epidemiology within the body", adding the explanation that conventional epidemiology, which used members of society as its material for study, could be extended to include other units such as societies of organs or of cell populations within the body. Regarding "cellular epidemiology", he pointed out that all the cells of the body are potential candidates for tumour formation; cancers, both spontaneous and induced, corresponding to almost every type of cell have been recognised. The site incidence of tumours is variable, suggesting that cells are not exposed equally or that they differ in susceptibility. Steiner stated that the interplay of these factors was a subject for study in cellular epidemiology.

GEOGRAPHICAL DISTRIBUTION OF CANCER

Observations regarding the incidence of cancer in different countries of the world have given us important information, not only about its actual prevalence but also about the sites in the body which are affected in patients of various nationalities.

Valuable work has been carried out by the Commission on Epidemiology and Prevention of the International Union Against Cancer. In 1966, as a result of their studies the UICC published *Cancer Incidence in Five Continents*. Following the Ninth International Cancer Congress in Tokyo the Commission formed a new Committee on Cancer Incidence, which decided that a second volume of that work should be published. This was prepared by the distinguished editors Doll, Muir and Waterhouse and published in 1970. The magnitude of the work is shown in the Introduction by Sir Richard Doll, who states that data are reported for 58 populations, 34 more than were included in Volume 1. Separate figures for the frequency of cancers of different histological types are included because, as he points out, cancers in any one organ may have many different causes and different causes may give rise to different histological varieties, so that variations in cancer incidence between different populations might be accentuated when tumour histology is considered in addition to the site of origin. This publication, which was an outstanding historical landmark, resulted from an enormous international effort and collaboration.

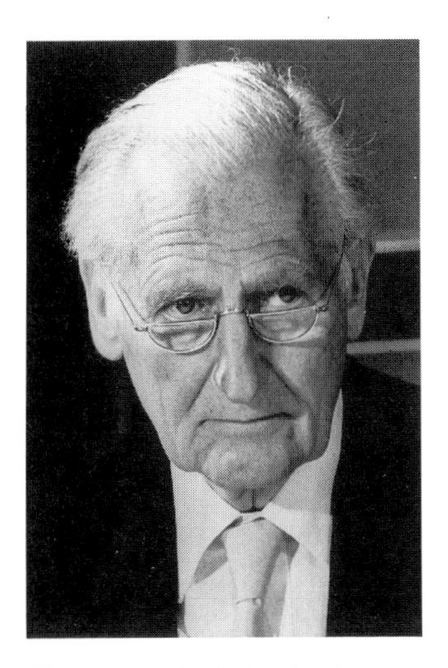

Figure 18.1 Sir Richard Doll.

The present author read with great interest the reference in the Preface to the work of his erstwhile friend George Oettlé, who had died. Oettlé was Director of the Cancer Research Unit of the South African Institute for Medical Research and the editors state that he was well known "for his demonstration, in conjunction with Dr John Higginson, that it was possible to obtain accurate cancer incidence figures for populations which lacked accurate mortality data. He inspired the collection of the new data for South African populations that are recorded here."

Information about the total annual mortality caused by cancer in England and Wales as well as about the mortality caused by cancer in different sites of the body has been made available in the Registrar-General's excellent *Statistic Review*. Data are also given regarding cancer mortality by age and sex. According to Stocks *(1958)*, this information has enabled cancer mortality trends to be assessed. In his article, which is copiously illustrated with tables and graphs, Stocks describes age-related mortality trends for all cancers except leukaemia and lymphadenoma, and also the trends for cancer affecting the main sites in the body. With regard to the first group, he states that the age-specific graphs show a general upward trend of male rates, apart from a period of stability between ages 50 and 65 from about 1925 to 1945, which is also shown by the cohort curves.

He states that female cancer rates have fallen continuously since 1915 for ages 40–60 and since about 1930 for higher ages. On the other hand, at early ages the rates have tended to rise.

The trends of cancer mortality in the main sites of the body are very instructive. Special reference is made to cancer of the lung and bronchus, where the trends are in remarkable contrast to those for other cancer sites.

Stocks states that for males the death rates at every age over 35 years increased continuously throughout the whole period from 1911 to 1954. Female rates behaved similarly, except that the increase began at a later date and the curves still had not flattened out (in 1958) except for ages under 40 years.

Special varieties of cancer

Burkitt's lymphoma

A malignant tumour arising in the jaws of African children was described by Burkitt *(1958–59)* and was recognised as a distinct clinical entity at Mulago Hospital in Uganda. Burkitt reported 38 cases of its occurrence and stated that in Uganda it was the commonest tumour in children aged between 2 and 14 years. In most patients it commenced in the region of the alveolar process of the maxilla or mandible, and the first symptom was the loosening of the deciduous molar teeth, which soon became embedded in the tumour. The tumour grew rapidly, causing gross deformity of the face, and later invaded the eye orbit, with resultant proptosis and then destruction of the eye.

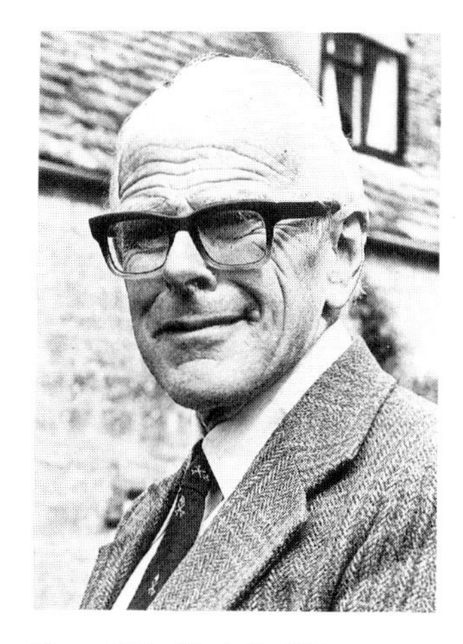

Figure 18.2 Denis Burkitt.

Less commonly the patient presented with a tumour which was high in the maxilla and invaded the eye orbit early on. The regional lymph nodes were not involved unless secondary infection had occurred in the tumour, but tumour metastases were found in many organs.

The histological appearance, initially described by O'Conor and Davies *(1960)*, was that of a highly malignant tumour, which in some cases resembled a lymphosarcoma; in many cases small tumour giant cells were present, similar to those seen in Hodgkin's disease.

Regarding the treatment of patients with early disease, Burkitt states that several years previously radical excision of the tumour was performed when this was feasible, but there had been tumour recurrence in the only patient who was traced, and surgical treatment was no longer advised. Radiotherapy was not available, but it was found that chemotherapy with nitrogen mustard administered intravenously caused temporary regression of the tumour.

Since this original description of the tumour by Burkitt, it has been recognised internationally as Burkitt's lymphoma and been of considerable

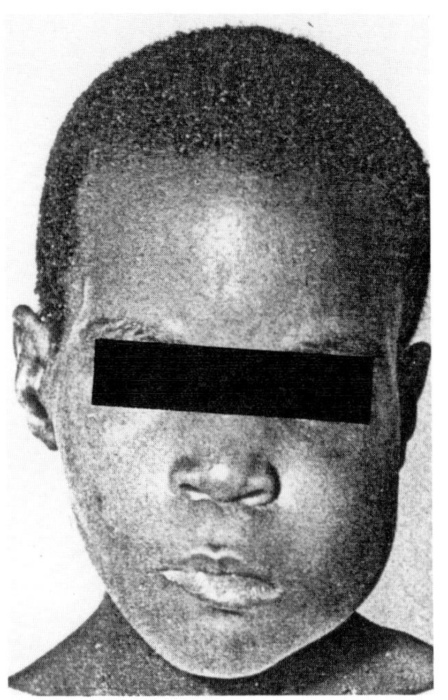
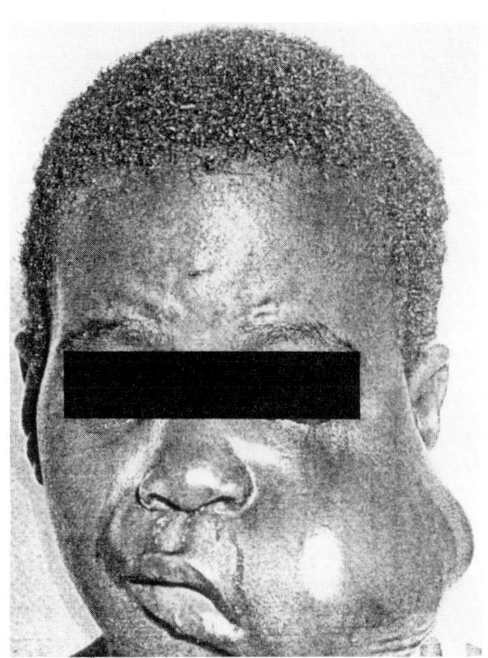

Figure 18.3 *Left:* A 10-year-old Ugandan girl with Burkitt's lymphoma in the left upper jaw. *Right:* This photograph taken 8 weeks later illustrates the rapid rate of growth.

interest to researchers and clinicians. Malignant lymphoma in African children is both a clinical syndrome *(Burkitt and O'Conor, 1961)* and a pathological entity *(O'Conor, 1961)*. The tumour was identified not only as a lymphoma, but also as a distinctive form of lymphoma *(Wright, 1963)*.

Epidemiological observations have shown that there is a geographical incidence pattern, which indicates a dependence on climatic factors and seems to implicate a biological agent *(Burkitt, 1962)*. Further study of the geographical distribution has indicated the close relationship between the areas where the tumour is endemic and those areas in which malaria is hyperendemic *(Kafuko and Burkitt, 1970)*. Burkitt stated that it was recognised that malaria was the factor that was delineated by the geographically limited climatic factors in the pathogenesis of this tumour.

Investigations regarding the aetiology of Burkitt's lymphoma were carried out by Harris *(1964)*, who concluded that the tumour probably results from a bizarre host reaction towards a common arthropod-borne virus, or a group of arthropod-borne viruses. He stated also that the intervention of chemical carcinogens in the environment or in food could not be excluded at that time.

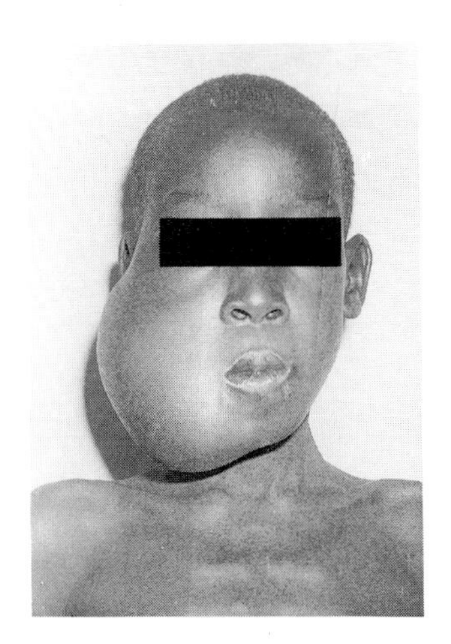

Figure 18.4 A 6-year-old boy with Burkitt's lymphoma in the right maxilla and right mandible.

An outstanding feature of the behaviour of Burkitt's lymphoma is the spectacular regression that can occur with chemotherapy with oral methotrexate, and especially with the administration of cyclophosphamide, which results in marked tumour regression and the patients remaining symptom-free for a period of more than a year. It has been found that alkylating chemicals and actinomycin D, which are used for the treatment of larger tumours, are more potent but tumour regression is only of short duration.

Naturally, Burkitt's lymphoma has continued to attract considerable interest, especially regarding its aetiology and treatment. Burkitt and Hutt *(1977)* stated that the current hypothesis concerning aetiology at that time was that hyperendemic malaria and the Epstein–Barr or other viruses were co-factors in the pathogenesis of the disease. They quoted Wedderburn,

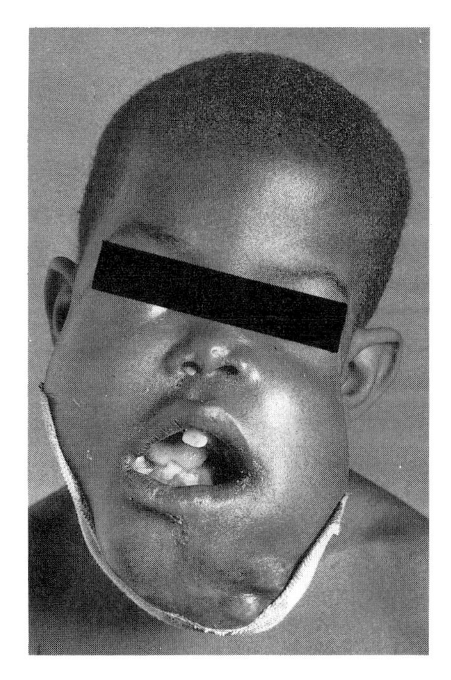

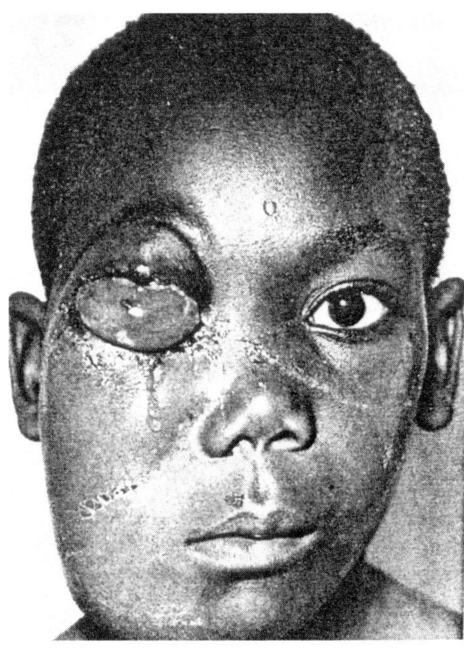

Figure 18.5 *Left:* A 4-year-old boy with Burkitt's lymphoma in the right and left maxillae and the right and left mandibles. *Right:* Burkitt's lymphoma with orbital presentation and deposits in the maxilla and mandible of a 6-year-old boy.

who stated that the experimental evidence provided by the study of oncogenic viruses in mice suggests that malaria might produce its effect by immunodepression.

At the present time we can pose the question as to whether Burkitt's lymphoma is the first cancer in humans discovered to be of virus causation.

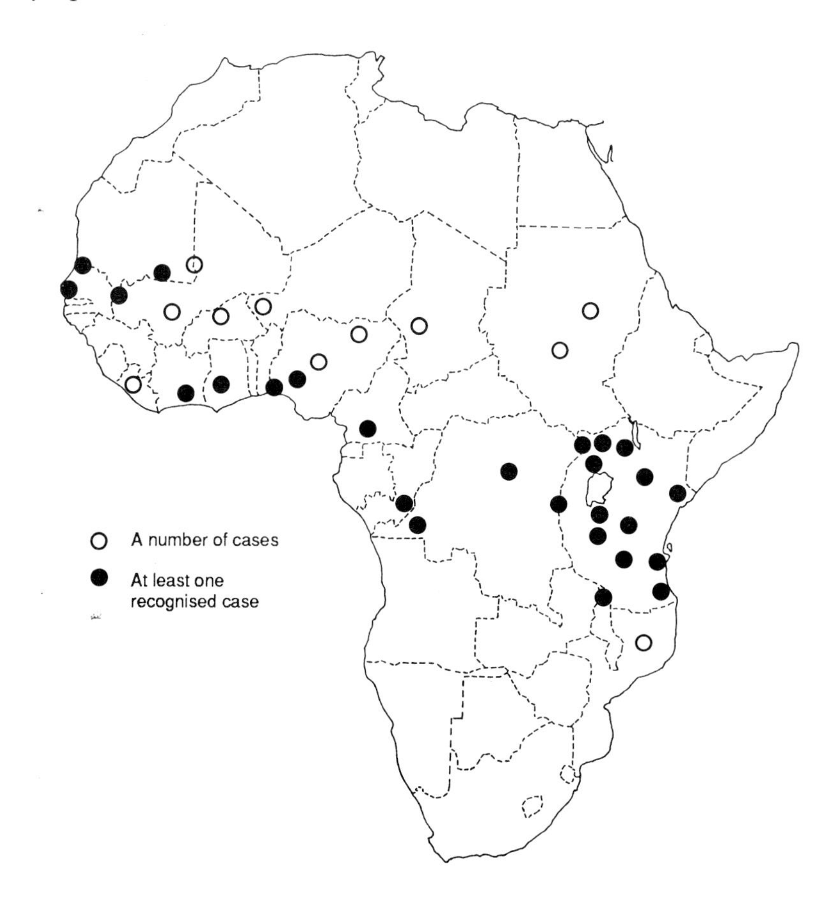

Figure 18.6 Geographical distribution of Burkitt's lymphoma.

Cancer of the liver

According to Berman *(1958)*, whose work on the subject is well-known, primary carcinoma of the liver is the most challenging cancer problem in Africa. His descriptions of its occurrence in Bantu natives of South Africa *(Berman, 1940)* attracted considerable attention, which was largely directed towards finding aetiological clues.

The disease usually affects young adults, especially males; indeed, in a series of 270 cases reported by Berman, all the patients were under 40 years old. He pointed out that the disease is rare in white people but common in people with pigmented skin. He described *(1940, 1941)* its features and the morbid anatomy, including microscopical appearances, in a series of 54 cases. In 39 cases both hepatic lobes were affected; in 19 cases the right lobe was affected, and in just one case the left lobe. In 24 cases the tumour was a hepatocellular carcinoma and in one case a cholangiocellular carcinoma. It is important to note that all the livers affected by carcinoma showed evidence of interlobular cirrhosis. Berman considered that the hepatomas were unicentric rather than multicentric in origin. Extrahepatic metastases were present in 31 of the 54 cases.

Regarding the aetiology of the tumours, Berman *(1941)* suggested four possibilities:

(1) Liver cirrhosis. This was present in all the 25 cases he examined personally and in 16 out of 29 cases at another hospital. He stated that liver cirrhosis was present in 405 out of a series of 555 cases of primary liver carcinoma which were reported in the literature.

(2) Parasite infestation. In these natives helminthiasis is frequently present. Berman found the ova of *Schistosoma haematobium* at autopsy in the bladder of 24 cases in the series of 54.

(3) Syphilis. The Wassermann reaction was positive in only eight out of 36 cases.

(4) Haemochromatosis. In all the cases which Berman examined there was a strong haemosiderin reaction, especially in the cirrhotic areas

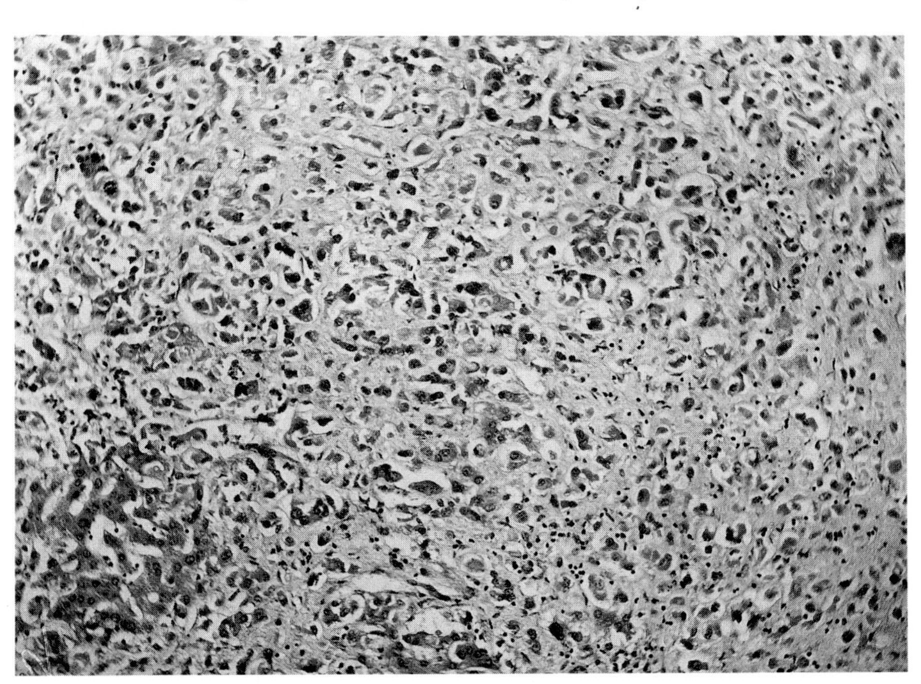

Figure 18.7 Histopathology specimen showing carcinoma in cirrhosis of the liver.

of the liver. Haemochromatosis occurs more frequently in South Africa than in Europe and more often in Bantu natives than in white people. It is always accompanied by cirrhosis of the liver.

All African native races consume alcohol from their early childhood and this fact is of interest in relation to the early age at which liver carcinoma develops.

Another possibility is keloid diathesis. In the Bantu races considerable connective tissue hyperplasia occurs after even only slight superficial wounds and it is possible that the liver reacts to injurious factors in a similar way.

Berman reviewed the whole subject in detail in 1958. He stressed the need for more research, as much of the evidence regarding the aetiology of the disease was circumstantial and the reason for the remarkable sensitivity of the African liver to cancer had still not been elucidated. He explained that in cirrhotic livers, environmental factors, in addition to malnutrition, are required for carcinogenesis to occur, but no naturally occurring carcinogens analogous to "butter yellow" or the other chemicals used in producing experimental liver cancer had been reported. He stated that as it seemed likely that the disease was preventable, research regarding the diets, habits and customs of African populations was necessary, in addition to searching for carcinogens. Furthermore, he considered that the solution of the problems relating to this unique tumour would illuminate the whole problem of cancer.

The incidence of primary cancer of the liver occurring in negroes of the United States of America was investigated by Kennaway *(1944)*. He compared his data with those concerning negroes in Africa but found no definite indication that American negroes had the same high incidence of liver cancer as African negroes, which demonstrates that the disease is not of purely racial character and might be due to some identifiable extrinsic factor. There is a difficulty which is caused by including cancer of the gall-bladder in the data concerning liver cancer.

Kennaway stated that cancer of the liver can be induced easily in the rat and mouse by compounds which are given in their food and furthermore that the diet is a controlling influence in this particular variety of carcinogenesis. He felt that similar compounds might be present in the African foodstuffs.

Cancer in relation to habits and customs

The accumulation of information about the relationship between cancer and various habits and customs has been of value both in increasing our knowledge of cancer aetiology and in helping to prevent cancer in certain sites of the body. The cancer prevention programmes used today place considerable emphasis on life-style, which includes habits and customs. Reference is made in the following paragraphs to some earlier important work on this subject.

Cancer in India

The prevalence in India of certain varieties of cancer which are associated with habits and customs has attracted much interest for many years. The

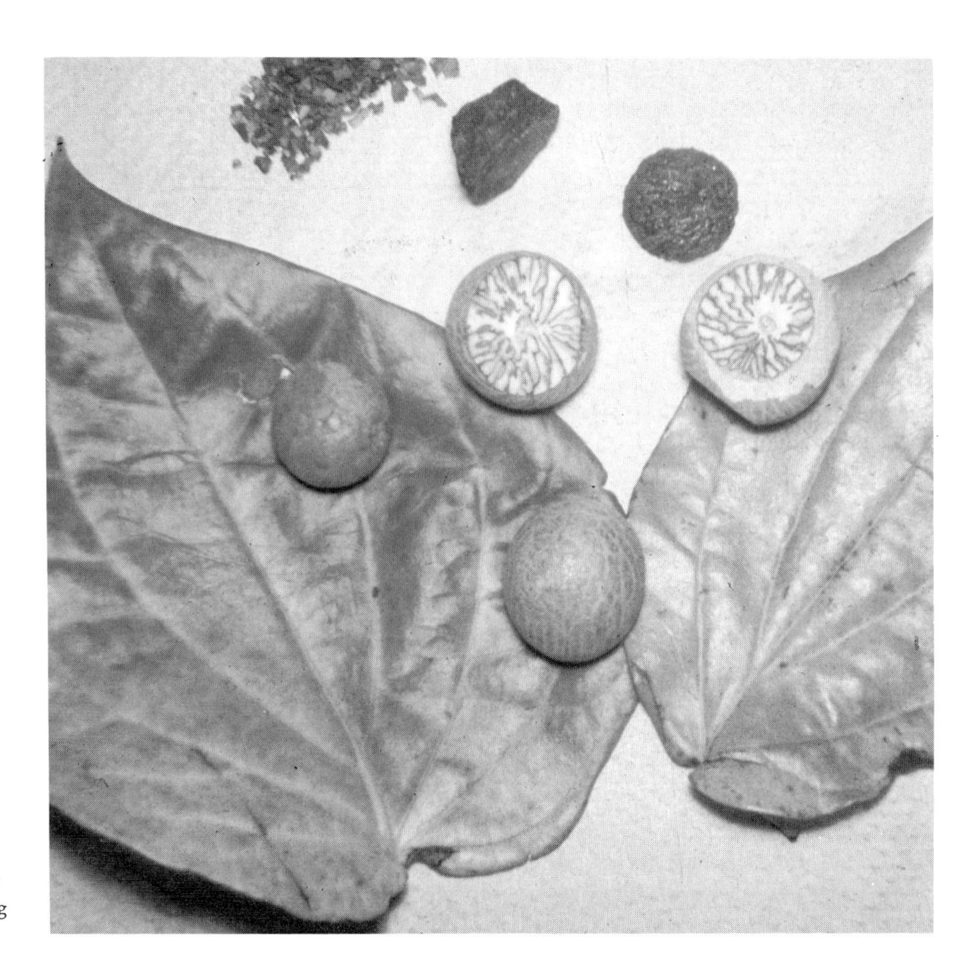

Figure 18.8 The betel nut and leaf associated with the habit of chewing tobacco in India.

subject was dealt with by Khanolkar *(1958)*, who stated that cancer of the lower lip was the most common variety of buccal cancer in certain parts of India and that the high incidence was associated with the habit, especially among men, of slowly sucking a mixture of tobacco and lime called Khaini, which at frequent intervals during the day was deposited in small amounts in the lower gingivolabial groove and gradually swallowed.

Cancer of the buccal aspect of the cheek is believed to stem from the habit of chewing tobacco, with or without betel leaf or betel nut, but it is considered that it is the variety of the tobacco which is the causative agent. Khanolkar stated that chewing betel probably inhibits the development of buccal cancer. He also reported the association of cancer of the hard palate with the habit of reverse smoking with the burning end of the cigarette or chutta placed inside the mouth.

He stated that cancer of the base of the tongue and tonsil was suggestive of an association with smoking local cigarettes (bidi), which are made by rolling tobacco flakes in a dried leaf of a variety of Bauhinia or Diospyros, and that cancer of the base of the tongue and hypopharynx appeared to be associated with the combination of smoking bidis and chewing tobacco.

There are two varieties of cancer of the unexposed parts of the skin which are peculiar to India and are associated with particular customs. These were described by Khanolkar *(1958)*, who referred to the original observations made by A. Neve in 1900 and E. F. Neve in 1924. These authors found a prevalence of squamous cell epithelioma of the skin of the lower part of the abdomen or thighs in the people of Kashmir, which they associated with the use of the kangri, an unglazed earthen pot packed with smouldering maple (chinar) leaves which natives place close to the abdomen to keep themselves warm. The heat causes severe erythema of the adjacent skin. Khanolkar pointed out that it was doubtful whether these mild burns were the entire cause of the cancer, for there might be carcinogenic substances in the smoke of chinar leaves and changes might occur in epidermal cells because of the recurrent inflammation every winter.

Khanolkar also described another skin cancer, called "dhoti cancer", which is associated with wearing a cotton cloth to cover the lower part of the body. This cloth, called the "dhoti" for men and the "sari" for women, is tied tightly round the waist, one end being carried under the groin and fixed on the back. Poorer people are obliged to work, bathe and sleep with the dhoti firmly attached to the loins. After many years this causes skin changes and occasionally carcinoma of the skin of the loin or groin.

Epidemiology of other tumours

There is a considerable amount of information about this subject, from which aetiological clues have been obtained and prevention programmes developed. It has been documented by Raven and Roe *(1967)* in their book on cancer prevention and an extensive literature is available for study. Brief reference is made here to certain cancers to illustrate their epidemiology.

Cancer of the nasopharynx

Incidence varies in different countries and races. Tumours of the nasopharynx are uncommon in the UK but occur frequently in the Chinese in many areas of the Far East, both inside and outside China. A genetic or racial susceptibility has been considered, but in their review of specific cancer incidence sites Higginson and MacLennan *(1973)* state that the aetiology of the disease is unknown and an association with herpes virus is uncertain.

The Paterson–Kelly syndrome

This syndrome is regarded as a precursor of carcinoma of the mouth, pharynx, especially the postcricoid region, and the oesophagus. It occurs in women and is characterised by the presence of dysphagia and anaemia. A detailed review was made by Raven *(1958)*, who referred to the original descriptions given by both Kelly and Paterson in 1919 (hence the name "Paterson–Kelly syndrome"). Raven *(1967)* quoted Wynder and Fryer, who noted the geographical incidence of the syndrome and of carcinoma of the hypopharynx in Sweden and stated that both conditions were more common in northern latitudes. They concluded that the excess of cancer of the upper alimentary tract in Swedish women over that in British, Danish and American women could be partly accounted for by the high incidence of the Paterson–Kelly syndrome in Sweden.

Carcinoma of the oesophagus

The incidence of this tumour has a very wide geographical distribution which has been noted by many authors. The subject is dealt with in detail by Oettlé *(1967)*, who mentioned, with others, the association of oesophageal carcinoma with smoking tobacco and drinking alcohol. The tumour is frequent in the Transkei area of South Africa and Oettlé states that it is much more common in the Bantu who brew alcoholic beverages in paraffin tins or drums than in those who use clay pots or calabashes for this purpose. He pointed out that differences in risk in adjacent areas, such as southern and northern Transkei, strongly suggest an adventitious causative agent.

Carcinoma of the stomach

This disease is found very frequently in many countries and the subject has been extensively studied. Burkitt and Hutt *(1977)* called attention to the high incidence rates in Iceland, Finland, parts of Russia, Japan, Chile and Colombia. Higginson and MacLennan *(1973)* stated that there had been a striking decrease in the incidence rates in the USA since 1935 and more recently in parts of Europe (these authors quoted Haenszel (1958) for the USA and Segi and Kurihara (1966) for Europe).

The subject of cancer in Iceland, where health records have existed since 1760, was dealt with by Dungal *(1958)*. He stated that cancer, particularly of the stomach, was the chief cause of death in Iceland for both men and women and that the increase in gastric cancer was higher than in most other countries, except possibly Japan. He considered that aetiological agents for the disease in Iceland must be sought in the environment, particularly in the food eaten; he discussed the latter subject in detail.

Higginson and MacLennan *(1973)* state that gastric carcinoma is almost certainly caused by environmental factors, since its incidence in emigrants decreases towards that prevalent in the country to which they emigrate, as seen in Japanese emigrants to the USA. They observe that although heated fats, fish diets and high cereal consumption have been suggested as aetiological factors, no consistent association has been found to explain the high frequency in different geographical areas and that nearly all studies show an inverse relationship with the consumption of dairy produce. Burkitt and Hutt *(1977)* suggest that one possible aetiological factor is the nitrate content of the soil, which is very high in the mountainous areas of Colombia, where the highest rates of gastric cancer are found.

Carcinoma of the colon and rectum

A helpful contribution to the epidemiology of carcinoma of the large bowel was made by Burkitt *(1973)*, who stated that in his study particular attention was paid to the close association of tumours of the large bowel with other, non-infective diseases of that organ, such as benign polyps, diverticular disease and ulcerative colitis. He observes that no other variety of cancer is so closely associated with Western civilisation and especially with the Western pattern of diet; in fact all the available evidence suggests that this bowel disease is dependent on environmental rather than on genetic factors. He discusses the environmental factors in detail, stressing that the most important is the quantity of unabsorbable fibre in the food, and presents the hypothesis that fibre deficiency is associated with faecal arrest, which is responsible for the proliferation of bacteria and their degradation of bile salts to carcinogens.

The literature about the epidemiology of tumours in other specific sites is considerable and is not included here, as sufficient evidence of the importance of the subject and its contribution to oncological knowledge has already been presented.

EPIDEMIOLOGY AND THE CAUSATION OF CANCER

Epidemiological studies have made valuable contributions to our knowledge of cancer causation and can confidently be expected to make more in future years. Reference is made here to the instructive article by Day and Muir *(1973)*, who appended a useful list of references. They emphasised the importance of considering how far each identified risk factor, or group of factors, can explain a disease's overall behaviour, which includes the following: geographic variation in incidence; differences in incidence between racial groups; the age-distribution of the tumour; sex differences; and familial incidence and space-time clustering. They discussed in detail both the behaviour of the disease itself and the relationship to the disease of the environment and the individual.

Statistical studies in the causation of cancer

The discipline of statistics is essential in epidemiological studies and, as Bennett *(1978)* stated, statistical expertise is required in the final analysis of the data and in the planning and execution of any study. A medical statistician should therefore always be consulted in the planning phase of epidemiological investigations.

Special reference is made here to Stocks' *(1958)* studies on the causation of cancer. He called attention to the lack of previous serious statistical study on that subject, which had meant that findings by some careful observers had been entirely forgotten for many decades, instead of being followed up. He gave as examples the work of Stern in Verona in 1842, who showed that the incidences of breast cancer and celibacy were associated, and that of Haviland, who in 1868 observed that cancer death rates in England and Wales seemed to be related to the kind of soil or subsoil on which people lived. Stocks had shown in 1924 that in Switzerland the distribution of cancer of the digestive tract and the distribution of goitre were connected in some way. He also stated that it might be necessary to wait a long time before some other discovery drew attention to the original observation that these diseases appear to be connected and that when considered together they begin to throw light on cancer causation.

He demonstrated the use of statistics in dealing with cancer causation from the viewpoints of heredity; sex and age incidence; occupation; marriage and childbearing; food and drink; soil and water. He also described in some detail the connection, shown by statistical studies, between tobacco smoking and air pollution and death rates from cancer of the bronchus, lung and pleura in England and Wales. He stated that in every investigation heavy cigarette smoking appeared to increase the risk of cancer of the lung and bronchus.

TOBACCO AND CANCER

Epidemiological and other investigations have produced important and strong evidence that smoking tobacco produces cancer in different organs of the body. In fact, we are now recognising the "tobacco cancers". Lung cancer is the commonest of these dangerous diseases which constitute an enormous challenge to preventive medicine at the present time. The mortality from lung cancer caused by smoking tobacco has now reached the seriousness of an epidemic and has become a matter of concern, both nationally and internationally, to governments and many other official bodies, who give warnings and advice about the tobacco habit and its serious dangers. Official reports on the subject were issued more than 20 years ago by the Royal College of Physicians of London *(1962)* and the Advisory Committee of the Surgeon General of the US Public Health Service *(1964)*; they contain detailed discussions of this major threat to public health. The organisation called "Ash" (Action on smoking and health) has for many years carried out important active work to control and eliminate the tobacco cancers; their splendid effort includes the regular publication and circularisation of an Information Bulletin. Special attention is called to the "Smoking and Health Bulletin", the issues of which are published at regular intervals and distributed internationally by the US Department of Health and Human Services, Office on Smoking and Health, Rockville, Maryland. This publication contains sections dealing with all aspects of the subject and has a complete subject index.

Early observations and developments

Stocks *(1958)* reported that nearly 50 years ago it was observed that the mortality rates from lung cancer in men up to the age of 65 were twice as great in large towns as in rural districts in England and Wales and that later the urban excess had increased even more. He also referred to workers in Germany and Holland who had found smaller proportions of non-smokers and larger proportions of heavy-smokers amongst men with lung cancer by comparing the tobacco-smoking habits of men with and without lung cancer.

Important contributions on the subject of lung cancer and tobacco-smoking were made by Doll and Bradford-Hill *(1952, 1964)*, whose initial articles should be studied in detail in order to appreciate the magnitude, methodology and results of their outstanding work. In their first study, which was limited to patients drawn mainly from London and the adjacent counties and which they reported in 1950, they concluded that smoking is a factor in the production of lung carcinoma. Subsequently they extended their investigation to other parts of the country and made more detailed inquiries into smoking habits. Nearly 5000 hospital patients were interviewed by four specially appointed almoners during the years 1948–1952 and the questions covered a wide range, including the patients' smoking habits. The authors concluded that there is a real association between smoking and lung carcinoma. They did not argue that tobacco smoke contributes to the development of all cases of lung carcinoma, that it is the sole cause of the increased death rate in recent years, or that it wholly explains the difference in the mortality rate between town and country.

Later *(1964)* they published their important article on the relationship between mortality and smoking, which embodied observations made by British doctors over a period of 10 years. The size of their investigation is shown by the fact that nearly 41 000 medically qualified men and women were observed for 12 years. During the first 10 years 4597 men and 366 women in the series died and their deaths were analysed in relation to their previously reported smoking habits. The authors state that the most pronounced association with smoking is shown by cancer of the lung, for which the annual death rate rises linearly in men from non-smokers to light smokers to medium smokers to heavy smokers, which indicates that there is no smoking threshold which must be reached before the death rate from lung cancer shows a response. They point out that in men who have given up cigarette smoking the death rate from lung cancer falls substantially and continues to fall step by step the longer smoking has ceased. They state that in women the few deaths which occurred during their study show only an association between smoking and lung cancer. In these articles by Doll and Bradford-Hill there are many important details for study and also a valuable list of literature references.

The connection between tobacco-smoking and lung cancer rightly attracts considerable attention from researchers, clinicians and all who are concerned with community health. Epidemiological and research studies were summarised by Pike and Roe *(1967)*, who cite the observation made by Wynder, Lemon and Bross, and also by Rele, that lung cancer rates in communities where smoking is forbidden are very much lower than in neighbouring communities where it is allowed. They state that the very large increase in death rates from lung cancer in many countries over the last 50 years has occurred in close association with large increases in *per capita* cigarette consumption. They also call attention to the relationship between the risk of lung cancer and the quantity and manner of tobacco consumption; the latter includes the habit of inhaling, the length of the butt of the cigarette, and pipe and cigar smoking.

The tobacco cancers

At the present time the consumption of tobacco by smoking is considered to be associated not only with lung cancer, but also with cancer in other organs, including the mouth, larynx, pharynx, oesophagus, pancreas, urinary bladder and the cervix uteri. Efforts are continuously increasing to persuade people, especially the young, not to start smoking tobacco and to advise and help smokers to give up this habit which is so dangerous to health. The subject of passive smoking is being stressed, together with the risks to children and others in "smoking homes", in transport, and at work. It is advisable that no pregnant woman should smoke. However, it can be very difficult to overcome the tobacco habit while tobacco is available. The view is gaining support in the UK and other countries that the cultivation of tobacco should cease, for that is the only real and logical solution to this dangerous world-wide problem.

AIR POLLUTION AND LUNG CANCER

The possible role of atmospheric pollution in the development of lung cancer has attracted considerable attention. This subject was discussed by Waller *(1970)*, who stated that all the evidence indicates that air pollution cannot be an important factor when compared with the risk of cigarette smoking. Regarding air pollution, he referred to studies of lung cancer in emigrant groups of people. For example, one investigation in the USA indicates that British-born people who have emigrated there have lower death rates from lung cancer than their compatriots whom they have left behind, whereas Norwegians, who have relatively low rates in Norway, experience somewhat higher rates in the USA. According to Waller, the implication is that something in the environment has affected people earlier in life, and exposure to pollution in the UK, which has been worse than in most other countries, might have contributed to the high death rates of those who have spent all, or even part, of their lives here. He pointed out that emigrants form selected parts of the population when these rates are considered.

Griffith *(1963)* described the different carcinogens in the atmosphere which might have a carcinogenic action on the human respiratory system and indicated the variety of further studies necessary to clarify the problem. In any case, the importance of smoking tobacco in relation to various forms of cancer must remain supreme.

CONCLUSION

The science of epidemiology has grown rapidly during recent decades. Expansion will continue in the future, so more clues concerning the aetiology of different oncological diseases will be found. The contribution of epidemiology to oncology is already most impressive and it has played a vital role in the inauguration of programmes of cancer prevention, in addition to the marked increase of knowledge. Research must continue in all aspects of epidemiology. The recent report by Muir *(1985)* illustrates the great value of a multinational approach in epidemiological studies of cancer aetiology.

REFERENCES

Advisory Committee of the Surgeon General of the US Public Health Service (1964). *Smoking and Health*. Public Health Service Publication No. 1103. US Government Printing Office, Washington

Bennett, A. E. (1978). Clinical epidemiology. In Raven, R. W. (ed.) *Foundations of Medicine — A Students' Guide*, pp 1–13. Heinemann Medical Books, London

★Berman, C. (1940). The clinical features of primary carcinoma of the liver in the Bantu races of South Africa. *South African J. Med. Sci.*, **5**, 92–109

★Berman, C. (1940). Primary carcinoma of the liver in the Bantu races of South Africa. *South African J. Med. Sci.*, **5**, 54–72

★Berman, C. (1941). The pathology of primary carcinoma of the liver in the Bantu races of South Africa. *South African J. Med. Sci.*, **6**, 11–26

(★ These articles were abstracted in *Cancer Res.* (1941), **1**, 176, 177 and 915)

Berman, C. (1941). The etiology of primary carcinoma of the liver with special reference to the Bantu races of South Africa. *South African J. Med. Sci.*, **6**, 145–56. (Abstracted in *Cancer Res.* (1942), **2**, 591–2)

Berman, C. (1958). Primary cancer of the liver in Africa. In Raven, R. W. (ed.) *Cancer*, Vol. 3, pp 228–39. Butterworth & Co., London

Burkitt, D. (1958–1959) A sarcoma involving the jaws of African children. *Br. J. Surg.*, **46**, 218–23

Burkitt, D. (1962). Determining the climatic limitations of a children's cancer common in Africa. *Br. Med. J.*, **2**, 1019–23

Burkitt, D. (1969). Etiology of Burkitt's lymphoma. *J. Natl. Cancer Inst.*, **42**, 19–28

Burkitt, D. (1973). Carcinoma of the colon and rectum. In Raven, R. W. (ed.) *Modern Trends in Oncology*, Part 1: Research Progress, pp 227–41. Butterworth & Co., London

Burkitt, D. and Hutt, M. (1977). Epidemiology. In Raven, R. W. (ed.) *Principles of Surgical Oncology*, pp 205–26. Plenum Medical Book Company, New York and London

Burkitt, D. and O'Conor, G. T. (1961). Malignant lymphoma in African children. I. A clinical syndrome. *Cancer*, **14**, 258–69

Day, N. E. and Muir, C. S. (1973). Aetiological clues from epidemiology. In Raven, R. W. (ed.) *Modern Trends in Oncology*, Part 1: Research Progress, pp 29–59. Butterworth & Co., London

Doll, R. and Bradford-Hill, A. (1952). A study of the aetiology of carcinoma of the lung. *Br. Med. J.*, **2**, 1271–86

Doll, R. and Bradford-Hill, A. (1964). Mortality in relation to smoking. Ten Years' observations of British doctors. *Br. Med. J.*, **1**, 1399–1410 and 1460–7

Doll, R., Muir, C. and Waterhouse, J. (1970). *Cancer Incidence in Five Continents*, Vol. 2. Distributed for the International Union Against Cancer by Springer-Verlag, Berlin, Heidelberg and New York

Dungal, N. (1958). Cancer in Iceland. In Raven, R. W. (ed.) *Cancer*, Vol. 3, pp 262–71. Butterworth & Co., London

Griffith, G. W. (1963). Atmospheric pollution and lung cancer. In Raven, R. W. (ed.) *Cancer Progress 1963*, pp 86–94. Butterworth & Co., London

Harris, R. J. C. (1964). Aetiology of Central African lymphomata. *Br. Med. Bull.*, **20**, 149–53

Higginson, J. and MacLennan, R. (1973). The world pattern of cancer incidence. In Raven, R. W. (ed.) *Modern Trends in Oncology*, Part 1: Research Progress, pp 9–27. Butterworth & Co., London

Kafuko, G. W. and Burkitt, D. (1970). Burkitt's lymphoma and malaria. *Int. J. Cancer*, **6**, 1–9

Kennaway, E. L. (1944). Cancer of the liver in the negro in Africa and America. *Cancer Res.*, **4**, 571–7

Khanolkar, V. R. (1958). Cancer in India in relation to habits and customs. In Raven, R. W. (ed.) *Cancer*, Vol. 3, pp 272–80. Butterworth & Co., London

Muir, C. S. (1985). Etiology of cancer. The value of a multinational approach. In Fortner, J. G. and Rhoads, J. E. (eds) *Accomplishments in Cancer Research 1985. General Motors Cancer Research Foundation*, pp 108–23. J. B. Lippincott Co., Philadelphia

O'Conor, G. T. (1961). Malignant lymphoma in African children. II. A pathological entity. *Cancer*, **14**, 270–83

O'Conor, G. T. and Davies, J. N. P. (1960). Malignant tumors in African children, with special reference to malignant lymphoma. *J. Pediatr.*, **56**, 526–35

Oettlé, A. G. (1967). The oesophagus. In Raven, R. W. and Roe, F. J. C. (eds) *The Prevention of Cancer*, pp 90–8. Butterworth & Co., London

Pike, M. C. and Roe, F. J. C. (1967). Bronchi and lungs — tobacco. In Raven, R. W. and Roe, F. J. C. (eds) *The Prevention of Cancer*, pp 170–80. Butterworth & Co., London

Raven, R. W. (1958). The Paterson–Kelly syndrome. In *Cancer of the Pharynx, Larynx and Oesophagus and Its Surgical Treatment*, pp 16–26. Butterworth & Co., London

Raven, R. W. (1967). The Paterson–Kelly syndrome. In Raven, R. W. and Roe, F. J. C. (eds) *The Prevention of Cancer*, pp 82–5. Butterworth & Co., London

Royal College of Physicians (1962). *Smoking and Health*. Pitman, London

Steiner, P. E. (1958). Epidemiology of cancer. In Raven, R. W. (ed.) *Cancer*, Vol. 3, pp 173–83. Butterworth & Co., London

Stocks, P. (1958). Cancer mortality trends in England and Wales. In Raven, R. W. (ed.) *Cancer*, Vol. 3, pp 184–207. Butterworth & Co., London

Stocks, P. (1958). Statistical investigations concerning the causation of various forms of human cancer. In Raven, R. W. (ed.) *Cancer*, Vol. 3, pp 116–71. Butterworth & Co., London

Waller, R. E. (1970). Tobacco and other substances as causes of respiratory cancer. In Raven, R. W. (ed.) *Symposium on the Prevention of Cancer*, pp 17–28. Heinemann Medical Books, London

Wright, D. H. (1963). Cytology and histochemistry of the Burkitt lymphoma. *Br. J. Cancer*, **17**, 50–5

CHAPTER NINETEEN

Endocrinology

Endocrinology is an important basic science in oncology, which continues to make a valuable contribution both to our knowledge of the aetiology and behaviour of the oncological diseases and to the treatment of patients, especially those with carcinoma of the breast and prostate. We now believe that these tumours, and possibly others, are under hormonal control, but we do not yet understand the mechanisms which are responsible. The latter are the object of considerable research today, and when they are understood it will be possible to manipulate them in a meaningful way for the benefit of patients and even to prevent carcinoma of the breast and prostate.

The endocrine system plays a vital role in regulating the normal development of various organs and systems of the body. It is therefore logical to assume that it is also closely linked with any abnormal growth, including neoplasia. This possible link has been the object of clinical observation and scientific research investigation for more than 100 years. Although important progress has been made, much more work remains to be done to clarify the whole subject.

DISTURBANCES IN THE ENDOCRINE SYSTEM

Disturbances in different components of the endocrine system can cause profound pathological changes in the body. Addison in 1855 published a clear description of the disease which now bears his name (Addison's disease), entitled *On the Constitutional and Local Effects of Diseases of the Suprarenal Capsules*. There are many other relationships which have long been recognised; for example, the fact that tumours of the pituitary gland cause acromegaly and hypothyroidism in cretins.

Throughout this century relationships with neoplasia have aroused enormous interest. Recently various clinical syndromes have been described which are caused by hormones actively secreted by tumours; for example, hypercalcaemia, hyperglycaemia and hyperuricaemia. These syndromes are dangerous and threatening to the patient's life, so early recognition and treatment are essential. Hormonal treatment of carcinoma of the breast and prostate is carried out routinely today, with impressive results.

As the endocrine system is linked so closely with neoplasia and hormonal therapy of various kinds has an important role in the general management and treatment of patients with oncological diseases, it is mandatory for the oncologist to possess a sound knowledge of endocrinology.

HISTORICAL CONTRIBUTIONS

The author's main objective in this chapter is to delineate the important historical contributions which endocrinology has made to oncology and to demonstrate the close association that exists between these disciplines. Special emphasis is placed on those endocrine glands and hormones that have been proved to be closely linked with malignant tumours.

THE OVARY AND OESTROGENS

The recognition of the hormonal functions of the ovary is based on the pioneer experimental work carried out by Marshall and Jolly *(1906)*, who demonstrated that oestrus can be induced in spayed dogs by injecting them with extracts of ovaries removed from another dog during oestrus, or by the implantation of oestrous ovaries into the peritoneum.

They discovered that the ovary produces two different hormones and that the secretion which causes oestrus is not the same as the hormone from the corpus luteum.

Adler *(1912)* reported that oestrus occurs in guinea-pigs when they are injected, either intramuscularly or intravenously, with extracts or press juices from whole ovaries or corpora lutea. Later, Allen and Doisy*(1923)* discovered that liquor folliculi from the sow's ovary causes oestrous-like changes in the rat's vagina. The hormone which was thought to cause these changes was variously called theelin, oestrin, and folliculin. It was isolated by Doisy, Thayer and Veler *(1930)* in crystalline form from the urine of pregnant women, and this compound became known as oestrone.

Following this original research, numerous oestrogens, both natural and synthetic, have been recognised. The highly active synthetic oestrogen compound, stilboestrol, introduced by Dodds, Goldberg, Lawson and Robinson *(1938)*, is now widely used clinically, especially in the treatment of patients with carcinoma of the prostate and for certain elderly patients with breast carcinoma. An advantage of using this compound is that it can be administered orally, and it is a satisfactory substitute for the natural oestrogens.

The sources of oestrogen

The ovary is the principle source of oestrogen, but we now know that it is also elaborated by other organs, including the adrenal glands. The ovarian output of oestrogen is regulated by a pituitary–ovary control mechanism, for hypophysectomy arrests the output and causes atrophy of the ovary. In healthy women the formation of an abundant quantity of oestrogen is intermittent and regulated by the pituitary–ovary control mechanism. The latter can be upset by either an excess or a deficiency of oestrogen, or by a derangement of the function of the pituitary gland.

Experimental research has been carried out concerning the effect of hypophysectomy on various tumours. It was shown by Korteweg and Thomas *(1939)* that breast cancer in mice continued to grow after hypophysectomy, but at a reduced rate.

The placenta

The placenta is known to secrete a considerable quantity of oestrogen, but this hormonal supply can have only a minimal action in the causation of neoplasms, since pregnancy occurs at infrequent intervals. In addition, pregnancy is usually followed by a lengthy period of lactation, during which there is a reduced output of oestrogen.

The adrenals

The removal of the ovaries and testes of animals does not suppress the output of oestrogen and it is believed that this hormone is also secreted by the adrenal glands. Furthermore, it seems that the adrenals acquire an increased capacity to secrete oestrogen after gonadectomy in either sex, and after the ovaries have ceased to respond to the follicle-stimulating hormone (FSH), i.e., after the menopause.

This information has been applied clinically in the treatment of patients with breast carcinoma by oophorectomy or ovarian radiation. The realisation that the supply of oestrogens is not cut off by these techniques led to the introduction of other modalities, including bilateral adrenalectomy, hypophysectomy and pituitary gland radiation. More recently further progress has been made in the treatment of breast carcinoma through the production of anti-oestrogen compounds such as Nolvadex (tamoxifen) and aminoglutethimide. These compounds are now used extensively, particularly Nolvadex, which is given to patients with any stage of the disease, alone or combined with other treatment. Consequently, the operations of oophorectomy, adrenalectomy and hypophysectomy are now performed less frequently. The anti-oestrogen hormones are important, for we recognise that after the ablation of the ovaries oestrogen is elaborated by the adrenals. In males, the testicle is the chief source of oestrogen, which is thought to be produced by the Sertoli cells.

The elimination of oestrogen

The metabolites of oestrogen are eliminated from the body through the alimentary and renal systems. Burrows and Horning (with whom the present author discussed the relevant experimental work at the Chester Beatty Research Institute in London) showed in their instructive book *(1952)* that oestrogen is excreted by the liver and flows with the bile into the duodenum, where a quantity is reabsorbed into the portal venous system and so returned to the liver. Whilst much is known about the amounts of oestrogen that appear in the urine daily, we do not understand the effect of kidney diseases on the urinary output. The fate of the remaining quantity of oestrogen is not precisely known.

The book by Burrows and Horning contains a chapter on the chemistry and metabolism of oestrogens written by C. W. Shoppee, a research scientist who was well known to the present author, and it gives the latter pleasure to recall the other's outstanding work. The author acknowledges that he has also received much valuable information from Burrows' book *Biological Actions of Sex Hormones (1949)*.

The liver and oestrogens

Shoppee considered that the liver is the principle site for the inactivation of oestrogens by enzyme oxidation, which depends upon the competence of the liver functions. These can be undermined in various ways *(Burrows and Horning, 1952)*. For example, when experimental rats are fed on a low-protein diet, liver cirrhosis develops, leading to consequent inability to inactivate oestrogens.

In humans with liver cirrhosis, gynaecomastia caused by excessive oestrogen can occur. It is known that the liver must receive an adequate supply of vitamin B complex to be able to inactivate oestrogen. Excessive circulating oestrogen due to liver incompetence was reported by Davies *(1948, 1949)* amongst the Bantu races of Africa, in whom fatty degeneration and cirrhosis of the liver are common, and it is interesting to note that Davies found that breast cancer in males was more frequent in Bantus than in Europeans.

Further clinical evidence was reported by Glass and his colleagues *(1940)*, who examined 14 males with chronic liver disease who showed signs of excessive oestrogenic activity, including atrophy of the testicles in all cases and gynaecomastia in eight. Their urinary assays showed a diminution in androgen content and rapid excretion of oestrogen in a free form, which indicated that the liver had failed to conjugate oestrogen.

The introduction of the subject of liver function into the broader topic of the metabolism and elimination of oestrogen is of academic interest and clinical significance. More research is still required in this connection.

EXPERIMENTAL RESEARCH ON OESTROGENS AND CANCER OF THE BREAST

Oestrogens can induce hyperplasia and tumours in the organs of several animals used in experiments. Whilst this carcinogenic property is recognised, we know that oestrogen has carcinostatic effects in some patients with carcinoma of the breast or prostate.

It is probable that the impressive results published by Beatson *(1896)* and others (described later) regarding the treatment of advanced breast carcinoma by oophorectomy attracted the attention of research scientists to the relationship between oestrogens and breast carcinoma. This clearly illustrates the value of constant feedback of information between the clinic and the laboratory.

The experimental work of Lathrop and Loeb *(1919)* showed that when oophorectomy was performed in female mice, of several different strains, before they reached the age of 6 months, there was a marked decrease in the incidence of breast cancer. Although the procedure did not entirely prevent this disease, it appeared later than in non-spayed mice. Spaying mice over the age of 6 months did not prevent the development of breast cancer.

Loeb *(1919)* also showed the differences between early and late spaying in mice. If it was done between the ages of 3 and 5 months, breast cancer was almost entirely prevented. When it was done between the 5th and 7th months, the incidence of cancer was reduced and when the disease did appear it was at a later average age than in non-spayed mice. Spaying after the age of 8 months had no appreciable effect on the incidence of breast cancer in these animals.

It is interesting to interpolate here the clinical observations made with regard to circumcision and carcinoma of the penis. This tumour is unknown in the Jewish race, who perform circumcision on the 8th day after birth, but it does occur in others who carry out the operation later, chiefly between the ages of 3 and 15 years.

Further experiments were carried out by Cori *(1927)*, who spayed mice of strain 3, 78% of the females of which normally develop breast cancer. Forty-nine animals spayed at the age of 2–6 months lived to the age of 19 or more months, and breast cancer occurred in only five animals. Thus spaying in the first 6 months of life reduced the incidence of breast cancer in these animals from 78% to 10%.

Cori then performed a second experiment by spaying 100 mice of the same strain, aged between 15 and 22 days; 86 mice were alive at the end of 10 months, 60 reached the age of 20 months and no animal developed breast cancer. At 20 months breast tumours had appeared in 74% of the untreated control mice of the same strain.

Murray *(1928)* not only confirmed the earlier experimental results but also provided additional evidence of the importance of oophorectomy in the control of breast cancer. He worked with a strain of mice where spontaneous breast cancer eventually developed in 80% of the untreated breeding females, but was unknown in untreated males. He removed the gonads from 210 4–6-week-old mice of each sex and then subcutaneously transplanted an entire ovary from a sister animal in the abdominal region of each male. He found that 38 (18%) of these males developed breast cancer, whereas no castrated male without an ovarian transplant did so.

Experiments with synthetic oestrogens

Experimental methodology changed from observing the effects of oophorectomy to studies on the use of synthetic oestrogens in animals.

Lacassagne *(1932)* administered at weekly intervals a solution of crystalline oestrone benzoate 0.03 mg dissolved in sesame oil to five young mice, three males and two females, aged between 10 and 18 days. These animals belonged to a strain in which about 72% of untreated females eventually developed spontaneous breast cancer, but the males were not affected. Breast cancer developed within 6 months in the three male mice and two separate tumours occurred in one animal. It also developed in one of the two females, at the early age of 4 months.

These results have been confirmed by other researchers who have induced breast cancer in both castrated and non-castrated male mice by the administration of synthetic oestrone.

The time scale during which the breasts of animals are subjected to effective supplies of oestrogen was investigated by Burns and Schenken *(1940)*. They found that a maximum effect was obtained with treatment lasting 16 weeks, and that continuous administration of oestrogen beyond this period caused no greater incidence of breast cancer.

Thus, experimental work has shown that early oophorectomy in mice can prevent breast cancer and that the administration of synthetic oestrogen in amounts greater than the physiological level can cause breast cancer in animals.

GENERAL ASPECTS OF HORMONES AND NEOPLASIA

The author has already referred to the book on oestrogens and neoplasia by Burrows and Horning *(1952)*, a splendid team of researchers who greatly enriched our knowledge of this subject. In the Foreword, Charles Huggins wrote: "The authors present many complex data which they skilfully integrate in a holistic approach which deserves the thanks of all workers in cancer and endocrinology."

Burrows and Horning explained that oestrogenic neoplasia is a special pathological entity, whether benign or malignant, and endocrine tumours have been induced in several organs. They are produced by an incessant and prolonged supply of the hormone over a long period of many years, and not by a temporary over-abundance of it.

To support this opinion they quoted the original observations of Lipschutz *(1950)*, who worked on the induction of fibromas and fibromyomas in guinea-pigs and showed that the administration of oestrogen over a long period produced tumours in the uterus and other abdominal organs. Normally there is a rhythmical output of oestrogen and the histological effects are reversed soon after the end of each period of secretion. When the oestrogen supply becomes incessant, neoplasms eventually appear as a result of the derangement of the rhythm, and the quantity of oestrogen required for this change is not large.

Oestrogens are only one of the factors that are necessary for the development of neoplasia; favourable circumstances are also required in special situations. Thus Burrows *(1949)* called attention to hereditary factors in the development of breast cancer and gave as an example the fact that female mice of different strains show wide differences in their liability to develop spontaneous breast cancer. Experiments have demonstrated non-genic and genic inherited agents. Regarding the non-genic hereditary virus ("milk factor"), Burrows cited the work of Lathrop and Loeb *(1919)*, who found that if mice with a high cancer incidence are crossed with mice with a low cancer incidence, the liability of the offspring to develop mammary cancer mainly follows that of the mother. The father's influence, though definite, is small and is contributed by the genes.

Lacassagne *(1932)* first observed that breast cancer is caused in male mice by oestrogen, if they belong to the strain in which the females have a high incidence of spontaneous breast cancer, that is, if they carry the mammary cancer virus in their tissues.

Burrows considered that there is little doubt that the "milk factor" is a virus and he used this term to mean a self-multiplying protein body which is small enough to traverse antibacterial filters and is able to multiply in the body. He suggested that it might be conveyed during lactation from mother to child, and until it is proved that such transmission does not occur, any mother whose family history suggests the presence of a trans-

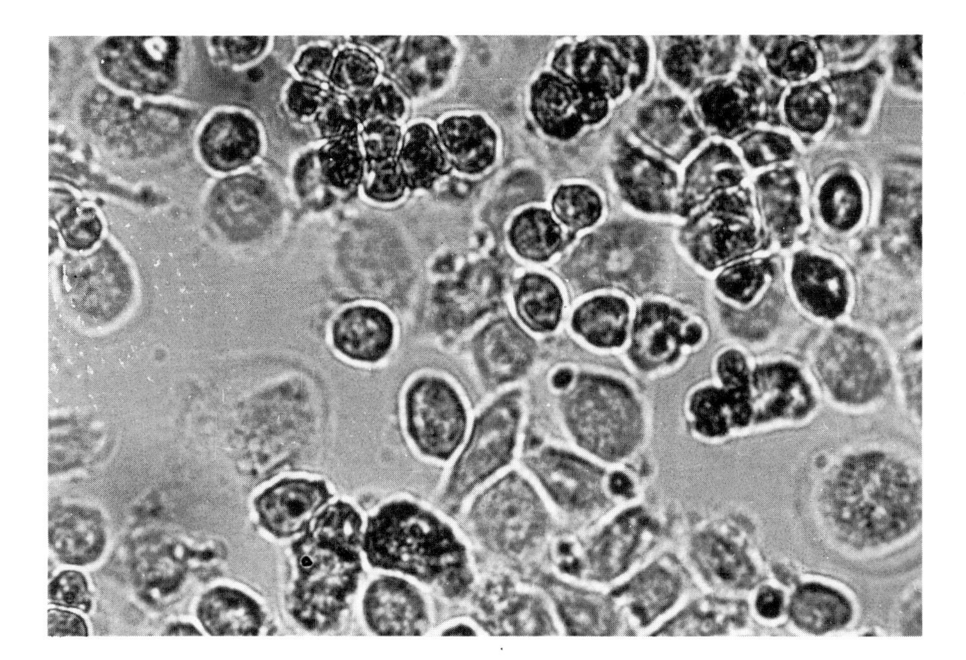

Figure 19.1 Human breast carcinoma cells growing in tissue culture without the addition of oestrogen to the medium (X 150). Note the scanty growth of cells which are very granular with large nuclei. The live cells are unstained.

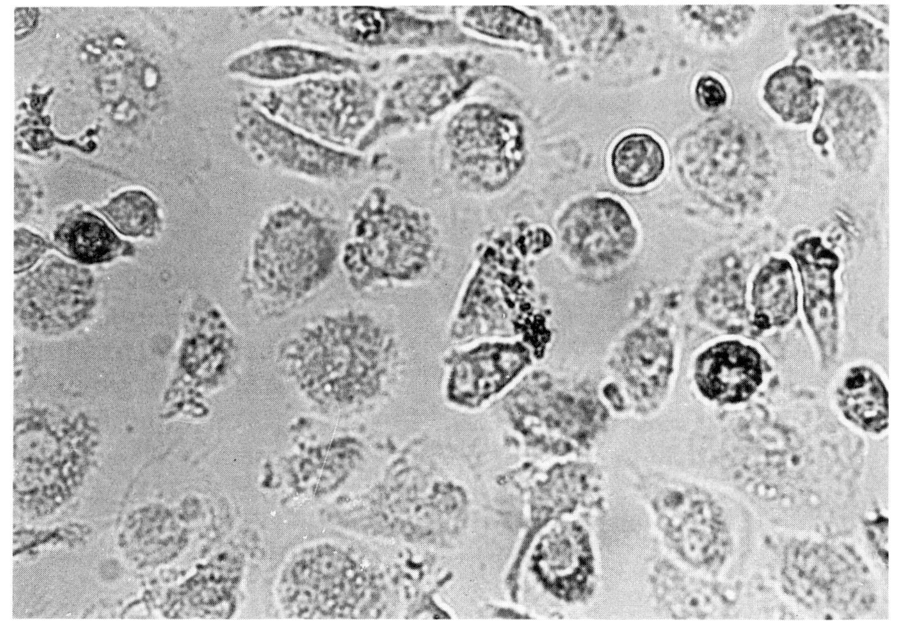

Figure 19.2 Human breast carcinoma cells growing in tissue culture with the oestrogen added to the medium (X 150). Note the high nuclear cytoplasmic ratio and the disorderly growth of the malignant cells. The live cells are unstained.

mittable milk factor of cancer ought not to breastfeed her female children.

This viral agent in the milk of mice was discovered by Bittner and is known as the Bittner virus *(Dmochowski, 1957)*.

The genic factor appears not to be of great significance when large numbers of mice are considered, but there is evidence that it does exist, for there is a paternal influence in the transmission of a liability to breast cancer, and this must be genic.

Oestrogenic neoplasia

Burrows described oestrogenic neoplasia as a gradual development through the successive stages of tissue hyperplasia to benign neoplasia and finally to malignant neoplasia. He considered that early tissue changes are reversible

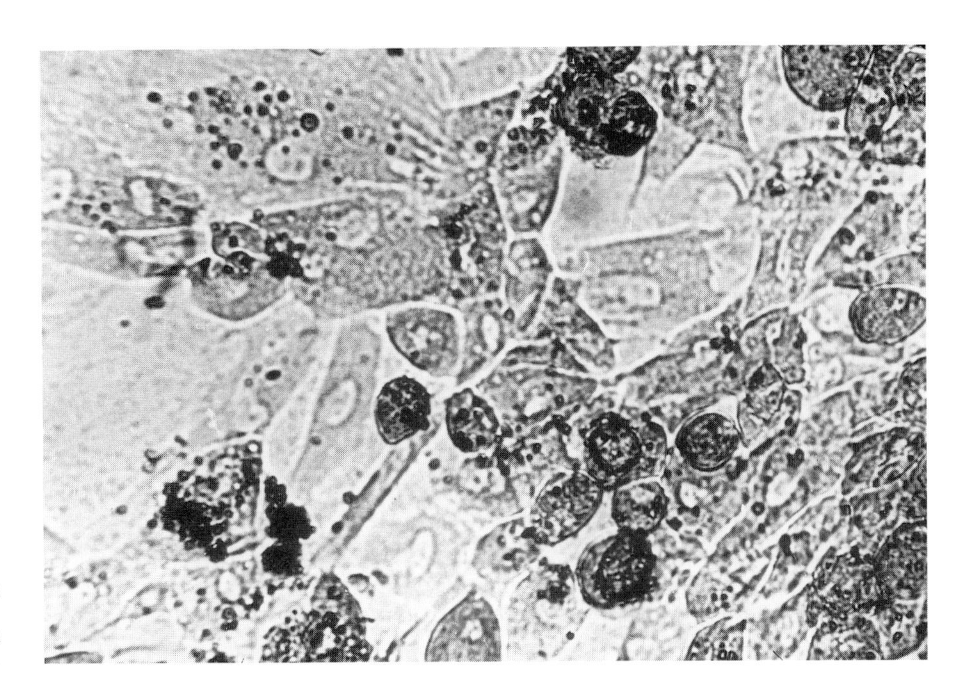

Figure 19.3 Human breast carcinoma semiconfluent subculture of tumour cells growing with the addition of oestrogen to the medium (X 135). Note the high nuclear cytoplasmic ratio, disorderly growth and the early formation of a mound.

and a complete cure will follow if the excess supply of oestrogen is checked and that cessation in the growth of a benign tumour can be effected in the same way. Thus by detecting and arresting an incessant output of oestrogen in early reproductive life, oestrogenic neoplasia might be prevented in later years.

The question can be posed as to whether the same processes are active in the breast, causing a fibroadenoma or carcinoma. A fibroadenoma is distinguished by possessing a fibrous capsule and there is no cellular invasion of the surrounding stroma. A carcinoma has no fibrous capsule and its outstanding feature is stromal infiltration and invasion of lymphatic and blood vessels. An atrophic scirrhous carcinoma is slow-growing and practically non-invasive, having a good fibrous tissue stromal barrier. This variety of breast carcinoma has a relatively good prognosis, in contrast to anaplastic carcinomas, which have a negligible fibrous stromal reaction and which invade contiguous tissue and lymphatic and blood vessels, causing lymph node and visceral metastases; the prognosis for these is poor.

Resistance in cancer

Our knowledge of host resistance in cancer is increasing and we now recognise both systemic and stromal resistance to neoplasms. In systemic resistance a competent immune system is necessary and there are feedback mechanisms to restrain invasive tissue enzymes. In this connection the hormonal status of certain tumours must be considered.

Stromal resistance results in the formation of a fibrous capsule around benign tumours, but in general the collagenous barrier to the neoplasm varies. There is resistance to invasion from intercellular ground substance. The surrounding lymphocytic response is greatest for slow-growing tumours. We are learning more about the role of vitamin C (ascorbic acid) in maintaining the integrity of the intercellular matrix and tissue resistance to malignant tumour invasion. This vitamin stimulates the formation of new collagen and inhibits the activity of invasive tumour enzymes, in addition to potentiating the immune system as a whole.

Burrows pointed out the different degrees of malignancy in breast carcinoma and that some tumours might continue to utilise oestrogen, which means that it is possible to check the disease temporarily by cutting off the supply by oophorectomy or other methods. However, hormonal control of breast carcinoma is seldom permanent; the resumption of activity is attributed to the oestrogen which is secreted by the adrenal glands, aided perhaps by the ability of the carcinoma to progress without oestrogen, which means that the tumour is hormone-independent.

Oestrogen receptors

Since the early work described above was done our knowledge about hormones and their relationship with neoplasia has continued to grow.

The mechanism of action of steroid hormones at a subcellular level is attracting considerable research interest today. The subject was reviewed by Williams *(1977)*, who was well known to the present author. He described a number of cell types in the body which are normally under the complete control of steroid hormones. The organs and tissues concerned are the primary and secondary sex organs and perhaps to a lesser degree the liver and kidneys.

The notable discovery of oestrogen receptors by Jensen and colleagues *(1967)* in uterine and vaginal tissues and later in breast and other tissues represented an important advance with valuable clinical connotations. Their initial work has been greatly expanded and we now recognise specific receptor sites for androgen, progestogen and corticosteroids. Attention is drawn to the review by Jensen and De Sombre *(1972)*.

Oestrogen receptors are cytoplasmic substances which bind to the oestrogen and then transfer it into the cell nuclei where its function is exercised. Williams stated that human breast tumours contain two different types of oestrogen receptor sites, with high and low affinity, respectively, for oestrogen. The high-affinity sites are considered to be involved in the cellular control process, while the low-affinity sites are apparently less specific in their action and are perhaps concerned with the steroid transport mechanism.

The methodology used several years ago showed that about 50% of primary breast carcinomas contained oestrogen receptors, but now our more sensitive methods show that 70–80% contain them. There is a high response rate to hormonal therapy in tumours with a high-level assay, and a low rate in tumours with a low-level assay.

Oestrogen receptor assays and prognosis

The oestrogen receptor status of the primary tumour is a useful marker of its biological aggressiveness, and assays of the receptor indicate tumour hormonal responsiveness and the likelihood of tumour recurrence and metastases. Oestrogen receptor assays are carried out routinely in patients with breast carcinoma when the tumour is removed, to obtain guidance regarding hormonal treatment. Increasing attention is also being given to the hormonal profile of patients with hormone-related tumours. This is a new parameter, which is used in addition to the staging method to determine treatment and assess prognosis.

CLINICAL ASPECTS OF HORMONES AND BREAST CARCINOMA

The original concept that the prognosis for young women with breast cancer might be improved by performing oophorectomy was conceived by Schinzinger in 1889, but it appears that he never carried out that treatment.

The work of Beatson

A historic event occurred on 20 May 1896, when George Thomas Beatson of Glasgow read before the Edinburgh Medico-Chirurgical Society his paper, "On the treatment of inoperable cases of carcinoma of the mamma: suggestions for a new method of treatment with illustrative cases". This article, which was published in the same year *(Beatson, 1896)*, included the details about one patient with local recurrent breast carcinoma and two patients with advanced primary breast carcinoma. The histopathology of the tumours was described by R. M. Buchanan and confirmed the clinical diagnosis of carcinoma.

The patients were treated by bilateral oophorectomy, which resulted in a remarkable regression of the disease. Beatson was greatly impressed and wrote: "We must look in the female to the ovaries as the exciting cause of carcinoma, certainly of the mamma, in all probability of the female generative organs generally, and probably of the rest of the body. I have felt for some time that the parasitic theory of cancer is an unsatisfactory one in many ways, and that in directing all our energies to working it out we are losing time and searching for what will never be found simply because it does not exist."

In his general thesis Beatson stressed three points, as follows: "There seems evidence of the ovaries and testes having control in the human body over local proliferations of epithelium; that the removal of tubes and ovaries has effects on the local proliferation of epithelium, which occurs in carcinoma of the mamma and helps in the tendency carcinoma has to fatty degeneration, and that this effect is best seen in cases of carcinoma in young people, a class of case where local removal of the disease is often unsatisfactory." In conclusion he stated: "I am not in a position to replace the old plan of local removal — which no doubt brings many disappointments, but has had of late years many encouraging results — by a new and untried method. All I feel is that there are grounds for belief that the aetiology of cancer lies not in the parasitic view, but in an ovarian and testicular stimulus, and that the whole subject requires careful working out. I need hardly say that if that view is found correct it must materially modify our present lines of treatment."

These opinions expressed so clearly by Beatson, together with his clinical observations, doubtless made a strong impact on the views held by the medical profession at that time. He demolished the parasitic theory of cancer causation and substituted the hormonal theory of breast carcinoma and other malignant tumours too. His work and opinions justifiably aroused tremendous interest, for they were of profound importance. Fundamental discoveries about hormones and neoplasia have since been made which have enriched our knowledge of the aetiology of malignant diseases and provided material help in the clinical care of patients.

The 70th Annual Meeting of the British Medical Association was held on 29 July–1 August 1902 in Manchester. In the section of surgery, time was devoted to "A discussion on the treatment of inoperable cancer", which was presided over by Henry Morris, Senior Surgeon to the Middlesex Hospital and the Cancer Department in London. Beatson took part in the discussion, stating his opinion on oophorectomy in advanced breast carcinoma as follows: "It must be admitted that in many of the cases the effects of this procedure on the local manifestations of the disease are transient and that fresh nodules appear. It is equally certain, however, that, notwithstanding this, there has been in a large number of cases an improvement in the general health, with a relief of pain and a disappearance of uncomfortable sensations generally. This has been remarked on by more than one operator. Further, in a certain number of cases the beneficial effects of the operation have been more permanent and there are patients, the subject of inoperable mammary cancer, in whom the disease has disappeared and who have remained well some years after oophorectomy. I am anxious that oophorectomy in inoperable mammary cancer should be judged entirely on its own merits. The treatment has been placed before the profession because I felt they should judge its effects themselves, and if, in their opinion, after a fair trial, it is found wanting, then I hope it will be abandoned and forgotten."

More than 80 years have now elapsed since Beatson's statement, but this treatment has neither been forgotten nor abandoned. The ovary and its secretions still remain in the central position in our understanding and management of breast carcinoma, for this is an endocrine problem.

The experience of other surgeons

The subject of breast cancer was discussed at the meeting of the Royal Medical and Chirurgical Society in London on 24 January 1905. Hugh Lett (later Sir Hugh Lett, who became President of the Royal College of Surgeons of England), Surgeon to the London Hospital, presented his analysis of a series of 99 cases of inoperable breast cancer treated by oophorectomy, in which there was a very marked improvement in 23.2% and a distinct, though less marked, improvement in 13.1%. Thus 36.3% of these cases benefited materially and one patient was alive and well 5 years later. Lett found that the most favourable age for this treatment was 45–50 years; he did not consider that the postmenopausal state was a contraindictaion but thought that after the age of 50 years the operation was scarcely worth doing.

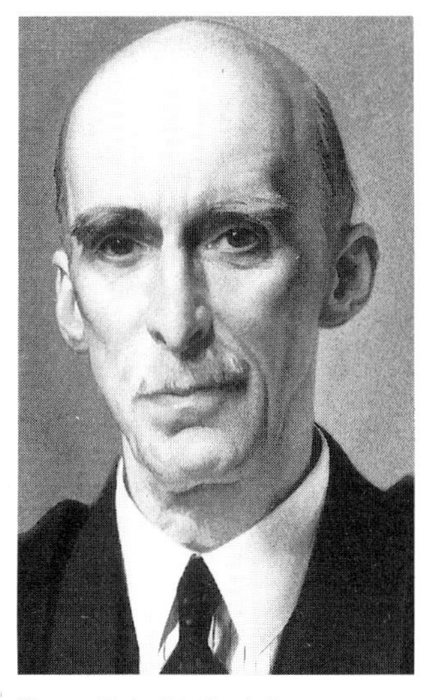

Figure 19.4 Sir Hugh Lett.

At the same meeting W. Bruce Clarke mentioned a patient with an inoperable breast carcinoma who had been treated by oophorectomy and who was well 5 years later, and said that all the patients he had treated in this way had benefited.

In the discussion, Stanley Boyd stated that his conclusions from treating a smaller number of cases coincided with those of Lett and that the chronic cases showed the best results. He did not consider "... that oophorectomy as a primary operation was advisable, but in two or three instances he had used the combination method — removing the breast and ovaries — with

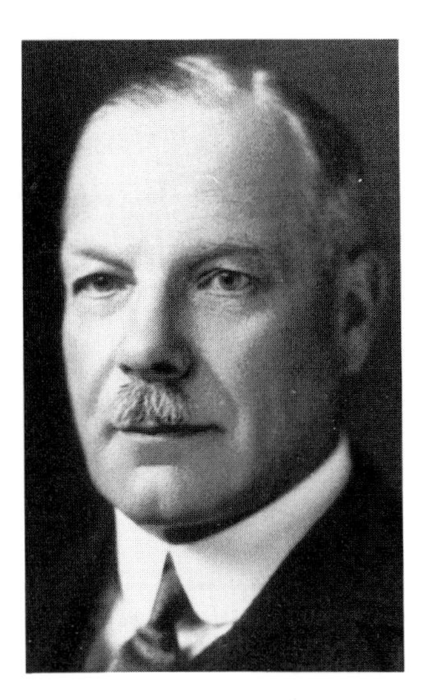

Figure 19.5 W. McAdam Eccles.

results which he did not think could have been obtained by removal of the breast alone".

This work of Boyd appears to be the first example of the treatment of carcinoma of the breast by combined mastectomy and oophorectomy, a method which was adopted by other surgeons at a later date. The present author recalls a number of patients he treated in this way, all of whom were in the high risk group.

Other prominent surgeons took part in the discussion on 24 January 1905. One of them, W. McAdam Eccles, Surgeon to the Royal Hospital of St Bartholomew in London, considered that much might be learned from the microscopical examination of the ovaries which had been removed from patients, and he mentioned a case with extensive cancer treated by oophorectomy where all the nodules atrophied except one or two small ones, and the patient lived for 26 months after the oophorectomy and for 35 months after the removal of the primary tumour.

Pearce Gould, Surgeon to the Middlesex Hospital, stated "... that his experience of the results of this operation had not been so favourable as those of Mr Bruce Clarke and he had seen but one case with a striking result. Sections of the atrophic growth showed considerable fibrosis and atrophy of the cell elements. It was clear that there were physiological means by which the disease could be arrested, and he looked forward to the time when these physiological means would be known and rightly applied."

This was a visionary statement by Gould concerning the "physiological" control of breast carcinoma, which is very relevant today. We continue to seek a complete understanding of hormone control mechanisms and methods to manipulate them, with the objective of preventing and curing breast carcinoma.

For many decades after the impressive work mentioned above, though oophorectomy in the treatment of breast carcinoma was not forgotten it did not receive the attention it merited. It was brought to the notice of the present author by Sir Holburt Waring, Senior Surgeon to the Royal Hospital of St Bartholomew in London (who later became President of the Royal College of Surgeons of England), when the author was Waring's resident house-surgeon at St Bartholomew's Hospital.

In his book *The Surgical Treatment of Malignant Disease (1928)* Waring stated that he had practised oophorectomy for breast carcinoma for several years and had found that in 20–30% of the patients the primary tumour diminished in size and sometimes even disappeared, and that secondary tumours became much smaller. However, favourable results appeared to be only temporary, as after 2–4 years tumour reactivity occurred, with fatal outcome. He stated that the best results seemed to be achieved in premenopausal women and mentioned ovarian radiation as part of the radiotherapy régime for inoperable and advanced breast carcinoma. This allusion to "ovarian radiation" made 60 years ago is surely very impressive.

A personal experience

The present author recorded in detail his experience in treating a patient with disseminated carcinoma of the breast with oophorectomy in 1949. At that time oophorectomy was seldom practised and largely forgotten as a method of treatment for breast carcinoma. The patient was referred to the author by a surgical colleague who asked if he could possibly recommend any treatment for her advanced disease. After the clinical examination the patient made the crucial statement that all her tumours increased in size prior to menstruation. The author immediately recalled Waring's observation, made 20 years before, regarding the treatment of breast carcinoma by oophorectomy and he decided to perform bilateral oophorectomy. The operation was followed by a most impressive regression of the disease. The following is the case-record, which the author published with clinical photographs *(Raven, 1950)*.

Case-record. Female aged 50 years, married with two children, had noticed 2 years ago a swelling in the right pre-auricular region; 9 months ago a painless swelling appeared above the inner end of the left clavicle and 4 months ago she noticed a large lump in her left breast and a small lump in the outer side of the left arm. Other similar lumps had appeared in the skin of the right shoulder, chest wall and right loin.

Her menstrual periods commenced at the age of 16 years; the cycle varied from 21 to 26 days; the duration was 7 to 8 days. During the last 2 years blood clots were present in the menstrual discharge. All the tumours increased in size prior to menstruation.

On clinical examination the patient's general nutritional condition was good. The following tumours were noted. Right pre-auricular 3.4 × 2.2 cm; left supraclavicular 5 × 2.2 cm; left breast, upper inner quadrant 3.5 cm diameter, attached to skin and fascia. There were hard fixed lymph nodes in the left axilla and multiple metastatic tumours were present in the skin over the right shoulder, left arm, chest wall and right loin. The right breast and right axilla were normal and no abnormality was detected in the abdomen. Radiograms of the chest, dorsal and lumbar spine and pelvis showed no metastases. A mild degree of anaemia was present. Operation: bilateral oophorectomy and excision biopsy of the skin tumour of the right shoulder for histopathology.

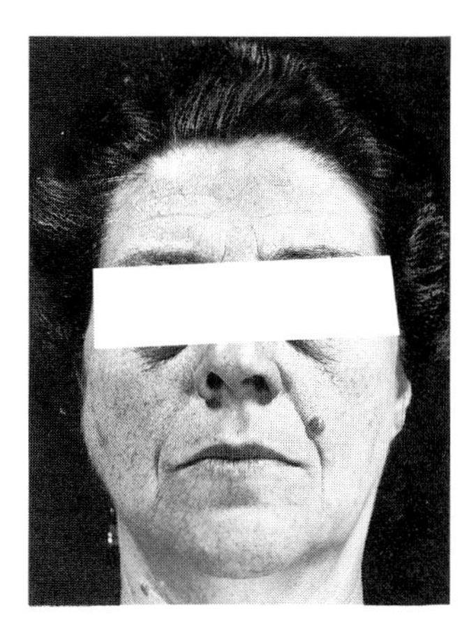

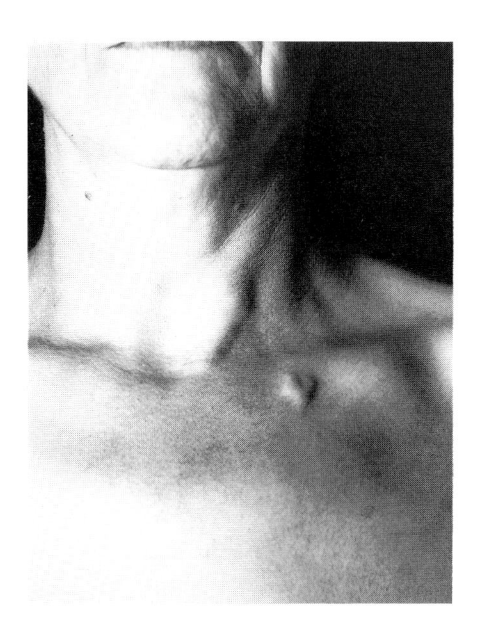

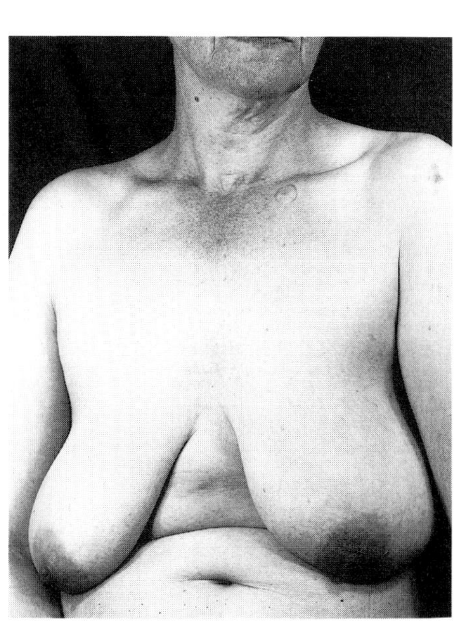

Figure 19.6 Clinical photographs of a female patient aged 50 with disseminated breast carcinoma, showing *above* a right pre-auricular tumour, *bottom left* a skin metastasis below the left clavicle and *bottom right* the enlarged left breast caused by a spheroidal cell carcinoma.

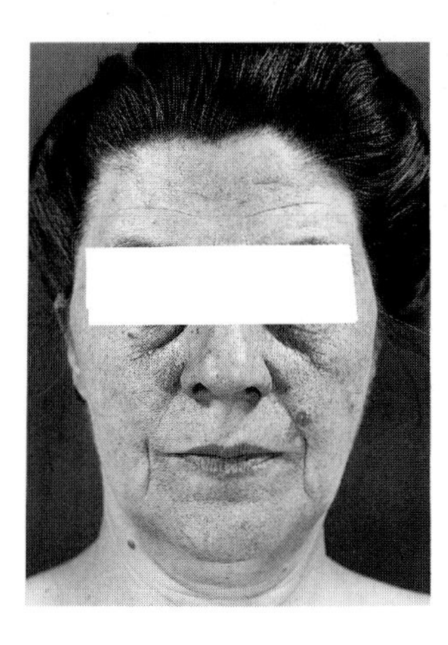

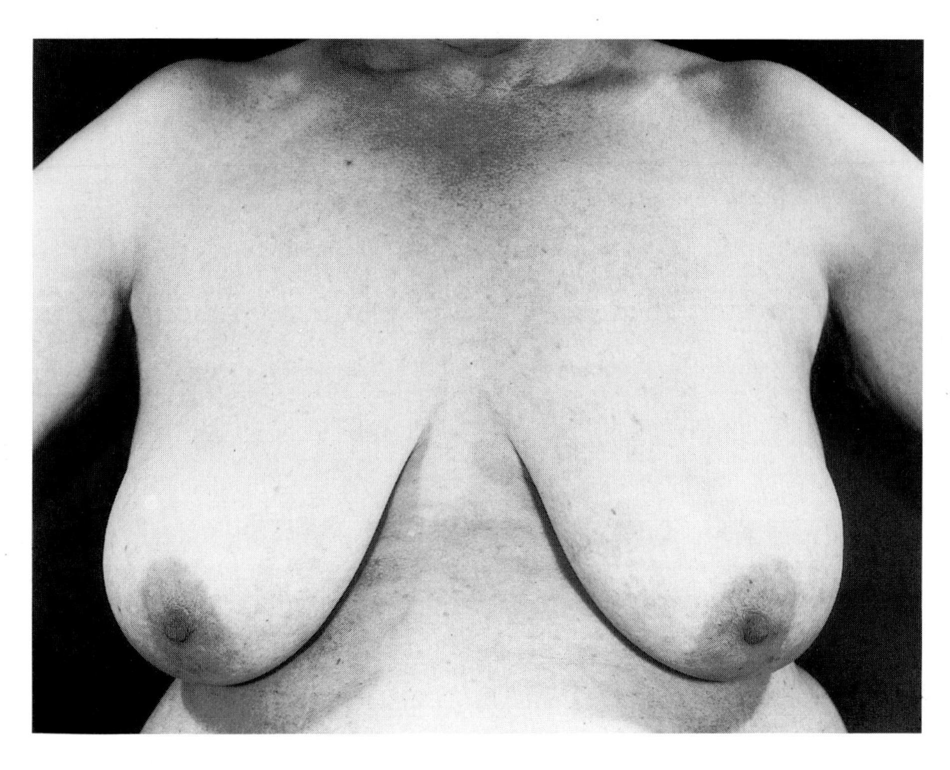

Figure 19.7 The patient in Figure 19.6, after bilateral oophorectomy. *Above:* Complete regression of the pre-auricular tumour 1 year and 10 months after the operation. *Right:* Regression of the primary carcinoma in the left breast and of the skin metastasis below the left clavicle 1 year and 4 months after the operation.

Histopathology: One ovary was enlarged with a cyst present 2.5 × 2 cm, containing watery fluid, and it had a thin lining of luteal cells. The other ovary was of normal size, but there was a wide, ill-defined zone of theca cell formation; otherwise it was normal.

The skin nodule was a spheroidal cell carcinoma with cells arranged in compact groups and narrow cords and there were isolated cells in the subcutis and deep layers of the dermis.

The postoperative results were carefully observed as follows: After 41 days the tumours were smaller and some skin tumours had disappeared. After 111 days the right pre-auricular tumour had disappeared, leaving a hollow area. The left breast carcinoma became very soft and smaller, at 2.5 cm diameter.

Six months later there was a residual area of slight thickening in the left breast, a small lymph node in the left axilla and an area of thickening in the skin of the left arm.

Seven months later all the tumours had disappeared; the tissues of the left breast were soft, pliable and normal; no lymph nodes in the left axilla; all the skin tumours had disappeared and the face was normal.

Subsequent course: The patient remained well for 2½ years, when the right axillary lymph nodes enlarged and were excised. Histopathology showed anaplastic polyhedral carcinoma.

The patient continued to be well until 3½ years after oophorectomy, then an enlarged right supraclavicular lymph node and small skin tumours appeared. These tumours regressed with methyl-testosterone therapy and the author noted that the patient looked younger than formerly. There was no clinical evidence of primary or disseminated breast carcinoma.

5½ years following oophorectomy a cyst 4 cm in diameter developed in the left breast. Later the patient's general condition began to deteriorate, with osseous and soft tissue metastases present. Bilateral adrenalectomy was then performed. Histopathology of the adrenal glands showed no abnormality.

The disease continued to progress and because there had been such an impressive response to oophorectomy and androgen therapy, it was agreed that a neurosurgeon should perform a hypophysectomy, but the patient died 2 days after the operation.

Autopsy showed the presence of disseminated breast carcinoma in many organs, soft tissues and bones. Histopathology showed a highly cellular carcinoma in the left breast, invading the lymphatics and venules, with focal haemorrhages and areas of fibrosis.

The survival period of this patient with disseminated breast carcinoma from oophorectomy to death was 7½ years.

Conclusions regarding breast carcinoma and oophorectomy

The evidence cited from various authorities demonstrates that tumour regression can result from oophorectomy for advanced and disseminated breast carcinoma. It occurs in about 30% of patients and the best responses are in premenopausal women. In some patients the response is quite dramatic, as in the author's patient reported above who lived for 7½ years after her oophorectomy.

We do not yet understand why only so few patients respond to the operation and why tumour regression is not permanent. The historical observations mentioned here are very important from both the academic and clinical viewpoints, for this initial work led to the development of the modern methods of synthetic hormonal treatment of breast carcinoma and a better understanding of the disease.

PROPHYLACTIC OOPHORECTOMY IN BREAST CARCINOMA

The encouraging results of oophorectomy in advanced and disseminated breast carcinoma suggested its possible role in preventing recurrent and metastatic disease after mastectomy for earlier disease.

Prophylactic oophorectomy and ovarian radiation were carried out by Nissen-Meyer *(1965, 1967)*, who explained that the term "prophylactic castration" is inadequate because oophorectomy is not expected to prevent recurrent disease but perhaps it will delay recurrences and prolong the total survival time for patients who are not cured by the primary surgical and radiation treatment. "Primary castration", therefore, is a more adequate term. Nissen-Meyer came to the following conclusions regarding this modality. After the natural menopause the ovaries might continue to produce hormones, in some patients for periods probably more than 10 years, and this ovarian function might stimulate the growth of breast carcinoma tissue, thus shortening the patient's life. Ionising radiation might suppress ovarian function, for primary ovarian radiation reduces the growth-rate of tumour tissue in patients with recurrent disease. The disease-free interval is on average increased by about 1–2 years in postmenopausal patients up to the age of 70 years. The total survival time is longer in groups of patients treated with "prophylactic" castration than in groups treated with "therapeutic" castration.

BREAST CARCINOMA IN CASTRATED WOMEN

There is considerable interest in the incidence of breast carcinoma which develops in women who have undergone oophorectomy for another condition, and reference is made to the work of Dargent *(1949)* on this subject. He found that in a series of 2000 patients with breast carcinoma 32 (1.6%) had previously undergone castration. He pointed out that this incidence was higher than that of carcinoma occurring during pregnancy, of which there were 21 cases (1.05%), or in males (16 cases — 0.8%). Although breast carcinoma is rare in castrated women, it does occur, so oophorectomy is not an absolute protection against it. The present author has had four patients with breast carcinoma who had undergone previous oophorectomy.

In Dargent's series of cases the interval between castration and the onset of breast carcinoma was from 2 months to 24 years and the number of patients over 60 years old was significantly high. When castration had been performed in women aged between 40 and 50, when the amount of circulating folliculin is considered to be significant, breast carcinoma generally appeared late. Only four of the 32 patients who developed breast carcinoma after castration survived for 10 years without recurrent disease.

It is important to note that oophorectomy and a radical mastectomy for carcinoma in one breast cannot prevent a carcinoma developing in the other breast. This is exemplified by the following case-history of a patient under the present author's care.

Case-record. A female aged 39 years underwent a left radical mastectomy and oophorectomy for a carcinoma (stage 2) in the left breast. Histopathology showed an infiltrating polygonal cell carcinoma with metastases in one axillary lymph node. The ovaries showed no abnormality. The patient remained well until 20 years later, when she developed a carcinoma in the right breast, for which a modified radical mastectomy was performed.

Histopathology revealed an invasive carcinoma composed of fairly uniform cells showing considerable glandular differentiation. The tumour was invading into fat; the mitotic rate appeared slow. No metastases were present in the axillary lymph nodes. Oestrogen receptor: 111.3 fmol per mg cyt prot. ER positive.

ADRENALECTOMY

Bilateral adrenalectomy as treatment for disseminated breast carcinoma was described first by Huggins and Bergenstal *(1952)* and they successfully carried out this operation which was made possible when cortisone acetate became available for replacement therapy. In addition to performing it in patients with advanced breast carcinoma they also performed it in patients with carcinoma of the prostate and reported that some disease regression occurred in both cases. Thus in their initial series of patients undergoing this treatment, two out of six patients with advanced breast carcinoma showed improvement, one moderately benefited, but three had no tumour regression. There were four cases of advanced prostate carcinoma which had become reactivated following its previous control with anti-androgen therapy and in these cases they observed some, or all, of the following

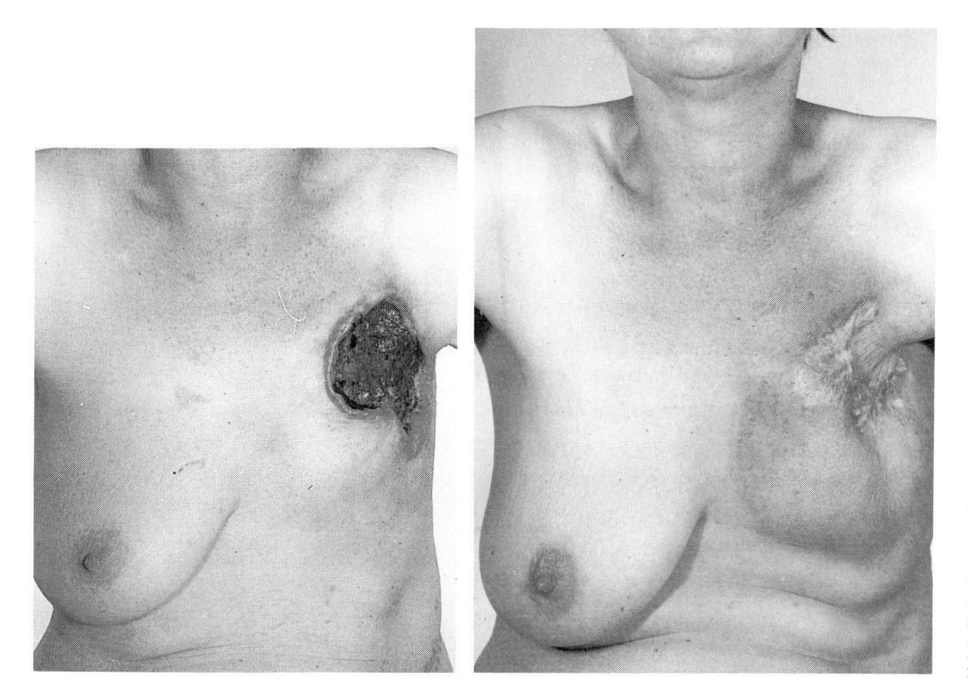

Figure 19.8 *Left:* A female patient with an advanced carcinoma of the left breast, which was treated with radiotherapy and bilateral adrenalectomy. *Right:* The treatment resulted in complete tumour regression and the patient is well 6 years later, with no recurrent or metastatic breast cancer.

effects: relief of intractable bone pain, a gain in body weight, a reduction in the levels of acid phosphatase, which had been considerably raised, a reduction in thermocoagulable proteins, an increase in total serum proteins, an increased haemoglobin and erythrocyte content of whole blood, and shrinkage of the primary carcinoma. No improvement was found in two cases. The patients were observed over periods extending from 2 to 9 months.

In a large series of cases of advanced breast carcinoma treated by bilateral adrenalectomy by the present author, 50% of the patients experienced significant benefit and some had remarkable improvement, including the

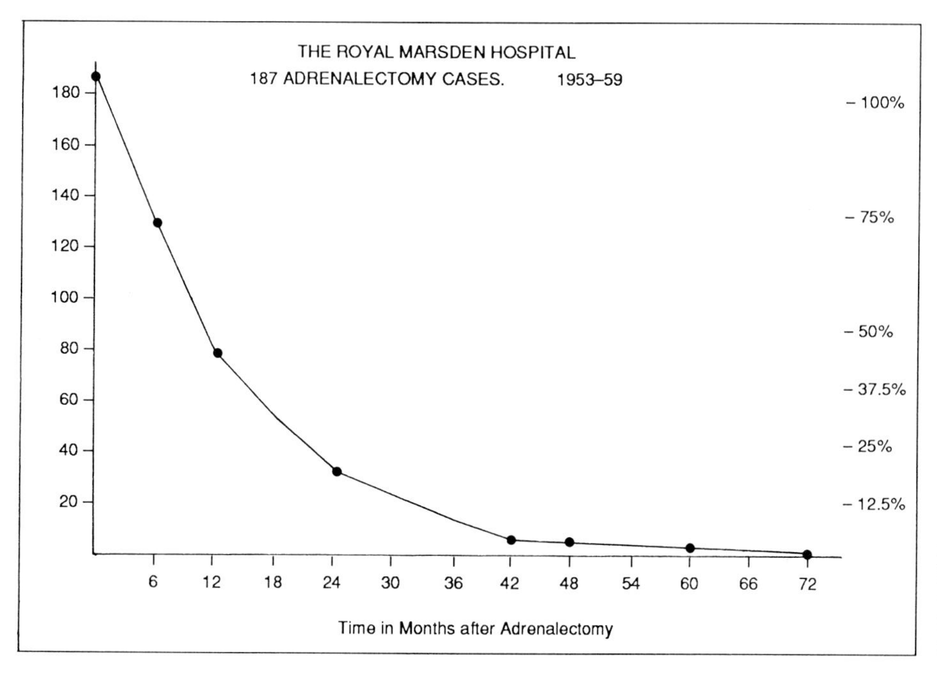

Figure 19.9 The survival results in a series of 187 patients with disseminated breast carcinoma treated by bilateral adrenalectomy at the Royal Marsden Hospital.

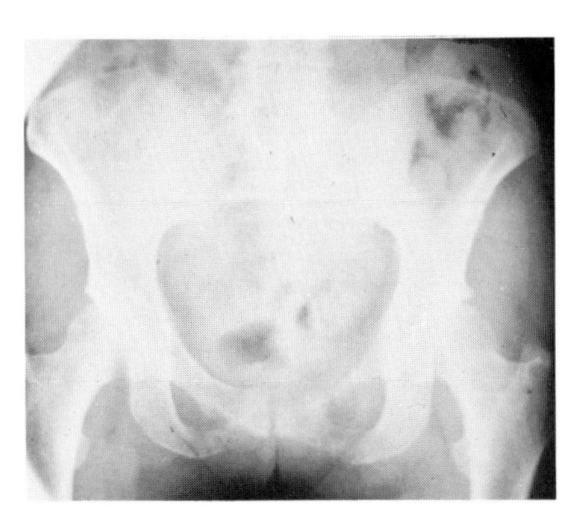

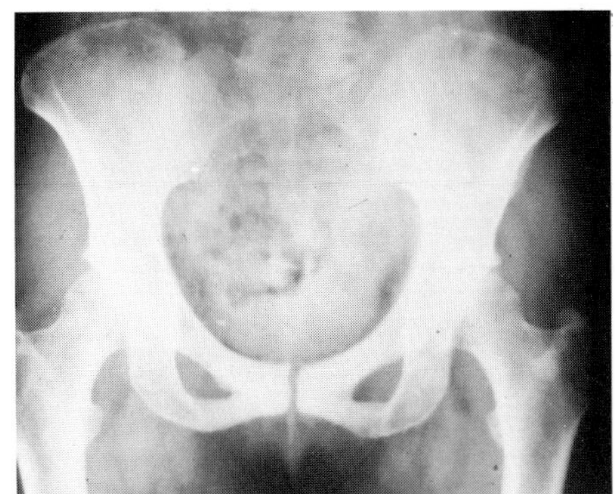

Figure 19.10 *Left:* Radiograph of the pelvis of a 47-year-old female patient who developed disseminated carcinoma of the breast 3 years after undergoing a right radical mastectomy. Extensive metastases in both pubic and ischial bones have caused a pathological fracture. *Right:* Radiograph of the same patient 5 months after bilateral oophorectomy and bilateral adrenalectomy, showing recalcification and healing of the fracture. The patient was pain-free and fully ambulant.

amelioration of pain and increased periods of survival. The disease was controlled for as long as 11 years. Other patients with recurrent breast carcinoma in the soft tissues of the chest wall enjoyed a marked regression of their tumours, which lasted up to 17 years.

The best results occurred in patients with osseous metastases: pathological fractures healed, recalcification of bones took place and severe bone pain was quickly relieved. Several patients had large ulcerating carcinomas of the breast and it was impressive to observe the tumour regression and the healing of the affected tissues.

Visceral metastases in the lung and liver are more resistant and show little or no response to adrenalectomy.

At the present time bilateral adrenalectomy is performed less frequently for metastatic breast carcinoma, due, undoubtedly, to the development and clinical use of synthetic hormones, especially Nolvadex (tamoxifen), aminoglutethimide and megestrol acetate, in addition to the availability of chemotherapy.

HYPOPHYSECTOMY

The removal of the pituitary gland as treatment for advanced breast carcinoma was performed first by Luft and Olivecrona *(1951)*. The present author visited Stockholm to discuss this method of treatment with the latter, a well-known neurosurgeon, and had the opportunity to witness him perform a hypophysectomy by the transcranial route.

Luft and Olivecrona *(1959)* also reported the results achieved by hypophysectomy in 59 patients with disseminated breast carcinoma who had not previously undergone bilateral adrenalectomy. There were four operation deaths and eight other patients were not evaluated for other reasons, so in all only 47 patients were evaluated. A remission induced by hypophysectomy occurred in 27 (57%), while in 20 cases no response was observed. The effects of the treatment in the group of patients with remission lasted for approximately 17 months. Luft and Olivecrona stated that it was not certain at that time whether hypophysectomy would induce a remission in a higher percentage of patients than adrenalectomy or combined adrenalectomy and oophorectomy. They thought that the course of the disease in patients with metastases in the brain, or extensively in the liver, would most probably not be altered by hypophysectomy and that women over 60 years of age probably would not respond.

Since beneficial effects have followed both bilateral adrenalectomy and hypophysectomy in advanced breast carcinoma, the problem arose as to which operation should be done. The present author has advocated bilateral adrenalectomy because the operation mortality was lower and replacement therapy was easier to carry out.

The operation of hypophysectomy was simplified by using the trans-nasal trans-sphenoidal route of approach, which is less traumatic for the patients, who are already suffering from the effects of disseminated breast carcinoma.

After the recognition of the value of surgical hypophysectomy, radiation hypophysectomy was developed, which made use of external and internal sources of radiation. Thus techniques were designed for the implantation of radon seeds, radioactive gold (^{198}Au) and radioactive yttrium (^{90}Y) into the pituitary gland. This subject was clearly described by Forrest *(1959)*.

Like adrenalectomy for advanced breast carcinoma, both the operation of hypophysectomy and radiation hypophysectomy are carried out much less frequently today, due to the development of hormonal therapy using synthetic hormones.

EARLY CLINICAL EXPERIENCE WITH SYNTHETIC HORMONES

Initial interest in the treatment of advanced breast carcinoma with synthetic oestrogens was stimulated by the discovery that they have a growth-retarding effect under certain circumstances. Haddow and colleagues *(1944)* reported a series of 73 patients with advanced cancer of different organs who were treated with the synthetic oestrogens triphenylchlorethylene, triphenylmethylethylene, and stilboestrol. Of the 22 patients with advanced breast cancer who were treated with triphenylchlorethylene, usually in doses of 3–6 g per day, 10 had a significant, but temporary, retardation, or even partial regression of the tumour. In one patient there was a prolonged arrest of the tumour.

Thirty cases of advanced malignant disease of other varieties were similarly treated, but only two cases—carcinoma of the bladder and carcinoma of the prostate—showed undoubted partial regression. Of the four cases of breast cancer and three cases of Hodgkin's disease that were treated with triphenylmethylethylene, usually by intramuscular injection, only one case of breast carcinoma showed even a temporary favourable response.

The same workers treated 14 cases of breast carcinoma with stilboestrol, which was given by intramuscular injection or orally for several months; five patients had alterations in their tumour similar to those observed with triphenylchlorethylene.

Serial biopsies for histopathology examination were carried out in a few cases where the tumour showed a marked clinical response. The histological changes included diminished mitosis, variations in staining and necrotic changes of a type which did not resemble those caused by radiation.

Pearson and his colleagues *(1955)* reported that the combined results of several clinics using oestrogens in the treatment of breast carcinoma showed that objective remissions of the disease occurred in 44% of the patients. The average duration of the remissions was 8 months, with a

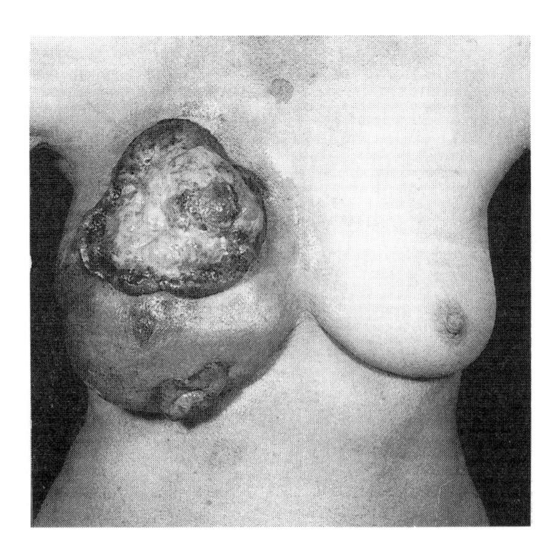
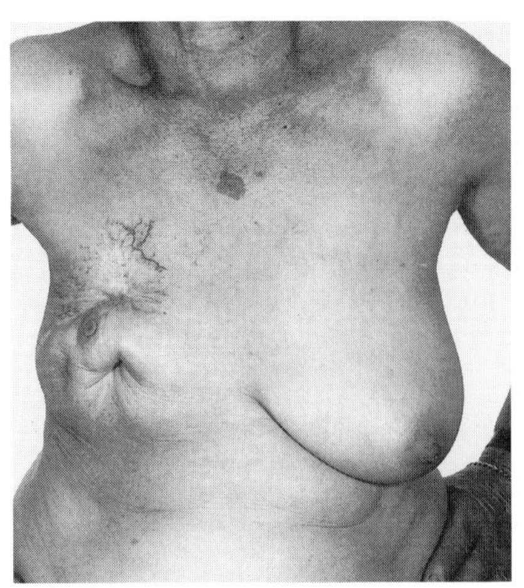

Figure 19.11 *Left*: A 71-year-old female patient with an advanced ulcerating carcinoma of the right breast. *Right:* Radiotherapy with a tumour dose of 5800 rads and administration of ethinyloestradiol and thyroid extract resulted in complete tumour regression, and ulcer healing occurred. The patient is well 15 years and 8 months later and has no recurrent or metastatic breast carcinoma.

median duration of about 4½ months. These authors stated that in approximately 50% of cases breast carcinoma is oestrogen-dependent, so that the administration of oestrogen in this group of patients is a potential hazard. The mechanism of the beneficial effects of oestrogens is not yet known, but at that time it was thought that they exerted a depressant action on the hypophysis.

ANDROGENS

The chief function of androgens is to stimulate the development and activity of the male reproductive organs. Experiments were carried out originally by John Hunter *(1794)*, which demonstrated the hormonal function of the testes. He showed that the rudimentary spur of a hen grew into a good masculine spur when it was transplanted into the leg of a cock, whereas the small spur of a young cock underwent no similar development when it was implanted in the leg of a hen. Hunter also called attention to the facts which indicated that the accessory male genital organs depended for their development, and probably for their existence, on the testes.

The testes are the main source of androgens, but experimental work has demonstrated that it is also produced by the ovary, and even in large amounts when ovarian tumours are present. Burrows *(1943)* described an excess of androgen which was secreted by ovarian tumours classified as arrhenoblastomas, thecomas, or granulosa cell tumours.

Androgen can also be elaborated by the adrenal glands. Hypertrophy of the adrenal cortex and some adrenal tumours in females, or in males before the onset of puberty, often cause virilism and in such cases an excess of androgen has been detected in the urine *(Simpson and colleagues, 1936)*.

Androsterone was isolated in crystalline form by Butenandt *(1931)*.

Inactivation and excretion of androgens

Androgens are rapidly inactivated in the body and excreted in the urine as substances with a reduced androgenic potency. Experimental investigations have demonstrated that androgen is inactivated in the liver *(Danby, 1940; Biskind, 1940)*.

It has been shown that oestrogen is a metabolic product of androgens, for it was found by Steinach and colleagues *(1936)* that the administration of androsterone to rats was followed by an increased excretion of urinary oestrogen and this occurred in both castrated and normal rats, which proved that the transformation does not occur in the testes. An increased output of oestrogen has been found in the urine of man after the administration of androgen *(Steinach and Kun, 1937)*.

Clinical application

The prostate

Carcinoma of the prostate is probably the most androgen-dependent tumour, and its treatment is designed to remove or neutralise androgens. Bilateral orchidectomy was shown by Huggins and Hodges *(1941)* to give a high remission rate and it is used frequently today, often combined with oestrogen therapy and radiation locally to the prostate. Hormonal profiles are established for the patients, to give guidance in endocrine therapy. Unless there are contraindications, prostatectomy is performed in patients with an early carcinoma of the prostate. Nesbit and Baum *(1950)*, reporting on the results of castration in prostatic carcinoma, showed that 31% of the patients survived 5 years.

Attention was called by Wang and Bulbrook *(1977)* to a new and potent anti-androgen called cyproterone acetate. This is now used in the treatment of patients with carcinoma of the prostate with encouraging results.

The breast

The treatment of carcinoma of the breast with androgen compounds has aroused considerable interest for nearly 50 years. The compound testosterone propionate was used by Loeser *(1939)* and by Ulrich *(1939)*, when it was established that androgen therapy can cause remissions in patients with advanced breast carcinoma.

Shimkin *(1957)* reported his results with a series of more than 450 females who were treated with androgens — primarily testosterone propionate — and stated that androgen therapy is indicated for premenopausal and menopausal patients with advanced breast carcinoma that is not amenable to radiotherapy. He reported that beneficial subjective effects are obtained in more than 50% of patients treated, but objective effects are obtained in only 10–15% of osseous metastases and in 10–25% of soft tissue metastases. The duration of improvement in patients that respond can vary from several weeks to more than 2 years. Side-effects can be serious when large doses of androgens are administered.

The present author can support these clinical observations from his own experience of the treatment of advanced breast carcinoma with testosterone phenylpropionate and later with the compound fluoro-hydroxy-methyltestosterone (Ultandren). The latter was produced by introducing a fluorine atom and a hydroxyl group into the methyltestosterone molecule. It is also known as fluoxymesterone and considered to be five times more potent in androgenic and anabolic activity than methyltestosterone. An added advantage is that it is fully active when given orally.

The considerable interest, around 30 years ago, in androgen therapy for advanced breast carcinoma is shown by the introduction of several new compounds. Mention is made of 19-norandrostenolone phenylpropionate (Durabolin), whose pharmacological effects were studied when it was found that phenyl propionic esterification enhances the activity and extends the duration of the effect of testosterone. This substance possesses much greater anabolic activity and minimal androgenic potency. It was pointed out by the present author *(Raven, 1959)* that in the treatment of breast carcinoma the nitrogen- and calcium-anabolic properties of the androgens are likely to be more important than their anti-oestrogenic effects. It was noted that when a response is achieved the patients with bone metastases experience pain relief and improvement in their general condition.

The use of androgenic hormones in the treatment of breast carcinoma has now diminished to a considerable extent and has been superseded by the use of more effective hormones which have been developed.

CLINICAL EXPERIENCE WITH NOLVADEX (TAMOXIFEN)

Reference was made earlier in this chapter to the use of Nolvadex (tamoxifen) in patients with breast carcinoma and the encouraging results which are being achieved at the present time. It is not the author's intention to deal here with this important new method of treatment, but attention is called to the publication by Patterson, Edwards and Battersby *(1981)* which followed a Symposium on the Progress of Endocrine Therapy for Breast Cancer held in Tokyo in 1981. In their booklet these authors give a detailed account of the clinical development and use of tamoxifen and comparisons with other forms of endocrine therapy for breast carcinoma, and they append many valuable references to the literature on the subject. The compound has been available internationally as a palliative treatment for breast cancer since the middle 1970s. The authors state that a summary of clinical trial data involving 3089 patients shows an overall objective response rate of 33%, with more than 50% of tumour regression. The good prognostic factors for a response are age, prior hormone responsiveness, oestrogen-receptor positive tumours and dominant soft tissue disease. Tamoxifen is now usually considered to be the first choice in hormone therapy for postmenopausal women with breast carcinoma, even those with osseous metastases. The side-effects are usually mild and the authors state that only 2.5% of the patients treated have been unable to tolerate this therapy.

Nowadays tamoxifen is used not only for advanced breast carcinoma but also in the continuing care of breasts which have undergone surgical treatment for earlier disease.

CANCER OF THE PROSTATE

The original observations connecting the testes with the genital organs were made by John Hunter in 1786. He noted that atrophy of the prostate followed castration and that the seminal vesicles were much smaller in eunuchs. However, if only one testicle was removed and the remaining testicle was normal, atrophy of the seminal vesicles did not occur. Hunter observed that before puberty there are few distinguishing features between males and females and that the special sex features appear mostly at puberty.

When her reproductive life has ended, the female loses some of her feminine characteristics and tends to become more masculine, or more like a hermaphrodite. He also observed that birds and mammals with a pronounced and limited breeding season have remarkable variations in the size and appearance of the gonads and accessory genital organs at different times of the year.

The subject was clarified by Berthold *(1849)*, who stated that the testes exerted their action, both generally and specifically, upon the body by some specific substance elaborated by testicular tissue. He also postulated that this substance is transported by the bloodstream to the extragonadal tissues.

From these classical concepts that normal tissue growth is regulated by a specific chemical substance there has now emerged the complicated subject of the hormonal control of neoplasia.

Castration in hypertrophy of the prostate

The first results following castration in hypertrophy of the prostate were reported by White on 28 May 1895 at a meeting of the American Surgical Association in New York *(White, 1895)*. He divided his communication into three sections: theoretical, clinical results and experimental results. With regard to the causation of prostatic hypertrophy, he gave evidence linking this abnormality with testicular function which produced some chemical substance. He stated, "It was the apparent analogy between the uterine and prostatic growths which led me to the investigation that resulted in my suggesting this operation to the profession." His analogy can be summarised as follows. The prostatic vesicle is the analogue of the sinus genitalis in the female — the uterine and vaginal cavities. The prostate and uterus are strikingly similar in structure, and would be almost identical if the tubular glands found in the inner walls of the uterus were prolonged into its substance. The histology of the growths, from small encapsulated tumours, easily shelled out, polypoid growths intimately connected with the uterus or prostate, up to enormous growths which far exceed the original bulk of the organ itself, is identical. Or there may be in either case a general hypertrophic enlargement affecting the whole organ. Lastly, the disturbances occur at about the same time in the sexual life of the two sexes, that is, during the latter half of the reproductive period. This ends sooner in the female than in the male, and accordingly we find the growths appearing in the former at a somewhat earlier age.

In his clinical section White tabulated the history of a series of 111 cases of prostatic hypertrophy treated by different surgeons with different methods. He stated, "The theoretical objections which have been urged against the operation of double castration have been fully negatived by clinical experience, which shows that in a very large proportion of cases (thus far in approximately 87.2 per cent) rapid atrophy of the prostatic enlargement follows the operation."

The third section was devoted to White's experimental work on dogs. In nearly every case where the vas deferens was tied or divided on both sides, he found that, without much testicular change, there was commencing atrophy of the prostate, with considerable weight loss. He thought that his experiments needed confirmation, as the absence of corresponding testicular change seemed to make the results somewhat anomalous, but he felt it was possible that the inclusion or severance of small, but important, nerves might account for the effect on the prostate. He also found that ligation of the vascular components of the spermatic cord, or of the whole cord, produced prostatic atrophy, but only after first causing disorganisation of the prostate.

Acid phosphatase in cancer of the prostate

Acid phosphatase was one of the earliest biological markers to be discovered in patients with cancer and it is a useful test for carcinoma of the prostate, especially when osseous metastases have developed. The following is the usual serum profile, including the reference range. Acid phosphatase (total) up to 3.0 units; acid phosphatase (prostatic) up to 1.0; prostatic acid phosphatase up to 3.5 ng per ml (measured by radioimmunoassay). In patients with prostatic carcinoma and osseous metastases all the values are raised.

Serum acid phosphatase falls after castration or oestrogen therapy. The test is therefore not only diagnostic, but also gives an indication of prognosis and response to treatment.

ECTOPIC HORMONE PRODUCTION BY TUMOURS

This subject is of fairly recent development and is included here not only because of its importance and interest, but also to demonstrate the wide ramifications of endocrinology in oncology.

During all its stages of development from the occult to dissemination a malignant tumour can cause metabolic disturbances with systemic effects by its capacity to secrete certain hormones. The clinical manifestations of these disturbances are now recognised as syndromes and the metabolic abnormalities can be measured in the blood and urine. Such syndromes can be very serious and even threaten the life of the patient, so they must be recognised and treated effectively at once. They are seen in patients with many varieties of cancer.

This subject was dealt with by Ellison and Neville *(1973)*, who stated that the ectopic production of hormones had clinical connotations, but they might also be important in the detection and screening of neoplasms, and as markers in monitoring their treatment. In their review they listed ectopic hormone production, the clinical syndromes and tumour sites.

The clinical syndromes include hypercalcaemia, hyperuricaemia, hypokalaemia, hyperglycaemia, the inappropriate antidiuretic syndrome and others. Their symptomatology and treatment have been reviewed by the present author *(Raven, 1986)*.

ONCOLOGY AND ENDOCRINOLOGY IN THE FUTURE

In this chapter an indication has been given of the immense contribution which has been made during past decades by the science of endocrinology to the theory and practice of oncology. The relationships between hormones and normal tissues and neoplasia are of fundamental importance. The discoveries that certain tumours are hormone-dependent have resulted in new methods of treatment; for example, hormonal therapy for carcinoma of the breast and prostate. Many problems still remain to be solved, so laboratory and clinical research must continue. It is likely that other tumours will be found to be related to hormones and we need to understand hormonal control mechanisms. The solutions will not only be valuable in the treatment of tumours, but are likely to give us a clearer understanding of their aetiology and nature and thus lead to their prevention.

Whilst today we can survey the past with interest and admiration for all that has been accomplished for patients with cancer, we look forward with confidence into the future, knowing that light will continue to be shed on our unsolved problems.

REFERENCES

Addison, T. (1855). *On the Constitutional and Local Effects of Diseases of the Suprarenal Capsules*. S. Highley, London

Adler, L. (1912). *Arch. Gynäkol.*, **95**, 349

Allen, E. A. and Doisy, E. A. (1923). An ovarian hormone. *J. Am. Med. Assoc.*, **81**, 819–21

Beatson, G. T. (1896). On the treatment of inoperable cases of carcinoma of the mamma: suggestions for a new method of treatment with illustrative cases. *Lancet*, **2**, 104–7 and 162–5

Berthold, A. P. (1849). Transplantation der Hoden. *Arch. Anat. Physiol. Wissensch.-Med. Berlin*, 42–6

Biskind, G. R. (1940). Inactivation of methyl testosterone in castrated male rats. *Proc. Roy. Soc. Exp. Med. Biol.*, **43**, 259–61

Boyd, S. (1900). On oophorectomy in cancer of the breast. *Br. Med. J.*, **2**, 1161–7

Burns, E. L. and Schenken, J. R. (1940). Qualitative studies on relationship between estrogen and mammary gland carcinoma in C3 H mice. *Proc. Soc. Exp. Biol. Med.*, **43**, 608–10

Burrows, H. (1943). Nomenclature of hormone-producing tumours of ovary. *J. Obstet. Gynaecol.*, **50**, 430–2

Burrows, H. (1949). *Biological Actions of Sex Hormones* (2nd edn). Cambridge University Press

Burrows, H. and Horning, E. S. (1952). *Oestrogens and Neoplasia*. Blackwell Scientific Publications, Oxford

Butenandt, A. F. J. (1931). Ueber die chemische Untersuchung der Sexualhormone. *Zeit. angew. Chem.*, **44**, 905–8

Clarke, W. B. (1905). Case of a woman 5 years after oophorectomy for inoperable cancer (case demonstrated at a meeting of the Royal Medical and Chirurgical Society). *Lancet*, **1**, 228

Cori, C. F. (1927). Influence of ovariectomy on spontaneous occurrence of mammary cancers in mice. *J. Exp. Med.*, **45**, 983–91

Danby, M. (1940). Formation and destruction of male hormone by surviving organs. *Endocrinology*, **27**, 236–41

Dargent, M. (1949). Carcinoma of the breast in castrated women. *Br. Med. J.*, **2**, 54–6

Davies, J. N. P. (1948). The cause of primary hepatic carcinoma. *Lancet*, **2**, 474–5

Davies, J. N. P. (1949). Sex hormone upset in Africans. *Br. Med. J.*, **21**, 676–9

Dmochowski, L. (1957). The part played by viruses in the origin of tumours. In Raven, R. W. (ed.) *Cancer*, Vol. 1, pp 214–305. Butterworth & Co., London

Dodds, E. C., Goldberg, L., Lawson, W. and Robinson, R. (1938). Introduction of stilboestrol, the first synthetic oestrogen. *Nature*, **141**, 247–8

Doisy, E. A., Thayer, S. and Veler, C. D. (1930). The preparation of the crystalline ovarian hormone from the urine of pregnant women. *J. Biol. Chem.*, **86**, 499–509. (Preliminary communication in *Am. J. Physiol.* (1929), **90**, 329–30)

Eccles, W. McAdam (1905). Discussion on an analysis of 99 cases of inoperable carcinoma of the breast treated by oophorectomy. *Lancet*, **1**, 228

Ellison, M. L. and Neville, A. M. (1973). Neoplasia and ectopic hormone production. In Raven, R. W. (ed.) *Modern Trends in Oncology*, Part 1: Research Progess, pp 163–81. Butterworth & Co., London

Forrest, A. P. M. (1959). Radiation hypophysectomy. In Raven, R. W. (ed.) *Cancer*, Vol. 6, pp 274–91. Butterworth & Co., London

Glass, S. J., Edmondson, H. A. and Soll, S. N. (1940). Sex hormone changes associated with liver disease. *Endocrinology*, **27**, 749–52

Gould, P. (1905). Discussion on an analysis of 99 cases of inoperable carcinoma of the breast treated by oophorectomy. *Lancet*, **1**, 1

Haddow, A., Watkinson, J. M., Paterson, E. and Koller, P. (1944). Influence of synthetic oestrogens upon advanced malignant disease. *Br. Med. J.*, **2**, 392–8

Homberger, F. and Fishman, W. A. (eds) (1953). *The Physiopathology of Cancer*. Hoeber-Harper, New York

Huggins, C. and Bergenstal, D. M. (1952). Inhibition of human mammary and prostatic cancers by adrenalectomy. *Cancer Rev.*, **12**, 134–41

Huggins, C. and Hodges, C. V. (1941). Studies on prostatic cancer: effect of castration, of oestrogen and androgen injection on serum phosphatases in metastatic carcinoma of the prostate. *Cancer Res.*, **1**, 293–7

Hunter, J. (1786). A description of the situation of the testes in the foetus, with its descent into the scrotum. In *Observations on Certain Parts of the Animal Economy* (4th edn). London

Hunter, J. (1794). *A Treatise on the Blood, Inflammation, and Gun-shot Wounds*. Printed by John Richardson, for George Nicol, Bookseller to His Majesty, Pall-Mall, London

Jensen, E. V., De Sombre, E. R. and Jungblatt, P. W. (1967). Estrogen receptors in hormone responsive tissues and tumors. In Wissler, R. W., Dao, T. L. and Wood, S., Jr (eds) *Estrogenic Factors Influencing Host-Tumor Balance*, p 15. University of Chicago Press, Chicago

Jensen, E. V. and De Sombre, E. R. (1972). Mechanism of action of female sex organs. *Ann. Rev. Biochem.*, **41**, 203

Korteweg, R. and Thomas, F. (1939). Tumor induction and tumor growth in hypophysectomized mice. *Am. J. Cancer*, **37**, 36

Lacassagne, A. (1932). Apparition de cancers de la mammelle chez le souris mâle, soumis à des injections de folliculine. *Compt. Rend. Acad. Sci.*, **195**, 630–2

Lathrop, E. A. C. and Loeb, L. (1919). Further investigations on the origin of tumors in mice: the tumor rate in hybrid strains. *J. Exp. Med.*, **29**, 475–500

Lett, H. (1905). An analysis of 99 cases of inoperable carcinoma of the breast treated by oophorectomy. *Lancet*, **1**, 227

Lipschutz, A. (1950). *Steroid Hormones and Tumors.* Williams and Williams, Baltimore

Loeb, L. (1919). Further investigations on the origin of tumors in mice. VI. Internal secretions as a factor in the origin of tumors. *J. Med. Res.*, **40**, 477–96

Loeser, A. A. (1939). Male hormone in the treatment of cancer of the breast. *Acta, Unio Int. Contra Cancrum*, **4**, 375

Luft, R. and Olivecrona, H. (1953). Experiences with hypophysectomy in man. *J. Neurol.*, **10**, 301

Luft, R. and Olivecrona, H. (1959). Hormone treatment of carcinoma of the breast — hypophysectomy. In Raven, R. W. (ed.) *Cancer*, Vol. 6, pp 265–73. Butterworth & Co., London

Marshall, F. H. A. and Jolly, W. A. (1906). Contributions to the physiology of mammalian reproduction. *Phil. Trans. Roy. Soc.*, **B198**, 99–141

Murray, W. S. (1928). Ovarian secretion and tumor incidence. *J. Cancer Res.*, **12**, 18–25

Nesbit, R. M. and Baum, W. C. (1950). Endocrine control of prostatic cancer: clinical and statistical survey. *J. Am. Med. Assoc.*, **143**, 1317–20

Nissen-Meyer, R. (1965). Castration as part of the primary treatment for operable female breast cancer. A statistical evaluation of clinical results. *Acta Radiol., Stockholm*, **Suppl. 249**, 1–133

Nissen-Meyer, R. (1967). The role of prophylactic castration in the therapy of human mammary cancer. *Eur. J. Cancer*, **3**, 395–403

Palmer, J. F. (ed.) (1887). *The Works of John Hunter*, Vol. 4, p 49

Patterson, J. S., Edwards, D. G. and Battersby, L. A. (1981). *A Review of the International Clinical Experience with Tamoxifen.* Clinical Research Medical Products Planning and Medical Department, Imperial Chemical Industries Pharmaceutical Division, Macclesfield, Cheshire

Pearson, O. H., Li, C., Maclean, J. P., Lipsett, M. B. and Wood, C. D. (1955). Management of metastatic mammary cancer. *J. Am. Med. Assoc.*, **159**, 1701–4

Raven, R. W. (1950). Cancer of the breast treated by oophorectomy. *Br. Med. J.*, **1**, 1343–5

Raven, R. W. (1959). The results of hormone treatment in disseminated carcinoma of the breast. In Raven, R. W. (ed.) *Cancer*, Vol. 6, pp 292–334. Butterworth & Co., London

Raven, R. W. (1986). Metabolic syndromes. In *Rehabilitation and Continuing Care in Cancer*, pp 153–62. Published on behalf of the International Union Against Cancer by Parthenon Publishing Group, Carnforth

Shimkin, M. B. (1957). Hormones and neoplasia. In Raven, R. W. (ed.) *Cancer*, Vol. 1, pp 161–213. Butterworth & Co., London

Schinzinger, A. (1889). Über Carcinome mammae. *Zentr. Org. Ges. Chir.*, **29**, 55

Simpson, S. L., De Fremery, P. and Macbeth, A. (1936). The presence of an excess of "male" (comb-growth and prostate-stimulating) hormone in virilism and pseudo-hermaphroditism. *Endocrinology*, **20**, 363–72

Steinach, E., Kun, H. and Peczenik, O. (1936). Beiträge zur Analyse der

Sexualhormonwirkungen. *Wren. klin. Wzchr.*, **49**, 899–903

Steinach, E. and Kun, H. (1937). Transformation of male sex hormones into substance with action of female hormones. *Lancet*, **2**, 845

Ulrich, P. (1939). Testosterone (hormone mâle) et son rôle possible dans le traitement de certain cancers du sein. *Acta, Unio Int. Contra Cancrum*, **4**, 377

Wang, D. Y. and Bulbrook, R. D. (1977). Endocrinology. In Raven, R. W. (ed.) *Principles of Surgical Oncology*, pp 227–61. Plenum Medical Book Company, New York and London

Waring, Sir Holburt J. (1928). *The Surgical Treatment of Malignant Disease*. Humfrey Milford. Oxford University Press, London

White, J. W. (1895). The results of double castration in hypertrophy of the prostate. *Ann. Surg.*, **22**, 1–80

Williams, D. C. (1977). Steroid hormones and cancer. In Raven, R. W. (ed.) *Principles of Surgical Oncology*, pp 157–77. Plenum Medical Book Company, New York and London

CHAPTER TWENTY

Immunology

Immunology is a complex basic science which has important relationships with oncology and these are becoming increasingly apparent. Immunological reactions are being studied in relation to the nature, development, diagnosis and even the treatment of cancer, and we now speak of immunoprophylaxis, immunodiagnosis and immunotherapy of the malignant diseases. Researchers and clinicians are paying ever-increasing attention to these subjects today, whereas some 30 years ago, when cancer research was expanding rapidly, there was but little work being carried out on immunological relationships with cancer.

However, a very helpful review was written by Green *(1958)*, which contained an extensive survey of the literature on the subject. In discussing antigenic change in the cancer cell he stated that no specific tumour antibody had been detected, but there was evidence that during the growth of transplanted tumours iso-antibodies were present to the normal iso-antigens in the tumour. This indicated the possibility that the progressive growth of a spontaneous tumour, when transplanted, might be due to lack of iso-antigens. Green discussed the biological evidence of immunological change in carcinogenesis and concluded that it shows that chemical carcinogenesis has an immunological background.

He included in his review the problem of the resistance of the body in human cancer, which has immunological connotations. He stated that the theory of antigenic loss provided a reason for invasion and metastasis, but little was known of the mechanism for the removal of normal cells, and homologous and autologous tissue immunity was only beginning to be understood. He thought it was reasonable to assume that the biological behaviour of the malignant cell was due to a failure of certain cells in the invaded tissue to identify it as a wandering displaced cell and that on this basis there was no difficulty in assuming there is resistance to cancer. He stated that the type of resistance the cancer cell evoked would be determined by its immunological structure and that the more readily it was identified, the more easily it would be disposed of. The effectiveness of the disposal mechanism probably varied considerably in different patients.

In the conclusion of his survey Green stated that immunological factors obviously pervade every aspect of cancer and cancer is itself an expression of an immunological change.

LATER DEVELOPMENTS

The role of immunological reactions in controlling cancer has become more clearly understood during recent years, following investigations which demonstrated that immune rejection reactions occur with experimental animal tumours which are similar to those which cause tissue graft rejections. The subject was reviewed by Baldwin *(1977)*, who stated, in addition to the foregoing experimental evidence, that laboratory tests for tumour-immune reactions have identified specific responses against some human tumours. Furthermore, there is some evidence suggesting that immunological reactions might be responsible for the control of cancer by the host. This interesting aspect of the subject is considered in greater detail.

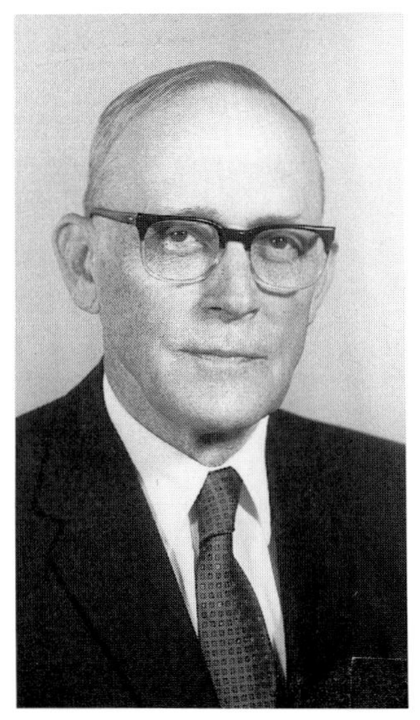

Figure 20.1 Warren H. Cole (1898–).

Spontaneous regression of human cancer

The fact that certain cancers in patients have regressed spontaneously either temporarily or permanently has interested researchers and clinicians for many years. With the growth of our knowledge about immunological responses in patients with cancer, we can now surmise that such reactions might be responsible for the spontaneous control of tumours.

An important book on this subject by Everson and Cole *(1966)* has aroused considerable interest and the present author acknowledges his indebtedness to its contents for the following information. Everson and Cole reviewed a large number of cases of spontaneous regression of cancer which were reported in the world literature during the years 1900–1965. They accepted a total number of 176 cases with adequate documentation, including histological confirmation of cancer, as possible examples of spontaneous regression of cancer. The commonest tumours concerned were hypernephroma (31 cases), neuroblastoma (29 cases), malignant melanoma (19 cases), choriocarcinoma (19 cases), bladder cancer (13 cases), soft tissue sarcoma (11 cases) and bone sarcoma (eight cases). The least frequent cancers were of the larynx, lung, pancreas, thyroid and tongue.

The phenomenon of cancer recrudescence many years after excision of the primary tumour has also been observed by clinicians. Good examples include patients who develop metastases 20 or more years after undergoing mastectomy for breast cancer and patients treated for ocular malignant melanoma who develop hepatic metastases many years later. These patients have "dormant" cancer cells which are under immunological control and we do not yet understand this mechanism or the reason why the cells suddenly become active.

Some patients have cancer metastases which regress after removal of the primary tumour, a good example being patients with hypernephroma. There are also patients with asymptomatic malignant tumours, such as carcinoma of the prostate, where the disease is quiescent.

It is obvious that more knowledge is required about immunological reactions and cancer before cause–effect immunology mechanisms can be implicated and explained in all these clinical examples.

Human cancer and immune deficiency states

This particular subject was dealt with by Currie *(1973)* in a more extensive review of human cancer and immunology. He stated that patients with immune deficiency conditions showed an increased incidence of malignant disease and gave good examples of this association, including patients with agammaglobulinaemia who showed an increased incidence of leukaemia and patients with the Wiskott-Aldrich and Chediak Higashi syndromes who had an increased incidence of lymphoreticular tumours. In addition, he stated that patients who were undergoing intensive immunosuppression, especially with antilymphocyte serum, had a tendency to develop malignant disease of the lymphoreticular system. He pointed out that the relationship between immune deficiency and cancer is not straightforward, for immune deficiency patients should develop tumours of all tissues rather than those of the lymphoid system, which are the targets of immune suppression.

There is an increasing number of people who have an immune deficiency state. These include patients who have undergone a kidney, liver, heart or other transplantation and who were immunologically suppressed to receive the organ. Certain therapeutic modalities such as radiation and corticosteroid administration are immunosuppressive. A recent example of immunodeficiency is in patients with AIDS and it is thought that they are more likely to develop cancer.

In general, it is accepted that persons with primary immune deficiency are susceptible to the onset of malignant disease. Much more laboratory and clinical research is required to measure and assess the "resistance" to cancer which is mediated immunologically, so that the appropriate treatment can be given to strengthen the defence mechanism of the body or avoid its impairment.

IMMUNODIAGNOSIS

The immunodiagnosis of various types of cancer is of practical importance today and researchers and clinicians are rightly giving it more attention. The subject was discussed by Baldwin *(1977)*, who described two concepts on which cancer immunodiagnosis is based and which have been verified in several specific instances.

The first concept is that patients with cancer can recognise neo-antigens on their tumour cells, which leads to the development of cellular and humoral responses against these neo-antigens which can be detected in various ways. Baldwin states that cellular immunity can be detected *in vitro* by the cytotoxicity of peripheral blood lymphocytes for cultured cells, or by the leukocyte migration test which measures the capacity of tumour cells or extracts to inhibit leukocyte migration in an appropriate medium. Cell-mediated immunity can also be detected by the capacity of patients to elicit delayed hypersensitivity responses against purified tumour antigen extracts injected intradermally.

In describing these tests Baldwin cites the work which was done by Cochran and colleagues *(1974)* and Herberman *(1974)*. He points out that the tests show that a patient responds immunologically to new antigens which are associated with a developing cancer, and therefore help in the diagnosis. At the present time, however, none of them have developed to a stage where they can be used routinely, except perhaps in serological studies of Burkitt's lymphoma and other cancers associated with the Epstein–Barr virus.

The second concept described by Baldwin is that human tumours secrete into the blood and other body fluids tumour-associated substances which can be detected and measured quantitatively by immunological techniques.

These tumour-associated substances belong to a class of antigens, now known as oncofoetal antigens, which are present in cancer cells and also in foetal tissue at certain stages of development. Outstanding examples are an alpha-fetoprotein which is secreted by hepatocellular carcinoma and a carcinoembryonic antigen which is associated with carcinoma of the colon and rectum. These antigens can be identified by immunoassay and thus have value not only in the diagnosis of primary tumours but also in the evaluation of prognosis for patients with metastatic and recurrent disease.

Carcinoembryonic antigen

Carcinoembryonic antigen, known as CEA, was identified by Gold and Freeman *(1965)*, who reported that at least two common, qualitatively tumour-specific antigens or antigenic determinants were present in adenocarcinomas of the human colon. They carried out further investigations to determine whether the antigens which are specific for colonic adenocarcinomas could be detected in other adult human tissues or in human embryonic and foetal tissues at different stages of gestation.

The results of their experiments with adult human tissues showed that only primary and metastatic carcinomas originating in other digestive system organs — oesophagus, stomach, duodenum, pancreas and rectum — contained components identical to the colonic tumour-specific antigens. The authors concluded that the tumour-specific antigens in cancers of the digestive system are determined by the site of origin of the tumours, as they found that metastases to the colon, pancreas or liver from carcinoma of the ovary or prostate showed no cross-reactivity with the colonic tumour-specific antigens. They also excluded the possibility that the tumour-specific antigens are products of an interaction between a growing, invasive mass and the surrounding normal tissue of the digestive system, or that they are related to exogenous contamination by enteric viruses. They found that carcinomas of the colon and rectum contained higher concentrations of tumour-specific antigens than carcinomas of the oesophagus and stomach.

They also considered the possibility of some relationship between the tumour-specific antigens of cancer of the digestive system and the embryonic development of the human gastrointestinal tract and its functionally related derivatives, the liver and pancreas. They investigated various tissues of foetuses between 2 and 8 months gestation and demonstrated that the antigens which, in the adult, were specifically localised to entodermal digestive system cancers were present also in the digestive organs of foetuses between 2 and 6 months of gestation.

Their results support the possibility of a distinct relationship between the system-specific tumour antigens and certain embryonic tissue components of the human digestive system. They named the common antigenic constituents "carcinoembryonic" antigens of the human digestive system and stated that during the embryonic and foetal processes of differentiation, specialisation and organisation in human gestation the entodermal tissue of the digestive system appears to contain specific antigenic components which disappear towards the later stages of gestation and which normally do not reappear during adult life. However, during the anaplastic changes associated with malignant transformation they reappear as tumour-specific antigens which are absent from comparable normal adult tissue.

This article by Gold and Freeman also contains an extensive list of references to the literature on carcinoembryonic antigens.

At the present time CEA measurements are of practical value in the diagnosis of metastatic and recurrent carcinomas, especially colonic and rectal carcinomas which follow surgical excision of a primary tumour, and in monitoring the treatment of secondary tumours, but the CEA test is relatively insensitive as far as regards the diagnosis of early primary carcinomas.

Alpha-fetoprotein

Alpha-fetoprotein is another tumour-associated foetal protein which is attracting considerable interest at present. Increased levels are found in the serum of patients with hepatocellular carcinoma. However, it is not a specific test for this carcinoma, since increased levels are also found in patients with other liver diseases, including hepatitis and cirrhosis, as well as in pregnant women, though the levels in these conditions are lower than in liver carcinoma.

Field *(1973)* stated that there is some evidence that the level of alpha-fetoprotein is linked with the actual mass of neoplastic tissue which is present; the same applies to CEA. The test may be helpful in the diagnosis of a liver mass and may provide additional evidence of the presence of a teratoblastoma. He also pointed out that primitive gonadal tumours have been reported to induce circulating alpha-fetoprotein. He stated that false negatives are common with this test, perhaps because of the insensitivity of the available techniques.

IMMUNOTHERAPY

During recent years researchers and clinicians have paid considerable attention to the possibility of cancer immunotherapy and much scientific research is being done on the subject. However, at the present time we cannot really speak of cancer immunotherapy.

Non-specific immunotherapy carried out by the administration of immunological adjuvants such as BCG and *Corynebacterium parvum* to stimulate a host response has produced variable effects in experimental tumour systems, including no response, regression, and even increased tumour growth. In his review of the subject Alexander *(1983)* states that in humans systematic administration has no effect, but local injection into skin tumours frequently leads to their disappearance and an associated intense local inflammatory reaction. He points out that the mechanism invoked is of great interest for it shows in a clinical setting that inflammatory cells release cytotoxic substances which can eradicate tumour cells and that there is evidence that a product released by T-cells belonging to the class of lymphotoxins is responsible for the selective killing of some types of cancer cells at sites of inflammation.

In his discussion of new immunological approaches to cancer treatment he states that tests should be done to determine whether a useful response might be induced by monoclonal antibodies produced in the laboratory and by clones of specific T cells grown *in vitro*, which are directed against antigens associated with the cancer cell but do not evoke a host response because they are not novel to the host. It might be possible for monoclonal antibodies to deliver anti-cancer substances directly into a tumour.

In his valuable review of human cancer and immunology Currie *(1973)*, when discussing immunotherapy, pointed out that the immune response appeared to be incapable of destroying large numbers of cancer cells, but it had been shown in animal experiments that immunotherapy techniques could destroy a limited number of cells. He suggested, therefore, that immunotherapy might play a vital role as adjunctive treatment to surgical excision, radiotherapy and chemotherapy, as these can cause a marked reduction in tumour size. After tumour debulking by these means, the use of immunotherapy, which must be carefully controlled, might be beneficial for a small amount of residual tumour.

An approach to cancer immunotherapy which has possible value is adoptive immunotherapy. Baldwin *(1977)* stated that in principle it should be possible to transfer immune factors from cancer patients in disease remission to a tumour-bearing host. At that time, however, there were practical difficulties. Animal experiments with tumours transplanted into syngeneic hosts showed that immunity can readily be transferred with lymphoid cells, but in humans transferred lymphoid tissue provokes an immune response in the recipient which may cause its rapid destruction. He mentioned alternative methods which involved the administration of immunological mediators, such as transfer factor and tumour immune antiserum.

The subject was discussed in detail by Rosenberg *(1985)*, who described several theoretical advantages of adoptive immunotherapy. He pointed out that if immune cells with anti-tumour reactivity could be developed, the marked specificity and sensitivity of immune reactions could make cells capable of attacking tumours but not normal tissues, giving resultant low treatment morbidity. The adoptive transfer of immune cells should not cause immunosuppression and probably would not require complete host immunocompetence, since competent immune cells would be transferred. Finally, because specificity would be high and morbidity low, adoptive immunotherapy could be combined with the other treatment modalities of surgery, radiotherapy and chemotherapy.

Rosenberg cited a new approach to raising immune lymphoid cells with anti-tumour reactivity in the mouse and also in humans, by generating immune cells by the incubation of normal lymphocytes in the lymphokine interleukin-2 (IL-2). They were capable of lysing fresh murine or human tumours, but they were not lytic for normal cells. These cells were called lymphokine-activated killer (LAK) cells. Rosenberg and colleagues carried out extensive studies in the mouse and showed that the adoptive transfer of LAK cells in conjunction with recombinant IL-2 can mediate the regression of established metastases in the lung and liver from various tumours in various mouse strains. This technique is a possible new approach to immunotherapy in human cancer and the results of further investigations are awaited with great interest. The initial results from the clinical trials which were reported by Rosenberg are encouraging. He stated that nine out of 22 patients have experienced objective responses, including patients with melanoma, renal cell cancer, colorectal cancer and lung adenocarcinoma. One patient with multiple subcutaneous melanoma nodules had a complete regression and was still disease-free 9 months after treatment. The other eight patients had a partial regression of disease.

In conclusion we can hope that in the future cancer immunotherapy will develop from this early stage. The possible risks to patients at the present time must not be overlooked. It is obvious that much more research and more clinical investigations are necessary for further progress to be made in this treatment modality.

IMMUNOPROPHYLAXIS

The prevention of cancer by immunological techniques has not escaped our attention, for it is an exciting concept. At the present time, however, no method of immunisation against the malignant diseases is available. If in the future it becomes possible to vaccinate people against cancer, as is done for other dangerous diseases, such as smallpox, the benefits will be enormous.

Harris *(1970)* called attention to the future of that which he termed "genetic engineering" and the possibility of "designing" vaccinating agents to confer immunity against a range of oncogenic DNA viruses without these agents being dangerous. He pointed out that we shall not be able to make this a practicable possibility until we have increased our knowledge of the relationship between oncogenic viruses and the cells which they transform.

REFERENCES

Alexander, P. (1983). Immunological aspects of malignant disease. *Cancer Forum*, **7** (2), 60–2

Baldwin, R. W. (1977). Immunology of malignant disease. In Raven, R. W. (ed.) *Principles of Surgical Oncology*, pp 279–301. Plenum Medical Book Company, New York and London

Cochran, A. J., Grant, R. M., Spilg, W. G., Macrie, C. E., Ross, C. E., Hoyle, D. E. and Russell, J. M. (1974). Sensitization to tumour associated antigens in human breast carcinoma. *Int. J. Cancer*, **14**, 19–25

Currie, G. A. (1973). Human cancer and immunology. In Raven, R. W. (ed.) *Modern Trends in Oncology*, Part 1: Research Progress, pp 127–43. Butterworth & Co., London

Everson, T. C. and Cole, W. H. (1966). *Spontaneous Regression of Cancer.*

W. B. Saunders, Philadelphia and London

Field, E. J. (1973). Immunological diagnosis of cancer. In Raven, R. W. (ed.) *Modern Trends in Oncology*, Part 1: Research Progress, pp 183–208. Butterworth & Co., London

Gold, P. and Freeman, S. O. (1965). Specific carcinoembryonic antigens of the human digestive system. *J. Exp. Med.*, **122**, 467–81

Green, H. N. (1958). Immunological aspects of cancer. In Raven, R. W. (ed.) *Cancer*, Vol. 3, pp 1–41. Butterworth & Co., London

Harris, R. J. C. (1970). Viruses and cancer. In Raven, R. W. (ed.) *Symposium on the Prevention of Cancer*, pp 80–6. Heinemann Medical Books, London

Herberman, R. B. (1974). Delayed hypersensitivity skin reactions to antigens on human tumors. *Cancer*, **34**, 1469–73

Rosenberg, S. A. (1985). A new approach to the treatment of cancer using the adoptive transfer of lymphokine activated killer cells and recombinant interleukin-2. In Fortner, J. G. and Rhoads, J. E. (eds) *Accomplishments in Cancer Research. General Motors Cancer Research Foundation*, pp 131–51. J. B. Lippincott Co., Philadelphia

CHAPTER TWENTY-ONE

Genetics

The importance of genetics in general medicine is fully recognised today and the significance of this science in oncology is becoming increasingly apparent with the growth of our knowledge about the genetic code and genetic mechanisms. Thirty years ago the subject of genetics and cancer was reviewed in detail by Koller *(1957)*, who appended an extensive list of references to earlier work, including the classical studies of Hansemann published from 1890 to 1906. He described three methods of approach for the solution of the intricate problem of genetics and cancer, using the knowledge which was available three decades ago. These included (1) an analysis of the cellular chromosomes and genes which form the physical basis of heredity, and comparison of their behaviour in normal and malignant cells; (2) a survey of the data obtained from the study of experimental tumours, where, as he pointed out, analyses of spontaneous and induced animal tumours, especially in mice, have shown that the origins of mammary carcinoma, lung adenocarcinoma and leukaemia are under genetic control.

From such experiments much information has been obtained about the role and the complexity of the hereditary factors involved in tumour development. (3) He also called attention to the possibility of a hereditary basis for human cancer, which is indicated by the available records of the pedigrees of families where several members have had cancer, often at the same site.

He discussed in detail the behaviour of chromosomes and genes during the development of cancer and stated that the transformation of a normal cell into a cancer cell is caused by a breakdown in the genetic control of cell division, which can be initiated by different agents, resulting in uncontrolled cell multiplication. He described the various features shown by the genetic material of the malignant cell and discussed their possible role in the genesis of cancer.

In his section dealing with genetics and experimental tumours Koller stated that the establishment of inbred strains in mice made it possible to investigate the roles of genetic constitution and the environment in cancer development. Differences in the incidence and types of tumours developed in the various strains are fundamentally genetic. The susceptibility of mice to cancer is inherited, but the genetic background is complex.

Regarding the subject of heredity and human cancer, Koller stated that a genetic basis is suggested by the published pedigrees which show a high incidence of particular cancers in members of one family and he cited cancer of the breast, uterus and stomach, and leukaemia as examples. We now know that certain rare neoplasms are genetically inherited. Members of families with familial disease who desire to have offspring may seek guidance from genetic counsellors. The most outstanding example of familial cancer is retinoblastoma, which occurs in the eye of children and can be bilateral.

Retinoblastoma is a highly malignant tumour. According to Ashton *(1958)*, it is bilateral in 20–30% of cases and the tumour in the second eye develops simultaneously with or several months after the tumour in the first eye affected. Ashton discussed the influence of heredity and pointed out that the majority of retinoblastomas arise sporadically, but the influence of heredity is well shown in other cases. He quoted several examples of familial incidence from the literature, as follows. Newton reported 10 out of 16 children affected in one family and Bell collected 36 pedigrees where retinoblastomas occurred in two generations in two or more siblings. Reese showed that the likelihood of a second sibling developing retinoblastoma is remote and probably about 1%, but the progeny of survivors with retinoblastoma are very likely to succumb to it; in his series nine out of 10 children of six survivors developed bilateral retinoblastoma. Ashton concluded that this tumour probably arises as an expression of a spontaneous gene mutation, which once acquired may be transmitted to the offspring as an irregular dominant trait.

The subject of genetic susceptibility to cancer was dealt with most clearly and helpfully by Bodmer *(1985)*, who included references to the literature. Regarding retinoblastoma, he stated that up to 40% of cases occurred as a definite dominantly inherited trait and he described the chromosomal, genetic and molecular studies regarding this tumour.

Bodmer also discussed familial polyposis coli, which is a dominantly inherited disease where there is a high incidence of progression to the development of one or multiple carcinomas. He pointed out that the primary genetic defect and the location of the gene in the human genome still remain unknown. The linkage between familial polyposis coli and carcinoma of the colon and rectum is of great clinical importance, because early investigations of the offspring of affected families will establish early diagnosis, leading to the removal of the polyps, or even the whole colon, and thus prevent carcinoma.

BREAST CANCER

Considerable interest has continued in the possible genetic susceptibility of the female offspring of women with breast carcinoma, so that, if this susceptibility is confirmed, they can be placed in a high-risk category and accordingly observed clinically for breast abnormalities. More work on the subject is still necessary to reach a final conclusion. Thus Holm and colleagues *(1982)* stated that there is little support for the view that genetic factors are significant in the aetiology of breast cancer.

This subject was discussed in detail by King *(1982)*, who explained that the investigation of the genetics and epidemiology of breast cancer in families illustrates the approach and objectives of genetic epidemiology. This particular discipline is the study of the interaction of genetic and environmental, cultural and behavioural influences on the distribution of diseases in human populations. King stated that consistent epidemiological evidence probably indicates that the single factor which increases the risk of breast cancer in a woman most dramatically is the presence of breast cancer in her immediate family, especially if more than one relative has had the disease, or a relative has had bilateral breast cancer, or cancer at an early age.

According to Anderson *(1977)* and Ottman *(1980)*, quoted by King, there is analytical evidence that perhaps 15% of breast cancer in Caucasian women in the USA is attributable to familial factors. King explained that from analysis of individual families where breast cancer is very common we can estimate the proportion of familial risk that is consistent with inheritance of genetic susceptibility to disease. She stated that this investigation was proceeding.

The importance of reaching a conclusion concerning genetic susceptibility to breast cancer is obvious from the clinical and other viewpoints. However, at the present state of our knowledge it seems that any such susceptibility is small.

GENETICS AND CHEMISTRY

The association of sciences in oncology has led to a major medical advance in recent years and it is of absorbing interest to see the developments in the exact sciences such as physics and chemistry and then subsequent fundamental contributions to the biological sciences. This theme was discussed by Chargaff *(1979)* in the context of the chemical basis of genetics. He stated that genetics is one of the youngest sciences — dating from 1900 when Gregor Mendel's observations were rediscovered — and that the initial exponents did not think in terms of chemistry. However, when the gene was defined as the unit of heredity and it was recognised that it was probably localised in the chromosomes, the attention of the chemist was necessary to investigate its chemical structure, which was thought likely to be a protein. Chargaff called attention to the careful research carried out by Avery and colleagues which led to the recognition that the hereditary units, the genes, were composed of DNA. This was followed by research on the composition of DNA, including the purines and the pyrimidines.

The identification of the DNA molecule as the gene material was an event of great historic importance. Hotchkiss *(1979)* has described the "DNA Revolution" which followed during the years 1930–1956. Horowitz *(1979)* stated that the discovery and elucidation of the connection between genes and proteins represented one of the major accomplishments of science in the 20th century, which has clearly illuminated the fundamental organisation of living systems. We now understand that every organism has a genetic heritage.

GENETICS AND CANCER

In the broadest terms cancer is a disease of the cell and is characterised by abnormal cellular division; consequently, the chemical mechanisms of normal and abnormal cell division are of exceptional importance. This subject was reviewed in a most instructive manner by Davidson *(1957)*, who also gave an extensive list of references to earlier work. He described in detail the chemistry of cell components, including the structure of the two main types of known nucleic acids, the ribonucleic acids (RNA) and the deoxyribonucleic acids (DNA). The RNA are abundant in the cell cytoplasm and present in small amounts in the nuclei, whilst the cell nuclei are composed mainly of DNA and protein, with small amounts of RNA, lipids and inorganic constituents. Davidson also discussed the function of DNA in heredity.

The subject of the biochemistry of cancer induction was dealt with by Griffin *(1957)*, who stated that cancer is caused by the changes induced in the metabolism and composition of normal cells by a carcinogenic stimulus. Investigators have considered that derangements in enzyme patterns, protein or ribonucleic acid composition might result in the formation of a type of cell where the alteration or change might be a permanent and unique feature. The carcinogenic stimulus might also cause changes in the deoxyribonucleoprotein or chromatin. During cancer induction the mechanism controlling cell division is removed.

These concepts held 30 years ago about the cellular changes in cancer are of much historic interest, especially when considered in the light of present genetic research and the new knowledge of cancer genetics that has accrued. As Bodmer *(1982)* states, cancer is a genetic disease at the cellular level, but not with a major inherited component. Inherited susceptibility to cancer might involve DNA repair deficiencies and differences in immune response mechanisms and in the metabolism of chemical carcinogens. In his comprehensive and most helpful review, with modern references, of the subject of cancer genetics Bodmer discusses likely future important developments, including the use of linked genetic markers to identify well-defined genetic susceptibility to different cancers and high-risk groups in families. He cites the example described by King of the linkage of the glutamate pyruvate transaminase enzyme marker to breast cancer. He stresses the important future objective of identifying the particular genes which are involved in determining inherited susceptibilities and establishing their functions and mechanisms. He states that we already understand something about a relatively high proportion of the basic genetic functions existing in the human genome and that eventually we shall know the whole DNA sequence of the human genome and understand its functional units. Finally, he states that by using recombinant DNA techniques with epidemiological and genetic studies the genetic contribution to the initiation and progression of cancers at the germ line and somatic cell levels will be understood.

The subject of DNA polymorphism and the recent applications of DNA technology to human genetics was dealt with in detail by White *(1982)*, who stated that a number of new human genetic markers were available for further study and that more would be identified. He also discussed the subject of oncogenes which have in common either an aetiological role in, or a close association with transformation and tumorigenesis and might therefore play a role in inherited tumour predispositions, in addition to other forms of carcinogenesis.

Baserga *(1985)* discussed the evidence indicating a considerable amount of overlapping between cell cycle-dependent genes, oncogenes, growth factors and receptors for growth factors. Hypothetically these four sets of genes are involved in cell cycle progression and any alterations in them can alter growth regulation. Baserga pointed out, however, that this does not mean cancer, but it could be the first step towards neoplastic transformation. The alteration might be a mutation of the genes or an overexpression of them. Research continues on this important subject of the role of genes and alterations in their structure or expression in altered regulation of cell growth.

An important and interesting review of oncogenes and cancer by Weber and McClure *(1987)* describes three features, as follows: mutation, when the *ras*-proto-oncogene might become oncogenic by a single point mutation which results in an amino acid substitution in the gene product which might alter the phenotype of the cell. Carcinogens might act by causing mutations at specific sites on cellular proto-oncogenes.

The same authors describe amplification, which means the repeating of the DNA sequences leading to overexpression of the gene product. They also define chromosomal translocation, as the transfer of a gene from its normal position to a position on another chromosome. This occurs consistently with certain tumours.

They discuss the possible clinical applications of future oncogene research, which they think will be considerable. They state that oncogenes are not the cause of cancer, but that proto-oncogenes encode proteins essential for normal cell growth and that these, when altered, contribute to the malignant phenotype. The authors visualise the possibility of specific anti-oncogene treatment with a monoclonal antibody, or a drug designed to compete for the altered oncogene product without affecting the normal protein. In the meantime, they call attention to the clinical value of the new method of classifying tumours by characterising the genes associated with particular stages of different tumours, so that tumours are typed and staged by oncogene expression. In this way, they state, there will be new approaches to prognosis, imaging for tumour metastases and possible screening of tissue sections for cancer cells.

This aspect of the subject was dealt with by Fischinger *(1987)*, who states that the clinician now has more parameters with which to identify a tumour and so can develop a new molecular pathology to discriminate amongst similar tumours and consequently select the most appropriate treatment. He cites the tumour neuroblastoma, where the degree of amplification of one oncogene is a good clue to total response to treatment and survival. He postulates the formation of an atlas of oncogene expression for common tumours in the future as our knowledge grows. He also states that the nature of oncogene products with their altered growth factors or receptors for these factors allows new approaches to be made in the design of specific agents for specific tumours.

REFERENCES

Anderson, D. E. (1977). Breast cancer in families. *Cancer*, **40**, 1855–60

Ashton, N. (1958). Malignant tumours of the eye and adnexa. In Raven, R. W. (ed.) *Cancer*, Vol. 2, pp 599–616. Butterworth & Co., London

Baserga, R. (1985). Cell cycle genes and oncogenes. In Fortner, J. G. and Rhoads, J. E. (eds) *Accomplishments in Cancer Research*, pp 190–7. J. B.

Lippincott Co., Philadelphia

Bodmer, W. F. (1982). Cancer genetics. In *Cancer Surveys. Advances and Prospects in Clinical, Epidemiological and Laboratory Oncology*, pp 1–15. Published for the Imperial Cancer Research Fund by Oxford University Press

Bodmer, W. F. (1985). Genetic susceptibility to cancer. In Fortner, J. G. and Rhoads, J. E. (eds) *Accomplishments in Cancer Research*, pp 198–211. J. B. Lippincott Co., Philadelphia

Chargaff, E. (1979). How genetics got a chemical education. In Srinivasan, P. R., Fruton, J. S. and Edsall, J. T. (eds) "The origins of modern biochemistry—a retrospect on proteins". *Ann. N. Y. Acad. Sci.*, **325**, 345–60

Davidson, J. N. (1957). Chemical mechanisms of normal and abnormal cell division. In Raven, R. W. (ed.) *Cancer*, Vol. 1, pp 76–122. Butterworth & Co., London

Fischinger, P. J. (1987). A vision of the future — oncology in the year 2000. *International Cancer News (UICC)*, January 1987, pp 4–6

Griffin, A. C. (1957). Biochemistry of cancer induction. In Raven, R. W. (ed.) *Cancer*, Vol. 1, pp 123–60. Butterworth & Co., London

Holm, N. V., Hauge, M. and Jensen, O. M. (1982). Studies of cancer aetiology in a complete twin population: Breast cancer, colorectal cancer and leukaemia. In Bodmer, W. F. (guest ed.) *Cancer Surveys. Advances and Prospects in Clinical, Epidemiological and Laboratory Oncology*, Vol. 1, No. 1, pp 17–32. Published for the Imperial Cancer Research Fund by Oxford University Press, Oxford and London

Horowitz, N. H. (1979). Genetics and the synthesis of proteins. In Srinivasan, P. R., Fruton, J. S. and Edsall, J. T. (eds) "The origins of modern biochemistry — a retrospect on proteins". *Ann. N. Y. Acad. Sci.*, **325**, 253–6

Hotchkiss, R. D. (1979). The identification of nucleic acids as genetic determinants. In Srinivasan, P. R., Fruton, J. S. and Edsall, J. T. (eds) "The origins of modern biochemistry — a retrospect on proteins". *Ann. N. Y. Acad. Sci.*, **325**, 321–42

King, M.-C. (1982). Genetic and epidemiological analysis of cancer in families: breast cancer as an example. In Bodmer, W. F. (guest ed.) *Cancer Surveys. Advances and Prospects in Clinical, Epidemiological and Laboratory Oncology*, Vol. 1, No. 1, pp 33–6. Published for the Imperial Cancer Research Fund by Oxford University Press, Oxford and London

Koller, P. C. (1957). The genetic component of cancer. In Raven, R. W. (ed.) *Cancer*, Vol. 1, pp 335–403. Butterworth & Co., London

Ottman, R. (1980). Endocrinology and epidemiology of familial breast cancer. Ph.D. dissertation. University of California, Berkeley

Weber, J. and McClure, M. (1987). Oncogenes and cancer. *Br. Med. J.*, **1**, 1246–8

White, R. (1982). DNA polymorphism: new approaches to the genetics of cancer. In Bodmer, W. F. (guest ed.) *Cancer Surveys. Advances and Prospects in Clinical, Epidemiological and Laboratory Oncology*, Vol. 1, No. 1, pp 175–86. Published for the Imperial Cancer Research Fund by Oxford University Press, Oxford and London

CHAPTER TWENTY-TWO

Virology

Virology continues to attract the profound interest of oncologists all over the world and a considerable research effort is being devoted to this basic science.

For many decades researchers and clinicians have debated about the role of viruses in the development of cancer. Early work on the subject was limited because of lack of knowledge about the structure and function of the constituents of the individual cell, in addition to considerable ignorance concerning the properties of viruses.

A detailed review of the role of viruses in the origin of tumours was made by Dmochowski *(1958)*, who included a valuable list of references to the literature on the subject up to that date. He stated that Borrel in 1903 and Bose in the same year were the first to formulate the hypothesis that cancer was of viral origin because of the fact that viruses have a proliferative action on tissues. He also cited the work of Ellerman and Bang, who in 1908 discovered the viral nature of fowl leukosis.

The next important discovery was made by Rous *(1911)*, who described how a sarcoma of a fowl could be transmitted by small quantities of a cell-free filtrate to other susceptible fowls. The tumour was formed of a single type of cells which were very slightly differentiated, resembling young connective tissue cells and highly malignant, and which infiltrated contiguous tissues and metastasised through the blood stream, but rarely through the lymphatic system. Rous stated that when a small portion of the tumour was placed in a new and susceptible host, most of its cells survived, were vascularised, proliferated and apparently gave rise to all the new growth. In a resistant host the growth soon died and no tumour followed.

Rous pointed out that, following his results, the first tendency would be to regard the self-perpetuating agent which is active in the sarcoma of the fowl as a minute parasitic organism. However, he stated, another kind of agent had to be considered, for it was conceivable that a chemical stimulant elaborated by the malignant cells might be the cause of the tumour developing in another host and thus producing the same stimulant.

Important research was carried out by Shope *(1932)*, who described a condition like a tumour in a wild cottontail rabbit, which he found was transmittable to both wild and domestic rabbits, but not to guinea-pigs, white rats, white mice or chicks. This tumour had the general appearance of a fibroma.

He later stated that the properties of the agent which causes a tumour-like condition in rabbits had been tested experimentally and the conclusion had been reached that the agent was a filtrable virus. He pointed out that while the tumour-like condition and infectious myxomatosis differ markedly in their clinical and pathological appearances, they were found to be related immunologically.

In his extensive review of the subject Dmochowski *(1958)* quoted Duran-Reynolds, who described the properties which known viruses share with tumour-inducing agents. These include their requirement of living cells; their ability to act on a specific genetic substrate; their species or cell specificity which may undergo variation; their ability to remain latent for long periods; the differences in the lesions they produce according to whether they act on young or adult hosts; and their appearance in either a free or so-called "masked" form. Dmochowski made the important statement that viruses induce proliferative lesions which persist for a comparatively short time, while tumour-inducing viruses cause a continuous, unrestricted, malignant, proliferative change. Furthermore, inflammatory lesions develop in the host, with little resistance; when intermediate resistance is present a tumour may develop, whereas with strong resistance no lesions may develop (quoted from Duran-Reynolds and Shrigley).

During subsequent decades considerable research was carried out on oncogenic viruses, both in animals and humans. The subject was reviewed by Houchens and Bonmassar *(1977)*, who gave a comprehensive list of references on this subject in the literature up to that date. They referred to the work of Strauss and colleagues and pointed out the similar morphology of the human wart virus and the Shope rabbit papillomavirus. They also discussed some of the evidence that adenoviruses, herpesviruses and B and C-type RNA viruses could be human cancer viruses.

VIRAL ONCOGENESIS HYPOTHESES

Houchens and Bonmassar described the two major hypotheses put forward to explain the mechanism of viral carcinogenesis, both of which emphasise the relationship between the RNA tumour viruses and their host cells.

Protovirus hypothesis of Temin

This hypothesis postulates that the oncogenic virus acts through a provirus mechanism whereby the viral genome is incorporated into the nucleic acid of the host cell by virion-RNA-directed DNA polymerase. Any mechanism which disrupts the unstable protovirus can induce neoplasia. The cellular malignant transformation might not be accompanied by viral production, so there is difficulty in recovering oncogenic viruses from human tumours.

Viral oncogenic hypothesis of Huebner and Todaro

This second hypothesis states that the oncogenic or genetic information for cell transformation is incorporated in both germ cells and somatic cells of most vertebrates. The transmitted oncogenes are normally suppressed but could be expressed by proper stimulation from various carcinogens.

Warwick *(1973)* pointed out that one aspect of viral carcinogenesis that complicates the hypothesis that human cancers have a viral origin is that almost all tumour-inducing viruses hitherto investigated cause sarcomas or leukaemias, whereas the majority of human cancers are carcinomas. An exception is the mouse mammary tumour virus, which is an RNA virus which produces carcinoma *in vivo*, but not *in vitro*. Warwick observed that this implies that the virus has a highly specific action mechanism, possibly depending on the hormonal influence. It is doubtful whether a viral mechanism is responsible for the production of human breast cancer.

VIRUSES AND HUMAN ACUTE LEUKAEMIAS

Many attempts have been made to determine the mechanism or mechanisms of leukaemogenesis. The evidence was discussed by Goldberg and Goldin *(1973)*, who stated that a strong association might exist between human acute leukaemia and viruses but that all our knowledge up to that time was only suggestive, although the experimental results from the work on laboratory animals might be highly so. They cited the important success of tissue culture studies with Burkitt's lymphoma, which epidemiological studies had shown was linked to an infectious agent, and they stated that this was probably the human tumour most closely connected with a viral aetiological agent.

RECENT WORK AND REVIEWS

There has been an impressive growth in our knowledge of tumour virology during recent decades, so the literature about this subject has assumed a considerable size. No attempt is made here to refer to all the important articles and reviews, but the objective is rather to indicate, however briefly, the relevance of virology in the history of oncology and its enormous potential value in our understanding and treatment of human cancer.

In his review Waterson *(1982)* stated that the evidence of the importance of human viral oncogenesis was increasing, for in addition to benign tumours caused by viruses, such as the common skin wart, a type of human leukaemia had been reported to yield a retrovirus similar to the leukaemia viruses of other vertebrates, the human T-cell leukaemia virus. This had been isolated from patients with mycosis fungoides. Waterson pointed out that the viruses which cause animal tumours are either double-stranded DNA viruses or members of a group of RNA viruses called retroviruses because their RNA can be transcribed into DNA. The viral DNA is then integrated with the host-cell DNA and is replicated in step with it. Waterson explained that malignant transformation is closely correlated with this integration of the viral DNA.

He cited the following important information concerning viral oncogenesis: It has been shown that hepatitis B virus is a cause of primary hepatocellular carcinoma and that Epstein–Barr virus is a cause of Burkitt's lymphoma and nasopharyngeal carcinoma. Furthermore, cytomegalovirus might be involved in Kaposi's sarcoma, and human papillomaviruses might cause skin cancers. However, the close association of a particular tumour with a virus does not necessarily mean viral causation.

Waterson called attention to the fact that human wart viruses and papillomaviruses have for a long time been known to cause benign papillomas of the skin, larynx and anorectal region, and malignant change has been reported in laryngeal papillomas, genital warts and a rare form of skin papilloma-epidermodysplasia verruciformis *(Orth and colleagues, 1979).*

Horwich *(1984)*, writing on the subject of oncogenes and human cancer, showed how oncogene research has revealed important links between the disciplines of tumour virology, chemical carcinogenesis and chromosomal analysis, in the investigation of cancer aetiology. He also pointed out that the identification of some of the biochemical mechanisms associated with neoplastic changes might lead in future to the development of more specific methods of treatment.

He listed three important recent advances in our knowledge of neoplastic transformation, as follows: oncogenes that can cause malignant transformation of cells growing in tissue culture have been identified in, and isolated from, human tumour cell lines and tumour tissue. These cellular genes are closely related to the viral genes which cause a variety of tumours in animals. Advances have occurred in chromosome staining techniques, which have demonstrated recurring patterns of chromosomal aberrations, especially translocations, in a high proportion of tumours. The protein product of one cellular oncogene is very similar to a growth factor, a class of protein that is able to override some regulatory mechanisms which control cell proliferation.

Horwich explained that improvements in techniques of chromosomal banding and of tissue culture had shown that oncogenes are found at the exact break-points of translocation which are frequently found in certain tumours, and he described Burkitt's lymphoma as a striking example.

Research is proceeding to clarify the mechanism of malignant transformation affected by oncogene expression through its protein product. We need more knowledge of the important biochemical differences between normal and malignant cells. As Horwich pointed out, it is necessary to bring together the basic sciences of tumour virology, molecular biology, cytogenetics and clinical oncology for important advances to be made in the management of patients.

In his review of retroviruses and cancer genes, Bishop *(1984)* states that we do not understand the role played by cellular oncogenes and their protein products in the routine functions of normal cells but that they are suspected to be involved in cellular differentiation and perhaps are the clues to the control of normal development which will lead to further knowledge about carcinogenesis. He then states that proto-oncogenes might "represent the seeds of cancer within our cells" and that at least 11 different proto-oncogenes have been shown to be implicated in the production of spontaneous tumours. Multiple steps in carcinogenesis are necessary for the production of tumours and possibly other factors, in addition to oncogenes, are required. He cites the genesis of Burkitt's lymphoma by implicating infection with Epstein–Barr virus, translocation of a proto-oncogene and mutational activation of another oncogene. The search for more oncogenes must continue, using new methodology.

The role of oncogenes in the development of cancer was considered by Barbacid *(1985)*, who stated that transforming genes have been identified in about 15% of the most frequent varieties of human cancers, including carcinomas of the lung, colon and liver, in addition to certain leukaemias, and that most of the transforming genes are members of the *ras*-gene family. The activation of *ras* oncogenes, however, is not correlated with the development of any specific variety of human cancer and it might be that they are randomly activated during tumour progression as an indirect consequence of the genetic disarray of cancer cells. Barbacid pointed out that perhaps they are involved in only a relatively small percentage of tumours because their activation is dictated by the nature of the cancer-initiating agent or event and furthermore that they seem to play a basic role in cell proliferation. He stated that activated *ras* oncogenes are found in a variety of cell types, including those of epithelial (carcinomas), fibroblastic (sarcomas) and haematopoietic (leukaemias) origin.

HEPATITIS B VIRUS AND PRIMARY CANCER OF THE LIVER

In the chapter on epidemiology reference was made to primary cancer of the liver; other aspects of this important subject are considered here. Observations were made that there is a geographical association between the incidence of primary liver cancer and the prevalence of carriers of hepatitis B virus, which is common in Africa and Asia but rare in the Western world, where primary liver cancer is also rare.

The subject was dealt with in some detail by Prince *(1984)*, who stated that when sensitive serological tests were made there was a striking association between the hepatitis B surface antigen and hepatocellular carcinoma. He pointed out that infection with the virus precedes by many years the development of the carcinoma. He explained that the role of the hepatitis B virus could involve a direct oncogenic effect, or there might be a mechanism which depends upon an intervening stage of hyperplasia due to cirrhosis; however, he quoted evidence that cirrhosis does not appear to be a prerequisite.

The association of hepatitis B vaccine with hepatocellular carcinoma has important clinical connotations, especially the prevention of this dangerous tumour. A safe vaccine is now required to prevent infection with the virus and thereby reduce the incidence of hepatocellular carcinoma. Prince also called attention to the value of alpha-fetoprotein measurements, which become markedly abnormal during the period of early development of the carcinoma when it can be surgically excised.

Considerable research effort is now being put into the development of vaccines against viruses, not only those which cause hepatitis B but also those that are responsible for Burkitt's lymphoma and the serious AIDS, which might predispose the patient to develop malignant disease. With regard to hepatitis B virus infection, recombinant DNA vaccine is now available for human use.

CONCLUSION

No attempt has been made in this chapter to deal in detail with the basic science of virology in relation to oncology, for the subject is already very extensive and is expanding rapidly. It is interesting to contemplate the enormous growth in our knowledge since the discovery, by Ellerman and Bang in 1908, of the viral nature of leukosis in fowls and the pioneer work in 1911 of Rous, who showed that a sarcoma in a fowl could be transmitted by small quantities of a cell-free filtrate to other susceptible fowls.

It is safe to predict that with the new scientific methodology which is being used today and which is yielding exciting new knowledge regarding the mysteries of neoplasia, we are on the brink of important developments in our understanding of the oncological diseases, which will lead to active prevention and more efficacious therapy.

REFERENCES

Barbacid, M. (1985). The role of ras oncogenes in neoplastic development. In Fortner, J. G. and Rhoads, J. E. (eds) *Accomplishments in Cancer Research 1985. General Motors Cancer Research Foundation*, pp 179–87. J. B. Lippincott Co., Philadelphia

Bishop, J. M. (1984). Viruses, genes and cancer. Retroviruses and cancer genes. In Fortner, J. G. and Rhoads, J. E. (eds) *Accomplishments in Cancer Research 1984. General Motors Cancer Research Foundation*, pp 98–105. J. B. Lippincott Co., Philadelphia

Dmochowski, L. (1958). The part played by viruses in the origin of tumours. In Raven, R. W. (ed.) *Cancer*, Vol. 1, pp 214–305. Butterworth & Co., London

Goldberg, A. I. and Goldin, A. (1973). Antiviral agents in the treatment of acute leukaemia. In Raven, R. W. (ed.) *Modern Trends in Oncology*, Part 1: Research Progress, pp 243–68. Butterworth & Co., London

Horwich, A. (1984). Oncogenes and human cancer. *Br. J. Hosp. Med.*, **32** (5), 262–6

Houchens, D. P. and Bonmassar, E. (1977). Virology. In Raven, R. W. (ed.) *Principles of Surgical Oncology*, pp 263–78. Plenum Medical Book Company, New York and London

Orth, G., Jablonska, S. and Jarzabek-Chorzelska, M. (1979). Characteristics of the lesions and risk of malignant conversion associated with the type of human papillomavirus involved in epidermodysplasia verruciformis. *Cancer Res.*, **39**, 1074–82

Prince, A. M. (1984). Hepatitis B virus and primary liver cancer. In Fortner, J. G. and Rhoads, J. E. (eds) *Accomplishments in Cancer Research 1984. General Motors Cancer Research Foundation*, pp 110–18. J. B. Lippincott Co., Philadelphia

Rous, P. (1911). A sarcoma of the fowl transmitted by an agent separable from the tumor cells. *J. Exp. Med.*, **13**, 397–411

Shope, R. E. (1932). A transmissible tumor-like condition in rabbits. *J. Exp. Med.*, **56**, 793–802

Shope, R. E. (1932). A filtrable virus carrying a tumor-like condition in rabbits and its relationship to virus myxomatosis. *J. Exp. Med.*, **56**, 803–22

Warwick, G. P. (1973). Newer aspects of carcinogenesis. In Raven, R. W. (ed.) *Modern Trends in Oncology*, Part 1: Research Progress, pp 61–97. Butterworth & Co., London

Waterson, A. P. (1982). Human cancers and human viruses. *Br. Med. J.*, **284**, 446–8

APPENDIX

The Lymphatics of Selected Organs and Tissues

The dissemination of malignant diseases, especially carcinoma, is frequent and dangerous. In practice the presence of lymph node metastases is frequently the touch-stone for prognosis assessment and the staging system is based chiefly on the extent of lymphatic dissemination. The stage of the disease is correlated with the method of treatment. The technique of the monoblock operation for the removal of the primary tumour with its lymphatic metastases is based on a precise knowledge of the lymphatic system. This is necessary not only for the surgical oncologist, but also for the radiation oncologist when the fields of radiation therapy are planned.

The valuable work and detailed illustrations contributed by experts during past decades are of great historical interest and the present author felt they should be correlated and specially presented. To attain this objective he therefore sought the expert assistance of Miss (now Professor) Nancy Joy and she produced all the drawings in this appendix with meticulous technique.

We made a careful study of the descriptions given by the authorities we consulted (see the following references) and on the basis of these designed an anatomical framework of selected organs and tissues, with the regional lymph nodes in the positions shown in the illustrations of the authorities. The lymphatic vessel routes correspond to the written descriptions given by the authorities.

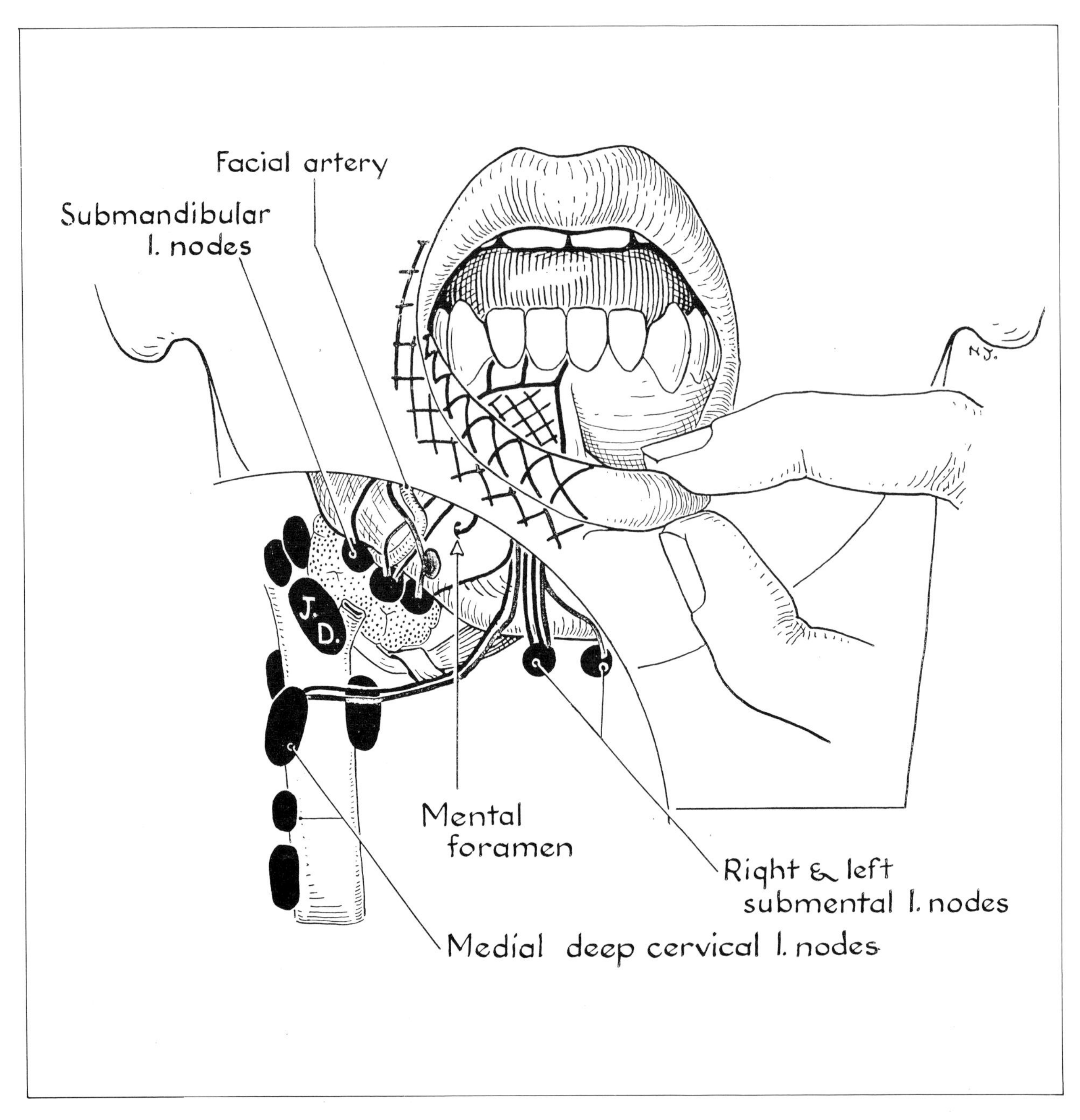

Figure A1 Scheme of the lymphatics of the lip. Based on the description by Poirier.

Cunningham describes an occasional median route from the lower gum to the submental lymph nodes. The route from the lingual side of the lip to the submental lymph node is exceptional. Routes from the medial part of the lip direct to the upper deep cervical lymph nodes are also exceptional. A route from the gingivo-labial groove enters the mental foramen of the mandible.

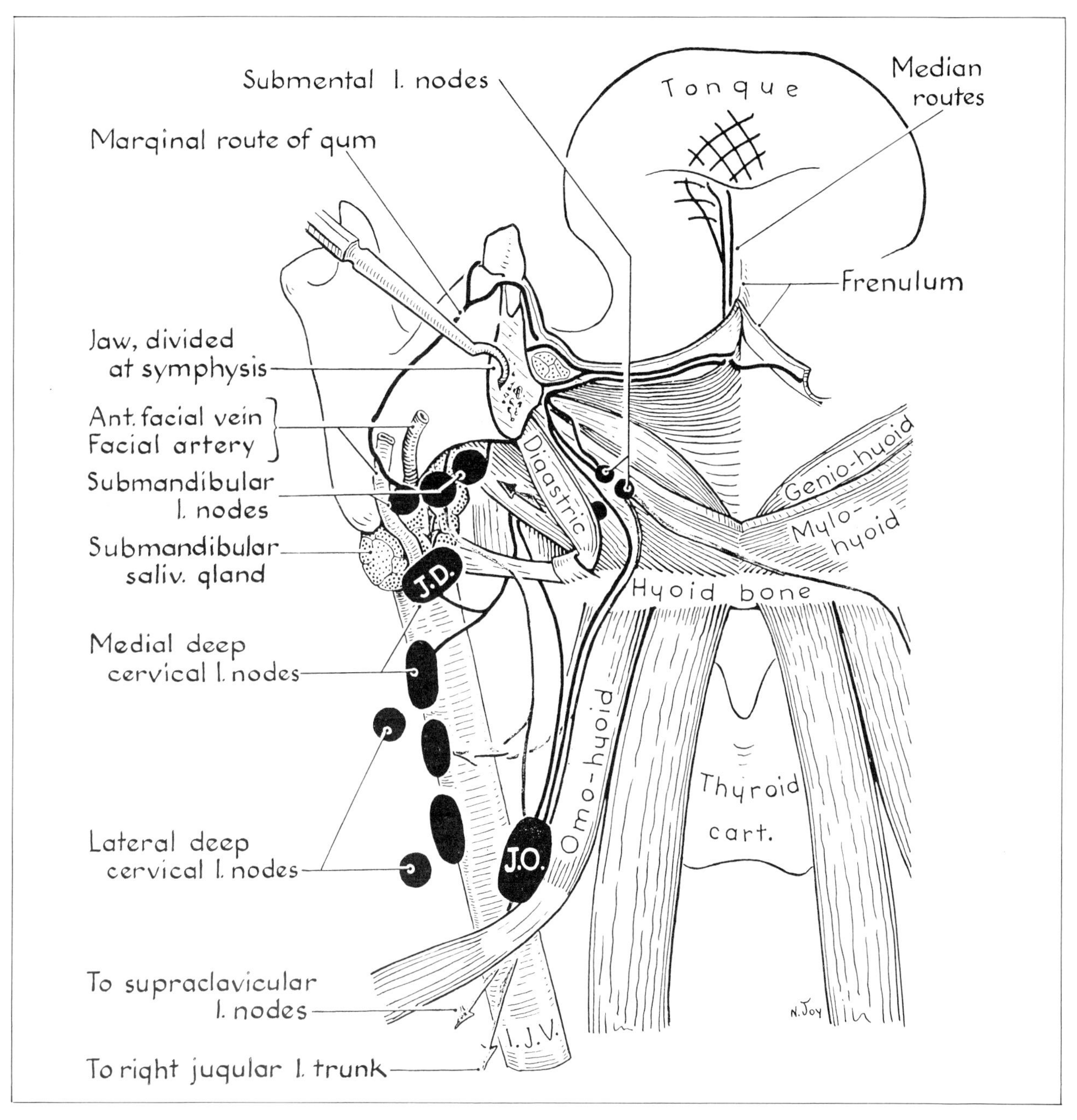

Figure A2 Scheme of the lymphatics of the mucous membrane of the tip of the tongue and afferent routes from the submental and submandibular groups of lymph nodes.

This diagram is based on the description by Jamieson and Dobson. No additional information is given by Poirier or Cunningham. Note the two routes from the tip of the tongue direct to the J.O. lymph node, one of which may pass superficial or deep to the central tendon of the digastric muscle. Jamieson and Dobson connect the submental and submandibular lymph nodes. Poirier describes the marginal route of the gum. Cunningham shows lymphatic vessels piercing the mylo-hyoid muscle at a distance from the periosteum of the mandible. Inconstant lymph nodes are found deep to and at the lower border of the submandibular salivary gland. There is an inconstant lymph node on the anterior belly of the digastric muscle on the route connecting the submental and submandibular groups of lymph nodes.

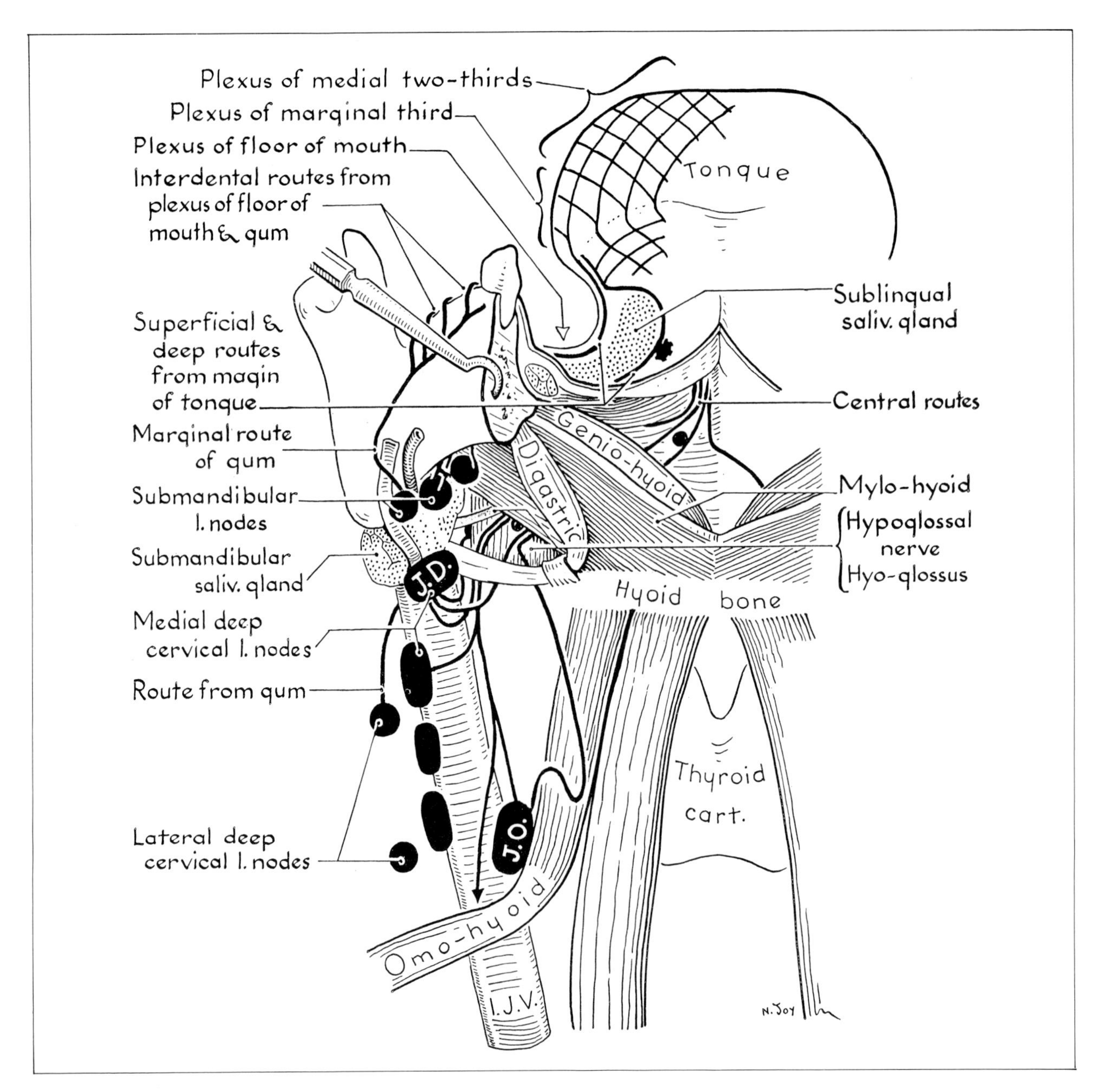

Figure A3 Scheme of the lymphatics of the mucous membrane of the anterior two-thirds of the tongue including the tip, draining directly to the regional lymph nodes. Based on the description by Jamieson and Dobson.

Poirier mentions the interrupting lymph nodes found beneath the sublingual and submandibular salivary glands. Cunningham mentions the small lymph node on the lymphatic route accompanying the lingual artery, and Jamieson mentions the lymph node on the route accompanying the hypoglossal nerve. Any lymphatic vessel which reaches, but does not enter, the J.O. lymph node passes on to the lymph nodes below the omohyoid muscle. Poirier states that the central lymphatic vessels may pass anteriorly or posteriorly to the central tendon of the digastric muscle.

Leaf and Küttner state that a lymph node is sometimes present on the internal surface of the submandibular salivary gland. Other lymph nodes are also inconstant at its lower border. Note that the mucous membrane lymphatic plexus is continuous over the whole surface of the tongue and also connects with the intramuscular lymphatic plexus. The communications between the various groups of lymph nodes are not shown.

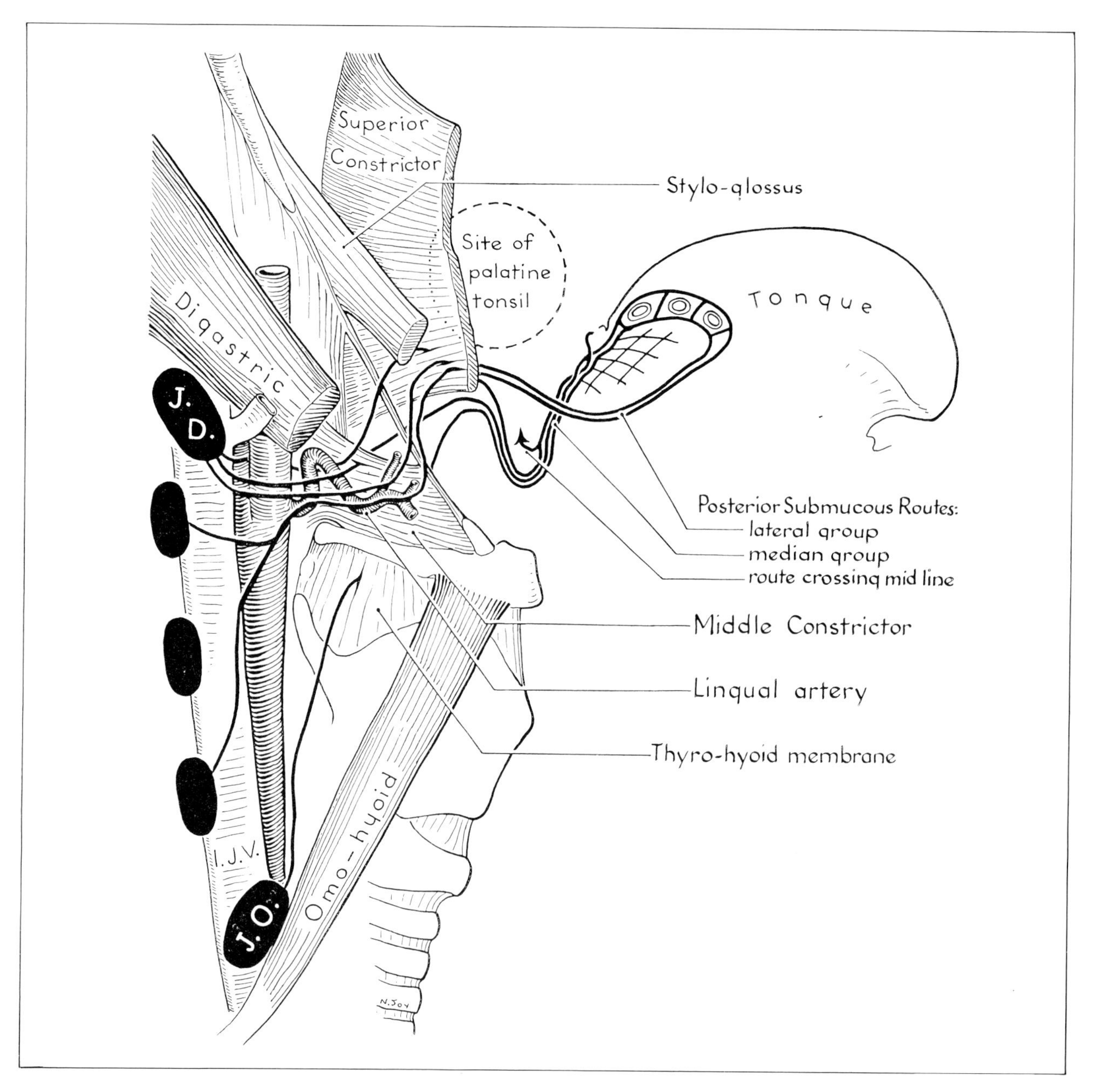

This diagram is based on the description by Poirier. Jamieson describes routes passing anterior and posterior to the external carotid artery to the median group of deep cervical lymph nodes. The median lymphatic vessels may bifurcate, and at the level of the glosso-epiglottic fold pass to the lymph nodes in either side of the neck.

Figure A4 Scheme of the lymphatics of the mucous membrane of the posterior third of the tongue.

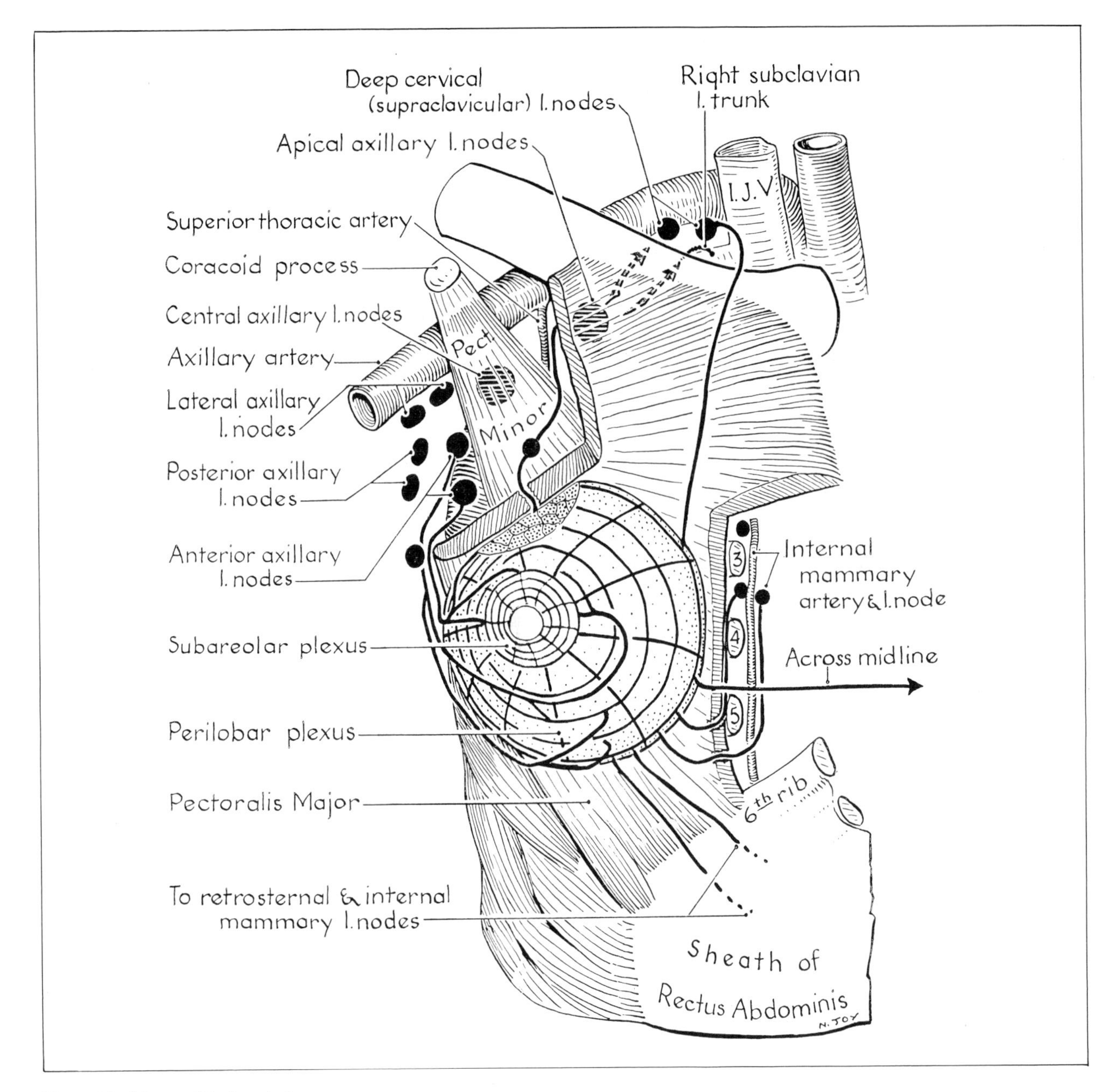

Figure A5 Scheme of the lymphatics of the breast.

This diagram is based on the description by Poirier. The anterior axillary lymph nodes are called "principal mammary lymph nodes" and lie on the third digitation of the serratus magnus muscle. Cunningham stresses that routes may drain directly to any subgroup of axillary lymph nodes, even to the lateral group along the axillary vein; this vein is omitted here to simplify the drawing. Cunningham also mentions three cutaneous routes not mentioned by Poirier: (1) to the lowest lymph nodes of the deep cervical group; (2) to the upper part of the sheath of the rectus abdominis muscle (apparent only in pathological cases which proceed to the retrosternal internal mammary lymph nodes); (3) irregular routes across the midline. Cunningham, in his surgical section, mentions diseased nodes in the retropectoral fascia between the pectoral muscles and above the pectoralis minor muscle on the first intercostal space in relation to the superior thoracic artery (the latter is not shown in the drawing).

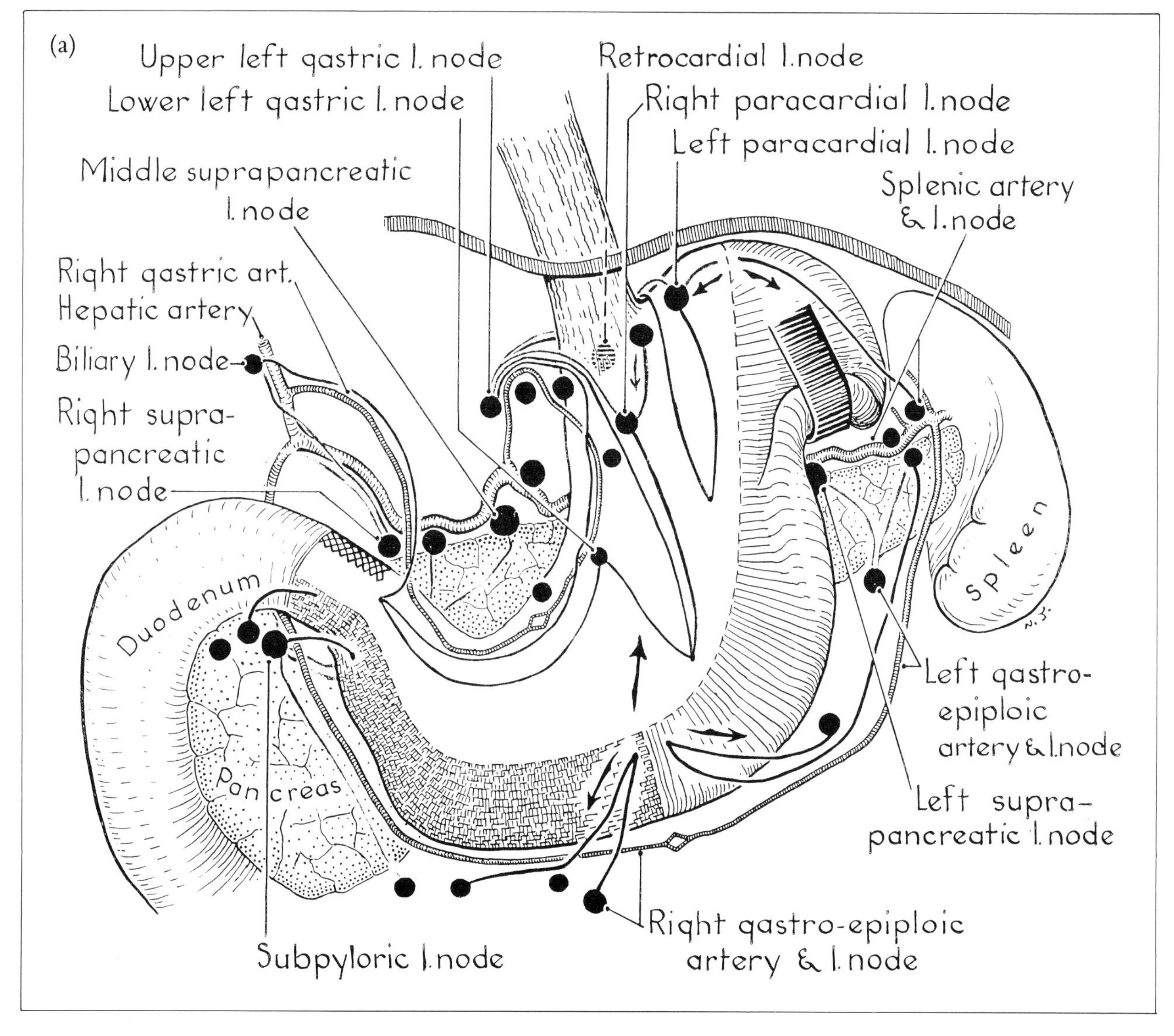

Figure A6(a) Scheme of the lymphatics of the stomach.

These drawings are based on a description by Jamieson.

Figure A6(a) shows the routes from the stomach and lower pyloric region. The pattern of lines dividing the areas is the same anteriorly and posteriorly, except at the pylorus. Jamieson describes the dividing line in the front of the stomach as dropping from the oesophagus; Poirier and Rowntree show it more to the left as we have placed it.

Figure A6(b) shows the routes from the pylorus and from the middle and right suprapancreatic groups. In this drawing the cisterna chyli and other details have been added from Cunningham's description. The pattern of drainage from the front of the pylorus is based on Poirier's diagram, but he does not state in his text where the central third drains. Cunningham in a diagram redrawn from Jamieson suggests the middle area is drained by the left gastric routes (Green, 9th edn, Figure 1164). Rouvière divides the pyloric area horizontally into two halves. Jamieson states that no observer has described lymphatic vessels ascending from the pyloric canal to reach the upper gastric lymph nodes near the upper border of the pancreas.

Lumbar and mesenteric nodes are secondary. Routes from the stomach

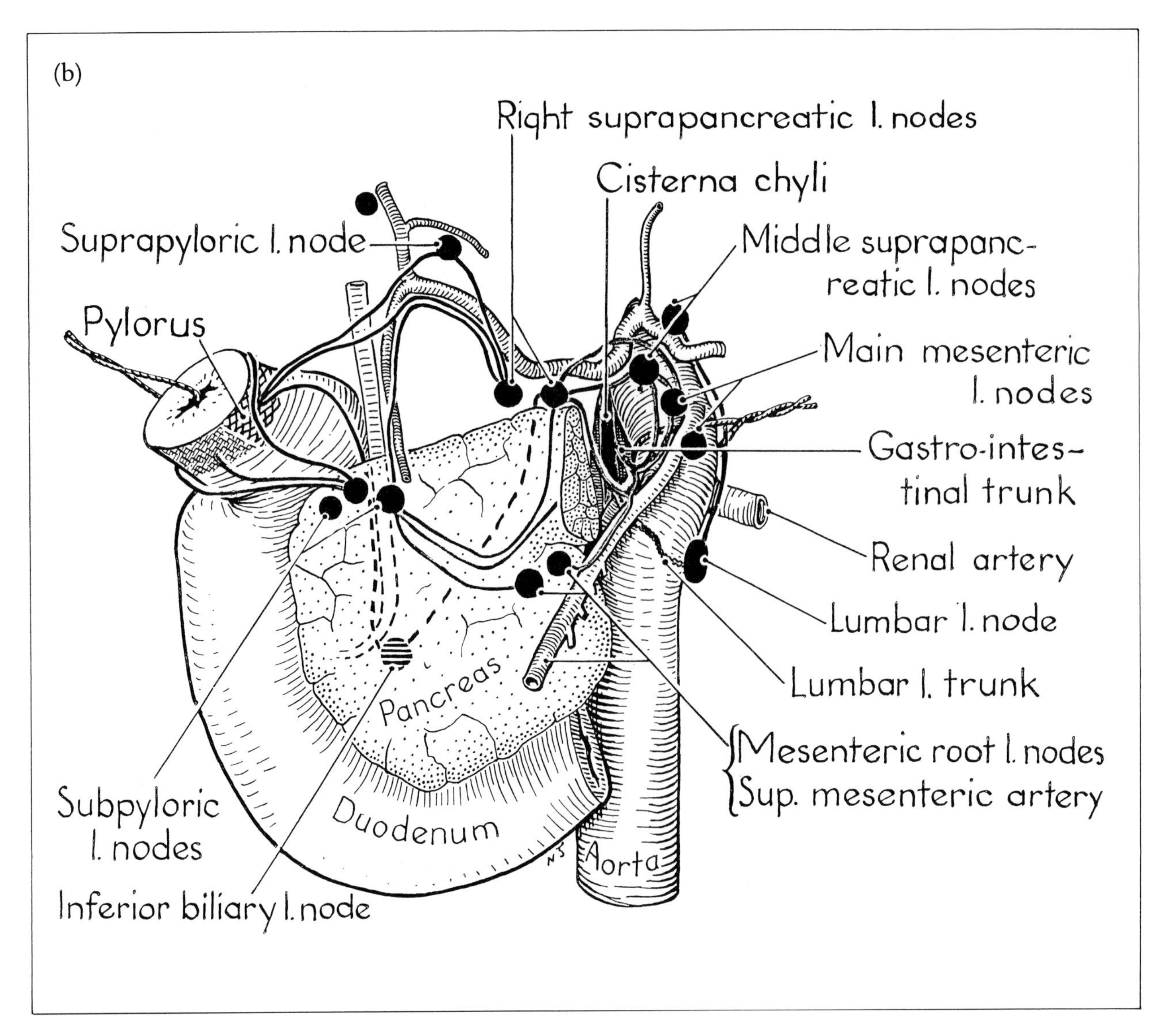

Figure A6(b) Scheme of the lymphatics of the stomach.

wall follow the arteries or veins to terminate in a node; node afferents are independent of blood vessels and terminate in the receptaculum chyli. An occasional route from the left to the right paracardial nodes is shown. Nodes in the gastrosplenic omentum are rare and inconstant. Jamieson considers that the subpyloric nodes he describes are the retropyloric nodes described by Poirier, and similarly the right gastro-epiploic is Poirier's subpyloric node. The suprapancreatic nodes communicate freely below the pancreas with the superior mesenteric nodes, the lymph flow being both ways and thence to the receptaculum chyli. The suprapancreatic nodes injected show a flow to a node just below the left renal artery and to a node between the aorta and inferior vena cava at a still lower level (not shown).

Jamieson describes a route passing from the posterior aspect of the pylorus to the lowest of the large and numerous biliary nodes posterior to the second part of the duodenum. Poirier states that aberrant nodes may be found in the great omentum along the descending borders of the right gastro-epiploic arch; these may be more than 5 cm distant from the greater curvature of the stomach.

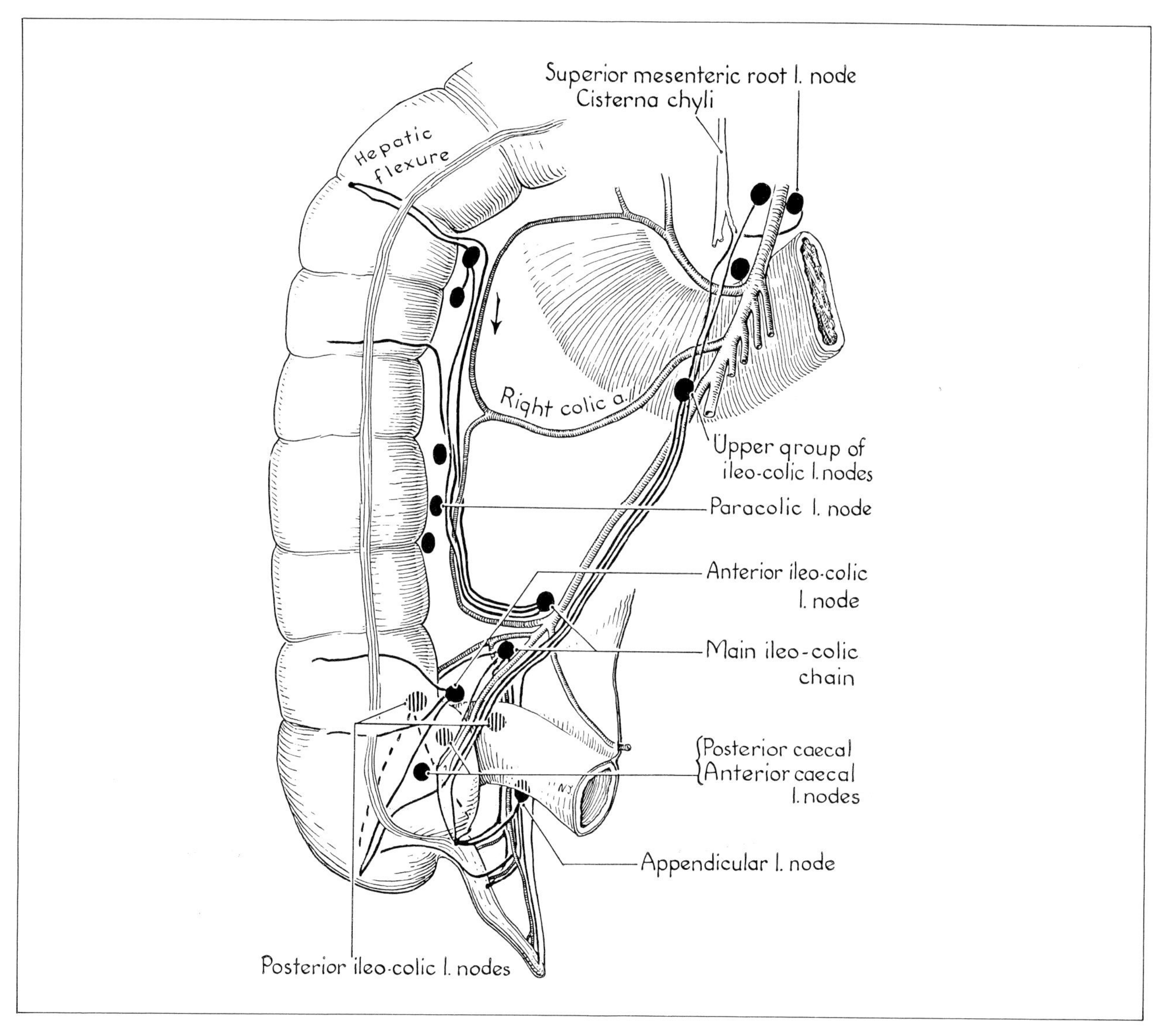

Figure A7 Scheme of the lymphatics of the appendix, caecum and ascending colon.

This diagram is based on a description by Jamieson and Dobson. When accessory appendicular arteries are present, lymph vessels from the proximal part of the appendix accompany them and are received by the posterior ileo-colic nodes. Lymph vessels from the posterior part of the base of the appendix are always interrupted by the nodes in the ileo-caecal angle. Rarely a lymph vessel may pass from the lowest part of the anterior caecal wall to a posterior ileo-colic node. Jamieson emphasises that the routes accompanying the right colic artery are occasional and always small. The posterior caecal nodes are usually covered with visceral peritoneum. Jamieson has not seen any communication between nodes of the caecum and appendix and nodes on the right common and external iliac arteries. He does not consider that a communication exists between lymphatics of the appendix and those of the uterus and ovaries. Nodes in, or near, the free border of the appendix and at the outer angle of the meso-appendix close to the caecum are prolapsed members of the posterior ileo-colic group and are always present in the meso-appendix. It is unusual to find caecal nodes below the lower margin of the ileo-caecal junction.

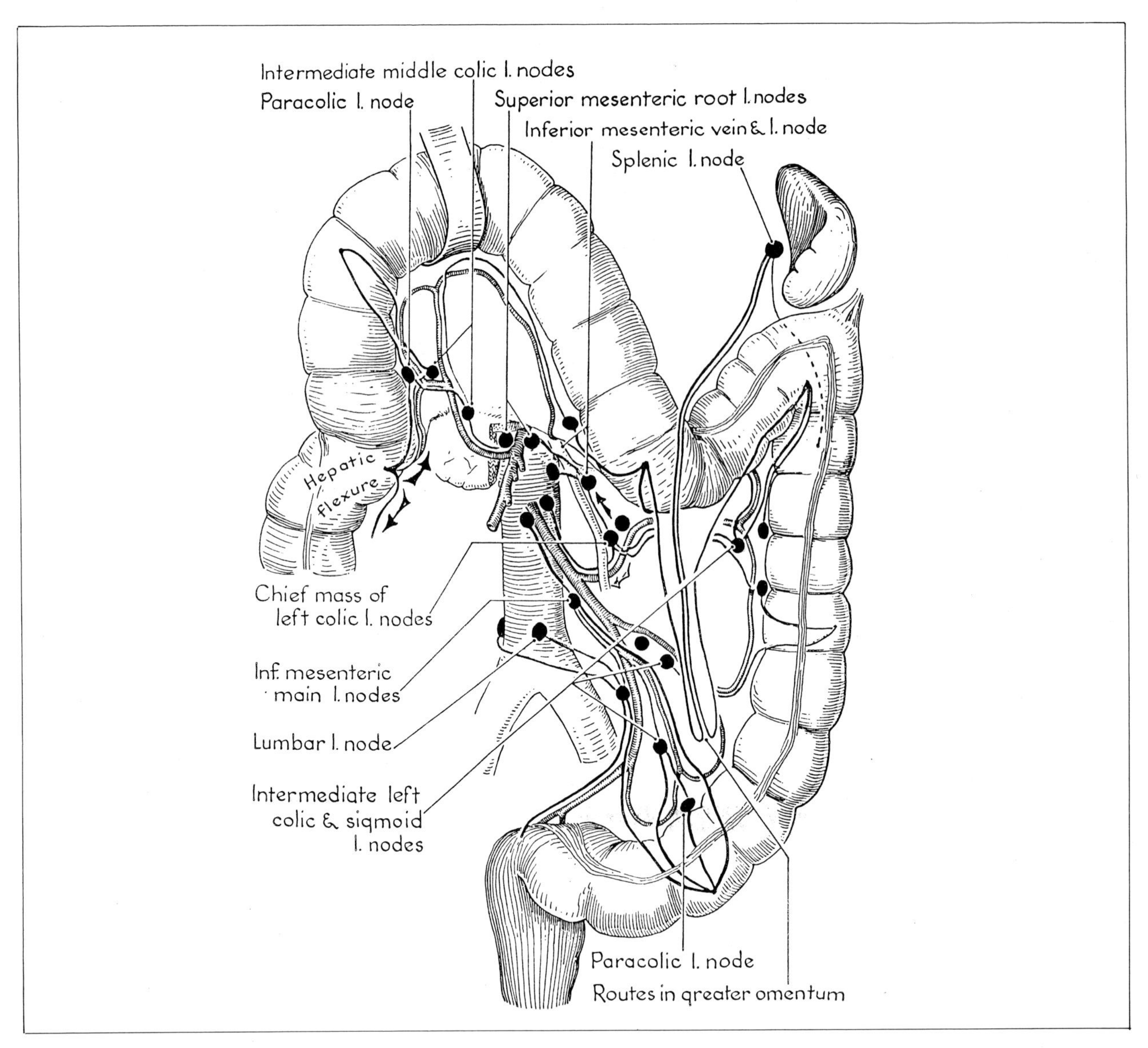

Figure A8 Scheme of the lymphatics of the transverse, descending and pelvic colon.

Jamieson states that the lymph vessels from the left third of the transverse colon and the splenic flexure which pass to the splenic node do not run with branches of the left gastro-epiploic artery to join lymph vessels proceeding from the stomach; they run in the great omentum transversely to the left, but at a lower level than the left gastro-epiploic vessels. On the other hand, Poirier states that lymphatics of the transverse colon communicate to a large extent with those of the great omentum, bringing them into relation with those of the inferior border of the stomach. There may be interrupting nodes in the great omentum. A route passes from the posterior aspect of the upper part of the descending colon to the splenic node. From the central portion of the transverse colon routes are not direct to intermediate nodes, but pass through the paracolic nodes. In the descending colon the routes go direct to intermediate nodes in one-third of persons. The efferents from the nodes around the inferior mesenteric veins pass to the lumbar nodes, superior mesentery root nodes and to nodes around the coeliac axis blood vessels. Jamieson considers there must be a communication between the nodes about the head of the pancreas and the great venous trunks.

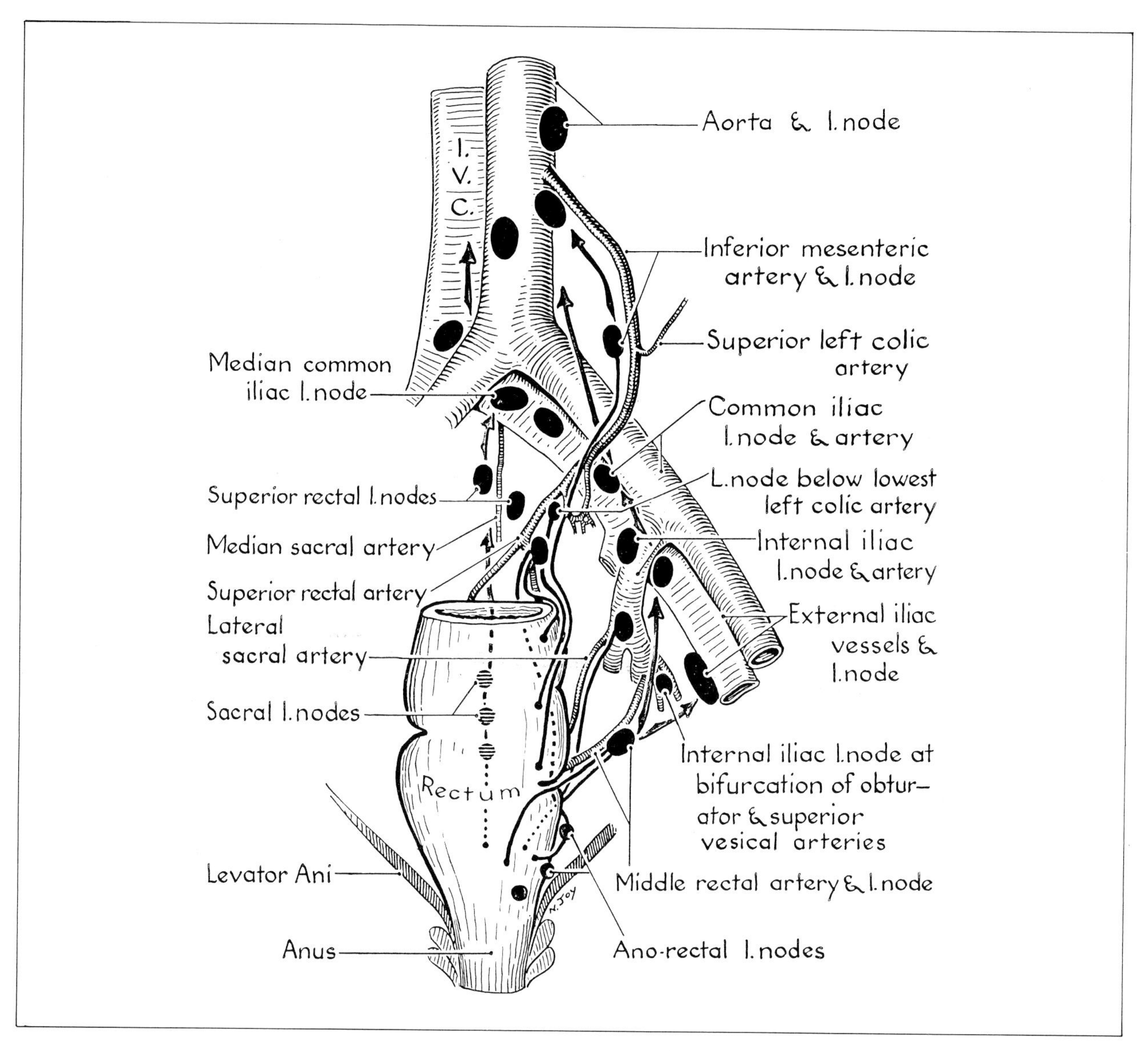

Figure A9 Scheme of the lymphatics of the rectum.

For the sake of simplicity only half of the rectum is shown. The diagram is based on a description by Cunningham and modified by additional information by Poirier. Cunningham in his surgical section gives more information than is given in the body of the text and describes a node below the lowest left colic artery. He also states that lymph vessels from the middle and upper parts of the rectum are interrupted by the pararectal nodes (these nodes are not shown). Poirier describes a route from below the third transverse fold to nodes with the superior rectal artery. Cunningham, in his surgical section only, describes routes starting between the third transverse fold and the ano-rectal junction accompanying the lateral sacral, median sacral, and middle rectal arteries. From there the lymphatic vessels enter the external, internal and median common nodes.

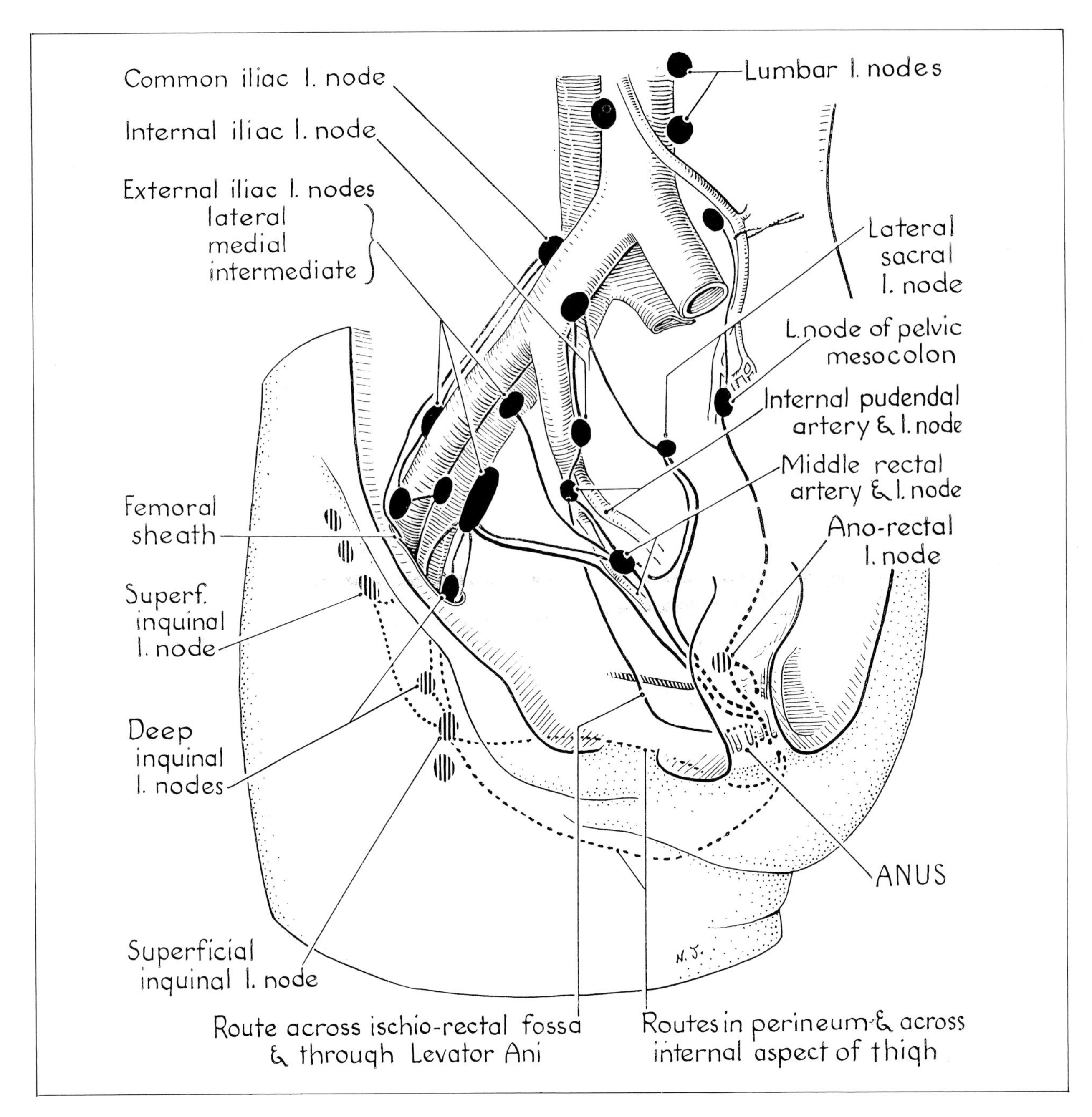

Figure A10 Scheme of the lymphatics of the anus.

This diagram is based on a description by Poirier. The nodes and routes are shown on the right side for simplicity. In addition, a route draining the mucous membrane which passes to a node in the pelvic meso-colon is shown. Occasionally routes accompany the inferior rectal branches of the internal pudendal artery and therefore pass behind the levator ani muscle.

The author gratefully acknowledges the valuable collaboration of Professor Nancy Joy, now in the Faculty of Medicine, University of Toronto, in this description of the lymphatics and thanks her for her skilful drawings.

REFERENCES

Cunningham, D. J. (1922). *Textbook of Anatomy*, 5th edn. Young J. Pentland, Edinburgh

Grant, J. C. B. (1948). *A Method of Anatomy* (4th edn). Baillière, Tindall and Cox, London

Green, T. H. (1900). *An Introduction to Pathology and Morbid Anatomy* (revised by H. Montague Murray), 9th edn. Henry Renshaw, London

Jamieson, J. K. and Dobson, J. F. (1920–21). The lymphatics of the tongue with particular reference to the removal of lymphatic glands in cancer of the tongue. *Br. J. Surg.*, **8**, 80–7

Leaf, C. H. (1898). *Anatomy of the Lymphatic Glands.* Archibald Constable & Co., London

Poirier, P. and Charpy, A. (1909). *Traité d'Anatomie Humaine*, Vol. 2: *Les Lymphatiques* (Poirier, P. and Cunéo, B.). Masson et Cie, Paris

Romaines, G. J. (ed.) (1972). *Cunningham's Textbook of Anatomy* (11th edn). Oxford University Press, London

Rouvière, H. (1932). *Anatomie des Lymphatiques de l'Homme.* Masson et Cie, Paris

Rouvière, H. and Vatelle, G. (1937). *Physiologie du Système Lymphatique.* Masson et Cie, Paris

ACKNOWLEDGEMENTS

For general assistance with facts and data in the compilation of the work:

The British Library, the Library of the Chester Beatty Research Institute, the Library of the Royal College of Surgeons of England, and the Library of the Royal Society of Medicine.

For illustrations:

Chapter 1
The British Library: Figures 1.1, 1.2, 1.3, 1.4, 1.5, 1.6, 1.7 and 1.8.
The President and Council of the Royal College of Surgeons of England: Figures 1.12, 1.13, 1.14, 1.15 and 1.16.

Chapter 3
The Librarian, Royal Marsden Hospital and Institute of Cancer Research: Figures 3.1, 3.2, 3.3, 3.4, 3.5, 3.6, 3.8 and 3.9.
Figure 3.7 is reprinted from *Nature* (1961), **191**, 430–2.
The President and Council of the Royal College of Surgeons of England: Figures 3.15, 3.16 and 3.17.
The Librarian of the Royal Beatson Hospital, Glasgow: Figures 3.10, 3.11, 3.13 and 3.14.

Chapter 4
Marie Curie Memorial Foundation: Figures 4.1, 4.2, 4.3, 4.4, 4.5, 4.6, 4.7, 4.8 and 4.9.
Cancer Relief: Figure 4.10.
Imperial Cancer Research Fund: Figures 4.11, 4.12 and 4.13 (supplied by Miss M. J. Gollyer).

Chapter 5
The Librarian, Royal College of Surgeons of England: Figures 5.1 and 5.2.

Chapter 7
Reprinted from publication by R. W. Raven by courtesy of Heinemann Publishers Ltd: Figures 7.2, 7.3, 7.4, 7.5, 7.6 and 7.7.
Courtesy of John Wright and Sons Ltd, *British Journal of Surgery*: Figure 7.10.

Chapter 8
Reprinted from *Foundations of Medicine* by R. W. Raven, courtesy of Heinemann Publications Ltd: Figure 8.9.

Chapter 12
The President and Council of the Royal College of Surgeons of England: Figures 12.2, 12.3, 12.6, 12.7 and 12.8.

Chapter 14
Courtesy of *British Journal of Surgery*: Figures 14.15, 14.16 and 14.17.

Chapter 16
Library of the Chester Beatty Research Institute: Figure 16.1.
Courtesy of Dr A. Holleb: Figure 16.3.

Chapter 17
Royal College of Surgeons of England: Figures 17.1 and 17.2.
Courtesy of *Journal of Cancer Research*: Figure 17.6.
Courtesy of *British Medical Journal*: Figures 17.7 and 17.10.
Courtesy of Cambridge University Press: Figure 17.8.
Library of Chester Beatty Research Institute: Figure 17.9.

Chapter 18
Courtesy of the Editor of *Cancer* and of D. P. Burkitt and G. T. O'Connor: Figures 18.3, 18.5 and 18.6.
Courtesy of D. P. Burkitt: Figure 18.4.

Chapter 19
Courtesy of Heinemann Publications Ltd: Figures 19.1, 19.2 and 19.3.
Courtesy of Butterworth Publishing Ltd: Figures 19.7, 19.8, 19.9 and 19.11.

Chapter 20
Courtesy of Dr A. Holleb: Figure 20.1.

INDEX